Nursing Approach to the Evaluation of Child Maltreatment

G.W. Medical Publishing, Inc.
St. Louis

This book is dedicated to:

The three deans at La Salle University School of
Nursing who over the past decade have encouraged our work.

Zane Robinson Wolf, PhD, RN, FAAN (1997-present)

Cynthia Flynn Capers, PhD, RN (1996-1997)
(Currently Dean, College of Nursing, University of Akron)

Gloria Ferraro Donnelly, PhD, RN, FAAN (1980-1996)
(Currently Dean and Professor, College of Nursing & Health Professions, Drexel University)

The incredible staff at the OUR KIDS Center in Nashville, Tenn.
The May 2001 roster is as follows:

Marti M. Rosenberg, BA, MBA, Executive Director
Deborah M. Bryant, MD, Medical Consultant
Sue Ross, MSN, PNP
Julie Rosof-Williams, MSN, FNP
Hollye Gallion, MSN, PNP
Maureen Sanger, PhD
Lisa Dupree, BS, MA, MSW
Phyllis Thompson, BSW, MSW, LCSW
Cate Loes, BS
Suzanne V. Petrey, BS, MS, MBA
Linda Patrick, BA
Carol Dozier
Karen Davidson

Nursing Approach to the Evaluation of Child Maltreatment

Eileen R. Giardino, PhD, RN, CRNP
Professor
La Salle University, School of Nursing
Nurse Practitioner
La Salle University, Student Health Center
Philadelphia, Pennsylvania

Angelo P. Giardino, MD, PhD, FAAP
Associate Chair—Pediatrics
Associate Physician-in-Chief
St. Christopher's Hospital for Children
Philadelphia, Pennsylvania
Associate Professor in Pediatrics
Drexel University College of Medicine
Adjunct Professor
La Salle University School of Nursing
Philadelphia, Pennsylvania

G.W. Medical Publishing, Inc.
St. Louis

Publishers: Glenn E. Whaley and Marianne V. Whaley

Design Director: Glenn E. Whaley

Managing Editors: Kristine Feeherty

Ann Przyzycki

Associate Editors: Grant Armstrong

Christine Bauer

Book Design/Page Layout: G.W. Graphics

Vicky Ho

Print/Production Coordinator: Charles J. Seibel, III

Cover Design: G.W. Graphics

Color PrePress Specialist: Terry L. Williams

Developmental Editor: Elaine Steinborn

Copy Editor: Elizabeth Hayes

Proofreader: Robert Saigh

Indexer: Jill Pulley

Printed in Canada

Publisher:

G.W. Medical Publishing, Inc.

77 Westport Plaza, Suite 366, St. Louis, Missouri 63146-3124 USA

Phone: (314) 542-4213 Fax: (314) 542-4239 Toll Free: 1-800-600-0330

http://www.gwmedical.com

Library of Congress Cataloging-in-Publication Data

Giardino, Eileen R.

  Nursing approach to the evaluation of child maltreatment / Eileen R. Giardino, Angelo P. Giardino.-- 1st ed.

      p. ; cm.

Includes bibliographical references and index.

  ISBN 1-878060-51-1 (pbk.)

 1. Child abuse. 2. Nursing.

  [DNLM: 1. Child Abuse--diagnosis. 2. Mandatory Reporting. 3. Nurse's Role. 4. Nursing Assessment--methods. 5. Physical Examination--methods. 6. Social Responsibility. WA 320 G4353n 2003]

I. Giardino, Angelo P. II. Title.

  RJ375.G53 2003

  616.85'8223--dc21

                                                    2003009800

CONTRIBUTORS

Eileen M. Alexy, MSN, RN, CS
Doctoral Candidate
Psychiatric Clinical Nurse Specialist
University of Pennsylvania, School of Nursing
Philadelphia, Pennsylvania

Marisa V. Atendido, MSN, CRNP
Nurse Practitioner
Children's Hospital of Philadelphia
Adolescent Care Center
Philadelphia, Pennsylvania

Kathleen M. Benasutti, MCAT, ATR-BC, LPC
Registered and Board Certified Art Therapist
Trauma Consultant
Treatment Research Institute at the University of Pennsylvania

Kathleen M. Brown, RN, CRNP, PhD
Adjunct Assistant Professor
University of Pennsylvania
School of Nursing
Philadelphia, Pennsylvania

Frank P. Cervone, Esq.
Executive Director
Support Center for Child Advocates
Philadelphia, Pennsylvania

Paul T. Clements, PhD, APRN-BC, DF-IAFN
Distinguished Fellow, International Association of Forensic Nurses
Psychiatric/Forensic Clinical Specialist
Assistant Professor
University of New Mexico, College of Nursing
Albuquerque, New Mexico

Sandra L. Elvik, MS, RN, CPNP
Assistant Medical Director
Child Abuse Crisis Center
Associate Professor of Pediatrics
UCLA School of Medicine
Harbor-UCLA Medical Center
Torrance, California

Diana K. Faugno, BSN, RN, CPN, FAAFS, SANE A/A
District Director
Pediatrics/Nicu
Forensic Health Service
Palomar Pomerado Health
Escondido, California

Eileen R. Giardino, PhD, RN, CRNP
Professor
La Salle University, School of Nursing
Nurse Practitioner
La Salle University, Student Health Center
Philadelphia, Pennsylvania

Angelo P. Giardino, MD, PhD, FAAP
Associate Chair—Pediatrics
Associate Physician-in-Chief
St. Christopher's Hospital for Children
Philadelphia, Pennsylvania
Associate Professor in Pediatrics
Drexel University College of Medicine
Adjunct Professor
La Salle University School of Nursing
Philadelphia, Pennsylvania

Holly M. Harner, CRNP, PhD, MPH
Assistant Professor
William F. Connell School of Nursing
Boston College
Chestnut Hill, Massachusetts

Stacey Lasseter, MSN, RN, SANE-A
Coordinator
Forensic Nursing Services
Forensic Nurse Examiners of St. Mary's Hospital
Richmond, Virginia

Anne Lynn, ACSW, MLSP
Project Director
Northeast Regional Children's Advocacy Center
Newtown, Pennsylvania

Frances M. Nadel, MD
Assistant Professor of Pediatrics
University of Pennsylvania School of Medicine
Attending Physician
Division of Emergency Medicine
Children's Hospital of Philadelphia
Philadelphia, Pennsylvania

Ann L. O'Sullivan, PhD, CPNP, FAAN
Professor of Pediatric Primary Care Nursing
Director, Family Nurse Practitioner Program
Director, Health Leadership Program
Director, Pediatric Nurse Practitioner Program
Co-Director, Center for Urban Health Research
University of Pennsylvania, School of Nursing
Philadelphia, Pennsylvania

Julie Pape, CPNP
Children's Hospitals and Clinics
St. Paul, Minnesota

Jennifer Pierce-Weeks, RN, CEN
Health Care Specialist
New Hampshire Coalition Against Domestic and Sexual Violence
State of New Hampshire SANE Program Coordinator
Department of Justice
Concord, New Hampshire
Sexual Assault Nurse Examiner, Pediatric
Dartmouth-Hitchcock Medical Center
Lebanon, New Hampshire
Sexual Assault Nurse Examiner, Adolescent/Adult/Pediatric
Valley Regional Hospital
Claremont, New Hampshire

Maureen Sanger, PhD
Psychologist
OUR KIDS Center
Nashville General Hospital
Assistant Professor of Pediatrics
Vanderbilt University School of Medicine
Nashville, Tennessee

Barbara Speller-Brown, RN, MSN, CPNP
Certified Pediatric Nurse Practitioner
Assigned to OUR KIDS Center
Nashville General Hospital
Vanderbilt University Medical Center
Nashville, Tennessee

Suzanne P. Starling, MD, FAAP
Medical Director, Child Abuse Program
Children's Hospital of The King's Daughters
Associate Professor of Pediatrics
Eastern Virginia Medical School
Norfolk, Virginia

Phyllis L. Thompson, LCSW
Licensed Clinical Social Worker
OUR KIDS Center
Nashville General Hospital
Vanderbilt University Medical Center
Nashville, Tennessee

FOREWORD

Child abuse and neglect constitutes a major problem that has an impact on over 1 million children in the United States each year. The safety of children is the responsibility of each member of society and reflects the values that social group places on the young. Yet many children in the United States remain unprotected or underprotected, exposed to abuse or neglect in a nation that leads the world in so many other areas. Clinicians Eileen Giardino and Angelo Giardino have done a superb job in providing guidelines for nurses to follow in protecting children.

Nurses interact with children, families, and caregivers daily and at all levels of care. They serve a major function in primary care situations, where most cases of abuse and neglect are detected. Therefore, it is appropriate that nurses be instrumental in equipping families and other caregivers for addressing child maltreatment issues.

If prevention of child maltreatment is the goal, then education is the principal means of achieving that goal. Educational interventions can be offered at every level of healthcare and in the course of the nurse's daily functions. This textbook prepares the nurse to present detailed, evidence-based information in the context of caring for families.

Identifying high-risk situations is key in breaking the cycle of abuse. The development of interventions that target families in crisis is an important step that can derail potential maltreatment and guide families to more constructive solutions to the problems they face. Nurses can be instrumental in offering a framework to help families during home visits, when children are brought for well-child care examinations or routine immunizations, when they are seen in school nurse's offices, or when they make emergency department visits, among other scenarios.

Once a child is abused or neglected, nurses may provide interventions that are designed to help children and families heal. Their role in this process can have long-term effects, helping a child move into adulthood without many of the scars from abuse that can prove debilitating if not addressed. The nurse, along with other healthcare providers, can make the difference between the child growing up damaged and potentially abusive and the child becoming a well-adjusted and loving parent.

The chapters offered in this book address the critical areas nurses must be aware of as they face the issues of child maltreatment and neglect. With these tools in hand, the nurse will be equipped to function as a positive instrument of change for families and, eventually, future citizens.

Ann W. Burgess, DNSc, FAAN, RN
Professor of Psychiatric Mental Health Nursing
Boston College School of Nursing
Chestnut Hill, Massachusetts

FOREWORD

As is true for every professional who interacts with children, nurses are mandated reporters and, thereby, must notify appropriate authorities when they encounter cases of child maltreatment. Therefore, they are responsible for understanding what constitutes abuse or neglect, what signs and symptoms are indicative of child maltreatment, what identifies families at risk for developing a pattern of child maltreatment, and how to intervene effectively. The nurse's focus must be on the safety and well-being of the child.

Nurses interact with other healthcare providers in rendering care for families and children, playing a major role in the healthcare team. Nurses may be considered the eyes and ears as they are often the first healthcare professionals who notice signs and symptoms suspicious for maltreatment. Therefore, it is essential that they be well prepared to identify problems and make accurate assessments of the cause. Their ability to obtain a complete history and perform a thorough physical examination may be crucial in exposing abuse or neglect. This is particularly true when they are functioning as clinical nurse specialists or nurse practitioners and in independent nursing centers. They also need to be sensitive to the various verbal, physical, and behavioral cues that alert one to the possibility of maltreatment. Suspicions that are raised must be thoroughly evaluated and the possibility that abuse or neglect is present must be considered along with other diagnoses.

This book offers the nurse the tools required to fulfill these roles. We begin with the basics: a definition of the problem of child abuse and neglect, the presenting signs and symptoms of child maltreatment, obtaining a complete history, and conducting an appropriate interview and physical examination. Then, we move through the various aspects that must be considered in greater depth, such as laboratory findings and obtaining appropriate forensic specimens, dealing with sexually transmitted diseases, considering appropriate differential diagnoses, documentation, and mental health problems, to list a few. The rare but fascinating Munchausen syndrome by proxy is outlined, along with information pertinent to sexual abuse of adolescents. How the nurse can effectively interact with other professionals is addressed, with full chapters on child protective services and legal issues that occur with child maltreatment cases. The special risks that children face with respect to the Internet are also explored. These chapters should equip the nurse to be a well-informed and effective guardian of children's health.

The practical information that nurses require is often outlined in special sections focused on nursing interventions. These discussions detail the hands-on actions that nurses can take in specific situations.

Healthcare professionals can only function well when they are given adequate, accurate information. This textbook offers in-depth, well-documented information that should help guide nurses to be exceptional providers of healthcare to the families they encounter each day. The editors are to be thanked for assembling a dedicated team of authors who offer their expertise in the important area of child maltreatment education for nurses.

Diana K. Faugno, BSN, RN, CPN, FAAFS, SANE-A/A
Escondido, California

PREFACE

"Suffer the little children to come unto me, and forbid them not: for of such is the kingdom of God." Mark 10:14

Children represent the future, and the value placed on the life of a child reflects the society's fundamental attitudes toward life. As members of society who have chosen to express these attitudes in very practical terms, nurses are in a unique position. The nursing profession aspires to convey the highest level of care to all patients. Laws in all 50 states recognize this responsibility to provide care and, as such, nurses are mandated to protect the most vulnerable children and are clearly defined as mandated reporters of child maltreatment. Many children in the United States are vulnerable, and they are exposed to abuse or neglect. It is, therefore, appropriate that nurses play an instrumental role in serving children and families because they are often the first healthcare professionals to have contact with them when they come for care.

Nurses involved in all areas of practice must first of all recognize that child maltreatment is possible and include it within the possibilities raised in generating a list of differential diagnoses. They must be familiar with the signs and symptoms that suggest maltreatment, be aware of the types of situations where child maltreatment may be seen, and certainly be attuned to the various presentations that may be seen. In particular, nurses must notice and correctly interpret the verbal, physical, and behavioral cues that point to child maltreatment or neglect.

The nurse's role in the evaluation of abuse and neglect is expansive and includes intervening in all of the aspects of preventing abuse or neglect; assessing the history, physical examination, laboratory and diagnostic data; observing family and cultural life, and listening to the child to obtain a clear picture; and managing the cases of children with the focus maintained on the best interests of the child. Ensuring that the child will be kept safe and protected from the risk of further harm is a key goal.

Maltreatment in any form is a crime and requires the involvement of various agencies and law enforcement personnel. Nurses must be aware of the steps to be taken and be able to interface with counterparts in other professions to best serve the child and family concerns. The policies and procedures of each healthcare facility or place of employment must be known and followed.

This textbook was written with the goals of informing nurses about their role as mandated reporters, instructing nurses in how best to carry out their responsibilities in this area, and aiding nurses to intervene effectively. To these goals, a group of contributors has been assembled who present extensive material in each relevant area.

Part One: Overview discusses the statistical data connected with child maltreatment and points out the various presentations that may be seen. It is important to keep this overall perspective in mind and maintain a sense of context.

Part Two: Healthcare Evaluation offers practical steps to follow in obtaining a history, conducting interviews, performing a physical examination, and obtaining appropriate laboratory studies and collecting forensic specimens. This section also addresses the issues of sexually transmitted diseases, conditions mimicking child abuse, and neglect. Each of these is defined and clear explanations of what is required are offered. The documentation needed to move forward with forensic or legal steps is also explained in detail.

Part Three: Related Issues offers to educate the nurse regarding concerns peculiar to child maltreatment and neglect. How to approach mental health issues and what to expect in the way of behavioral responses are outlined. Special procedures and considerations related to adolescence are elucidated. The relatively rare but often sensational Munchausen syndrome by proxy is explained so that nurses may be informed of this possibility in formulating a differential diagnosis. The roles played by child protective services, social services, and the legal system are discussed with respect to the nurse's interactions with these entities. Domestic violence may complicate cases of child abuse, and a chapter is devoted to clarify the nurse's role in these difficult cases. A thorough explanation of the dangers of the Internet is offered, along with the nurse's role in preventing the abuse and neglect of children.

Within the text and in several appendices are various available resources to support the nurse in dealing with the repercussions of child maltreatment. The extensive references used in each chapter may be valuable to nurses who want to learn more and explore various issues in greater depth.

Putting together a project such as this is a work of purpose that brings a great deal of professional satisfaction and, of course, involves a great deal of hard work on the many people involved in such a large project. We would like to thank the many contributors who took on an extra academic project and spent many hours researching and writing these chapters; the anonymous peer reviewers for each chapter who provided a second set of eyes and helped us identify areas for improved clarity; our respective schools and departments who provided the scholarly environment for us to conceptualize and complete the book; the many publishers of books and journals who graciously permitted us to incorporate valuable copyrighted material within the chapters; and, finally, to the dedicated professionals at GW Medical who consistently supported this project and made it go from idea to printed words on printed pages. With their attention to detail, this book became a reality.

We hope that each reader will come away from this text better equipped and more fully prepared to advocate for our children.

Eileen R. Giardino, PhD, RN, CRNP
Angelo P. Giardino, MD, PhD, FAAP
Philadelphia, Pennsylvania

TABLE OF CONTENTS

PART TWO: HEALTHCARE EVALUATION
CHAPTER 3: HISTORY AND THE HEALTHCARE INTERVIEW 49

CHAPTER 4: THE PHYSICAL EXAMINATION IN THE EVALUATION OF SUSPECTED CHILD MALTREATMENT: PHYSICAL ABUSE AND SEXUAL ABUSE EXAMINATIONS 69

Nursing Approach to the Evaluation of Child Maltreatment

G.W. Medical Publishing, Inc.
St. Louis

Chapter 1

THE PROBLEM OF CHILD ABUSE AND NEGLECT

Eileen R. Giardino, PhD, RN, CRNP

The safety of children is a responsibility that every society must take seriously. It is the role of adults to protect and nurture the young members so that they can develop into healthy and productive members of society. Unfortunately, for many American children, protection has not been achieved. The scope of child maltreatment is pervasive in society, and the profound consequences of its effects on individuals are far-reaching.

Nurses interact with children and their families and caregivers at all levels of healthcare. They educate people, intervene in primary care and institutional settings, and provide services to help children and families heal. It is important for nurses to have a clear understanding of what child abuse and neglect are, how to identify risk factors, and then how to intervene to provide competent and comprehensive healthcare for children who have experienced child abuse and neglect. This chapter discusses the problem of child maltreatment, offers a conceptual framework to help explain how and why specific types of child abuse and neglect occur, and then identifies the role of nursing in evaluating and treating child sexual abuse.

INCIDENCE: SCOPE OF THE PROBLEM

Approximately 1 million children in the United States are victims of child abuse and neglect. The US Department of Health & Human Services (USDHHS) collects and analyzes data yearly from reports of the states' child protective services (CPS) agencies in an effort to track the data on child abuse and neglect. The 1999 report shows that an estimated 826 000 children were victims of abuse and neglect (USDHHS, 1999). The rates of neglect, physical abuse, and sexual abuse per 1000 children in the population has declined over a 5-year period from 1995 to 2000, along with a comparable decline in the total crime rate since 1993 (USDHHS, 1999).

The following numbers indicate the trend in maltreatment rates according to specific types of abuse over the past 10 years for every 1000 children in the population (USDHHS, 1999):

— 2.5 per 1000 are physically abused (down from 3.5 in 1990)

— 1.8 per 1000 are sexually abused (down from 2.3 in 1990)

— 0.9 per 1000 are emotionally abused (up from 0.8 in 1990)

— 6.5 per 1000 are neglected (up from 6.3 in 1990)

See Figures 1-1 to 1-3 and Table 1-1.

FATALITIES

The number of child deaths caused by neglect or abuse over the past decade has increased. The rate of child fatalities in 1997 was 1.7 children per 100 000, or 1192 in the population. This figure was based on reports of 967 fatalities from only 41 states

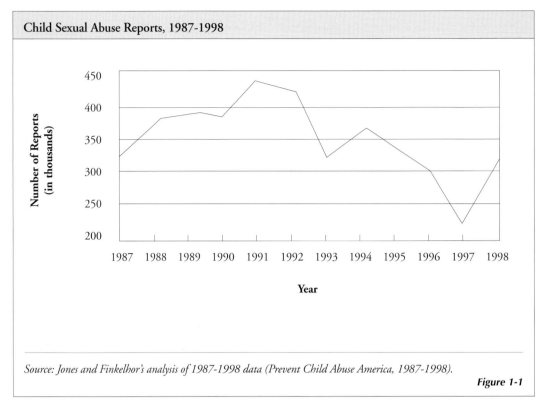

Child Sexual Abuse Reports, 1987-1998

Source: Jones and Finkelhor's analysis of 1987-1998 data (Prevent Child Abuse America, 1987-1998).

Figure 1-1

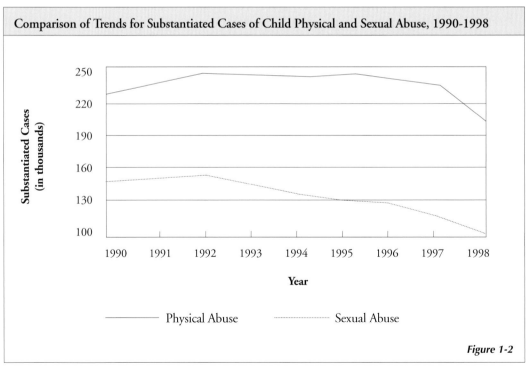

Comparison of Trends for Substantiated Cases of Child Physical and Sexual Abuse, 1990-1998

Figure 1-2

Figures 1-1 to 1-3. *Reprinted from Jones L, Finkelhor D.* The Decline in Child Sexual Abuse Cases. Office of Juvenile Justice and Delinquency Prevention Juvenile Justice Bulletin. *Washington, DC: US Dept of Justice, Office of Justice Programs; 2001. Available at: http://www.ncjrs.org/pdffiles1/ ojjdp/184741.pdf. Accessed March 11, 2003.*

Comparison of the Decline in Substantiated Cases of Child Sexual Abuse With Declines in Rates of Female Victimization by Intimate Partners, Total Violent Crime, Rape Victimization, Child Poverty, and Teen Births

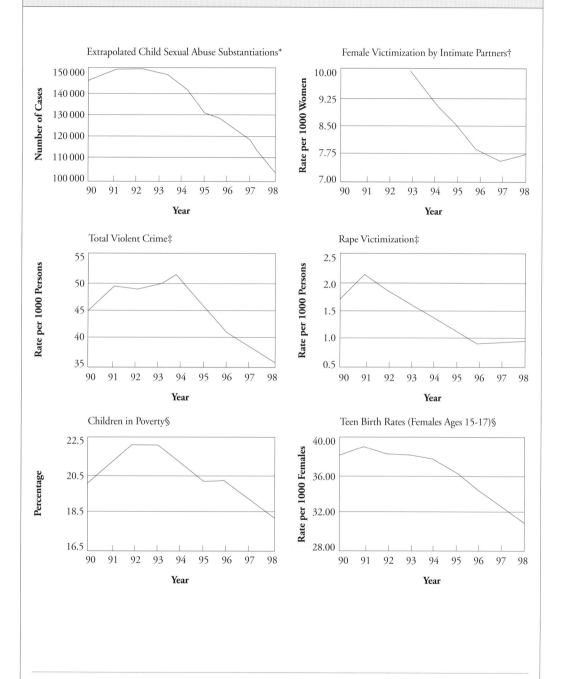

*Jones and Finkelhor's analysis of 1990-1998 data (US Department of Health & Human Services, 1992-2000).

†1993-1998 NCVS data (Rennison and Welchans, 2000). Data not available for 1990, 1991, and 1992.

‡1990-1998 NCVS data (Bureau of Justice Statistics, n.d.).

§1990-1998 data (Federal Interagency Forum on Child and Family Statistics, 2000).

Figure 1-3

Table 1-1. Victimization Rates: 1990-1999 SDC			
REPORTING YEAR	CHILD POPULATION	VICTIM RATE	ESTIMATED NUMBER OF VICTIMS
1990	64 163 192	13.4	860 577
1991	65 069 507	14.0	911 690
1992	66 073 841	15.1	994 655
1993	66 961 573	15.3	1 026 331
1994	67 803 294	15.2	1 029 118
1995	65 753 891	14.7	996 091
1996	64 235 441	14.7	955 786
1997	64 059 405	13.8	881 464
1998	69 709 448	12.6	903 395
1999	70 199 435	11.8	826 162

Reprinted from US Department of Health & Human Services. Child Maltreatment 1999: Reports From the States to the National Child Abuse and Neglect Data Systems. *Washington, DC: US Government Printing Office; 1999.*

(USDHHS, 1999). The number of fatalities known to have occurred from child maltreatment reported in 1999 was 1.6 children of every 100 000 children in the population, or a national estimate of 1100 child deaths. Children in the foster care system accounted for 22 fatalities, or 2.1% of the deaths (USDHHS, 1999). Child neglect (38.2%) was the most common form of abuse associated with child fatalities (USDHHS, 1999).

It is estimated that over half of the reports of child abuse and neglect (54.7%) were made by professionals who came into contact with the child or family (USDHHS, 1999). It is nursing's responsibility to have expertise in the area of child abuse and maltreatment because nurses are on the forefront of evaluating children and families in all settings.

CHILDREN WITH DISABILITIES

An increasing number of children in the United States have some type of disability, ranging from minor learning disabilities to severe developmental or physical problems. Advances in technology help children with certain physical, developmental, or genetic disorders survive and function to varying degrees in home environments (Goldson, 1998). The incidence of abuse in children with disabilities varies depending on specific parameters related to the type of disability. However, in 1991 the incidence of abuse in children with disabilities was nearly twice the rate for those without disabilities (USDHHS, 1993) **(Table 1-2)**.

COSTS OF MALTREATMENT

The direct and indirect expenses associated with child maltreatment are sizeable (Daro, 1988) and include costs related to low birth weight babies, infant mortality, special education, protective service, foster care, juvenile and adult criminality, and psychological services (Caldwell, 1992). The costs of immediate foster care and of longer-term placement were estimated to have a total cost of $1.1 billion for cases identified in 1983. Costs also are incurred within the juvenile justice system as a result of high-risk criminal activity associated with exposure to some forms of maltreatment (National Clearinghouse on Child Abuse and Neglect Information [NCCANI], 1998).

Lost productivity secondary to disabilities resulting from abuse and neglect costs were estimated to range from approximately $650 million to $1.3 billion per year using 1983 numbers (Daro, 1988). Regarding treatment programs, Daro (1988) estimated that if each case identified in 1983 were enrolled in a recognized treatment program, costs for such services could vary from $2.8 billion to $28 billion, depending on the professional level of the staff providing the care.

Table 1-2. Incidence of Child Maltreatment: Overall and by Whether or Not Children Have Disabilities

TYPE OF MALTREATMENT	INCIDENCE FOR ALL CHILDREN (PER 1000)*	INCIDENCE FOR ALL CHILDREN WITH DISABILITIES (PER 1000)†	INCIDENCE FOR ALL CHILDREN WITHOUT DISABILITIES (PER 1000)‡	RATIO OF INCIDENCE FOR ALL CHILDREN WITH DISABILITIES TO INCIDENCE FOR ALL CHILDREN WITHOUT DISABILITIES
Any maltreatment	22.6	35.5	21.3	1.67
Physical abuse	4.9	9.4	4.5	2.09
Sexual abuse	2.1	3.5	2.0	1.75
Emotional abuse	3.0	3.5	2.9	1.21
Physical neglect	8.1	12.3	7.7	1.60
Educational neglect	4.5	9.0	4.1	2.20
Emotional neglect	3.2	7.6	2.8	2.77

Estimates are from the Study of the National Incidence and Prevalence of Child Maltreatment (NIS-2).
†*Estimates were derived by multiplying column 1 by the ratio of percent of children with a specific type of maltreatment with disabilities to percent of children in the general population with disabilities.*
‡*Estimates in this column were derived by disaggregating the estimates in column 1, given the estimates in column 2.*

Adapted from US Department of Health & Human Services. A Report on the Maltreatment of Children With Disabilities. 105-89-16300. Washington, DC: US Government Printing Office; 1993.

Moving beyond these early projections, national spending on child maltreatment remains high. The National Call to Action, a coalition of national organizations working to implement a 20-year plan to decrease the prevalence of child maltreatment, presented data to the US Congress showing that in 1998, states reported spending $15.6 billion on child welfare, including prevention, investigation, out of home placement, and adoption (Wilson & Pence, 1999).

With enormous financial costs at stake, the federal government and professionals in the field called for the inclusion of cost effectiveness in child maltreatment program evaluations (Dubowitz, 1992). Most recently, professionals working on prevention strategies to protect children from child abuse and neglect have examined the costs and potential benefits associated with various prevention programs. The work of Olds, Hill, Mihalic, and O'Brien (1998) demonstrated that prenatal and infant nurse home visitation improved a wide range of maternal and child health outcomes in a cost-effective manner. Others have produced equally compelling cost analyses for prevention strategies. For example, Michigan estimated that direct and indirect expenditures for the nearly 16 000 children who were maltreated in fiscal year 1991 amounted to an estimated $823 million annually, whereas the cost of providing child maltreatment services to all first-time parents in that time period would have been $43 million—yielding a 19 to 1 cost advantage to prevention (Caldwell, 1992).

DEFINITIONS OF THE PROBLEM

Child abuse and neglect encompass various situations in which a parent or caregiver fails to provide for the health and well-being of a child. Abusive caregiver acts are those of commission or omission that have an injurious effect on the physical, psychosocial, or developmental well-being of the child. The results of abuse or neglect may end in physical or emotional harm, death, an act or failure to act that presents an imminent risk of serious harm, or sexual exploitation or abuse of the child (USDHHS, 1996, 2001a).

CATEGORIES OF MALTREATMENT

The broad categories of maltreatment include physical abuse, sexual abuse, emotional and psychological abuse, and neglect **(Table 1-3)**. Each category contains definitions for further clarification. Federal legislation also provides a basis for state definitions by identifying a minimum set of acts or behaviors that characterized maltreatment and defines specific acts considered physical abuse, neglect, and sexual abuse (USDHHS, 1996).

Physical Abuse

The definition of physical abuse is the infliction of physical injury as a result of acts that may or may not have intended to hurt the child. Physical injury may have occurred as a result of beating, punching, kicking, biting, burning, or shaking a child (USDHHS, 2001b). Physical abuse may result in serious injury by nonaccidental means and includes specific signs and symptoms such as bruises, burns, fractures, lacerations, or subdural hematoma. Injuries may have resulted from physical punishment or excessive discipline by the child's parent or caregiver (USDHHS, 2001a, 2001b). All states prohibit the physical maltreatment of children although the criminal statutes that define physical abuse vary. Some states define different levels of abuse depending on the type of harm inflicted on the child, and some speak to a parent or caregiver's failure to protect a child from harm inflicted by another (USDHHS National Center for Prosecution of Child Abuse, 1999).

Sexual Abuse

Sexual abuse is defined as any form of sexual exploitation of children. A central component of sexual abuse is the misuse of an adult's power relationship with a child

Table 1-3. Victimization Rates by Maltreatment Type: 1995-1999 SDC

YEAR/ PARAMETER	PHYSICAL ABUSE	NEGLECT	MEDICAL NEGLECT	SEXUAL ABUSE	PSYCHOLOGIC ABUSE	OTHER ABUSE
1995						
Population	66 509 741	55 509 741	44 901 943	65 551 752	61 164 114	55 428 857
Number of Victims	236 514	509 454	23 541	122 542	42 869	144 705
Rate	3.6	7.7	0.6	1.9	0.7	2.7
Number of States	48	48	31	46	40	35
1996						
Population	65 068 883	65 068 883	49 111 322	65 068 883	60 431 527	55 200 768
Number of Victims	224 697	493 158	23 412	117 058	55 199	157 827
Rate	3.5	7.6	0.5	1.8	0.9	2.9
Number of States	46	46	33	46	39	33
1997						
Population	58 452 893	58 452 893	42 190 820	58 452 893	55 874 790	48 171 022
Number of Victims	194 512	435 877	18 552	96 984	48 599	88 018
Rate	3.4	7.5	0.4	1.7	0.9	1.9
Number of States	43	43	30	43	38	29
1998						
Population	66 964 555	66 964 555	49 305 311	66 964 555	63 825 291	52 788 857
Number of Victims	195 891	461 274	20 338	99 278	51 618	217 640
Rate	2.9	6.9	0.4	1.5	0.8	4.1
Number of States	48	48	35	48	43	33
1999						
Population	67 421 449	67 421 449	48 311 250	67 421 449	65 892 458	49 715 250
Number of Victims	166 626	437 540	18 788	88 238	59 846	219 549
Rate	2.5	6.5	0.4	1.3	0.9	4.4
Number of States	49	49	38	49	48	33
Total	**1 018 240**	**2 337 303**	**111 631**	**524 100**	**258 131**	**827 739**

Note: Rates were based on the number of victims divided by the child population, multiplied by 1000. The numbers of victims are based on data from reporting states for that year.

Reprinted from US Department of Health & Human Services. Child Maltreatment 1999: Reports From the States to the National Child Abuse and Neglect Data Systems. *Washington, DC: US Government Printing Office; 1999.*

and betrayal of the child's trust by the older adult (Sgroi, 1982). Specific activities noted as sexual abuse include any sexual activities by an older person that involve a dependent, developmentally immature child or adolescent and that are for the sexual stimulation and/or gratification of that person or of other persons, such as in child pornography or prostitution. Specific activities include sexualized kissing, fondling, exhibitionism, masturbation, digital or object penetration of the vagina or anus, and oral-genital, genital-genital, and anal-genital contact (Faller, 1988; Kempe, 1978; Sgroi, 1982). Also included are rape, statutory rape, molestation, prostitution, and caregiver or interfamilial relationships. Guidelines define sexual abuse in this context as the persuasion, use, inducement, enticement, employment, and/or coercion of a child to engage in, or assist another person to engage in, sexually explicit conduct or simulation of such conduct in order to produce visual depictions of it (USDHHS, 1996).

Emotional and Psychological Abuse

Emotional abuse involves a pervasive pattern of interactions on the part of the parents or other child caregivers that cause or could cause emotional, behavioral, cognitive, or mental disorders. It is most often defined on the basis of signs in the child's behavior or condition rather than abusive situations. There are habitual abusive interactions that often occur on a continuum within the child's environment. Interactions such as comparisons, name-calling, belittling through comments, scapegoating, humiliating or isolating exchanges, and screaming and raging are part of the interactions included in emotional and psychological abuse. Some cases of emotional abuse may support CPS intervention. One example is the extreme use of bizarre forms of punishment, such as confining a child in a dark closet. Included also is psychological inaccessibility or the rejection of treatment for the child (NCCANI, 2001). It is often difficult to link the acts of the parent or caregiver to the child's behaviors or condition.

Child Neglect

Child neglect is failure on the part of the caregiver or the caregiving environment to provide for a child's basic needs (Dubowitz, Giardino, & Gustavson, 2000; USDHHS, 2001a). Neglect is further categorized as physical, educational, or emotional. A component of clinical judgment is required in assessing some forms of neglect because there may be a recognition of cultural values or considerations of poverty-related causes not to provide what might be considered the necessities of life (USDHHS, 2001a). Specifics of physical neglect include a parent or caregivers' abandonment, delay in or refusal to seek appropriate healthcare, inadequate supervision, expulsion from the home, and refusal to allow a runaway child to return home (USDHHS, 2001a). Individual state laws may exclude neglect resulting from poverty or religious beliefs or practices as constituting failure on the part of parents or legal guardians to provide necessary care. Controversial situations include parental refusal of medical treatment for a child on religious grounds when the child's life is threatened. Such cases are often subject to litigation between parents and CPS professionals. (See Chapter 8, Clinical Aspects of Child Neglect, for further discussion.)

Emotional neglect is characterized by caretaker behaviors that indicate inattention to a child's emotional well-being. Such actions as inattention to affection needs, failure to address or provide psychological care, and abusive behaviors to spouse or others in the presence of a child are examples of emotional neglect. Allowing a child to use alcohol or drugs may be included in this category. Finally, caregivers engage in educational neglect when they fail to address the child's educational needs. Actions such as failure to enroll children of mandatory age in school, allowing chronic truancy, or failure to attend to special educational needs may be categorized as educational neglect (NCCANI, 2001; USDHHS, 2001a, 2001c).

LEGAL, INSTITUTIONAL, AND PERSONAL DEFINITIONS OF ABUSE

Defining the term ***child abuse*** is difficult because of its multifaceted nature and the complex set of behaviors involved in the various forms of abuse (Ludwig, 1992). Definitions of child abuse are important because they guide individual, legal, and institutional responses to child abuse and neglect. Healthcare providers need to understand child abuse definitions and comply with the definitions contained in the state laws that govern their geographical areas of practice. The ongoing institutional, legal, and individual components should all be in accordance with local and state laws that define and govern the many aspects of abuse. Ludwig (1992) defines 3 separate aspects of abuse that may vary with individuals and time.

First, the ***legal*** definition of abuse states that abuse is what the law says it is. Legal definitions guide professional practice in that professionals must comply with laws at the local, state, and federal levels. Legal definitions are specific for different types of abuse such as physical abuse, sexual abuse, or physical neglect.

The second type of definition is termed ***institutional***; an organization defines specific aspects of child abuse and then reports accordingly (Ludwig, 1992). The practical interpretation of a state law may vary from one institution to the next. Organizational definitions of abuse or neglect are developed to encompass a broad range of presentations, etiologies, or clinical manifestations with which the organization deals (Azar, 1991; Bourne, 1979; Helfer, 1987; Ludwig, 1992). Organizational definitions guide policies and procedures in the context of institutional environments and involve policies and procedures for professional conduct and practice. A theme underlying all organizational definitions is that active or passive caregiver behaviors are harmful to the growth and development and/or the well-being of the child (Ludwig, 1992).

The third level of definition is termed ***personal***; each individual may have his or her own definition of acceptable parental or caregiver behaviors (Ludwig, 1992). A person's individual definition encompasses a personal framework for abuse and then guides the person's perspective and clinical judgments. Specific actions such as the reporting of abuse are linked to a person's personal definition. Experiences of child rearing, family life, socioeconomic status, and religious, racial, or cultural factors may cause variance in individual definitions (Ludwig, 1992). A conflict could arise when a parent accused of abuse and the nurse reporting abuse see the situation differently, as in a case involving corporal punishment.

Professional and individual definitions of abuse often focus on what a professional looks for or deals with in relation to abusive situations. For example, healthcare providers such as nurses usually focus on specific physical aspects of injury in order to uncover and then describe injuries, whereas law enforcement looks at aspects of the abuse that may provide evidence to determine the innocence or guilt of an alleged perpetrator (Giardino & Ludwig, 2002; Ludwig, 1992). The focus of the social worker is usually on the family system and its caregivers and how that system gives rise to a situation in which abuse occurs.

THE CHILD ABUSE PREVENTION AND TREATMENT ACT

Many state laws are based on the Child Abuse Prevention and Treatment Act (CAPTA) definitions although states' definitions vary from detailed to vague regarding specifics of abuse. CAPTA, as amended (USDHHS, 1996), supports individual state efforts to develop, run, expand, and increase community-based, prevention-focused efforts and family resource and support programs. CAPTA was enacted by Congress to ensure that child victims of abuse and neglect can receive a comprehensive approach through state resources to integrate multiple agencies such as social service, legal, mental health, education, and substance abuse agencies (USDHHS, 1996).

CAPTA lays the groundwork for the federal government to provide aid to states for the human, technical, and fiscal resources necessary to develop and implement child protection strategies. These resources are particularly needed in low-income communities (USDHHS, 1996). State grants fund the improvement of CPS systems through training programs for CPS workers and mandated reporters and help to improve services to disabled infants with life-threatening conditions (USDHHS, 1999).

THE IMPACT OF PHYSICAL ABUSE AND NEGLECT

A child experiences the effects of abuse and neglect immediately and then over potentially many years. Even when an abusive situation was short lived, the psychological effects of that trauma may be experienced time and again. The physical effects may also be long term with approximately 37% of maltreated children with injuries developing a disability (USDHHS, 1993). Nurses treat children and then adults who are survivors of all forms of child maltreatment; thus, an understanding of the dynamics of abuse and the impact it has on individuals and families is an important aspect to providing comprehensive care for people of all ages.

Children who experience physical abuse exhibit more physical injuries, neurological signs, scars, and skin markings than those not abused (Kolko, 1992). Brain dysfunction and death are also consequences. The behavioral effects of physical maltreatment and neglect lead to problems with poor school performance (Eckenrode, Laird, & Doris, 1991) and aggressive behavior (Dodge, Bates, & Pettit, 1990). Abuse can have long-term effects on the mental health of adult survivors. Mental health problems manifested include multiple personality disorder, posttraumatic stress disorder, dissociative disorders, and physical manifestations of headaches and pelvic pain (Glod, 1993). Although the majority of abuse survivors will not experience the most extreme impairment, a large number of victims experience some level of dysfunction (Berliner & Elliott, 1996; Briere, 1992; Erickson & Egeland, 1996; Kolko, 1996). Briere (1992) describes 3 stages of impact that maltreatment may potentially have on the child: (1) initial reactions, including alterations in normal development, pained affect, posttraumatic stress, and cognitive distortions; (2) an accommodation response to ongoing abuse that includes coping behaviors anticipated to increase safety and/or decrease pain; and (3) ongoing accommodation and long-term effects reflecting initial reactions and accommodations rooted in the ongoing coping responses. Understanding and then implementing therapeutic efforts focused on coping strategies of the child or adult can help support the healing process of the survivor (Briere, 1992). (See also Chapter 10, Mental Health Aspects of Child Survivors of Abuse and Neglect.)

CONCEPTUAL FRAMEWORKS

Conceptual frameworks can put aspects of child physical abuse, neglect, and sexual abuse into the greater perspective of the overall family and social systems. Abuse always takes place in the context of family and social systems that have broken down or failed to protect the child. Theoretical frameworks that explain the complex causes of abuse are helpful to the practitioner who may be the one to identify abusive situations or treat the individual child or family members. The following sections describe 4 different frameworks that put abuse into a greater sociological perspective.

The conceptual frameworks to be discussed deal with the phenomena of physical abuse, neglect, and sexual abuse. Although it is sometimes the case that a child who is sexually abused may also experience physical abuse and/or neglect, and vice versa, there still seem to be certain individual and family dynamics that lead a person to abuse in a specific manner. Dynamics of the phenomena suggest that physical and sexual abuse are separate phenomena with unique abuser patterns of behavior, etiology, and treatment modalities (Finkelhor, 1986; Jason, Williams, Burton, & Rochat, 1982).

THE EPIDEMIOLOGICAL FRAMEWORK

The epidemiological approach to child abuse and neglect builds an understanding for the short- and long-term effects of abusive processes on normal child development (Helfer, 1987). People raised in abusive situations may have sensory system modifications that make it difficult for them to process their environment in a healthy way. Therefore, a child who struggles with difficult family situations and unrealistic expectations learns from adults inappropriate and maladaptive ways to meet his or her needs throughout the life span (Helfer, 1987). In essence, abusive situations may continue because the child turned adult learned few healthy interaction skills and developed poor decision-making abilities.

Helfer (1973) describes 4 categories that help make up the potential for abuse, as follows: (1) how parents were raised; (2) ability of caregivers (families) to use other people to help them when they are stressed; (3) quality of relationship between parents; and (4) how parents view the child. The epidemiological approach accounts for how a person who develops an abusive caregiving style begins to feel out of control through the negative interactions of unmet needs, muted senses, and few choices. This leads to poor self-esteem, an inability to trust others, and a possible series of unhealthy decisions about friends and partners (Helfer, 1987).

THE ECOLOGICAL FRAMEWORK

Child physical maltreatment occurs when there is dysfunction between the adult and child. The incidence of child maltreatment seems to increase as stressors outweigh the supports that people have within their environment (Belsky, 1993). The ecological approach to the study of abuse and neglect identifies the multifaceted causes of child abuse and then works to integrate divergent viewpoints of the role of the child, patterns of family interaction, and cultural values and social stress in the etiology of child maltreatment (Belsky, 1980; Justice, Calvert, & Justice, 1985). The model recognizes that although abusing parents and caretakers may have developmental histories that predispose them to possible maltreatment of children, stress-producing forces from within the family (microsystem) and in the outside (exosystem) environment may increase the likelihood of conflicts between parents and child (Belsky, 1980).

In essence, abusing parents enter into the family microsystem with potentially predisposing histories to treat children abusively. Then, stress-producing forces within the family (microsystem) and forces from outside of the family (exosystem) further increase the possibility of abusive behavior through parent-child conflicts. Parental/caregiver response to such conflicts results in maltreatment (Belsky, 1980). The ecological model can serve as a guide for both the prevention of child abuse and neglect and the identification of at-risk families. The model can help nurses understand factors and forces within a family system that may predispose a person to acting on abusive tendencies. Healthcare providers who understand the dynamics of individuals with their microsystems and exosystems are better prepared to intervene with support.

LONGITUDINAL PROGRESSION MODEL FOR CHILD SEXUAL ABUSE

The phenomenon of child sexual abuse occurs when there is a breakdown of protective mechanisms within the child's sociological system. The failure of protective mechanisms in some cases of sexual abuse occurs in a relatively systematic manner (Finkelhor, 1984). Sexual encounters between adults and children often occur within predictable patterns and are described by 5 separate phases (Sgroi, Blick, & Porter, 1982) known as engagement, sexual interaction, secrecy, disclosure, and retraction. A practitioner's understanding of the dynamics of child sexual abuse enables more appropriate interventions.

Engagement Phase

In child sexual abuse, the perpetrator usually has an opportunity to engage in inappropriate behaviors because he or she has entrée to private interactions with the child. Often, the abuser is someone within the child's family circle or an adult who has access to the child through age-appropriate group activities (Sgroi, 1982). The perpetrator typically engages the child in sexual behaviors by first proposing interactions and activities that are acceptable and interesting to the child, such as going for ice cream or becoming a friend who meets psychological needs or provides material rewards (Sgroi, 1982).

Sexual Interaction Phase

In the sexual interaction phase, the perpetrator engages in sexually inappropriate behavior through activities such as undressing, exposing genitals, and touching. These activities may progress in the level of sexual interactions suggested and encouraged by the perpetrator. Fondling, masturbation, and penetration of the child's body in a variety of ways may be realized at this phase (Sgroi, 1982). In boys and girls, the mouth and anus are areas for possible penetration, while penetration of the vagina in females may progress from digital penetration. In general, the sexual interaction phase involves a series of inappropriate sexual expectations and activities required of the child. Successful perpetrators may be subtle in their coerciveness to persuade compliance. However, in many situations, often in family relationships, the child is threatened into compliance through force or threat of force (Sgroi, 1982).

Secrecy Phase

The desire of a perpetrator is to keep the age-inappropriate sexual activity a secret to the rest of the world. Secrecy allows repetition of the behaviors, maintains the lack of accountability and responsibility, and avoids the interference of and judgment by society of the abusive adult (Sgroi, 1982). Therefore, the perpetrator must persuade the child to keep the secret through direct or indirect coercion. Perpetrators encourage secrecy in many ways, often by offering rewards or bribes or using threats. A subtle threat may involve the perpetrator indicating disapproval of the child if the child does not comply, whereas an explicit threat is one by which the perpetrator indicates harm to the child or loved ones if secrecy is broken. The secrecy phase may last for weeks, months, or years and only ends when the child maltreatment comes to light (Sgroi, 1982).

Disclosure Phase

A child's disclosure of sexual abuse occurs in either an accidental or purposeful manner (Sgroi, 1982). ***Accidental disclosure*** occurs when external circumstances come into play that reveal a perpetrator's inappropriate sexual behaviors. The following are usual scenarios that occur in accidental disclosures:

— A third party observes child and perpetrator in inappropriate activity and tells someone else.

— Physical injury occurs to the child and is noted by an outside observer.

— Signs of a sexually transmitted disease (STD) are noted through evaluation of a new onset of symptoms in the child, such as irritation or penile or vaginal discharge.

— The child becomes pregnant.

— The child engages in age-inappropriate sexual activity in other settings, such as in school or with playmates, that indicates his or her exposure to developmentally inappropriate behaviors.

Accidental disclosure may precipitate a crisis within the family system because the child did not purposely set out to disclose the situation. Therefore, the clinician should be prepared to anticipate problems and foresee the need for crisis intervention when disclosure occurs (Sgroi, 1982).

Purposeful disclosure occurs when the child decides to tell another person about the sexual abuse. There are many reasons for sharing the secret with others, and these vary with the child's developmental level. A young child may want to share the experience, whereas an older child may want to end the abuse and escape family or individual pressure or release personal anger or frustration with the abusive situation (Sgroi, 1982). Disclosure often brings the child mixed emotions of relief, guilt, and disloyalty because the circumstances surrounding the abuse are complex and family relationships are likely to be affected and potentially disrupted.

Retraction Phase

After a child discloses sexual abuse and the events surrounding it, it is not uncommon for the child to recant the story. Family members are often overwhelmed by the situation and may want to forget about it (Sgroi, 1982). The perpetrator may exert direct or indirect pressure on the family and/or the child to induce guilt or fear that the family will be disrupted or destroyed as a result of legal actions taken against the perpetrator. This may be especially true if the perpetrator is the breadwinner of the family because incarceration will inevitably lead to financial loss for the family. Therefore, family members may pressure the child to retract the story and details of the abusive events. Family members may say that the child fabricated the details, and thus, the story can be dismissed as a flight of the imagination.

TRAUMAGENIC DYNAMICS MODEL FOR CHILD SEXUAL ABUSE

Models that explain the dynamics of how child abuse and neglect come to be in a family system are important because they help practitioners understand and identify those factors as seen in healthcare visits with children and their caregivers. Models provide frameworks that help to characterize the kinds of psychological injury that happen to a child who has been sexually abused. The Traumagenic Dynamics Model developed by Finkelhor and Browne (1985) describes how specific dynamics come together in a child to alter the child's cognitive and emotional being and distort aspects of worldview, self-concept, and ability to receive and give affection. The model describes 4 trauma-causing dynamics responsible for the child's psychological alterations called traumatic sexualization, betrayal, powerlessness, and stigmatization. The dynamics are used to assess child sexual abuse victims and then anticipate potential problems to which the child may be vulnerable (Finkelhor & Browne, 1985).

There may be common types of trauma to a person's psyche caused by physical, sexual, and emotional abuse and neglect. However, Finkelhor and Browne (1985) postulate that the trauma caused by sexual abuse is unique. They describe 4 dynamics that come together in the circumstances of sexual abuse.

Traumatic sexualization caused by sexual abuse is a process that shapes a child's sexual feelings and attitudes in a way that is developmentally inappropriate and interpersonally dysfunctional (Finkelhor & Browne, 1985). It is a complex process that occurs when a child is rewarded by a perpetrator for sexual behavior that is developmentally inappropriate or given attention or privileges for inappropriate behavior. Traumatic sexualization also occurs through the perpetrator's distortion to the child of the importance and meaning of a child's sexual anatomy and through misconceptions the child develops of sexual behavior and sexual morality. Furthermore, the child's mind begins to associate frightening memories and events to sexual activity (Finkelhor & Browne, 1985). A sexually traumatized child may demonstrate age-inappropriate sexual behaviors, along with a myriad of confusion surrounding his or her own sexual self-concept, and may experience difficult emotional associations with sexual activity (Finkelhor & Browne, 1985).

Betrayal occurs when an individual who should be a trusted person or one on whom a child is vitally dependent causes the child harm. The child may experience different levels of adult betrayal, one involving the person who actually molests the child and others involving family members who should have protected the child but perhaps failed to believe the story or take the child out of an abusive situation. The degree of betrayal experienced is affected by the child's relationship to the perpetrator, how much trust there was in the beginning between the two, and the possible disbelief of others when the child does disclose the abuse (Finkelhor & Browne, 1985). All of the situations experienced throughout abusive activities contribute to betrayal dynamics. One aspect of emotional trauma is the impairment the child may have in future relationships with adults and others to be able or willing to form trusting relationships.

Powerlessness is a process whereby the child attempts to halt the abuse or have it halted by others but is unable to do so. Over time, the child learns to feel disempowered or powerless to change situations (Finkelhor & Browne, 1985). He or she has a resultant loss of self-efficacy and feelings of powerlessness over his or her life. Child sexual abuse involves the invasion of a child's body space and territory, as well as coercion and manipulation that tend to cause feelings of entrapment and an inability to change situations. Powerlessness is a process that occurs to the psyche, inner being, and will of a child. Impaired coping strategies may result from this phenomena and manifest in symptoms such as phobias, nightmares, depression, clinging behavior, and running away (Finkelhor & Browne, 1985).

A child experiences *stigmatization* when negative connotations of the abusive behavior become incorporated into the child's psyche. These connotations include feelings of shame, badness, or guilt (Finkelhor & Browne, 1985). It is often the abuser who helps instill such thoughts and inferences through activities such as blaming or demeaning the child for the abusive behavior or conveying shame concerning the nature of the activity. Stigmatization comes from the child knowing that family and community consider certain sexual activity taboo. The term "damaged goods" has been applied to how a child victim of sexual abuse often feels that he or she is less than whole or is damaged in some way (Sgroi, 1982).

Children experience a myriad of emotional and psychological reactions to child sexual abuse. Circumstances such as how well or poorly the abuser treats the child, or keeping a difficult secret, reinforce the stigma of the abuse. Some manifestations of the stigmatization phenomena may be feelings of isolation or gravitation toward others who feel the same self-destructive behavior, depression, and suicide attempts. Victims of child sexual abuse often carry a great amount of shame and guilt for a long time and experience a low sense of self-esteem (Finkelhor & Browne, 1985).

The organizing framework of traumagenic dynamics helps healthcare providers understand possible outcomes in the emotional and physical development of child sexual abuse survivors. Manifestations may be seen at all stages of development and include age-inappropriate sexual behaviors such as masturbation or sexualized play with other children. The list of problems that adult survivors of child sexual abuse experience is lengthy. Survivors report flashbacks, inability to form intimate relationships with others, and a higher incidence of sexual victimization (Finkelhor & Browne, 1985). The more the nurse knows about the dynamics of child sexual abuse and the manifestations of abuse, the better able he or she is to deal with the problems that clients may have.

THE ROLE OF THE NURSE IN CHILD ABUSE AND NEGLECT

MANDATED REPORTING

Nurses as healthcare providers are mandated reporters of abuse in every state and the District of Columbia, along with other professionals who interact with children. It is important that nurses understand reporting laws in their specific state, the circumstances under which one reports abuse, and to whom reports are made (O'Toole, O'Toole, Webster, & Lucal, 1996; USDHHS, 2001b). Circumstances under which a nurse or other mandated reporter should report include when there is reasonable cause to suspect or believe that a child has been abused or neglected and when one observes a child subjected to circumstances or conditions that might reasonably result in abuse or neglect (Freed & Drake, 1999; USDHHS, 2001b). Nurses who have greater knowledge and expertise in child abuse and neglect are better reporters (Flaherty, Sege, Binns, Mattson, & Christoffel, 2000). (See Chapter 14, Legal Issues, for further discussion.)

DEALING WITH CHILD MALTREATMENT

Nurses' responsibility in dealing with child maltreatment emanates from the roles that emerge from the practice of nursing (Bridges, 1978). Nursing practice has been described in a multitude of ways and has been summarized by Bridges (1978) as comprising the following 2 functions:

1. Identification of the child's and family's needs around possible maltreatment

2. Provision of appropriate services to the child and family that focus on the safety and well-being of the child

Bridges (1978) further states that nurses' effectiveness as members of the multi-disciplinary team caring for the child and family depends on the following:

— Competency in understanding and performing nursing skills

— Perception and understanding of the nursing role and resultive expectations by the nurse and the other team members

— Body of knowledge and guidelines that govern nursing practice

The above points are applicable to nursing settings in which nurses may encounter children and families within both the traditional healthcare setting and the growing range of related settings in which nurses may practice. McCleery and Pinyerd (1988) have characterized the traditional settings in which the nurse may encounter children, as follows:

— Routine home visits by public health and home health nurses

— Clinic, office, or emergency department

— In-patient hospital units

— Schools and camps

With advanced practice nursing and the increase in clinical nurse specialists and nurse practitioners, there are many areas of practice in which nurses work collaboratively with physicians and other healthcare professionals or in independent settings such as nursing centers. In the area of sexual assault, nurses have assumed specialized roles in the evaluation and investigation of the victims of abuse and assault. Such nurses pursue additional training and may be designated forensic nurses called sexual assault nurse examiners (SANEs). SANEs evaluate victims by assessing the person, collecting forensic evidence, and documenting the findings of the evaluation (Ledray, 1999).

Pediatricians caution that the evaluation of suspected child sexual abuse requires particular attention to the developmental aspects of childhood and requires a comprehensive approach based on training in the care of children and the unique aspects of child sexual abuse (Finkel & DeJong, 2001). Nurses also participate in prevention, mental health, and research activities as they relate to child maltreatment.

RESEARCH PERSPECTIVES ON CHILD ABUSE AND NEGLECT

Ongoing research in child abuse and neglect is important because of the many problems that abuse is known to cause to individuals and society. Specific problems such as poor academic performance, delayed development, depression, delinquency, and substance abuse are known outcomes of some, while others demonstrate criminal and domestic violence and inappropriate sexual behaviors (Collaborative Studies Coordinating Center, 2001) in response to childhood traumas.

Nurses can become involved in many types of research to address the complex phenomenon of child abuse. Nurses have been on the forefront of home visitation as a way to educate parents and caregivers identified as at-risk families and prevent further abuse (Eckenrode et al., 2000; Olds et al., 1997). Much still needs to be determined concerning the efficacy of such initiatives and whether the outcomes justify the funding and future funding of such programs. Current home visitation programs provide new data for home visitation statistics, while longitudinal studies on those families that have been part of home visitation initiatives will help determine the effectiveness of the programs. It is important to determine the impact of specific types of abuse on the child's life, looking at longitudinal and developmental effects (Collaborative Studies Coordinating Center, 2001; Runyan et al., 1998) of child abuse on the child and the adult. Research based on the ecological perspective (Belsky, 1980, 1993) on abuse can help healthcare providers focus on the ways in which factors affecting individuals and their families and communities come together in the causes and consequences of maltreatment (Collaborative Studies Coordinating Center, 2001).

Outcome research on abuse and neglect shows that supportive, responsible people and systems can help decrease the harmful effects of child abuse on the child and future adult. It is important that the child be nurtured and supported in a safe environment to enhance the possibility of healing and normal development.

SUMMARY

The pervasive nature of child abuse and neglect in society is immense, and the effects of abuse and neglect are great on those children and adults who survive the trauma. Nurses have a grave responsibility to understand the issues involved in maltreatment and then to be prepared to advocate for children through direct clinical care provided to the child and family. As nurses grow in their knowledge of the types of maltreatment and the underlying causes, this provides for better identification of the problem, intervention, and eventually prevention efforts.

Later chapters outline the major aspects of the healthcare approach to the care of children suspected of having been abused or neglected, detailing the nurse's role in meeting the needs of these children and their families.

REFERENCES

Azar S. Models of child abuse: a metatheoretical analysis. *Crim Just Behav*. 1991;18:30-46.

Belsky J. Child maltreatment: an ecological integration. *Am Psychol*. 1980;35:320-335.

Belsky J. Etiology of child maltreatment: a developmental-ecological analysis. *Psychol Bull*. 1993;114:413-434.

Berliner L, Elliott D. Sexual abuse of children. In: Briere J, Berliner L, Bulkley J, Jenny C, Reid T, eds. *The APSAC Handbook on Child Maltreatment*. Thousand Oaks, Calif: Sage Publications; 1996:51-71.

Bourne R. Child abuse and neglect: an overview. In: Bourne R, Newberger E, eds. *Critical Perspectives on Child Abuse*. Lexington, Mass: Lexington Books; 1979:1-14.

Bridges CL. The nurses' evaluation. In: BD Schmitt, ed. *The Child Protection Team Handbook*. New York, NY: Garland Publishing; 1978:65-81.

Briere J. *Child Abuse Trauma: Theory and Treatment of the Lasting Effects*. Newbury Park, Calif: Sage Publications; 1992.

Caldwell R. The Costs of Child Abuse vs. Child Abuse Prevention: Michigan's Experience. Michigan State University website. June 12, 1992. Available at: http://www.msu.edu/user/bob/cost.html. Accessed December 16, 2002.

Collaborative Studies Coordinating Center. *LONGSCAN: Longitudinal Studies of Child Abuse and Neglect*. Consortium for Longitudinal Studies in Child Abuse and Neglect. 2001. Available at: http://www.bios.unc.edu/cscc/LONG/longdesc.html. Accessed July 28, 2001.

Daro D. *Confronting Child Abuse: Research for Effective Program Design*. New York, NY: The Free Press; 1988.

Dodge K, Bates J, Pettit G. Mechanisms in the cycle of violence. *Science*. 1990;250:1678-1683.

Dubowitz H. The diagnosis of child sexual abuse. *Am J Dis Child*. 1992;146:688-693.

Dubowitz H, Giardino A, Gustavson E. Child neglect: guidance for pediatricians. *Pediatr Rev*. 2000;21:111-116.

Eckenrode J, Ganzel B, Henderson C, et al. Preventing child abuse and neglect with a program of nurse home visitation. *JAMA*. 2000;284:1385-1391.

Eckenrode J, Laird M, Doris J. *Maltreatment and Social Adjustment of School Children. National Center on Child Abuse and Neglect*. Grant 90CA1305. Washington, DC: US Dept of Health & Human Services; 1991.

Erickson M, Egeland B. Child neglect. In: Briere J, Berliner L, Bulkley J, Jenny C, Reid T, eds. *The APSAC Handbook on Child Maltreatment*. Thousand Oaks, Calif: Sage Publications; 1996:4-20.

Faller K. *Child Sexual Abuse: An Interdisciplinary Manual for Diagnosis, Case Management, and Treatment*. New York, NY: Columbia University Press; 1988.

Finkel M, DeJong AR. Medical findings in sexual abuse. In: Reece R, ed. *Child Abuse: Diagnosis and Treatment*. New York, NY: Lippincott Williams & Wilkins; 2001:207-286.

Finkelhor D. *Child Sexual Abuse: New Theory and Research*. New York, NY: The Free Press; 1984.

Finkelhor D. *A Sourcebook on Child Sexual Abuse*. Beverly Hills, Calif: Sage Publications; 1986.

Finkelhor D, Browne A. The traumatic impact of child sexual abuse: a conceptualization. *Am J Orthopsychiatry*. 1985;55:530-541.

Flaherty EG, Sege R, Binns HJ, Mattson CL, Christoffel KK. Health care providers' experience reporting child abuse in the primary care setting. *Arch Pediatr Adolesc Med*. 2000;154:489-493.

Freed P, Drake V. Mandatory reporting of abuse: practical, moral, and legal issues for psychiatric home health nurses. *Issues Ment Health Nurs*. 1999;20:423-436.

Giardino A, Ludwig S. Interdisciplinary approaches to child maltreatment: accessing community resources. In: Finkel M, Giardino A, eds. *Medical Evaluation of Child Sexual Abuse: A Practical Guide*. 2nd ed. Thousand Oaks, Calif: Sage Publications; 2002:215-231.

Glod CA. Long-term consequences of childhood physical and sexual abuse. *Arch Psychiatr Nurs*. 1993;7:163-173.

Goldson E. Children with disabilities and child maltreatment. *Child Abuse Negl*. 1998;22:663-667.

Helfer R. The etiology of child abuse. *Pediatrics*. 1973;51:777-779.

Helfer R. The developmental basis of child abuse and neglect: an epidemiological approach. In: Helfer R, Kempe R, eds. *The Battered Child*. 4th ed. Chicago, Ill: The University of Chicago Press; 1987:60-80.

Jason J, Williams S, Burton A, Rochat R. Epidemiological differences between sexual and physical child abuse. *JAMA*. 1982;247:3344-3348.

Jones L, Finkelhor D. *The Decline in Child Sexual Abuse Cases. Office of Juvenile Justice and Delinquency Prevention Juvenile Justice Bulletin*. Washington, DC: US Dept of Justice, Office of Justice Programs; 2001. Available at: http://www.ncjrs.org/pdffiles1/ojjdp/184741.pdf. Accessed March 11, 2003.

Justice B, Calvert A, Justice R. Factors mediating child abuse as a response to stress. *Child Abuse Negl*. 1985;9:359-363.

Kempe C. Sexual abuse, another hidden pediatric problem: the 1977 C. Anderson Aldrich lecture. *Pediatrics*. 1978;62:382-389.

Kolko D. Characteristics of child victims of physical violence: research findings and clinical implications. *J Interpers Violence*. 1992;7:244-276.

Kolko D. Child physical abuse. In: Briere J, Berliner L, Bulkley J, Jenny C, Reid T, eds. *The APSAC Handbook on Child Maltreatment*. Thousand Oaks, Calif: Sage Publications; 1996:21-50.

Ledray LE. IAFN Sixth Annual Scientific Assembly highlights. *J Emerg Nurs*. 1999;25:63-64.

Ludwig S. Defining child abuse: clinical mandate—evolving concepts. In: Ludwig S, Kornberg A, eds. *Child Abuse: A Medical Reference*. 2nd ed. New York, NY: Churchill Livingstone; 1992:1-12.

McCleery JT, Pinyerd BJ. Nursing evaluation and treatment planning. In: Bross DC, Krugman RD, Lenherr MR, Rosenberg DA, Schmitt BD, eds. *The New Child Protection Team Handbook*. New York, NY: Garland Publishing; 1988:127-135.

National Clearinghouse on Child Abuse and Neglect Information. *Prevention Pays: The Costs of Not Preventing Child Abuse and Neglect*. Washington, DC: US Dept of Health & Human Services; 1998.

National Clearinghouse on Child Abuse and Neglect Information. *What Is Child Maltreatment?* National Clearinghouse on Child Abuse and Neglect Information. Available at: http://www.calib.com/nccanch/pubs/factsheets/childmal.cfm. Accessed May 8, 2001.

Olds D, Eckenrode J, Henderson CR Jr, et al. Long-term effects of home visitation on maternal life course and child abuse and neglect. *JAMA*. 1997;278:637-643.

Olds DL, Hill PL, Mihalic SF, O'Brien RA. *Blueprints for Violence Prevention, Book Seven: Prenatal and Infancy Home Visitation by Nurses.* Boulder, Colo: Center for the Study and Prevention of Violence, University of Colorado at Boulder; 1998.

O'Toole A, O'Toole R, Webster S, Lucal B. Nurses' diagnostic work on possible physical child abuse. *Public Health Nurs.* 1996;13:337-344.

Runyan D, Curtis PA, Hunter WM, et al. LONGSCAN: a consortium for longitudinal studies of maltreatment and the life course of children. *Aggress Violent Behav.* 1998;3:275-285.

Sgroi SM. *Handbook of Clinical Intervention on Child Sexual Abuse.* New York, NY: DC Heath and Company; 1982.

Sgroi SM, Blick L, Porter F. A conceptual framework for child sexual abuse. In: Sgroi SM, ed. *Handbook of Clinical Intervention on Child Sexual Abuse.* New York, NY: DC Heath and Company; 1982:9-37.

US Department of Health & Human Services. *A Report on the Maltreatment of Children With Disabilities.* 105-89-16300. Washington, DC: US Government Printing Office; 1993.

US Department of Health & Human Services. Child Abuse Prevention and Treatment Act, as Amended (October 3, 1996). 42 U.S.C. 5106g et seq. P.L. 104-235, October 3, 1996.

US Department of Health & Human Services. *Child Maltreatment 1999: Reports From the States to the National Child Abuse and Neglect Data Systems.* Washington, DC: US Government Printing Office; 1999.

US Department of Health & Human Services. *What Is Child Maltreatment?* National Clearinghouse on Child Abuse and Neglect Information. Available at: http://www.calib.com/nccanch. Accessed June 19, 2001a.

US Department of Health & Human Services. *Child Abuse and Neglect State Statutes Elements: Reporting Laws: Number 1: Definitions of Child Abuse and Neglect.* National Clearinghouse on Child Abuse and Neglect Information. Available at: http://www.calib.com/nccanch/pubs/stats01/define/index.cfm. Accessed June 8, 2001b.

US Department of Health & Human Services. *Child Abuse and Neglect State Statutes Elements: Reporting Laws: Number 2: Mandatory Reporters of Child Abuse and Neglect.* May 15, 2001. National Clearinghouse on Child Abuse and Neglect Information. Available at: http://www.calib.com/nccanch/pubs/stats01/mandrep.cfm Accessed July 6, 2001c.

US Department of Health & Human Services, National Center for Prosecution of Child Abuse. *Child Abuse and Neglect State Statutes Elements: Crimes: Number 34: Physical Abuse.* Washington, DC: National Clearinghouse on Child Abuse and Neglect Information; 1999:1-29.

Wilson C, Pence D. How should child protective services and law enforcement coordinate the initial assessment and investigation? In: Dubowitz H, DePanfilis D, eds. *Handbook for Child Protection Practice.* Thousand Oaks, Calif: Sage Publications; 1999:101-104.

Chapter 2

PRESENTATION AND OVERVIEW OF THE EVALUATION OF CHILD MALTREATMENT

Sandra L. Elvik, MS, RN, CPNP
Eileen R. Giardino, PhD, RN, CRNP
Angelo P. Giardino, MD, PhD, FAAP

The healthcare practitioner who evaluates children and families sees many presentations for child abuse and neglect, ranging from the most obvious, pathognomonic situations to subtle, occult injuries or high-risk situations that are only uncovered because of a high index of suspicion and meticulous medical evaluations. Additionally, forms of maltreatment related to sexual abuse and exploitation may only present with nonspecific behavioral concerns. They are referred to as nonspecific complaints because they represent behaviors that might be seen in children experiencing other serious situations, such as parental divorce or moving to a new location, and are not necessarily specific to maltreatment. Often, however, the nurse is among the first healthcare professionals to have contact with the maltreated child. Therefore nurses involved in all areas of practice must recognize the signs and symptoms that may suggest maltreatment, as well as be familiar with situations in which child maltreatment is seen. Regardless of the practice setting, all healthcare providers must be attuned to the many faces of child maltreatment and be sensitive to verbal, physical, and behavioral cues that alert to the possibility of maltreatment. Nurses and other healthcare providers must then work to evaluate these suspicions and findings in light of the following child- and family-specific information:

— Historical details provided

— Physical signs uncovered

— Laboratory and diagnostic testing data received

— Family background/cultural practices observed

— The child's expected developmental level and abilities

The best interests of the child and families are served by a healthcare provider who has a low index of suspicion for the possibility of child maltreatment and who generates broad differential diagnoses that consider child abuse and neglect and its various forms as a possible explanation for what is before him or her. In the early years of professional study of child maltreatment, Sgroi (1975) recognized that a prerequisite for healthcare providers diagnosing sexual abuse is their willingness to consider that it exists. When abuse or neglect is not part of a differential diagnosis, a healthcare provider is not likely to rule in or out that diagnosis.

Child maltreatment in any form is a crime, and there are mandatory reporting laws in all 50 states that direct the steps to take when a child comes to a professional with findings that suggest child abuse or neglect (US Department of Health & Human Services [USDHHS], 2002). Child abuse reporting laws clearly define mandated reporters, who by virtue of their work with children are obligated to alert appropriate authorities of suspicions concerning abuse and neglect. Nurses are mandated reporters in all 50 states. State laws and regulations vary from state to state on such items as time parameters for reporting, format for the report, and how and when law enforcement is involved. It is important for nurses and other healthcare providers to familiarize themselves with the outline of the law under which they are practicing, as well as the policies and procedures at their place of employment and practice. (See Chapter 14, Legal Issues.)

The healthcare evaluation of child maltreatment is best done in a multidisciplinary manner with each discipline contributing its expertise in the process (Giardino & Ludwig, 2002). The role of nurses in evaluating abuse and neglect is far-reaching and includes intervening in all aspects of the prevention, evaluation, and treatment of children who have been abused. The advanced practice nurse has assumed major areas of responsibility in collaboration with physician colleagues around the following areas of child abuse evaluation:

— Interviewing the child for the medical history

— Examining the child for physical findings and collecting forensic evidence when appropriate

— Ordering and interpreting appropriate laboratory and diagnostic tests

— Observing interactions between child and family

— Generating differential diagnoses

— Carefully documenting the findings of a complete healthcare evaluation

The diagnostic approach to a child suspected to have been abused or neglected relies on the clinical process of taking a history, performing a physical examination, and obtaining laboratory findings to allow the differential diagnosis, which includes a wide variety of conditions, and ends with a diagnostic impression and development of the treatment plan. This chapter provides an overview of the healthcare evaluation process related to possible forms of child maltreatment seen by the practicing nursing professional focusing on physical abuse, sexual abuse, and neglect.

OVERVIEW: PRESENTATIONS AND EVALUATION

PHYSICAL ABUSE

Eighteen percent of the nearly 1 million annual substantiated reports for child maltreatment can be categorized as physical abuse (Peddle & Wang, 2001). Physical abuse is diagnosed when a child sustains an injury inflicted by a parent, caregiver, or anyone else in a position of authority over the child. Injuries from physical abuse may present in various ways to the healthcare provider. The injury may initially be obvious or occult and only discovered later in the comprehensive evaluation. Ludwig (1999) suggests a "building block" approach in which each block represents a component of the healthcare evaluation and the blocks build on each other **(Figure 2-1)**. As the blocks are stacked, the growing tower may rise to a "concern threshold" where the data gathered suggest the need for further consideration of child maltreatment, or the block tower may exceed the concern threshold and cross the reporting threshold, requiring the healthcare provider to make a report to the child protective services (CPS) agency. Each component of the healthcare evaluation provides information represented by a block. The stack of blocks increases until it reaches the point at which concern for possible abuse either arises or is confirmed.

Physical injuries may present incidentally during complete examinations done for routine well-child care evaluations or during acute illness visits. Injuries may be so severe that the child presents moribund and is in need of emergency medical care and resuscitation. Some children present with fatal injuries and cannot be saved. Additionally, a child may present over time, with a pattern of injuries that suggests repeated abuse over a time period.

Presentation of a child with the diagnosis of possible physical abuse is a medical emergency. The healthcare evaluation of a child suspected to be physically abused should be undertaken immediately. The healthcare provider's goals are to assess and treat the child who has a potential inflicted injury and to ensure that the child will be kept safe and protected from risk of subsequent injury.

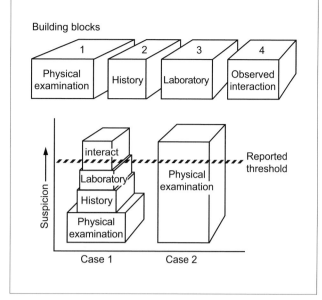

Figure 2-1. *Building a level of suspicion. Reprinted with permission from Ludwig S. Child abuse. In: Fleisher GR, Ludwig S, eds.* Textbook of Pediatric Emergency Medicine. *4th ed. Philadelphia, Pa: Lippincott Williams & Wilkins; 1999:1680.*

Once a child comes for care of an injury, the healthcare provider completes a thorough healthcare evaluation to diagnose the extent of injury and the mechanism by which it resulted. A complete healthcare evaluation in the face of possible maltreatment includes the following components:

— History from child and caregiver, including the periods before, during, and after the injury occurred

— Physical examination to evaluate obvious injury and possible hidden injuries

— Laboratory and diagnostic testing as appropriate for possible findings

— Observation of the child and caregiver interaction throughout the healthcare episode, noting caregiver-child communication and caregiver responses to the child's needs

— Meticulous documentation of the entire evaluation, beginning with the initial presentation for care and concluding with a diagnostic impression

Obtaining a history for an injury can begin with simply asking the question, "What happened here?" or, "How did the injury happen?" in an open-ended, nonthreatening manner. This approach gives the verbal child and/or caregiver the opening needed to provide details of how the injury occurred. Based on the response to this question, other questions related to the injury may be asked and documented (Farley & Reece, 1996). This information may or may not be accurate. The healthcare provider considers the history in light of the rest of the physical examination and then determines the plausibility of the mechanism of injury offered. If the presentation, history, and injury do not seem concordant or have characteristics that do not make sense, the level of suspicion is raised to the point of reporting the information to CPS.

Careful documentation of the caregiver's account at the time of presentation is essential because it is possible that an abusive caregiver's initial report will change over time as the seriousness of the situation becomes clearer (Elvik, 1998). It is important for the healthcare professional to carefully document the time and content of statements made by the parent/caregiver in the medical record so that it can then be shared with other professionals involved in the case. Discrepancies noted during the evaluation are an important component in the overall evaluation. (See Chapter 3, History and the Healthcare Interview, for details on interviewing children and caregivers.)

Presentations and subsequent evaluations of injuries with the following characteristics are among the most worrisome for possible child maltreatment:

— *Magical injuries in the young child:* two-month-old with femur fracture or skull fracture but no one witnessed any trauma that would provide an injury mechanism.

— *Changing history of the injury over time:* initial mechanism of injury that was offered changes in subsequent interviews to what are thought to be more plausible stories or to descriptions that may account for injuries that have been newly uncovered.

— *History incongruous with injury seen on physical examination:* history of minor trauma in the face of massive injury.

— *History implausible for injury:* mechanism of injury does not explain the injury found on examination.

— *Developmentally incompatible history:* child not developmentally capable of doing what caregiver said he or she did to get the injury observed.

— *Self-inflicted trauma history:* child threw himself into bathtub of scalding hot water.

— *Young sibling or playmate blamed for serious injury:* eighteen-month-old sibling blamed for massive intracranial injury found in 6-week-old brother.

— *Delayed presentation/late medical care:* caregiver brings child for care of injury long after a reasonable caregiver would have sought healthcare assistance.

Differentiating Accidental From Inflicted Injuries

As the child's injuries are examined, the healthcare provider should pay special attention to the location of the injury, the injury pattern, the mechanisms that could plausibly explain the injury seen as opposed to the one that is described by the caregiver on presentation, and the developmental level and capabilities of the child. Children and adults can be injured accidentally despite reasonable precautions taken in the environment, but careful evaluation of the injury is necessary to determine an

Table 2-1. Typically Accidental Versus Possibly Nonaccidental Injury Sites	
TYPICALLY ACCIDENTAL	POSSIBLY NONACCIDENTAL
Forehead	Scalp
Elbow	Behind ears
Knees	Neck
Shins	Axillae
Iliac crest	Inner thighs
	Webs of fingers/toes
	Genitalia

accidental (noninflicted) versus an inflicted mechanism. In the context of a case that is possibly physical abuse, several types of injuries are discussed, specifically bruises, burns, skeletal fractures, and central nervous system (CNS) injury.

Bruises

Bruising is the most common soft tissue injury seen in childhood, and bruises are a nearly universal finding on the routine well-child examination. However, certain characteristics invoke more concern for possible inflicted trauma. These characteristics are related to the location of the bruises, the shape of the bruises, and the amount and extent of the bruising.

In active children, accidental bruises are generally seen over areas with a bony prominence, such as the knees and shins. The forehead and chin are other sites of accidental trauma, especially in toddlers who are learning to walk and run. Inflicted trauma may at times cause bruising in protected (clothed) areas of the body that would be viewed as uncommon in accidental trauma. Injuries seen in "hidden" or protected body areas are of significant concern and may be easily overlooked during an examination. Hidden areas include the neck, axillae, abdomen, back, and inner thighs, which are more difficult to reach **(Table 2-1)**.

There are countless ways to inflict bruising injuries on a child's skin, including use of hands and objects. Pinches and slaps by the caregiver may or may not leave patterned markings. Additionally, some objects used to injure children have characteristic shapes that, when forcefully applied

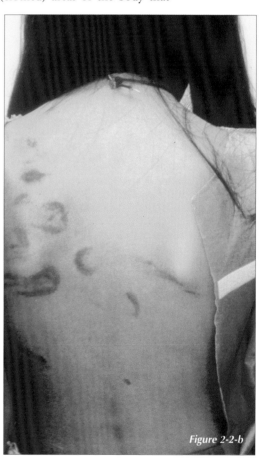

Figure 2-2-b

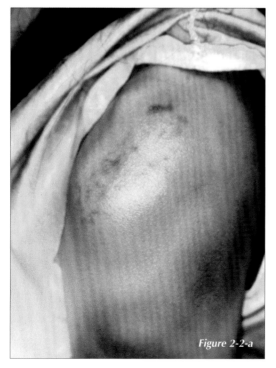

Figure 2-2-a

Figure 2-2. (a) *Nine-year-old Asian girl. The history was that the biological father became angry with the child for getting a "bad" grade on a test. (The grade was a "B," and the father wanted the child to get "straight As.") The father began punching the child with his fist but soon tired and grabbed a hanger. This is the child's shoulder and upper arm.* **(b)** *The child's back. Note the fixed loop marks, which are consistent with the child's history of being hit with a hanger. (No court case was conducted; the father confessed to the beating and was sent to jail.)*

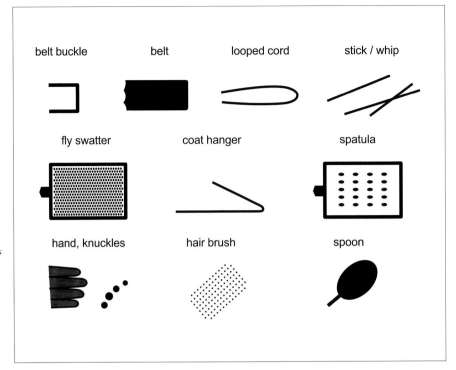

Figure 2-3. Marks from objects that bruise. Reprinted with permission from Johnson CF. Inflicted injury versus accidental injury. Ped Clin North Am.1990;37:803.

against the child's skin, leave characteristic geometric markings **(Figure 2-2-a and -b)**. Patterned bruising on the child's skin makes the identification of the implement used to harm the child possible. The nurse should describe in detail the pattern of the injury, including shape, dimensions, pattern, and coloring variability (such as areas of normal skin interspersed with reddish-blue linear markings). **Figure 2-3** illustrates shapes of commonly used objects that may be employed to bruise children.

Child abuse typically occurs longitudinally and represents a pattern of caregiving behaviors over time that result in the child's injury. Indication of ongoing battering of the child raises the concern of physical maltreatment. The child may have a large amount of bruising and/or the bruising may be composed of crops of bruises of different ages. Caution is needed when attempting to date bruises based on their color (Schwartz & Ricci, 1996). In general, bruises undergo a series of color changes from the reddish-blue seen in the immediate phase to the yellowish-brown seen during final stages of resolution (Wilson, 1977). Exact times for bruise changes to occur cannot be determined because they are quite variable and the literature does not support certainty in actual dating (Schwartz & Ricci, 1996). However, healthcare providers can compare bruises on a specific child and determine the age of the injury based on color changes. At best, healthcare providers should only give broad ranges of how old they suspect different bruises are in comparison to others.

Cultural factors must also be considered. Families who have emigrated from other parts of the world bring with them certain traditions. Besides foods and celebrations of particular holidays, there are customary forms of health and healing that may differ from those of traditional Western practices. The healthcare provider should consider the child's cultural background because the folk healing practices common to some cultures may leave characteristic marks on a child's skin (Feldman, 1997). Some Asian families practice *cao gio*, or "coining," in which a coin is rubbed over the area of pain or illness. The friction from the rubbing of the coin results in petechiae and bruising, usually over the ribs and chest. "Cupping" is a practice used in some parts of China since the third century BC; it involves lighting a match into a small round "cup" made of glass, bamboo, ceramic, or metal. Once heated, the cup is applied quickly to the skin. The heating and cooling creates a partial vacuum as the cup sticks tightly to the skin, and this suction-like action creates a bruise that resembles a circular burn. Several cups may be applied at any one time to a particular part of the body for the purpose of increasing blood circulation and promoting healing (Feldman, 1997).

Some skin findings may raise concern for possible abuse but on evaluation are found to have a nonabusive cause. For example, a Mongolian spot is a skin finding commonly mistaken for abuse **(Figure 2-4)**. This blue-black macule is seen on the skin, most often over the sacrum, of many darker skinned children. Other youngsters have small circular spots scattered over the skin. A nurse concerned about the identification of this birthmark can review birth records, previous histories, and prior examinations. If the assessment for abuse is benign and the child is felt to be safe, the examiner can schedule a 2-week follow-up visit to re-examine the skin. During the interim time, a bruise would be expected to fade, whereas the Mongolian spot would remain constant. Mongolian spots usually lighten after the first few years of life.

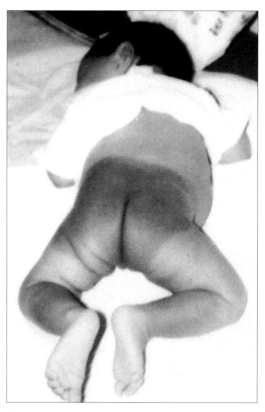

Figure 2-4. *Mongolian spots. This is a 4- to 5-month-old who was seen in the failure-to-thrive clinic. The lesions are Mongolian spots. Because they are so extensive, most people think they are bruises.*

For bruise assessment, the nurse examiner considers a broad differential diagnosis that includes organic disorders that can cause the child to bruise or injure easily. (See Chapter 7, Differential Diagnosis: Conditions That Mimic Child Maltreatment, for a discussion of differential diagnosis.) A number of hematological conditions can cause easy bruising, and an appropriate laboratory workup may reveal the presence of such conditions and explain certain bruises **(Table 2-2)**.

After completing a history, physical examination, and review of laboratory and diagnostic testing, the nurse and other collaborating healthcare professionals weigh the possibility that the bruising is likely to have occurred in the way the caregiver described. They draw on knowledge of the general mechanism of injuries, the developmental level of the child, and the consistency of the history provided, then compare these impressions with observation of the child's actual injuries.

Burns

Burns are a common soft tissue injury seen in children and have significant public health implications related to prevention efforts. Burns may be minor, severe, and at times fatal, with significant potential to disfigure the child's appearance. Important factors to consider when the child has a burn include the location of the burn, shape and pattern of the burn on the skin, and extent of the burn. Matching the history offered with what the examination reveals is an essential responsibility for the healthcare provider.

Table 2-2. Medical Conditions Presenting With Skin Lesions That May Be Confused With Child Maltreatment	
Connective tissue	Ehlers-Danlos syndrome
Genetic	Osteogenesis imperfecta (OI) (bruises with fractures)
Hematological	Leukemia, von Willebrand's disease, idiopathic thrombocytopenic purpura (ITP)
Infectious	Meningococcemia
Pediatric	Physical abuse, sexual abuse

Various kinds of burns are possible based on how they occur. For example, hot liquids may come in contact with the child's skin causing ***scalding burns***. Scalding burns are further subdivided into ***splash burns***, in which the liquid spills or pours onto the skin, and ***immersion burns***, in which the child's skin is submerged in the hot liquid. ***Contact burns*** are seen when a hot object comes in contact with the child's skin. Characteristic shapes or patterns may be left on the child's skin depending on the shape of the object, temperature, and amount of time the object is in contact with the child's skin. (**Figure 2-5** demonstrates the shapes of commonly used objects that may be employed to burn children.) Open-fire–flame burns and electrical burns are also possible but less commonly seen in the context of physical abuse.

Certain presentations of a burned child that raise particular concern for possible abuse are as follows:

— Implausible history for burn based on child's development (**Figure 2-6**), age of the burn, and appearance of the burn

— No history offered for burn; child just found to have a burn (magical)

— Caregiver who was watching child is not present during the healthcare evaluation of the child

— Sibling or playmate blamed for child's burn

— Pattern that suggests the child was restrained during injury

— Delay in seeking healthcare

— Presence of other injuries

— Signs and symptoms of neglectful caregiving, including poor hygiene, malnutrition

— History of previous injury

Given the history and physical examination of a child with a scalding burn, the healthcare provider must consider what would be reasonable to expect on examination given the caregiver's report about how the burn occurred. Children are naturally curious and explore their environment in a developmentally appropriate manner. As a result, they may attempt to pull objects that contain hot liquids off of stoves, tables, and countertops. If a 2-year-old presents with a history of having

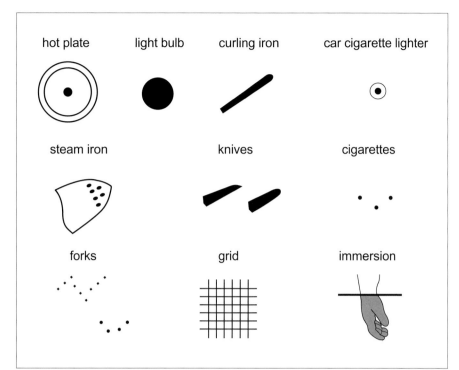

Figure 2-5. *Marks from objects that burn. Reprinted with permission from Johnson CF. Inflicted injury versus accidental injury. Ped Clin North Am.1990;37:807.*

walked over to the stove and pulled a pot of boiling water onto himself, the expected burn from such a mechanism would have a characteristic shape made as the hot liquid fell on the child's skin. One could expect the liquid to hit the child's face, neck, and shoulder as he looked up and was reaching to pull the pot off the stove. The hot liquid then would be expected to pour down the child's skin, most likely involving the reaching arm, chest, and back, cooling as it spreads across the skin, with the most distal end being the least severely burned. The initial point of contact has the most serious burn. As the hot liquid layers out over the skin and cools, one would expect the edges to be less severely burned **(Figure 2-7)**. If examination reveals a circular burn on the child's back, this is inconsistent with the mechanism described in the history. The findings would be more consistent with a hot liquid being thrown at the child rather than a spill or pouring. Such a discrepancy should raise concerns about physical abuse using a hot liquid and requires reporting to the CPS agency.

Immersion burns are among the most serious burns seen in children and carry a high rate of morbidity and mortality when they result from abuse. Forced immersion burns often have a characteristic pattern that is formed as the abusive caregiver uses physical strength to hold the child in contact with the hot liquid, often hot bath water. As the child is plunged into the hot liquid, she typically tries to recoil from the hot liquid, but cannot overcome the larger, more powerful caregiver. If the child held by her arms is plunged into the scalding hot liquid buttocks or feet first, the child instinctively attempts to pull the legs up to attempt escape. In the classic abusive immersion burn, the buttocks are submerged and pressed against the container holding the hot liquid. In such a case the skin of the child's anterior thigh comes in close approximation with the femoral area skin as the child struggles against the attack and effectively seals out the hot water and results in sparing of that skin. The skin of the central portion of the buttocks may be held forcefully against the surface of the container, which is potentially cooler than the scalding hot liquid. This scenario leads to a central area of protected skin on the buttocks, the "hole in

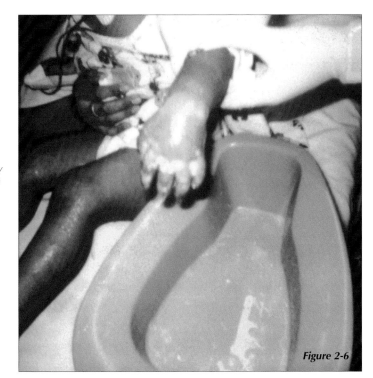

Figure 2-6. *Inflicted liquid burn of a 2-year-old boy. The biological father initially gave a history that the child climbed onto a stool next to the sink, turned on the hot water, and checked it with his hand, causing the burn. The nurse directed the detective to return to the home and take a picture of the child next to the sink. Even on the stool, it was clear that the child could not reach the faucet to turn on the water. Eventually the father confessed to holding the child's hand under the water as a punishment for something the child had done wrong.*

Figure 2-7. *Accidental liquid burn. This 2-year-old pulled a hot liquid from the stove onto himself. The burn was accidental, but serious.*

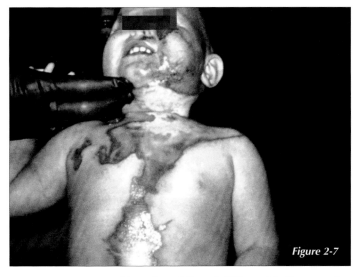

doughnut" pattern. In forced immersion burns, there are often sharp lines of demarcation between burned and unburned skin in a stocking and glove type of pattern, which forms as different parts of the child are held in place in the scalding water. These sharp lines of demarcation are not expected in an accidental immersion because the child, if not force-fully held in place, would splash around, trying to get out of the water **(Figures 2-8 to 2-10).**

In evaluating scalding burns, the healthcare provider must consider a broad list of differential diagnoses because skin conditions may initially appear similar to burns. (See Chapter 7, Differential Diagnosis: Conditions That Mimic Child Maltreatment, for a discussion of the differential diagnosis.)

Skeletal Fractures

Fractures in the long bones are common injuries in children, especially as they grow older and become involved in sporting activities, but skeletal injuries are also frequently seen in physically abused children. Other than clavicle fractures that occur during birth, skeletal fractures in infants and young children should raise concerns about possible maltreatment. Healthy bones are strong, and a fair amount of force is required to break a child's bone, especially the relatively large femur. Histories for injury with the inconsistencies already described are of concern with abusive fractures as well. The presence of long bone fractures and histories of minor trauma or unwitnessed falls in the nonwalking infant should be highly suspect. The child's developmental abilities must always be considered in evaluating the plausibility of an injury mechanism leading to a skeletal fracture. Other bones besides the long bones may be fractured during maltreatment, with the most worrisome fractures being those of the rib and skull. Because of the forces required to generate long bone fractures and the risk of other associated injuries, infants who have such fractures without a reasonable, witnessed mechanism of injury are considered at risk for potentially life-threatening injury. Therefore, CPS should be notified for an immediate evaluation to prevent reinjury to the child.

Skeletal fractures in young children are not always obvious initially and may be uncovered only during a thorough healthcare evaluation. Because of this, the American Academy of Pediatrics (AAP, 2000) recommends a skeletal survey be done for children under age 2 years who are being evaluated for possible physical abuse. The AAP (2000) defines the skeletal survey as a complete set of radiographs with examination of each bone for possible fracture. The specific radiographic views contained in a skeletal survey include the following:

—Anteroposterior views of the appendicular skeleton:

> — Humeri
> — Forearms
> — Femurs
> — Lower part of legs
> — Feet

— Oblique and posteroanterior views of the hands

— Lateral views of the axial skeleton, along with the additional views contained in parentheses:

> — Cervical spine
> — Lumbar spine (lateral)
> — Thorax (plus anteroposterior view)
> — Pelvis (anteroposterior view, including mid and lower lumbar spine)

— Frontal and lateral views of the skull bones

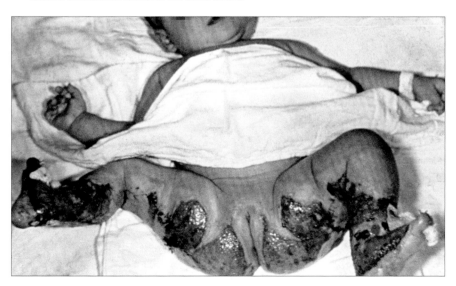

Figure 2-8.
Immersion burn. The child appears to be 10 to 12 months old. Of interest are the areas of sparing where the body was "folded" up to protect the skin as much as she could. (Contributed by James Williams, MD; Stockton, Calif.)

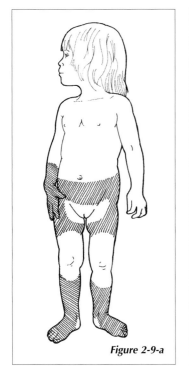

Figure 2-9-a

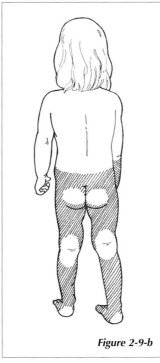

Figure 2-9-b

Figure 2-9. *(a) and (b) Hole in doughnut pattern of immersion burns on a child forced into a bathtub of hot water. (c) How the hole in doughnut pattern of immersion burns is produced.*

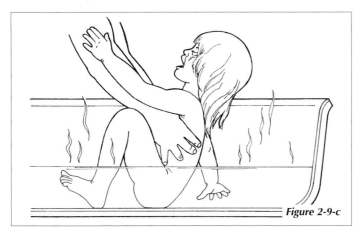

Figure 2-9-c

Many different types of fractures are defined by the location of the break on the bone. All fracture types have been seen in child maltreatment-related inflicted injuries, although some patterns are more commonly associated with child maltreatment than are others (Launius, Silberstein, Luisiri, & Graviss, 1998). Fractures associated with physical abuse are discussed in Chapter 4, The Physical Examination in the Evaluation of Suspected Child Maltreatment: Physical Abuse and Sexual Abuse Examinations. The skills of knowledgeable pediatric radiologists are invaluable in identifying fractures and in assessing potential mechanisms and risk of abuse-related trauma. Additionally, the healthcare provider may be asked to help investigators date when the fracture may have occurred.

It is possible to date skeletal injuries within a relatively certain time frame based on a combination of factors related to tissue formation and bone healing (Cooperman & Merten, 2001; Islam, Soboleski, Symons, Davidson, Ashworth, & Babyn, 2000). Dating involves being able to recognize the following: soft tissue changes, visibility of fracture line, callus calcification, and ossification of new periosteal bone (Launius et al., 1998). Along with those factors, the younger the bones of infants, the more rapidly the fracture may heal. Each of the 4 phases of healing indicates specific aspects of healing that can be viewed via radiography. For example, periosteal bone formation occurs in the second phase of healing and begins to occur after injury approximately 7 to 10 days in infants and 10 to 14 days in older children. In general, more precise dating can occur when there is a shorter time period between injury and the dating process (Cooperman & Merten, 2001). (See Chapter 4, The Physical Examination in the Evaluation of Suspected Child Maltreatment: Physical Abuse and Sexual Abuse Examinations.)

Whenever a healthcare provider is considering child maltreatment in the context of skeletal fractures, a broad list of differential diagnoses should be assessed, including all relevant medical conditions. A common differential diagnosis when considering skeletal fracture is osteogenesis imperfecta (OI), a genetic disorder affecting the formation of collagen that has various characteristic manifestations. The presence of these manifestations should be explored during the healthcare evaluation. (See Chapter 7, Differential Diagnosis: Conditions That Mimic Child Maltreatment, for a discussion of differential diagnosis of fractures.)

Central Nervous System Injury

Among the most serious patterns of injuries identified in maltreated children are the inflicted brain injuries and subsequent CNS impairment seen with the shaken baby syndrome or shaken impact syndrome (SBS/SIS). Brain injuries seen in SBS/SIS result from the application of rotational forces to the child's head and neck. These were initially described as "whiplash shaken baby syndrome" to capture the "to and from" movement of the child's head as the child was violently shaken (Duhaime, Christian, Rorke, & Zimmerman, 1998). Rotational forces are distinct from the low-velocity translational forces seen in common household falls. Infants, with their relatively large heads, weak neck muscles, and relatively strong spinal ligaments, when violently shaken to and fro, may sustain serious injuries to the brain and its associated vascular and neural connections, which may result in significant impairment.

The presence of a subdural hematoma (SDH) is a classic manifestation of SBS/SIS, and SDHs may be of different ages, appearing radiographically as both chronic and acute. SDHs are often associated with retinal hemorrhages and occasionally, but not necessarily, with other injuries, including various other intracranial findings. Whether the injuries to the brain in SBS/SIS require an injury mechanism, that is, the impacting of the child's head against a fixed surface, remains a debate in

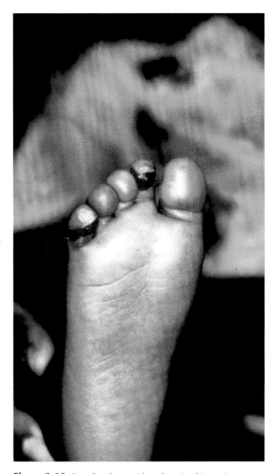

Figure 2-10. *Branding burn with a changing history in a 15-month-old boy. Three different histories were given by the mother to CPS, the emergency department physician, and the child abuse team. The history told to the nurse was that the mother ran the bath water but was out of the room for "just a minute" while the tub filled. She turned off the faucet but didn't check the temperature of the water. She put the child into the tub and as his toes entered the water he pulled his feet back and screamed. Only 2 toe pads of the right foot and one toe pad of the left foot were involved. The child also had a number of scars on the back of his thigh. No other burns were noted. The children were removed from the home when it was later discovered that the mother's boyfriend was the suspect.*

the professional literature. From a clinical evaluation and overall investigation perspective, the child is viewed to have been violently attacked, whether by shaking alone or shaking plus the impact of his or her head against a fixed surface. Regardless of the ultimate outcome of this scientific inquiry, the fact remains that the injury is inflicted and not accidental.

Children who sustain injury from SBS/SIS are typically young, almost always under age 2 years, with many younger than age 6 months (Berkowitz, 1995; Duhaime et al., 1998; Duhaime & Partington, 2002). In the less severe cases, symptoms on presentation include irritability, lethargy, and poor feeding, while more severe cases include apnea, seizures, and unresponsiveness (Monteleone & Brodeur, 1998). Histories offered by abusive caregivers are often misleading and inaccurate. Physical examination typically finds neurological impairment referable to the brain injury; approximately 50% present with severe impairment (Duhaime et al., 1998). Other physical findings may be present, with 65% to 95% of shaken babies having retinal hemorrhages (Duhaime & Partington, 2002; Reece & Sege, 2000). A smaller percentage have skull, rib, and/or long bone fractures. It is common to find no extracranial injuries, and this should not be viewed as evidence for nonabusive injury. Laboratory and diagnostic imaging demonstrates that a child with CNS injury often has bloody cerebrospinal fluid and imaging studies demonstrating SDH. The differential diagnoses for SDH in an infant with no witnessed injury are limited, so abuse is usually at the top of the list. Children with this injury have sustained a serious, life-threatening injury and require appropriate medical evaluation and treatment as well as CPS reporting and investigation. (See Chapter 13, Child Protective Services and Child Abuse, for discussion.)

Minor household falls are frequently offered as reasons for the severe injury. The consensus among experts in the field is that severe life-threatening injuries from common household falls are uncommon (Chadwick, Chin, Salerno, Landsverk, & Kitchen, 1991; Monteleone & Brodeur, 1998). The more suspicious the history offered initially, the more classic are the findings for shaken baby; the more severe the injuries, the higher is the suspicion for inflicted trauma.

Dating the age of a head injury has strong implications for the medical evaluation and an ensuing investigation of the injury by CPS and possibly law enforcement. Magnetic resonance imaging (MRI) can distinguish between fresh blood in an acute SDH and older blood that is undergoing resorption in subacute and chronic SDH. There is debate around the significance of finding both acute and chronic SDHs. The analysis of these debates requires an extensive literature review. However, there are several key clinical points on the presentation of a child who has sustained an SBS/SIS associated injury. It can be said with a high degree of certainty that traumatic, acute SDH, associated with brain swelling and severe neurological impairment (including death), is associated with the following (Duhaime et al., 1998):

— Injury from major mechanical forces

— Presentation with symptoms rapidly and with no long lucid period between injury and onset of symptoms as contrasted with a slowly evolving epidural hemorrhage

— No occult subclinical injury occurring "out of the blue" in an otherwise healthy infant

CHILD FATALITY

Each year approximately 2000 children die as a result of child maltreatment—approximately 5 children per day (National Clearinghouse on Child Abuse and Neglect Information, 2001a, 2001b). Some children come to the emergency medical services system seriously injured with catastrophic, life-threatening CNS and thoracoabdominal injuries. The more obvious battering cases are typically identified as inflicted injuries. More commonly however, children die from subtle forms of neglectful caregiving. In the year 2000, of the 1.71 children of every 100 000 children in the population who died from abuse or neglect, 34.9% of those children died from neglect only, whereas 27.8% died from physical abuse only (Administration for Children and Families, 2002). The percentage of children who die from neglect is greater than other forms of reported deaths from types of abuse.

Correct identification of child fatalities associated with maltreatment may be difficult depending on the circumstances surrounding their presentation and on a number of associated factors in a given community. Healthcare providers may have an impact on the accuracy in accounting for the number of child maltreatment fatalities and should be aware of how to ensure an appropriate response to child fatalities that result from child maltreatment. The following broad systemic issues are identified as underlying the ambiguity in maltreatment-related child fatalities:

— Variation in the way child deaths are reported, leading to inaccurate reporting of the number of children who die from child maltreatment

— Lack of national standards for child death investigations and child autopsies

— Variation in the manner in which CPS, law enforcement, and medical examiners handle the investigative process

— Use in many states of elected coroners who are not required to have medical training or child maltreatment training (rather than medical examiners who are physicians)

In response to these concerns, state and local governments have empaneled multidisciplinary child fatality review teams that review all cases of child death in a given locality. Teams seek to identify causes of death and need for systemic reforms to prevent similar deaths. They also facilitate system improvements around enhancing investigations in the future while trying to build broad coalitions between the disciplines and agencies involved (Kolilis, 1998).

Perhaps one of the more difficult areas to understand about maltreatment versus noninflicted causes of natural death is sudden infant death syndrome (SIDS). SIDS is diagnosed when no other explanation fits the unexpected death of an infant under age 1 year after a complete investigation, including autopsy, death scene investigation, and review of clinical history has been conducted (Kairys, 2001). To assist in distinguishing SIDS from fatal child abuse, the AAP issued a policy statement that seeks to clarify several key points about these 2 scenarios (Kairys, 2001). SIDS is more common than infanticide and is the most common cause of death between ages 1 and 6 months. Approximately 90% of SIDS deaths occur by age 6 months, with the peak incidence between 2 and 4 months. The etiology of SIDS is not understood and has been associated with various factors, as follows:

— Prone sleeping position

— Sleeping on a soft surface

— Maternal smoking, antepartum and postpartum

— Bundling and overheating of the child

— Delayed or absent prenatal care

— Young maternal age

— Prematurity

— Low birth weight

— Male gender

In 1992 the AAP recommended that infants be placed on their back to sleep (Kattwinkel, 2000). Campaigns to decrease infants sleeping in a prone position (e.g., "Back to Sleep") have been associated with an approximately 50% decrease in prone sleeping and an approximately 40% decrease in SIDS deaths. The AAP is clear, however, that despite some of the uncertainty around this syndrome, SIDS is a diagnosis of exclusion and should only be made after thorough investigation and medical admission that the death is completely unexplained (Kairys, 2001). Specifically, criteria to attribute an infant death as SIDS include the following:

— Complete autopsy is done, including cranium and cranial contents, and autopsy findings are compatible with SIDS.

— No gross or microscopic evidence of trauma or significant disease process.

— No evidence of trauma on skeletal survey.

— Other possible causes of death are adequately ruled out, including meningitis, sepsis, aspiration, pneumonia, myocarditis, abdominal trauma, dehydration, fluid and electrolyte imbalance, significant congenital lesions, inborn metabolic disorders, carbon monoxide asphyxia, drowning, or burns.

— No evidence of current alcohol, drug, or toxic exposure.

— Thorough death scene investigation and review of the clinical history are negative for abuse.

The AAP Committee on SIDS (Kairys, 2001) concluded with recommendations on the evaluation of sudden unexplained infant deaths. The AAP encouraged healthcare providers to be rigorous in pursuing the medical evaluation and contributing to the investigation, while maintaining a supportive approach to the parents because of the uncertainty surrounding the case and their stress and bewilderment at the loss of the child (Kairys, 2001). (A complete report is available at www.aap.org/policy/re0036.html.)

SEXUAL ABUSE

Sexual abuse accounts for approximately 11% of child maltreatment cases annually, and it is recognized as a significant health problem affecting the well-being of a relatively large number of children (at least 108 000 children in 1998) (USDHHS, 1988). The following are some of the ways in which sexual abuse presents to the healthcare provider:

— Purposeful disclosure by the child that inappropriate sexual activity is occurring (Sgroi, Blick, & Porter, 1982).

— Accidental discovery in which a third party (other than child or perpetrator) observes or suspects inappropriate sexual activity and reports it or when another child victim discloses the perpetrator's behavior.

— During medical evaluation for genital signs or nonspecific physical symptoms leading to the discovery of genital trauma, sexually transmitted disease (STD), or other findings suggestive of sexual abuse. Because of heightened recognition of sexual abuse, parents are more attuned to genital complaints, especially from their daughters.

— During medical and mental health evaluation for nonspecific behavioral complaints leading to the discovery of sexual abuse.

Table 2-3 identifies specific and nonspecific physical and behavioral complaints of sexual abuse.

Sexual abuse is a unique form of child maltreatment separate from physical abuse, which typically occurs over time by a perpetrator known to the child and/or family. The most important component of the sexual abuse evaluation has proved to be the information collected from the child and caregivers during the medical interview or history-taking process. During history taking the child is likely to disclose the inappropriate activity that has been occurring while in the care of the perpetrator. The physical examination in cases of child sexual abuse is often without specific findings

---

Table 2-3. Identification of Sexual Abuse

PHYSICAL COMPLAINTS	BEHAVIORAL COMPLAINTS
Specific	**Specific**
— Genital injury: bruises and lacerations	— Explicit descriptions of sexual contact
— Rectal laceration, fissures	— Inappropriate knowledge of adult sexual behavior
— STDs	— Compulsive masturbation
— Pregnancy	— Excessive sexual curiosity, sexual acting out
Nonspecific	**Nonspecific**
— Anorexia	— Excessive fears, phobias
— Abdominal pain	— Refusal to sleep alone, nightmares
— Enuresis	— Runaways
— Dysuria	— Aggressive behavior
— Encopresis	— Attempted suicide
— Evidence of physical abuse in genital area	— Any abrupt change in behavior
— Vaginal discharge	
— Urethral discharge	
— Rectal pain	

Reprinted with permission from Ludwig S. Child abuse. In: Fleisher GR, Ludwig S, eds. Textbook of Pediatric Emergency Medicine. *4th ed. Philadelphia, Pa: Lippincott Williams & Wilkins; 1999:1685.*

(Adams, Harper, Knudson, & Revilla, 1994; Bowen & Aldous, 1999; Kerns & Ritter, 1992; Reichert, 1997). (See Chapter 4, The Physical Examination in the Evaluation of Suspected Child Maltreatment: Physical Abuse and Sexual Abuse Examinations, for discussion of the physical examination.) However, many families and some relatively uninformed professionals may mistakenly think that the physical examination will provide evidence to confirm the child's allegation and inappropriately may place too much emphasis on the presence or absence of findings.

When a child is being evaluated for possible sexual abuse, it is critical for the nurse and other healthcare professionals to remember that the physical examination does not usually reveal findings of either acute or chronic trauma (Adams et al., 1994; Bowen & Aldous, 1999; Kerns & Ritter, 1992). However, laboratory findings positive for STDs or forensic evidence indicating the presence of sperm or seminal products in the prepubertal child are usually indicative of sexual abuse (Christian, Lavelle, DeJong, Loiselle, Brenner, & Joffe, 2000).

How a child discloses may be problematic. The perpetrator forcing the child victim to keep the "secret" is nearly universal behavior in child sexual abuse. Coercion may be implicit, as in subtle threats that if the secret is disclosed, then the child may be left alone without friends, or explicit, by direct threats to the safety of the child or family (Sgroi et al., 1982). Even after disclosure the child may be ill-prepared for the maelstrom of activity and emotions that ensue from the people involved and may be overwhelmed by the events that occur in the course of investigating the situation. This includes the involvement of CPS and law enforcement, the need for a medical examination that may be perceived as stressful, and perhaps the arrest of someone known and potentially valued by the family.

Children often feel helpless when in the midst of a sexually abusive situation. The sense of helplessness arises from the child's realization that the people and environment that were supposed to protect the child failed to do so. As a result, the child may lose faith that disclosure of sexual abuse would serve to make things better at home. Additionally, after disclosure occurs, the child may be subjected to pressure from family members and other caregivers to recant and retract the disclosure in an effort to return life to the way it was before the abuse came to light (Sgroi et al., 1982). These circumstances place the child in a difficult position and account for the observation that disclosures of sexual abuse often may go through a cycle during the investigation and aftermath in which the child retracts the disclosure and then discloses again.

Nonspecific Behavioral Complaints

Presenting symptoms that suggest the need for a sexual abuse evaluation are often nonspecific behavioral complaints that span the entire continuum of emotional and behavioral symptomatology. They vary from externally oriented symptoms, such as various forms of acting out, including aggression and delinquent-type behaviors, to

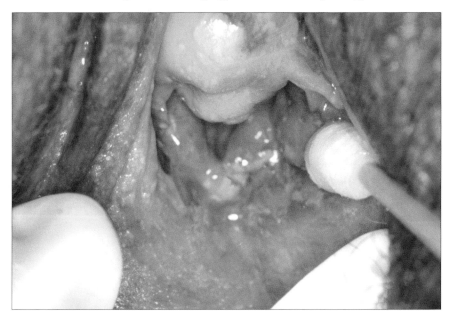

Figure 2-11. *Adolescent with abnormal genital examination demonstrating chronic abuse. This 17-year-old girl lived with her mother and stepfather in another state but regularly visited her biological father and stepmother. On visits to the father, the girl complained of a chronic vaginal discharge. The stepmother took her to several clinics, all of which told the girl the discharges were normal at her age; no cultures were done. During a visit to her father the girl finally disclosed years of sexual abuse by her stepfather and her stepbrother, which included ongoing vaginal and anal penetration. On examination, there was a minimal amount of hymenal tissue. The applicator demonstrated a hymenal defect that ran through the hymen to its base and is consistent with a healed tear. Her vaginal culture was positive for* Trichomonas *and* Chlamydia *organisms. Her serological test results were positive for syphilis and human immunodeficiency virus (HIV). She was referred to a specialty clinic for HIV-positive patients, where she was noncompliant with medications. She was reportedly having sex with her current boyfriend without barrier protection. It was unclear whether she had shared her immune status with her partner. Soon after that she turned age 18 years and was lost to follow-up.*

internally focused symptoms, such as appearing withdrawn, feeling depressed, and becoming suicidal. The behavioral and emotional manifestations are nonspecific in that they also can be seen in other stressful situations that the child may experience, such as the loss of a parent, parental divorce, or diagnosis of a serious illness. Thus, no specific behavioral symptom automatically implies that a child has been sexually maltreated. Nonspecific behavioral complaints include the following:

— Extremes of activity ranging from hyperactivity to withdrawal

— Poor peer relationships

— Regressing to behaviors from an earlier developmental stage

— Enuresis/encopresis

— Fear of adults who were liked formerly

— Poor school performance

— Sexualized play/promiscuity

— Excessive/compulsive masturbation

— Sexual aggression toward playmates or younger children

— Running away

— High-risk/delinquent behaviors

— Suicidal gestures/suicide attempts

Nonspecific Genital Complaints

Nonspecific genital complaints may also be presenting symptoms of child sexual abuse. These genitally focused signs and symptoms may be directly related to the genital manipulation that occurred during the abuse, or the signs and symptoms could be related to the child's increased focus on the anogenital area as a result of age-inappropriate sexual contact imposed on him or her by the perpetrator (**Figure 2-11**). The evaluation of genital complaints may present unique challenges for both the child and the healthcare provider. Healthcare providers commonly overlook genital and anal areas in a well-child examination even though sound clinical practice would promote assessing the genital area at every visit (Ladson, Johnson, & Doty, 1987; Lentsch & Johnson, 2000). Healthcare providers should familiarize themselves with normal anatomical changes that occur throughout the child's life by routinely examining the anogenital area and documenting findings from these specific areas during each healthcare visit.

Some nonspecific complaints can be confused with sexual abuse. For example, vulvovaginitis is the most common pediatric gynecological diagnosis seen in a primary care setting (Sifuentes, 1996). Presenting problems generally fall into 3 categories: erythema, discharge, and spotting/blood in the diaper or underwear.

Genital erythema is a common finding in the prepubertal female. Most often the redness is associated with nonsexual etiologies. The healthcare provider must ask the caregiver about the hygiene habits practiced by the child and family. Chemical irritation occurs from harsh soaps used for bathing or laundry detergents that leave a residue in the child's underwear. Frequent bubble baths or the use of a harsh product in the water, such as dishwashing soap, can also be a culprit and cause a chemical irritation and subsequent signs and symptoms (Elvik, 1998).

Mechanical irritation may be characterized by maceration of the skin, as in diaper dermatitis, and can be caused by tight-fitting clothing and nylon underpants. Girls

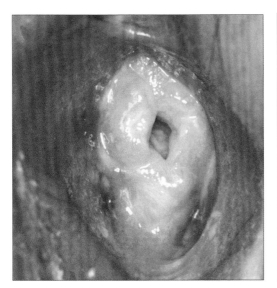

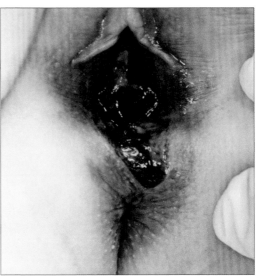

Figure 2-12. *Adolescent with normal redundant hymen. This 13-year-old Tanner stage 3 girl has a normal hymen reflecting increased estrogen effect. Note the white substance in the labia minora, which is normal physiological leukorrhea.*

Figure 2-13. *Prepubertal child with evidence of acute sexual assault. A 2-year-old girl had blood in her diaper. The history given by the mother and aunt was that the child had sustained a straddle-type injury on the padded arm of an overstuffed chair. The laceration transected the hymen completely at the 6 o'clock position and ran through the vaginal floor, then through the perineum and into the anus. This injury required surgical intervention. It was later discovered that the uncle had vaginally penetrated her; the aunt and the child's mother tried to protect him. He was eventually convicted, and because of the mother's actions, the child was placed into a foster home. The child was later relinquished by the mother and adopted by the foster mother.*

who spend a great deal of time in wet bathing suits for swimming or in leotards and tights for ballet are prone to this as well (Emans, Laufer, & Goldstein, 1998).

There are 2 times in a young girl's life when a vaginal discharge may be viewed as normal. First is the newborn period, when white or blood-tinged exudates may be noted around the vaginal opening. This occurs in response to the systemic withdrawal of the mother's estrogen from the baby. A second time a vaginal discharge would be expected is approximately 6 to 12 months before the onset of menses (Sifuentes, 1996). Some girls at this time may experience a white discharge called physiological leukorrhea **(Figure 2-12)**. This may continue for several years. Once menstrual cycles are well established, pubertal young women may notice a cyclical change of secretions, from clear/mucoid to white (Emans et al., 1998).

There are other nonabuse-related causes of vaginal discharge that the clinician should consider **(Table 2-4)**. Poor hygiene may lead to a vaginal discharge that appears whitish-yellow. Girls frequently wipe from the perianal area toward the genitalia after a bowel movement, bringing bacteria into this sensitive region. Autoinoculation of pathogenic bacteria is also possible, especially with organisms from the respiratory tract during an illness. A symptom pattern composed of vaginal discharge, erythema, and anal pruritus should lead the healthcare provider to suspect infestation with pinworms *(Enterobius vermicularis)*.

Any vaginal discharge in a prepubertal girl, from scant to copious and from clear to purulent, warrants cultures for infectious agents, including STDs. Gonorrhea is notorious for presenting as a purulent discharge in the prepubertal girl (Ingram, Everett, Flick, Russell, & White-Sims, 1997). The discharge associated with

Table 2-4. Causes for Vaginal Discharge

CONSISTENCY	COLOR	CAUSE
Thin	White/yellow	Chemical irritation *Chlamydia trachomatis*
Thin	Clear/white	Physiological
Cheesy	White	*Candida*
Thick, profuse	Green/yellow, purulent	*Trichomonas* *Neisseria gonorrhoeae*
Moderate	Brown, bloody	Foreign body *Shigella*

Chlamydia organisms is usually less impressive than that of gonorrhea. (See Chapter 6, Sexually Transmitted Diseases in the Setting of Maltreatment, for discussion of the STDs in child maltreatment.)

Blood in the diaper or underwear is cause for alarm in the parent and healthcare provider **(Figure 2-13)**. The nurse's primary objective is to locate the source of the bleeding and determine whether it is vaginal, urethral, or anal. Frank vaginal bleeding in a prepubertal child calls for an expedient gynecological referral, although several nonsexual means of spotting are possible. For example, urethral prolapse may present as a beefy-red mass of varying size that can cover the vaginal opening, giving the appearance of a traumatized hymen. It is often accompanied by mucosal ulceration and bleeding and is most common in African American girls (Abrams & Lewis, 1954). Small masses of prolapsed mucosa may resolve with simple symptomatic treatment, including warm sitz baths and attention to proper hygiene. Large masses of prolapsed mucosa, on the other hand, may be difficult to manage. Those that do not resolve themselves after 3 days of sitz baths should be referred to a pediatric urologist for further evaluation and management.

Prepubertal girls occasionally present with a brown, blood-tinged, foul-smelling vaginal discharge. Although this may be a sign of shigellosis, the most common etiology for this is a retained vaginal foreign body. The primary cause is overzealous wiping, resulting in small pieces of toilet tissue deposited in the vagina. The foreign body acts as a direct irritant and also plays host to a myriad of bacteria that make the genital mucosa friable and prone to bleeding. Careful examination of the area is necessary, and lavage of the area is a mainstay of diagnosis and treatment (Emans et al., 1998; Giardino & Christian, 1997). One of the authors (Elvik) has experience with removing pieces of carpet fiber from the vagina of a very young child who presented with genital erythema, edema, and a bloody, foul-smelling discharge. The child responded well when the fibers were gently lavaged from the vaginal vault, using warm saline solution via an infant feeding tube.

Genital bruising and external lacerations may result from straddle injuries that can occur when a female child falls onto an object such as the crossbar of a bicycle or a bar of a jungle gym. The hard, fixed object forcefully sandwiches the tissues of the genitalia between it and the pubic bone, causing bruising of the labia majora and

Table 2-5. Presentation of Neglect		
PROVISIONAL	DEVELOPMENTAL	SUPERVISIONAL
Failure to provide basic needs, including shelter, food, clothing, education, immunizations, healthcare	Preventing normal growth and development by curbing normal exploration	Placing a child in a situation that may result in serious injury or death
	Having unrealistic expectations of a child's ability	Leaving a very young child in the care of a sibling who is too young or immature to provide adequate care
	Keeping a child restrained	

minora and lacerations with bleeding. Straddle injuries rarely cause trauma to the vagina and hymen (Berkowitz, 1996a). (See Chapter 7, Differential Diagnosis: Conditions That Mimic Child Maltreatment, for a discussion of the differential diagnosis of genital findings.)

NEGLECT

Neglect, defined as a pattern of caregiving that does not adequately meet the needs of the developing child, has been recognized in the past less than physical and sexual abuse (Dubowitz, Giardino, & Gustavson, 2000). However, neglect is the single most common type of maltreatment, accounting for over 53% of reported and substantiated cases of abuse (USDHHS, 1999). There are typical presentation patterns for the various types of neglect, although the signs and symptoms related to neglect are often more subtle than those seen in physical abuse and, to some extent, sexual abuse. Neglect often presents in an insidious manner, over time, with the child's needs being inconsistently met in various dimensions, such as nutrition, healthcare, development, and supervision.

The legal definition of neglect varies from state to state. From a presentation perspective, however, the healthcare provider may identify neglect using the following 3-part categorization system (Cantwell, 1997) **(Table 2-5)**:

— ***Provisional neglect:*** the caregivers are not able to give the child basic necessities such as food, clothing, shelter, and healthcare.

— ***Developmental neglect:*** the caregivers do not provide the child with an appropriately stimulating environment.

— ***Supervisional neglect:*** the caregivers do not adequately protect the child from environmental hazards, thus risking injury and placing the child at times in imminent danger and risk.

The evaluation of a child for possible neglect requires careful attention to all the components of the healthcare process, including history over time, physical examination, appropriate laboratory and diagnostic studies, and observation of parent-child interactions. (See Chapter 8, Clinical Aspects of Child Neglect, for a discussion of child neglect.) The record should reflect meticulous documentation of what is heard and seen, as well as what attempts have been made to address problems and what the results have been. The evaluation is focused on the child's present needs and how the caregivers attempt to meet those basic needs. In the primary care setting, neglect often presents over time and becomes clear as a pattern of caregiving emerges that inconsistently meets the child's needs. Nurses have close contact with the child and caregivers and are thus ideally suited to participate in the evaluation of the neglectful caregiving. (See Chapter 8, Clinical Aspects of Child Neglect, for a discussion of neglect and Chapter 7, Differential Diagnosis: Conditions That Mimic Child Maltreatment, for a discussion of the differential diagnosis for failure to thrive.)

Provisional Neglect

Parents are expected to provide the basic needs for their children, such as food, shelter, clothing, nurturance, schooling, and health and dental care. Caregivers may intentionally deprive a child of these things or be so distracted by their own problems that they become inattentive to the child and the child's requirements. Caregivers may also be unable to understand the child's needs based on their own cognitive level or learning style or may be unable to marshal community or personal resources to meet their child's needs. Regardless of the underlying reason, the outcome is that the child's needs are not met satisfactorily.

One of the most common presentations of provisional neglect is failure to thrive (FTT). Children with FTT fall below the third to fifth percentile for height and/or weight, or show a drop in 2 percentiles between health visits (Berkowitz, 1996b). In FTT that results from neglect, often no organic cause can be associated with the small stature and weight of the child. Several medical conditions can predispose a child to be at low percentiles for these parameters. However, nurses can monitor a child's growth during each encounter, plotting the increments on a standardized growth curve to evaluate growth of the infant/child at regular intervals. Additionally, observing how the caregiver responds to the child's cues about hunger and the manner in which the caregiver provides the child with food can be very informative components of the evaluation.

Immunizations have become a controversial topic of concern in recent years. Some parents oppose the vaccines and are afraid of potential complications. Parents who have researched the pros and cons of vaccines and make a decision based on the information obtained contrast dramatically with parents whose inattention to the child's preventive healthcare needs causes them to "forget" to immunize their child. (See Chapter 8, Clinical Aspects of Child Neglect.)

Developmental Neglect

Children must be exposed to a large spectrum of activities and events to progress developmentally. From the earliest days, the baby learns about the environment by being held, by looking into an expressive face, and by hearing verbalizations from caregivers.

Physical examinations provide an opportunity to assess children for developmental neglect. Babies and children who have no other developmental complications or illness will interact with the examiner on some level. A child who experiences developmental neglect may demonstrate certain behaviors. These include the inability to make eye contact, resistance to being held, and inability to relate to the nurse at all during the evaluation. In such cases, discussion about these findings with the caregiver is critical. Be aware of parents who complain that the child is hyperactive or "into everything," especially when the child's behavior represents developmentally appropriate exploration of the child's surroundings. Such statements indicate that the parent may have unreal expectations of the child's capabilities, such as expecting an 18-month-old child to sit quietly in front of the television set for hours.

Supervisional Neglect

The ongoing development of a young child's new skills may present a challenge for the parent in terms of supervision and protection. The most conscientious parent can turn away for "just a minute," and the child can get into a deadly situation. When this happens and the child presents with injuries, the bruises and burns will have plausible explanations. Although such injuries may not constitute physical abuse, they are reportable as neglect in some states. The following case study is an example of supervisory neglect.

Case Study

CS was an 18-month-old girl brought to a small community emergency department with a deep, fresh, patterned burn to her left mandible. The hospital staff reported the injury as suspicious, and the family was escorted by CPS to a suspected child abuse and neglect (SCAN) team at another hospital.

The parents were in their late teens. When they arrived at the second hospital, they were tearful and visibly shaken. The child was crying as well.

The family had attended a barbecue earlier that day with some friends. Out of concern for their child's safety, the parents had placed her in her car seat and employed the safety restraints. Unfortunately, the car seat was close to a small hibachi-type barbecue grill that was on the ground, still hot from the afternoon meal. To free herself, the girl started rocking back and forth in the seat and flipped it on its side, landing the child on the barbecue grill. This had been witnessed by a number of people at the party. The child was immediately taken to the community hospital.

Although the injuries to the child were consistent with the mechanism described by the parents, and deemed not to have been inflicted, it was suggested that the social worker visit the home of the child and instruct the parents on diligent supervision and safety issues when dealing with a young child.

Supervision problems also arise when parents allow older siblings to watch younger ones during play or bathing. A number of tragic situations have developed when an older, but still immature, child is left to care for an infant.

A child who repeatedly presents with signs of neglect in provisional, developmental, or supervisory areas should be reported to the proper authorities, as should the child less than age 2 years who is alleged to be accident-prone. The nurse who regularly addresses the issues of safety, supervision, and normal development may protect a child from long-term disability or death.

SUMMARY

Although it may be difficult to believe that an adult is capable of injuring a small child, the nurse who cares for children must keep this possibility in mind whenever a young patient presents with an unusual injury. As with any presenting complaint, it is important to obtain a complete history and physical examination, with consideration of the differential diagnoses for the signs and symptoms. The nurse decides whether or not findings are suspicious based on knowledge and experience. Abuse and neglect cases are challenging and bring various conflicting emotions to all parties involved. However, to ignore child maltreatment or to deny its existence places a vulnerable child at risk for further abuse or death. Although nurses have legal mandates to encourage reporting child maltreatment, the care and safety of children should serve as an even greater motivation to become involved in these cases.

REFERENCES

Abrams M, Lewis KH. Prolapse of the female urethra in young girls. *J Urol.* 1954;72:222-225.

Adams J. The role of photo documentation of genital findings in medical evaluations of suspected child sexual abuse. *Child Maltreat.* 1997;2:341-347.

Adams J, Harper K, Knudson S, Revilla J. Examination findings in legally confirmed child sexual abuse: it's normal to be normal. *Pediatrics.* 1994;94:310-317.

Administration for Children and Families. *Child Maltreatment 2000: Table 5-6 Child Fatality Victims by Type of Maltreatment, 2000.* Washington, DC: US Dept of Health & Human Services; 2000. Available at: http://www.acf.hhs.gov/programs/cb/publications/cm00/table5_6.htm. Accessed December 17, 2002.

American Academy of Pediatrics. Diagnostic imaging of child abuse. *Pediatrics.* 2000;105:1345-1348.

Berkowitz CD. Pediatric abuse. New patterns of injury. *Emerg Med Clin North Am.* 1995;13:321-341.

Berkowitz CD. Child sexual abuse. In: Berkowitz CD, ed. *Pediatrics: A Primary Care Approach.* Philadelphia, Pa: WB Saunders; 1996a:411-415.

Berkowitz CD. Failure to thrive. In: Berkowitz CD, ed. *Pediatrics: A Primary Care Approach.* Philadelphia, Pa: WB Saunders; 1996b:415-420.

Bowen K, Aldous M. Medical evaluation of sexual abuse in children without disclosed or witnessed abuse. *Arch Pediatr Adolesc Med.* 1999;153:1160-1164.

Cantwell H. The neglect of child neglect. In: Helfer M, Kempe R, Krugman R, eds. *The Battered Child.* 5th ed. Chicago, Ill: The University of Chicago Press; 1997:347-373.

Chadwick DL, Chin S, Salerno C, Landsverk J, Kitchen L. Deaths from falls in children: how far is fatal? *J Trauma.* 1991;31:1353-1355.

Christian C, Lavelle J, DeJong A, Loiselle J, Brenner L, Joffe M. Forensic evidence findings in prepubertal victims of sexual assault. *Pediatrics.* 2000;106:100-104.

Cooperman D, Merten D. Skeletal manifestations of child abuse. In: Reece R, Ludwig S, eds. *Child Abuse: Medical Diagnosis and Management.* 2nd ed. Phildelphia, Pa: Lippincott Williams & Wilkins; 2001:123-156.

Dubowitz H, Giardino A, Gustavson E. Child neglect: guidance for pediatricians [review]. *Pediatr Rev.* 2000;21:111-116.

Duhaime AC, Christian CW, Rorke LB, Zimmerman RA. Nonaccidental head injury in infants: the "shaken-baby syndrome." *N Engl J Med.* 1998;338:1822-1829.

Duhaime AC, Partington M. Overview and clinical presentation of inflicted head injury in infants. *Neurosurg Clin N Am.* 2002;13:149-154.

Elvik S. Child maltreatment. In: Soud T, Rogers J, eds. *Manual of Pediatric Emergency Nursing.* St. Louis, Mo: Mosby; 1998:586-605.

Emans SJ, Laufer MR, Goldstein DP, eds. *Pediatric and Adolescent Gynecology.* 4th ed. Philadelphia, Pa: Lippincott-Raven; 1998.

Farley R, Reece R. Recognizing when a child's injury or illness is caused by abuse. In: *Portable Guides to Investigating Child Abuse, 1996.* Washington, DC: US Dept of Justice, Office of Justice Programs, Office of Juvenile Justice and Delinquency Prevention; 1996.

Feldman K. Evaluation of physical abuse. In: Helfer M, Kempe R, Krugman R, eds. *The Battered Child*. 5th ed. Chicago, Ill: The University of Chicago Press; 1997:175-220.

Giardino AP, Christian CW. Vaginal foreign bodies. In: Henretig F, King C, eds. *Textbook of Pediatric Emergency Procedures and Techniques*. Baltimore, Md: Williams & Wilkins; 1997:971-974.

Giardino AP, Ludwig S. Interdisciplinary approaches to child maltreatment: accessing community resources. In: Finkel M, Giardino A, eds. *Medical Evaluation of Child Sexual Abuse: A Practical Guide*. 2nd ed. Thousand Oaks, Calif: Sage Publications; 2002:215-231.

Ingram DL, Everett VD, Flick LA, Russell TA, White-Sims ST. Vaginal gonococcal cultures in sexual abuse evaluations: evaluation of selective criteria for preteenaged girls. *Pediatrics*. 1997;99:1-4.

Islam O, Soboleski D, Symons S, Davidson LK, Ashworth MA, Babyn P. Development and duration of radiographic signs of bone healing in children. *Am J Roentgenol*. 2000;175:75-78.

Johnson CF. Inflicted injury versus accidental injury. *Ped Clin North Am*. 1990;37:803.

Kairys SW. Distinguishing sudden infant death syndrome from child abuse fatalities (RE0036). *Pediatrics*. 2001;107:437-441.

Kattwinkel J. Changing concepts of sudden infant death syndrome: implications for infant sleeping environment and sleep position (RE9946). *Pediatrics*. 2000;105:L650-L656.

Kerns D, Ritter M. Medical findings in child sexual abuse cases with perpetrator confessions. *Am J Dis Child*. 1992;146:494.

Kolilis DM. Child fatality review teams. In: Monteleone JA, ed. *Child Maltreatment*. 2nd ed. St. Louis, Mo: GW Medical Publishing; 1998:509-530.

Ladson S, Johnson CF, Doty RE. Do physicians recognize sexual abuse? *Am J Dis Child*. 1987;141:411-415.

Launius G, Silberstein M, Luisiri A, Graviss E. Radiology of child abuse. In: Monteleone J, ed. *Child Maltreatment*. 2nd ed. St. Louis, Mo: GW Medical Publishing; 1998:31-58.

Lentsch KA, Johnson CF. Do physicians have adequate knowledge of child sexual abuse? The results of two surveys of practicing physicians, 1986 and 1996. *Child Maltreat*. 2000;5:72-78.

Ludwig S. Child abuse. In: Fleisher GR, Ludwig S, eds. *Textbook of Pediatric Emergency Medicine*. 4th ed. Philadelphia, Pa: Lippincott Williams & Wilkins; 1999:1680-1685.

Monteleone J, Brodeur A. Identifying, interpreting, and reporting injuries. In: Monteleone J, ed. *Child Maltreatment*. 2nd ed. St. Louis, Mo: GW Medical Publishing; 1998:1-29.

National Clearinghouse on Child Abuse and Neglect Information. *Child Fatalities Fact Sheet*. Washington, DC: US Dept of Health & Human Services; 2001a.

National Clearinghouse on Child Abuse and Neglect Information. *What Is Child Maltreatment?* Washington, DC: US Dept of Health & Human Services; 2001b.

Peddle N, Wang CT. *Current Trends in Child Abuse Prevention, Reporting, and Fatalities: The 1999 Fifty State Survey*. Chicago, Ill: National Center of Child Abuse Prevention Research, Prevent Child Abuse America; 2001.

Reece R, Sege R. Childhood head injuries: accidental or inflicted? *Arch Pediatr Adolesc Med*. 2000;154:11-15.

Reichert S. Medical evaluation of the sexually abused child. In: Helfer M, Kempe R, Krugman R, eds. *The Battered Child*. 5th ed. Chicago, Ill: The University of Chicago Press; 1997:313-328.

Schwartz A, Ricci L. How accurately can bruises be aged in abused children? Literature review and synthesis. *Pediatrics*. 1996;97:254-256.

Sgroi SM. Sexual molestation of children. The last frontier in child abuse. *Child Today*. 1975;4:18-21, 44.

Sgroi SM, Blick L, Porter F. A conceptual framework for child sexual abuse. In: Sgroi SM, ed. *Handbook of Clinical Intervention on Child Sexual Abuse*. New York, NY: DC Heath and Company; 1982:9-37.

Sifuentes M. Vaginitis. In: Berkowitz CD, ed. *Pediatrics: A Primary Care Approach*. Philadelphia, Pa: WB Saunders; 1996:279-282.

US Department of Health & Human Services. *National Study on the Incidence and Prevalence of Child Abuse and Neglect (NIS-2)*. Washington, DC: US Government Printing Office; 1988.

US Department of Health & Human Services. *Child Maltreatment 1999: Reports From the States to the National Child Abuse and Neglect Data Systems*. Washington, DC: US Government Printing Office; 1999.

US Department of Health & Human Services. *Child Abuse and Neglect State Statutes Elements: Reporting Laws: Number 2: Mandatory Reporters of Child Abuse and Neglect*. National Clearinghouse on Child Abuse and Neglect Information. Available at: http://www.calib.com/nccanch/pubs/stats02/mandrep.cfm. Accessed December 17, 2002.

Wilson E. Estimation of the age of cutaneous contusions in child abuse. *Pediatrics*. 1977;60:750-752.

Chapter 3

HISTORY AND THE HEALTHCARE INTERVIEW

Barbara Speller-Brown, RN, MSN, CPNP
Maureen Sanger, PhD
Phyllis L. Thompson, LCSW

The healthcare interview, or history-taking process, is an important component of the medical evaluation completed in the context of suspected child maltreatment. A child's caregiver or the communicating child provides the history in verbal, written, or sign language as necessary. When carefully documented, the history provides a record of what was described and explained when the child came for care to the healthcare setting. The history accomplishes the following for the overall evaluation:

— Lays the groundwork that frames the entire evaluation

— Suggests areas for detailed examination

— Assists in targeting laboratory and diagnostic testing

— Provides clues to possible diagnoses other than the one initially suspected

The history component of the health evaluation has become somewhat standardized and is traditionally composed of individual sections that contain specific information related to the problem. The following sections are each explained in the context of a complete history and physical examination:

— ***History of the present illness (HPI):*** provides an account of the problem(s) for which the child or caregivers are seeking care. It includes information to describe the reason the person is being evaluated. The HPI elaborates the details of the problem or symptom(s), such as the timing of the complaint, the location and setting in which the problem occurred, factors that aggravated or alleviated the problem, and other relevant information (the patient's response to the problem and the effect of the problem on the child's life) (Bickley & Szilagyi, 2003).

— ***Past medical history (PMH):*** includes childhood illnesses such as measles, chickenpox, or chronic conditions with which the child has been diagnosed and for which he or she has been treated if necessary.

— ***Birth history:*** includes relevant information concerning the mother's health during pregnancy, complications before or during delivery, birth order if a multiple birth, and birth weight of the child. Also included may be problems the child encountered with breathing, feeding, infections, or parent–child interactions such as bonding or early caregiving. The birth history also includes neurological or developmental problems the child may have experienced after birth (Bickley & Szilagyi, 2003).

— ***Social history:*** relevant for determining lifestyle issues of the child and family. It generally captures information about lifestyle issues relevant to the health and well-being of the family and risk factors for health and health maintenance issues of the family (Bickley & Szilagyi, 2003).

— ***Family history:*** explores disease patterns in the family and factors that may influence health risks for particular diseases. The family usually includes the child's parents, siblings, and grandparents. Aunts and uncles are of secondary importance. The amount of information gathered usually depends on the child's specific problem and the relevance of family disease patterns on the particular problem (Coulehan & Block, 2001). For example, a family history of alcoholism or drug abuse may be more important to maltreatment and neglect than diabetes or heart disease.

— ***Review of symptoms (ROS):*** generally documents relevant subjective information related to each of the major body systems. The purpose of the ROS is to ensure that other important symptoms the child may experience have not been missed (Bickley & Szilagyi, 2003). Each system can be introduced with questions such as "Has the child ever experienced any problems with hearing or ear infections?" or "Does Jane have any problems with breathing or allergies?"

In the setting of suspected child maltreatment, the history provided by the caregivers or the communicating child is seen as being an important part of the overall evaluation and feeds into the investigation. In alleged physical abuse the circumstances surrounding the injury are central to the history taking, whereas the description by the child about any inappropriate sexual activities becomes the focus in sexual abuse cases. Where neglect is suspected, the pattern of caregiving described by the caregivers and evident to the examiner is the target of the healthcare interview. The first section of this chapter discusses the history and interview in the setting of suspected physical abuse or neglect. The next section describes the central value and unique aspects of history taking in the context of the sexual abuse evaluation.

HISTORY AND INTERVIEWING IN CASES OF SUSPECTED PHYSICAL ABUSE OR NEGLECT

In pediatric practice, the caregiver typically provides the healthcare interviewer with the details of the history. This is especially true with infants, young children, children who are extremely frightened or fearful, and those who are severely injured or unconscious. However, older children who have mastery of some form of language are able to complement the caregiver history. When interviewing a child, the healthcare provider must remember the developmental level and communicative abilities of the child and the circumstances surrounding the interview (Bickley & Szilagyi, 2003; Lewis & Pantell, 1995). In dealing with children, attention should be paid to the setting and the environment in which the history and interview are conducted.

In cases of physical abuse in which the child comes for immediate care to the emergency department, the urgency of the child's medical condition will determine how much attention can be paid to modifying the setting to make it as quiet and private as possible. It is advisable to interview children when they are not hungry, sleepy, or otherwise physically uncomfortable. This can be accommodated to some extent in less urgent circumstances but may not be possible in more urgent situations in which critical care and life-saving interventions are necessary.

Establishing rapport with the child before discussion of the incident provides a good foundation for open dialogue. This can be done through various techniques that avoid intimidation by the examiner and creation of an imbalance of power. The interviewer should minimize the size differential between himself or herself and the child by getting on the same physical level. This may involve using a child's table and chairs or sitting at or below the child's line of sight. If possible, the interviewer should sit on a chair by the side of the bed or stretcher and position himself or herself in a comfortable spot from which the child can make eye contact. Standing over and looking down on the child is the least favorable position for the interview. Assuring the child that he or she is not in any trouble is essential.

WARM-UP AND GROUND RULES

At the beginning of the history-taking effort with the child, the healthcare provider should start with generic warm-up steps to establish a dialogue with the child. Introductions should be made, and a simple explanation of the role of the nurse as interviewer should be given to the child. Depending on the child's developmental and maturity level, it would be ideal to speak with the child at some point without the caregiver present as well.

To begin the interview process, the examiner first introduces himself or herself and tells the child who he or she is. The role of the examiner is to ask what may be difficult questions of the child while respecting the child's feelings. The examiner's job is to develop rapport with the child and put the child at ease while asking questions about difficult issues. The examiner also explains to the child an important rule: the child has the right to ask the examiner to stop at any time during the evaluation and examination, and the examiner will stop. If the interviewer fails to follow the rule, any trust established with the child will be forfeit.

It is important to keep questions and sentences simple when speaking with the child and to use words familiar to the child's vocabulary and understanding. For example, the interviewer should use the child's words for body parts, such as *belly* rather than *stomach*. Interviewers must not assume that their meaning of a word is the same as the child's and that pronunciation is consistent. Care must be taken when using pronouns like "he" or "she" and words like "there" and "that" because the child may be unable to follow the meaning of the scenario. Therefore, it may be clearer to use people's names or titles rather than pronouns to describe other people.

The preferred approach to the interview is to use open-ended, nonleading questions. This may be difficult because few children easily open up and give a narrative of the incident for the examiner to record. More often than not, the examiner must ask specific questions of a child depending on personality, developmental level, and willingness to talk. The interviewer first starts with general or neutral questions and then leads to more specific details. Allowing for the narrative and slowly moving to more specific questions when the child is having difficulty is appropriate to ascertain the information needed for a medical evaluation with appropriate evidence collection.

Typical questions that might help to establish rapport with the child include the following:

— What is your name? How old are you?

— Where do you live? Who lives with you? Who visits you?

— What are your mother's and father's names?

— What school do you go to? What grade are you in?

— What is your favorite subject? Your least favorite subject?

— What is your teacher's name? Who was your teacher last year?

— What makes you happy? Sad? Mad? Scared?

— What do you like best about the people you live with? Least?

— Why are you here today?

The child's developmental level should be assessed quickly and considered throughout the ensuing evaluation. The developmental history is used to ascertain when the child reached developmental milestones and if the child has any special needs. The child's developmental level is often a guideline for determining if the stated cause of the injury is consistent with the child's physical and psychological development. The child who is a slow developer may be a source of frustration to a caregiver and increase the risk for abuse (Giardino, Christian, & Giardino, 1997).

The child should be told that it is okay to answer, "I don't know" or "I don't understand," rather than guess a response. It is important to ask questions that encourage the child to give more than a "yes" or "no" answer and to avoid leading questions that start with "did" or "does." The healthcare provider should be aware of the child's nonverbal communication and must be patient, allowing the child ample time to respond to any question asked. The healthcare interviewer must encourage the child to be comfortable and must remain neutral in responding to the child's responses so as not to influence answers.

In suspected physical abuse, the history is important and is initiated by asking open-ended questions about what happened. Asking the child initially, "Why are you here today?" may help the child open up and relate his or her story. When a child is developmentally able to interact with the examiner, it is ideal to ask both the child and the caregiver separately and then compare the answers (Ludwig, 2000).

SPECIFIC HISTORY OF INJURY

At this point, the history-taking effort shifts to the events surrounding the reason for the present evaluation. With suspected child physical abuse, the child has sustained some sort of injury and may be upset and in discomfort. The nurse interviewer, therefore, should try to ask as few direct questions as possible but attempt to obtain the what, who, how, where, and when of the events surrounding the time that the injury occurred. This history taker should avoid "why" questions because they may imply blame to the child (Kolilis & Easter, 1998). However, the nurse and other healthcare providers must use clinical judgment in each of the questions asked. In some circumstances, asking the child, "Why do you think this happened?" may be entirely appropriate. It will depend on the unique circumstances of each individual case. In any event, the child requires ongoing reassurance that he or she is believed and not at fault for what happened.

Along with specific history about the child and the injury, the interviewer also observes the child's interactions with the caregiver(s). Behaviors and interactions that demonstrate indifference to the child's injuries, lack of support for the child, or lack of awareness of the seriousness of the injuries raise concerns for the stability of the relationship between adult and child (Giardino et al., 1997). Other concerning signs are a child who does not look to the caregiver for emotional support or a caregiver who belittles the child. Although these signs are not definite for abuse, they raise the level of suspicion (Giardino et al., 1997).

Questions for the caregiver and child that may be useful in completing a thorough history in the setting of possible physical abuse include the following:

— When did the injury occur? (date and time)

— Where did the injury occur? (location)

— Who had caregiving responsibility for the child at the time of the injury?

  1. Was that caregiver watching the child?

  2. Had that caregiver left the child in someone else's care?

  3. Did the caregiver witness the injury?

— What was happening during the time before the injury occurred?

— What was the response to the injury?

  1. What was the child's response?

  2. What was the caregiver's response?

  3. If someone else was watching the child, what has been his or her response? Is that person here with the child?

  4. What happened after the injury?

After completing the history of the present situation, the interviewer then moves on to the other components of the history. The interviewer questions the caregiver about the child's past medical history, birth history, social history, family history, and complete ROS. The data from these history components are then explored for findings or patterns that might suggest child maltreatment. Information from all of these sections of the history is important, particularly if there were prior incidents of injury, because it is essential to determine how the caregiver(s) responded to them.

At the end of the history-taking process, the interviewer should ask the child and caregiver if they have any questions. It is appropriate to comfort the child, but the healthcare provider should not make promises about what will happen to the alleged perpetrator in the case. Also, it is out of the healthcare provider's realm to know or discuss with the child to whom he or she will be discharged after the healthcare encounter because these decisions are not under the healthcare provider's complete control.

NEGLECT

In cases of neglect, the focus of the evaluation is on the patterns of caregiving the child receives. Neglect is a heterogeneous clinical entity, and its presentation, evaluation, and treatment are somewhat distinct from the manner in which physical abuse and sexual abuse are determined in the healthcare setting. In view of the ongoing nature in which neglectful caregiving manifests, the history-taking effort does not often hinge on one episode. Instead, multiple histories elicited over time during routine and sick visits are usually linked together to form a more comprehensive picture of how the caregiver(s) can meet the child's physical and emotional needs. In view of the more insidious nature of neglect, there is great value in history over time.

In thinking about the history taking in cases of possible neglect, it may be helpful for the nurse to think in terms of both generic and specific assessments. The generic assessment evaluates patterns of caregiving or symptoms that might suggest the need for further exploration. The specific assessment screens then build on the generic screens and focus on particular forms of neglect that may be suspected. Dubowitz, Giardino, and Gustavson (2000) reviewed generic and specific assessments. For generic neglect screening the following should be assessed:

— Circumstances related to the child's basic needs being met; whether actual or potential harm exists

— Patterns of neglect observed in the past or present; whether child protective services (CPS) has been involved

— Identification of possible contributing factors at the child, caregiver, family, and community levels

— Identification of strengths and challenges for the child, family, and community

— Information on previous interventions and their results

— Prognostic information related to motivation to change and availability of formal and information resources (Dubowitz et al., 2000)

The specific assessment then depends on what is uncovered during the generic screening and on the form of neglect suspected. In the healthcare setting, the nurse can focus on physical neglect, medical neglect, and failure to thrive (FTT). In looking at physical neglect, protection from avoidable environmental hazards is paramount and specific questions should explore the following:

— Poisonous or hazardous materials in easy reach of children

— Tobacco smoke exposure around children with respiratory conditions

— Presence of domestic violence

— Failure to use automobile restraints, smoke detectors, bicycle helmets

— Access to firearms

— Appropriateness of clothing for environmental conditions

    1. Perceptions of caregiver and child on clothing worn

    2. Whether others have made comments about clothing or have teased the child

In considering medical neglect, the specific assessment focuses most heavily on whether there is compliance or adherence with healthcare recommendations and whether noncompliance results in potential or actual harm to the child. Questions would revolve around the following:

— The child's condition and the relevance of the noncompliance

— Existence of barriers to care (i.e., insurance, transportation, skills)

— Whether the recommendations were clear

Finally, looking specifically at FTT, the history focuses on nutritional intake and patterns of the child's growth. Questions should include the following:

— Detailed dietary history

— Perceptions of feeding and meal times

— Barriers to acquiring food

— Understanding of caloric intake and appropriate food selections

Chapter 8, Clinical Aspects of Child Neglect, offers a complete discussion of the evaluation of neglect.

HISTORY AND INTERVIEWING IN CASES OF SUSPECTED SEXUAL ABUSE

Words from children and adolescents about their experiences of victimization are often the most significant evidence in cases of sexual abuse. Statements from children describing their molestation are key to identifying victims and intervening on their behalf. People rarely witness a child's molestation, offenders infrequently admit to an offense, and there is often no medical evidence to prove that sexual abuse has occurred. Healthcare providers encounter various situations that may raise suspicion about sexual abuse. Physical symptoms, behavioral difficulties, or comments from a child may warrant direct questioning about possible sexual victimization to determine whether maltreatment has occurred and what type of medical, mental health, or legal intervention is needed.

Nursing professionals gather information from children and adolescents about their health and well-being and whether or not they have been sexually abused. Pediatric healthcare providers are in an important position to obtain information from children by virtue of the relationship with their patients and the helping role they embody. Some children will reveal more information about their sexual contacts to medical professionals, when issues of their health may be at stake, than they will with caregivers or investigators. In addition, children's statements about abuse made to healthcare providers in the course of medical diagnosis and treatment may be admissible in court. Thus, it is incumbent upon healthcare providers to conduct skillful and developmentally sensitive interviews and to preserve the information through accurate and thorough documentation.

Guidelines for gathering information from children and adolescents, as well as their caregivers when sexual abuse is a concern, and procedures for documenting such information are presented in the following section. Although the discussion and examples focus on sexual abuse, these guidelines can be applied to questioning children about other forms of maltreatment as well.

OBTAINING INFORMATION FROM CAREGIVERS

An important first step in exploring concerns that a child may have been molested is to gather information from the child's caregiver. It is most appropriate that this conversation take place privately, without the child present, so the caregiver can speak freely and openly about his or her concerns and the caregiver's statements do not influence or contaminate what the child subsequently reports. Talking first with caregivers informs the healthcare provider about the basis for the sexual abuse concerns, as well as the child's physical, developmental, and mental health status. This information provides the framework for conducting a focused and productive medical history with the child. A detailed caregiver history may also guide diagnosis and treatment decisions.

The medical interview with the caregiver should include several elements pertaining to sexual abuse concerns and to the child's general physical, developmental, and mental health status **(Table 3-1)**. Questioning specific to sexual abuse should include the reasons the caregiver is concerned about molestation. When a child has made statements suggestive of sexual abuse, it is useful to know how the child's disclosure came about, whom the child has told, and the extent to which others have questioned the child. Eliciting from the caregiver his or her knowledge of the child's statements, information about the perpetrator (including name, relationship to the child, and age), and the types of sexual contact the child may have experienced may be critical to determining the child's need for medical evaluation, as well as the child's safety. The caregiver's knowledge of high-risk behaviors or conditions in the perpetrator, such as drug use, sexual promiscuity, and known sexually transmitted diseases (STDs) is also important (Jenny, 1996). In situations involving acute assaults, such information may guide medical decisions about providing prophylaxis to the child for infections or, in nonacute cases, may help determine the need to test for STDs.

Table 3-1. Gathering Medical History From Caregivers

HISTORY OF SEXUAL ABUSE CONCERNS

— When caregiver first became concerned and why
— Statements made by child suggestive of abuse
  — How statements came about
  — Who has questioned the child and how
  — Specific sexual acts described by child
  — Identity of the alleged perpetrator and relationship to child

CHILD'S SEXUAL HISTORY

— Prior allegations/investigations of sexual abuse
— History of consensual sexual activity
— Sexualized behaviors
— Exposure to sexual information/material

CHILD'S PHYSICAL HEALTH STATUS

— Significant past medical history
— History of anogenital abnormalities, injuries, infections, diagnostic procedures
— Results of past anogenital examinations

CHILD'S DEVELOPMENTAL HISTORY

— Past developmental concerns
— Current cognitive and communication skills
— Academic functioning

CHILD'S MENTAL HEALTH STATUS

— History of psychological difficulties
— Recent behavioral or emotional disturbances
— History of psychological evaluation/intervention
— Personal or family stresses
— Quality of peer relationships

FAMILY FUNCTIONING

— Family composition and relationships
— History of abuse, neglect, domestic violence
— Support and resources
— Ability to protect child

The healthcare provider should also explore the caregiver's knowledge of the child or adolescent's sexual history, including prior incidents of consensual and nonconsensual sexual activity, exhibition of sexualized behaviors, and exposure to sexual information and sexually explicit media. Inquiring about the child's sexual knowledge and the child's terminology for male and female private parts provides information that may be critical to understanding the history the child provides and ensuring that questions are asked using terms the child understands.

In regard to a child's general health status, it is helpful to discuss with the caregiver the child's past medical history, as well as current problems or symptoms. A thorough medical history may reveal patterns of injury, neglect, or FTT (Frasier, 1997). A report of past anogenital injuries, bladder or kidney infections, or episodes of unexplained vaginal or rectal bleeding may be of particular importance. A developmental history of the child, including the age at which motor and language milestones were reached, is also useful. Knowledge of a child's cognitive, speech, or language difficulties must be taken into account when questioning the child. Finally, eliciting information about patterns in the child's academic, social, behavioral, and emotional functioning may identify the existence of problems warranting mental health intervention and may yield data to help clarify the diagnostic picture.

Hearing caregivers talk about their children's suspected sexual abuse may evoke feelings in the healthcare provider ranging from sadness to shock to anger. Particularly difficult are situations in which it appears that the caregiver may have contributed to the circumstances that enabled the abuse, such as by exposing the child to a known perpetrator, by ignoring signs that abuse was occurring, or by failing to believe the child's disclosure of molestation. In all circumstances, healthcare providers should strive to maintain an objective, nonjudgmental, and nonblaming stance. This approach encourages an open exchange of information with the caregiver and establishes a productive working relationship that may lead to needed services for the child and family.

Caregivers concerned that their child may have been molested have many questions and look to healthcare providers for information, guidance, and support. One of their immediate concerns may be the nature of the anogenital examination. Caregivers often fear that the forensic medical evaluation will be painful and invasive and mistakenly believe the examination will determine conclusively whether or not their child has been molested. Correcting such misconceptions and sharing accurate information is important in allaying caregivers' anxieties and creating realistic expectations regarding the outcome of their child's examination.

Many caregivers request that they be present during their child's anogenital examination. Whereas preschool-age children often want and need their caregiver present during the examination for support and assistance, school-age children and adolescents may prefer to do the examination on their own. Allowing school-age children and adolescents to decide who is present during their examination can give the child a measure of control over the situation and demonstrates respect for their needs and preferences.

Caregivers should be told that information obtained from them and their child may be shared with CPS when there is reasonable cause to suspect that the child has been abused. Explaining to caregivers the dictates of state child abuse reporting laws and the importance of complying with the law may help caregivers understand and accept why reporting is necessary. Healthcare providers should also be knowledgeable about state statutes related to the issue of consent for the medical examinations of children for whom abuse is suspected. In some jurisdictions, examinations of children for suspected abuse can be conducted without the consent of the child's parent or legal guardian.

Whenever possible, it is important to inform caregivers of the nature and purpose of the medical evaluation and seek their assent and cooperation.

GATHERING MEDICAL HISTORY FROM THE CHILD

Obtaining medical history from a child or adolescent, particularly when there is concern about sexual abuse, is a challenging task and one that requires careful attention to the content and the process of the interaction. In regard to the content, healthcare providers' questions should focus on information relevant to medical diagnosis and treatment. It is not the place of medical professionals to conduct exhaustive investigative interviews that detail the dates, circumstances, and contexts of each reported episode of sexual touching. Such interviews are best left to specially trained CPS workers, forensic interviewers, and law enforcement investigators.

Healthcare providers must be sensitive to the process of gathering information from children about molestation. Many children have difficulty acknowledging or talking about their sexual victimization for fear of social and legal repercussions, shame or embarrassment, or threats by the perpetrator of harm if the child tells anyone. Approaching children and adolescents in an empathic and supportive manner and being sensitive to changes in a child's affect or behavior during questioning may increase the likelihood of eliciting information about abuse.

Table 3-2 outlines one approach to conducting a medical history with children and adolescents when there is concern about sexual abuse. Whenever possible, healthcare providers should conduct the questioning in a room that is quiet, private, and child friendly. Providers should talk with the child or adolescent alone, without caregivers present. Talking at eye level; maintaining a calm, accepting demeanor; and respecting the child's pace in providing information will set the stage for a productive exchange of information. Additional guidelines for questioning children are listed in **Table 3-3**. Obtaining a medical history from children involves 4 steps:

1. Establishing rapport with the child

2. Obtaining information about the child's general physical and mental health status

3. Inquiring about sexual abuse

4. Providing closure

Establishing Rapport

Establishing rapport with a child or an adolescent is a critical precursor to eliciting sensitive information about a child's experience of maltreatment. An important first step is to establish for the child what will occur during interaction with the healthcare provider, to help allay the child's anxieties or fears. The healthcare provider should introduce himself or herself and describe the evaluation process. Children should be told why questions will be asked and what will happen to the information provided. Specifically, children should be told in simple terms that the interview is for the purpose of medical diagnosis and treatment, for example, "I want to know about problems you've been having with your body, and about things that have happened to your body, so I can check to see if you're okay or need any medicine."

Once the healthcare provider establishes the purpose of the evaluation, he or she may ask the child or adolescent about general topics such as school, extracurricular activities, or hobbies. Inquiring about topics that are nonthreatening and of interest to the child helps put the child at ease, promotes verbal exchange, and builds the relationship between the child and interviewer. A child's conversation regarding general topics also provides the healthcare professional with important information about the child's

---

Table 3-2. Gathering Medical History From Children

RAPPORT BUILDING

— Create a comfortable, nonthreatening environment

— Establish that the purpose of the interview is for medical diagnosis and treatment

— Invite the child to ask questions and express feelings

— Encourage the child to correct wrong information or ask for clarification

— Be genuine and show concern

— Assess the child's cognitive and language skills

— Explain the importance of only talking about the truth

— Discuss limits of confidentiality

GENERAL HEALTH CONCERNS

— Inquire about health-related symptoms

— Ask about anogenital problems, discomfort, or concerns

— Inquire about changes in eating and sleeping patterns

— Assess recent academic, behavioral, and emotional functioning

— Inquire about medication use

SEXUAL ABUSE INQUIRY

— Establish the identity of and child's relationship to the perpetrator(s)

— Ask where the perpetrator touched the child and how

— Inquire about whether and how the child touched the perpetrator

— Ask about penetration, oral contact, and ejaculation

— Explore time frame of abuse, particularly the most recent incident

— Ask about prior history of consensual and nonconsensual sexual contact

CLOSING

— Elicit and respond to child's questions

— Let child know what will happen next

— Prepare child for anogenital examination

---

cognitive, language, and speech skills, so that subsequent questioning can be geared toward the appropriate developmental level.

During this phase, the healthcare provider can also lay the foundation for clear communication with the child and maximize the likelihood of obtaining accurate and reliable information. In gathering a history from a child about maltreatment, it is critical that efforts be made to elicit truthful reports from the child and to ensure that the manner and content of questioning neither pressure nor coerce the child to respond in specific ways, nor suggest information or answers to the child. Obtaining accurate reports from a child may be enhanced by telling the child the following (Reed, 1996):

1. It is important to tell the truth.

2. Not to guess but to admit when he or she is unsure of or does not know an answer.

3. It is okay to correct the interviewer's mistakes.

4. He or she has permission not to answer questions.

It is necessary to inform children about the limits of confidentiality during the initial phase of the interview. Children and adolescents should never be told or led to believe that the information they provide will remain private because a disclosure of abuse must necessarily be reported. Explaining to children and teenagers that their statements may be shared with others to ensure their safety and protection is critical for honest, informed communication with a child.

Eliciting General Health Concerns

Once adequate rapport is achieved and guidelines for clear communication are established, the healthcare provider may question the child or adolescent about significant past medical history and recent health problems or concerns. Such questioning focuses the child on issues related to his or her body. This is also a good time for the healthcare provider to learn the child's terms for various body parts, including the genital and rectal areas. The healthcare provider should inquire about any physical

---

Table 3-3. Interviewing Guidelines

INTERVIEWER SHOULD

— Make the child comfortable

— Interview the child alone

— Question in a nonthreatening manner

— Ask open-ended questions appropriate to the child's developmental level

— Use terms the child can understand

— Tell the child you believe him or her

— Allow the child to ask questions and express feelings

— Explain the examination process thoroughly and encourage questions

— Document immediately

INTERVIEWER SHOULD NOT

— Ask leading or suggestive questions

— Suggest the child was abused

— Promise not to tell

— React with negative facial or body language

— Act as if you do not believe the child

— Criticize the family

— Make a determination about the validity of the allegations

Adapted from Freese S. Child Sexual Abuse Impact and Aftershocks. St. Paul, Minn: Project Impact; 1989.

---

problems the child or adolescent is experiencing, as well as the presence of mental health difficulties. Symptoms such as sleep disturbances, behavioral regression, somatic complaints, anxiety, depression, fearfulness, irritability, aggressive conduct, and drug and alcohol use are common in children who have been abused (Kendall-Tackett, Williams, & Finkelhor, 1993). When healthcare providers discuss general health concerns with a child or an adolescent, they may uncover stressful or traumatic events the child has experienced, including molestation. If not, then it is appropriate to proceed to the next phase of questioning, which is inquiring specifically about sexual abuse.

Inquiring About Sexual Abuse

When questioning a child about sexual abuse, it is best to start with open-ended questions, which invite the child to provide a narrative account of his or her experiences. Such questions typically elicit the most accurate reports and are least likely to be misleading (Reed, 1996). Open-ended questions such as "Do you know why you're here today?" or "What happened?" will sometimes yield a disclosure from a child about abuse.

Sexually abused children are often reluctant to discuss their victimization and may be unwilling to volunteer information unless asked specific questions about possible abuse (Reed, 1996). If open-ended questions are not productive, the next step is to ask focused questions, which direct the child's attention to persons, actions, circumstances, body parts, or other relevant contextual information. The interviewer often has some idea of the circumstances surrounding the suspected abuse, based on the caregiver history, which will guide the kind of focused questions to be asked.

Faller (1990) explains that questions regarding abuse may be person-focused ("What is Uncle Johnny like?" or "What do you and Uncle Johnny do together?") or situation-focused ("Tell me about the time Uncle Johnny came to baby-sit."). Another type of focused question relates to the child's experience with or knowledge of body parts. Such questioning often follows naturally from the child's identification and naming of body parts ("Who has a pee pee? What is it for? Has anything happened to your pee pee?") (Faller, 1990). Alternatively, the interviewer may focus the child on information the child has already shared ("Did you tell your foster mom about something that happened before you came to foster care?" or "I know you told your teacher about something that happened to you. Tell me about that.") (Faller, 1999).

For some children, it may be necessary to resort to more close-ended questions such as multiple choice and yes/no questions ("Have you had touches on your body that you didn't like or that made you feel uncomfortable?" or "Has anyone touched your private parts?"). It is generally better to elicit the name of the perpetrator from the child ("Did someone touch your pee pee? Who?") than to name the person and see if the child agrees ("Did Uncle Johnny touch your pee pee?"). Although close-ended questions may be necessary when interviewing a child, they tend to produce information that is viewed as less accurate and reliable. Thus, when a child provides new information in response to a close-ended question, the interviewer should return to more open-ended questions to elicit further details, such as "What happened next?" or "Tell me more about that." It is always best to avoid asking a child leading questions about abuse. Leading questions suggest an answer ("Uncle Johnny touched your private with his penis, didn't he?") and may heighten the likelihood of false reporting by a child.

If a child indicates that he or she has been involved in inappropriate sexual contact, the healthcare provider should try to obtain specific pieces of information for the purpose of medical diagnosis and treatment, namely "Who?" "What?" and "When?"

Identifying who molested the child is critical for the protection of the child and helps guide decisions about the type of examination that may be needed and whether testing for STDs is indicated. For example, a 4-year-old girl who experienced penile-genital contact with an adult male may have different medical needs than a 4-year-old girl experiencing the same act by a 9-year-old boy. After a child has indicated that a particular person molested him or her, ask if anyone else has engaged the child in sexual activity because some children and adolescents will have been molested by more than one individual and some will have engaged in consensual sexual contact.

Information about what happened to the child should focus on the types and extent of sexual contact the child experienced. Specific information regarding the parts of the perpetrator's body that made contact with the child's body is essential for guiding decisions regarding examination of the child and interpretation of medical findings. Questions may include whether penetration of the child's mouth, vagina, or rectum occurred, if there was ejaculation, and whether the child experienced pain or bleeding after sexual contact.

It is important to determine when the incident(s) of sexual abuse occurred, as reported by the child. Of particular relevance is the time and date of the child's most recent sexual contact. A child or adolescent who has been sexually assaulted within the previous 72 hours may require a rape kit and may be eligible to receive prophylaxis for pregnancy and disease. (See Chapter 6, Sexually Transmitted Diseases in the Setting of Maltreatment, for a more complete discussion.)

If it is too difficult for the child to talk, the child may be offered other media with which to communicate, such as drawing or writing (Faller, 1999). Some children who appear too anxious or reluctant to verbalize their experiences may be able to draw or point on a picture of a person where or how the touching occurred. Other children may be willing to write down answers to questions about their molestation when they are unable to speak the words aloud. Children should never be coerced, bribed, or badgered to talk. If a child or an adolescent is unable or unwilling to share information, this should be respected and the sexual abuse inquiry terminated.

Providing Closure

The final step in the history-taking process is to provide the child with some closure. After responding to multiple questions and perhaps revealing sensitive and emotion-laden information, the child may need an opportunity to express his or her feelings and seek information from the healthcare provider. The experience of sexual abuse evokes many questions and issues for children and adolescents. These include concerns about the intactness and health of their bodies, fear of AIDS and other diseases, uncertainty about virginity, and confusion about sexual orientation. An open and honest discussion of these issues with a healthcare provider often can be enlightening and reassuring to children.

The examination itself is a source of anxiety and uncertainty for children and adolescents who will be undergoing a forensic medical evaluation. Healthcare providers can do much to allay these concerns by providing preparatory information to patients before their check-up. Children and adolescents benefit from knowing the specific procedures that will occur during the examination and how each component of the examination is likely to feel. When a colposcope is used, children and adolescents should be shown how this instrument works and how photographs that may be taken are used and stored. When healthcare providers take time to prepare children for genital examinations, often the result is patients who are more cooperative and who experience less anxiety during their check-ups (Finkel, 2002).

DEVELOPMENTAL CONSIDERATIONS

Although the guidelines in **Table 3-2** are broadly applicable to the pediatric population, it is essential that healthcare providers tailor their questioning to the developmental level of the child. Studies suggest that the quality of a child's report depends on the competence of the questioner to ask questions in language children can comprehend about concepts they can understand (Saywitz & Goodman, 1996). Following are some guidelines for questioning children of different ages about their experiences of abuse.

Questioning Preschool-Age Children

Obtaining reliable and understandable information from children between age 3 and 5 years is a formidable task. Although many preschoolers can provide accurate accounts of personally significant events, they may not be able to give an organized or consistent description of maltreatment incidents. They also may have limited capacity to describe events in detail (Sattler, 1998). Preschool-age children exhibit thinking that is egocentric and concrete. They focus on their own experiences and have difficulty understanding the viewpoints of others. Their language is simple and often literal. Thus, they may interpret questions about being touched on their private areas as including contact only with a hand or finger and not by a tongue or penis.

Most children age 3 years and older can label body parts, although their terms for the genital and rectal areas may be idiosyncratic and they may be unfamiliar with anatomically correct labels. A useful strategy for questioning preschoolers about sexual abuse is to have them label body parts on a picture of a person or on themselves. This strategy establishes the child's knowledge of and terms for various body parts, including private areas. The interviewer then asks about contact to the body using the anatomical terms the child understands.

A useful but controversial tool in talking with children about sexual abuse is the anatomically detailed doll. The American Professional Society on the Abuse of Children (APSAC, 1995) has established guidelines for the use of dolls. These dolls may best be used as an anatomical model to facilitate discussion of body parts and to identify the child's names for private parts. Dolls also act as a demonstration aid to assist the child in clarifying his or her statements about sexual touching (Faller, 1996). Use of the anatomically detailed dolls is not a diagnostic test, and the reaction of children to the dolls cannot be used to prove or disprove allegations of abuse. The fact that some children fail to demonstrate sexual activity with the dolls does not mean they have not been sexually abused, and conversely, the fact that they do show sexual activity does not mean that they have been sexually abused (Faller, 1996). Professionals who choose to use anatomically detailed dolls should be trained in their use and should be sure that their practice conforms to accepted guidelines (APSAC, 1995).

Many interviewers use anatomical drawings to help identify a child's labels for private parts and provide the child with another means of indicating (e.g., by pointing on the drawings) what type of sexual contact they experienced. Drawings, whether formal or informal, may be useful aides in communicating with young children and with children who are reluctant to verbalize the sexual contacts they have experienced.

Between ages 3 and 5 years, most children can respond accurately to "Who," "What," and "Where" questions. Therefore, questions about who touched their bodies, where on their bodies they were touched, and what the perpetrator did to their bodies are appropriate and generally within the developmental capacity of preschool-age children. Very young children cannot reliably answer questions about "When" or "How many" because they have not yet mastered the concepts of time or enumeration (Hewitt, 1999). Thus, providing details about when an abusive incident occurred, the timing of the most recent assault, or the number of abusive episodes is beyond the capabilities of children under age 6 years.

Although preschoolers are able to recall salient experiences accurately, they tend to recall only that information about which they are directly asked. Consequently, open-ended questions often yield little information from very young children; they need specific, direct questions to prompt their memories (Fivush, 1993). Concomitantly, very young children may be particularly susceptible to the effects of leading and suggestive questions, which can contaminate children's reports and undermine their credibility.

Keeping language simple and questions contained to one idea at a time is key to eliciting information from preschoolers. For example, instead of asking, "What did Johnny do after you left his house and drove to the farm?" ask, "Where did you go with Johnny? What did you do there?" Preschoolers may be reluctant to admit when they do not understand a question or do not know an answer. Young children may be helped to overcome this reluctance when encouraged to ask for clarification and when given permission to say, "I don't know" if they are unsure of an answer. Given the inherent difficulties and pitfalls of eliciting information from young children, questioning of preschoolers, if necessary, should be kept to a minimum.

Questioning School-Age Children

Between ages 6 and 12 years, children's thinking becomes more logical and their vocabulary expands rapidly. Consequently, school-age children may seem to understand adults' questions and provide responses that seem to reflect adult-like understanding of concepts. However, adult-like use of language does not necessarily reflect adult-like linguistic or cognitive capabilities (Walker, 1996). Children may use words before they really understand them. For example, the child who reports that "My uncle had sex with me" may not be referring to intercourse and may not be clear on what the word "sex" means. Thus, healthcare providers must clarify statements made by school-age children.

Compared with preschoolers, school-age children have a more developed sense of time. They can use words describing clock and calendar time, as well as duration, in seemingly appropriate ways. However, an adult-like concept of time may not be fully developed until children reach their mid-teens (Walker, 1996). It may be more useful, when questioning a school-age child about when an event occurred, to help the child place the event in relationship to a concrete event in the child's life, such as whether it happened during the school year or summer vacation, before or after Christmas, or in the daytime or nighttime.

School-age children are able to respond to open-ended questions and to provide a narrative account of their experiences, although healthcare providers often need to use focused or close-ended questions to elicit sensitive information from them. Because school-age children can think about the consequences of revealing a history of sexual abuse, they may be more reluctant than preschool-age children to share such information. It is useful, therefore, to attend to a child's nonverbal signals during questioning, particularly when inquiring about abuse. A child's change in behavior, voice level, or emotional expression or attempts to avoid or divert the interviewer when questions about abuse are broached may signal a problem, even if the child does not admit to victimization.

Questioning Adolescents

Developmentally, adolescents have adult-like cognitive and language skills and can accurately relate details of abusive experiences, including when the sexual contact occurred and the circumstances surrounding the abuse. Although they are capable of providing a narrative account of their victimization, they may be reluctant to do so out of shame, concern for the perpetrator, fear or mistrust of the legal system, concern about social embarrassment, or anxiety regarding parental response. A matter-of-fact discussion regarding the risks of sexual activity and the potential health-related benefits of identifying an STD, or providing STD and pregnancy prophylaxis, may encourage the adolescent to provide a truthful admission of sexual contact.

Adolescents may be particularly concerned with issues of privacy and confidentiality and want to know what the healthcare provider will do with the information obtained during the medical encounter. Whereas in many medical situations adolescents have a right to confidentiality when seeking healthcare, notably regarding contraception and pregnancy, such rights cannot be extended to experiences of abuse. The adolescent must understand the purpose of the evaluation and that, in situations in which abuse is suspected, the healthcare provider has a legal obligation to report information to the appropriate child welfare agency.

The general medical history from the adolescent should include menstrual history and use of contraception. Genital complaints, which may be symptomatic of an STD, should be elicited in a detailed review of systems (Frasier, 1997). A report of drug or alcohol abuse, depression, anxiety, eating disorders, self-injury, poor academic achievement, or problematic peer relationships may indicate a need for mental health services.

Questions about an adolescent's sexual abuse should identify the perpetrator and all forms of sexual contact that occurred, when the most recent incident occurred, whether the abuse occurred on more than one occasion, whether associated pain or bleeding occurred, whether and where ejaculation occurred, and whether a condom was used. Assess whether the adolescent understands terms such as ejaculation and condom and provide explanations when needed. In addition to eliciting information about an adolescent's sexual abuse experiences, it is imperative to ask about consensual sexual contacts as well. If a teenager reports having engaged in intercourse with a peer subsequent to having been raped, this will necessarily alter the interpretation of any positive findings from a forensic medical evaluation.

DOCUMENTATION

Although careful documentation is essential for quality patient care, recording observations or statements pertaining to child abuse has forensic significance as well. Healthcare providers' records detailing their questioning and examination of children may provide information that is critical to, and critically scrutinized by, the child protection, law enforcement, and legal systems. Timely, accurate, and comprehensive recording of conversations conducted with children and their caregivers about abuse is essential not only to preserve evidence but also to protect healthcare providers who may be called on to testify in court about their evaluations.

Most states allow medical professionals who have gathered information in the course of diagnosing and treating patients to testify in court about what patients reported to them. This exception to the hearsay rule, commonly referred to as the medical diagnosis and treatment exception, means that statements from children about abuse, when made in the course of diagnosis and treatment, may be admissible in court, whereas statements made to other individuals are considered hearsay and typically are not admissible (Myers, 1992).

The child's medical record should include several elements to increase the likelihood that the information obtained will meet the medical diagnosis and treatment exception to the hearsay rule. Healthcare providers should document, whenever possible, that the child

> ### Table 3-4. Components of Thorough Documentation of History of Child
>
> — Notation that child was informed that the purpose of questioning was for diagnosis and treatment
>
> — Statement that child was told the importance of providing accurate information
>
> — Record of questions used to elicit statements from child about abuse
>
> — Verbatim responses given by child about abuse
>
> — Observation of child's affect and demeanor during interview

was informed that the purpose of questioning was for medical diagnosis and treatment and that the child was told of the importance of providing accurate information. In addition, the information elicited and documented from the medical history of the child should be pertinent to effective diagnosis and treatment (Myers, 1992).

Healthcare professionals should take particular care in recording information obtained during their inquiry about abuse. Documentation should include the question or context that led to a particular response from the child, and statements by the child about abuse should be recorded verbatim (Dubowitz & Bross, 1992). It is important, as well, to record the child's affect and demeanor during questioning because it may be useful in assessing the credibility of the child's history and the child's response to the abuse (Dubowitz & Bross, 1992). **Table 3-4** summarizes information that should be included when documenting interviews with children about abuse. When written in a thorough, objective, and legible manner, using words that are easily understood by nonmedical professionals, the medical record should be useful to investigators, caseworkers, and attorneys and provide them with an accurate record of the child's statements and how they were elicited. A detailed record of such conversations will also be useful should the healthcare provider be called to testify several months or years from the time the information was gathered, when memory about the details of such conversations has long faded. Careful documentation thus has important implications for both the disposition of the child and the credibility and integrity of the healthcare provider.

TAKING ACTION

Once the healthcare provider has obtained information from a child and caregiver and has completed a medical examination of the child, decisions regarding diagnosis, treatment, and follow-up must be made. The American Academy of Pediatrics' Committee on Child Abuse and Neglect has published suggested guidelines to help healthcare providers determine when to report sexual abuse of a child based on a patient's history, physical examination, and laboratory findings (American Academy of Pediatrics, 1999). If, based on the medical history or examination, the healthcare provider has reasonable cause to suspect the child has been abused, the situation must be reported to the state agency mandated to investigate reports of child abuse and neglect. The need for medical or mental health follow-up should also be discussed with the family. Knowledge of community resources, including professionals specializing in the evaluation or treatment of sexually abused children, is necessary for the healthcare provider to provide appropriate guidance and referral.

Recommendations regarding further psychosocial evaluation or counseling may be indicated when information gathered by the healthcare provider is concerning, yet does not warrant a report to CPS. If the history obtained by the healthcare provider raises little or no concern about abuse, this impression should be shared with the family. In such cases, the most appropriate intervention may be for the caregiver and healthcare provider to monitor the situation and to convene again should new or additional concerns arise.

SUMMARY

Healthcare providers are often the gatekeepers to specialized medical, social, and mental health interventions for children and families. Conducting a thorough evaluation of a child when there is concern about abuse may be the critical first step in stopping the child's victimization and connecting the child and his or her caregivers with the services they need to deal effectively with their situation. The healthcare provider is an important link in the safety net created to identify and treat victims of abuse. It is the responsibility of healthcare providers to make sure this link is a strong one.

REFERENCES

American Academy of Pediatrics. Guidelines for the evaluation of sexual abuse of children: subject review. *Pediatrics.* 1999;103:186-191.

American Professional Society on the Abuse of Children. *Guidelines for Use of Anatomical Dolls During Investigative Interviews of Children Who May Have Been Sexually Abused.* Chicago, Ill: APSAC; 1995.

Bickley L, Szilagyi P. *Bates' Guide to Physical Examination & History Taking.* 8th ed. Philadelphia, Pa: Lippincott Williams & Wilkins; 2002.

Coulehan JL, Block MR. *The Medical Interview: Mastering Skills for Clinical Practice.* 4th ed. Philadelphia, Pa: FA Davis Company; 2001.

Dubowitz H, Bross DC. The pediatrician's documentation of child maltreatment. *Am J Dis Child.* 1992;146:596-599.

Dubowitz H, Giardino A, Gustavson E. Child neglect: guidance for pediatricians. *Pediatr Rev.* 2000;21:111-116.

Faller KC. Types of questions for children alleged to have been sexually abused. *APSAC Advisor.* 1990;3:3-5.

Faller KC. *Evaluating Children Suspected of Having Been Sexually Abused.* Thousand Oaks, Calif: Sage Publications; 1996.

Faller KC. Focused questions for interviewing children suspected of maltreatment and other traumatic experiences. *APSAC Advisor.* 1999;12:14-18.

Finkel M. Physical examination. In: Finkel M, Giardino A, eds. *Medical Evaluation of Child Sexual Abuse: A Practical Guide.* 2nd ed. Thousand Oaks, Calif: Sage Publications; 2002:39-98.

Fivush R. Developmental perspectives on autobiographical recall. In: Goodman G, Bottoms B, eds. *Child Victims, Child Witnesses: Understanding and Improving Testimony.* New York, NY: The Guilford Press; 1993:1-24.

Frasier LD. The pediatrician's role in child abuse interviewing. *Pediatr Ann.* 1997;26:306-311.

Freese S. *Child Sexual Abuse: Impact and Aftershocks.* St. Paul, Minn: Project Impact; 1989.

Giardino A, Christian C, Giardino E. Evaluation of abuse and neglect. In: Giardino A, Christian C, Giardino E, eds. *A Practical Guide to the Evaluation of Child Physical Abuse and Neglect.* Thousand Oaks, Calif: Sage Publications; 1997:23-59.

Hewitt S. *Assessing Allegations of Sexual Abuse in Preschool Children*. Thousand Oaks, Calif: Sage Publications; 1999.

Jenny C. Medical issues in sexual abuse. In: Briere J, Berliner L, Bulkley JA, Jenny C, Reid T, eds. *The APSAC Handbook on Child Maltreatment*. Thousand Oaks, Calif: Sage Publications; 1996:195-205.

Kendall-Tackett KA, Williams LM, Finkelhor D. Impact of sexual abuse on children: a review and synthesis of recent empirical studies. *Psychol Bull*. 1993;113:164-180.

Kolilis G, Easter R. The role of law enforcement in the investigation of child maltreatment. In: Monteleone J, Brodeur A, eds. *Child Maltreatment*. 2nd ed. St. Louis, Mo: GW Medical Publishing; 1998:421-433.

Lewis C, Pantell R. Interviewing pediatric patients. In: Lipkin M, Putnam S, Lazare A, eds. *The Medical Interview*. New York, NY: Springer-Verlag; 1995:209-220.

Ludwig S. Child abuse. In: Fleisher G, Ludwig S, eds. *Textbook of Pediatric Emergency Medicine*. 4th ed. Philadelphia, Pa: Lippincott Williams & Wilkins; 2000:1669-1704.

Myers J. *Legal Issues in Child Abuse and Neglect*. Newbury Park, Calif: Sage Publications; 1992.

Reed LD. Findings from research on children's suggestibility and implications for conducting child interviews. *Child Maltreat*. 1996;1:105-120.

Sattler JM. *Clinical and Forensic Interviewing of Children and Families*. San Diego, Calif: Jerome M. Sattler, Publisher; 1998.

Saywitz KJ, Goodman GS. Interviewing children in and out of court: current research and practice implications. In: Briere J, Berliner L, Bulkley JA, Jenny C, Reid T, eds. *The APSAC Handbook on Child Maltreatment*. Thousand Oaks, Calif: Sage Publications; 1996:297-305.

Walker A. *Handbook on Questioning Children*. Chicago, Ill: ABA Center on Children and the Law; 1996.

Chapter 4

The Physical Examination in the Evaluation of Suspected Child Maltreatment: Physical Abuse And Sexual Abuse Examinations

Eileen R. Giardino, PhD, RN, CRNP
Kathleen M. Brown, PhD, RN, CRNP
Angelo P. Giardino, MD, PhD, FAAP

Healthcare professionals play important roles in identifying, referring, and evaluating possible victims of child maltreatment. Physicians and advanced practice nurses are called upon to conduct the healthcare evaluation component of the suspected abuse investigation. The healthcare evaluation for suspected physical or sexual abuse requires a comprehensive history, thorough physical examination, appropriate laboratory and diagnostic studies, and observation of child and caregiver interactions. As the healthcare evaluation proceeds, the clinician initiates treatment for physical injuries or conditions that are uncovered and identified. Some of these conditions that require treatment may have resulted from the maltreatment, and the clinician uses information from the history, physical examination, laboratory/diagnostic assessment, and observation to make a judgment about the likelihood that the given findings were inflicted or abusive in etiology.

The physical examination of children suspected of having been maltreated represents an essential element of the comprehensive healthcare evaluation, as well as an important part of the overall maltreatment investigation. A thorough physical examination permits the healthcare provider to do the following:

— Search for and identify any physical injuries or conditions that require treatment

— Document physical findings at the time of the examination (using notes, drawings, and photographs)

— Obtain laboratory specimens and diagnostic studies where indicated

— Collect and preserve any forensic evidence

— Provide appropriate treatments directed at restoring health when findings or conditions are present

— Reassure child and family of ways to attain or restore health and well-being

Those who conduct the healthcare evaluation of a child suspected of abuse or neglect must be skilled in conducting the physical examination. The information gathered during the physical examination is eventually combined with findings generated during the other components of the healthcare evaluation, namely, the history-taking phase, assessment of laboratory and diagnostic data, and observations of caregiver and child interactions. The clinician then synthesizes all these data into a diagnostic impression. The data and the diagnostic impression become important pieces of information that are used by the broader investigative team as they conduct the overall maltreatment investigation, which occurs when child abuse or neglect is suspected.

This chapter focuses on how to conduct a comprehensive physical examination in the setting of suspected child maltreatment that is child sensitive and as health promoting as possible. The examination process and procedures to evaluate a child suspected of the various forms of maltreatment may be taxing on the child and caregivers. Therefore, the evaluation of a child suspected of having been maltreated requires that a healthcare professional exhibit patience, understanding, kindness, and support during the process of a full physical examination. This chapter is specific for physical examinations done in cases of suspected physical and sexual abuse. The issues surrounding the physical examination for suspected neglect are discussed in detail in Chapter 8, Clinical Aspects of Child Neglect.

GOALS AND FOCUS

The 3 major categories of child maltreatment are physical abuse, sexual abuse, and neglect. Each maltreatment category presents its own unique evaluation-related challenges to the clinician who is called on to determine the extent of the child's injury. The evaluation of a child who potentially has been physically abused tends to focus on the physical injuries present. It occurs in a thorough "head-to-toe" manner, looking for internal and external injuries consistent with the abuse (Jenny, 1996). The physical examination in the setting of suspected physical abuse includes a standard evaluation of each system accessible to the examiner, focusing on identifying any injuries, including those focused on in this chapter, that is, bruises, burns, skeletal trauma, and head trauma.

The goal of the physical examination of the child suspected of having been sexually abused is also done in a complete head-to-toe manner and seeks to determine if there are any physical injuries or forensic findings from the sexual abuse. Forensic findings include the perpetrator's body substances such as semen or saliva, materials such as hair, or clothing that may be used as evidence in the legal setting (Jenny, 1996). The search for forensic evidence during the physical examination often depends on the time period from which the suspected sexual abuse may have last occurred to the child relative to the time of the healthcare evaluation. If the suspected abuse occurred fewer than 72 hours from the time of the physical examination, then the examination may focus on the search for physical findings and the collection of forensic specimens that may still be present on or in the child's body, clothing, or other environmental materials such as linens or upholstery. Finding traces of forensic evidence is less likely when the abuse is suspected or known to have taken place more than 72 hours from the time of the physical examination; thus, the focus in this situation shifts from forensic evidence collection to the identification of possible physical findings.

The findings of the genital examination of children who have been sexually abused are often either normal or nonspecific (Adams, 2001; Adams, Harper, Knudson, & Revilla, 1994; Ludwig, 2000). This lack of physical findings should not be seen as ruling out sexual abuse but as the finding in a given case at the time of the physical examination. The relative paucity of definitive physical findings in cases of sexual abuse has its roots in the types of sexual contact that the perpetrator may have engaged the child in during the abuse, the length of time between the abuse and the disclosure and subsequent presentation to the healthcare setting for evaluation, and the relatively rapid healing observed in the mucous membranes of the child's anogenital tissues. Despite the expectation of few findings, a complete examination is necessary, however, because the child and family may have significant concerns about possible injury and findings that might suggest a nonsexually-related condition may be uncovered. (See Chapter 7, Differential Diagnosis: Conditions That Mimic Child Maltreatment, for discussion of conditions that may mimic child sexual abuse.) The paucity of physical findings in physical examinations done for suspected sexual abuse also reinforces the need for a comprehensive healthcare evaluation that goes beyond the physical examination and forensic evidence collection because a comprehensive evaluation searches for other possible indicators of abuse, such as specific historical information, nonspecific physical complaints, and nonspecific behavioral complaints common in the setting of sexual victimization (Ludwig, 2000).

Child neglect is the most prevalent form of child maltreatment. Signs of neglect manifest to the examiner either clearly, with very specific findings, or over a period in a more insidious manner. The comprehensive evaluation for neglect and specifics regarding the physical examination in cases of suspected neglect are described in more detail in Chapter 8, Clinical Aspects of Child Neglect.

EVALUATION VERSUS INVESTIGATION
The healthcare professional who conducts the physical examination is part of a healthcare team that often plays dual roles in the effort necessary to serve the child suspected of having been physically or sexually maltreated. The first and primary role of the healthcare provider is to evaluate the child's healthcare needs. The healthcare evaluation is well-defined and comprehensive when undertaken in the setting of suspected maltreatment. A complete healthcare evaluation includes a history, physical examination, laboratory assessment, and observations of the caregiver and child that lead to a differential diagnosis and diagnostic impression. The healthcare evaluation is oriented toward assessing the child's health status and then intervening to restore health where necessary with appropriate treatments.

A child maltreatment investigation goes beyond the healthcare evaluation and includes a broader assessment of the child's caregiving environment and the people and situations to whom the child is exposed. Such an investigation may occur as a result of information reported to child protective services (CPS) personnel or law enforcement officers by healthcare providers who suspect maltreatment after having completed an evaluation. Other individuals and mandated reporters, however, may trigger investigations, and these may lead to the request for a healthcare evaluation to search for findings that might indicate maltreatment.

A distinction exists between the healthcare evaluation and the investigation completed by CPS or law enforcement (Finkel, 2002b). The healthcare provider has specialized training in the medical evaluation and is trusted by the child and family. The clinician can help the child and family understand the need to answer difficult questions asked during the history and participate in the physical examination or specimen collection process that may be uncomfortable or embarrassing for the child. The clinician reports findings and information to investigative agencies and cooperates with the investigators. The child and family should see the healthcare provider as someone working with them to identify medical conditions, provide treatment modalities, and address health and wellness issues stemming from the abuse.

The healthcare information from the clinician's evaluation is central to the investigation process but is not the only component of the full investigation. Investigators are individuals from disciplines and agencies mandated by laws and regulations to explore allegations of suspected maltreatment. For example, law enforcement officers are an important component of the full investigative team. Law enforcement officers determine whether or not a crime has been committed and begin appropriate legal action toward holding the abuser responsible for his or her actions. CPS agencies and CPS workers, often social workers, ideally operate hand in hand with law enforcement agencies and police officers to protect children. CPS plays an important role in the investigation of child abuse, focusing on the families' functioning and ability to protect the child. CPS agencies provide necessary social support services to families in need and may ultimately need to remove children from caregiving environments determined to be unsafe.

The healthcare provider, in addition to conducting the healthcare evaluation, is viewed as one with unique skills directed at collecting and preserving forensic evidence key to the investigation of alleged child abuse. Here, the clinician participates with law enforcement, social services/CPS, and the courts to obtain evidence for the forensic investigative team.

Healthcare providers interact with other members of the investigation team as they share information from the healthcare evaluation. Other investigation team members include prosecutors, who are responsible for pursuing the court-related process that holds offenders accountable for illegal activities. Prosecutors seek evidence to support the prosecution of an alleged perpetrator, as well as clinician-generated information concerning findings of the medical evaluation that support the diagnosis of child maltreatment. The healthcare provider can also refer children evaluated for suspected child maltreatment to victim service agencies whose purpose is to provide counseling and support services for victims of any crime, depending on available services in a given community. Victim agencies often house trained forensic interviewers, counselors, and specialists who provide support to the child and family. Various disciplines come together to make the whole experience better for the child. They work together to help the child prepare for testifying in court and provide support persons to accompany the child to court.

THE PHYSICAL EXAMINATION IN CHILD MALTREATMENT EVALUATIONS

The evaluation and investigation of suspected child maltreatment is ideally undertaken as a multidisciplinary process (Giardino & Giardino, 2003). The findings from the physical examination of a child suspected of having been maltreated are important to the healthcare evaluation and the investigation of suspected abuse. The clinician must develop a comfort level with the potentially varying perspectives held by different team members about the information uncovered during physical examination.

The healthcare perspective is typically focused on supporting the child and caregivers, reassuring all involved, and restoring the health of the child, whereas the forensic perspective focuses on preserving and documenting evidence that will withstand court scrutiny. These perspectives require training and experience to understand the utility of each and how team members can work together to ensure that both the evaluation and investigation proceed in a way that will best serve each team members' focus and needs.

It is important that the healthcare provider know which of the team members to consult for assistance before, during, and after the physical examination when there are medical or forensic concerns related to the evaluation. The healthcare team members may provide consultations regarding medical and nursing concerns, while forensic concerns, such as photography and preservation of evidence, are best addressed by the more forensically oriented team members.

Clinical judgment and diagnosis in genital examinations for child sexual abuse can have far-reaching consequences. These include what can happen to those suspected or accused of the crime if incorrect findings and conclusions are reached (Kirschner & Stein, 1985). Also, examiners should understand that a normal examination or one without findings is common in children who have been sexually abused, so a normal examination does not rule out the possibility of sexual abuse (Adams, 2001; Adams et al., 1994; Hornor & McCleery, 2000).

PROFESSIONAL KNOWLEDGE ABOUT CHILD ABUSE EXAMINATIONS

Examining a child who has been physically or sexually abused is a science and an art. The science involves the theory and details related to what to examine and what the findings may signify. The art of completing an examination is learned through experience. The art of the examination is important because it helps the examiner gain cooperation from the child who may be hesitant and view the examination as threatening. It is a challenge to gain the cooperation and trust of the child, so that a complete examination can be performed without retraumatizing the child (Finkel & DeJong, 2001).

A healthcare evaluation of a child suspected of maltreatment necessarily includes a complete physical examination, in which each body system and structure is examined in a standard manner. In cases of physical abuse, special attention should be given to areas of suspected injury, such as the anogenital area. Routine pediatric visits should include an external genital evaluation and documentation of developmental staging of the breasts and genitalia using the Tanner stages; the evaluation of child sexual abuse requires this, as well as a more detailed external inspection of the genital and anal areas (Botash, 1997).

Clinician inspection of the anogenital area of prepubertal children, despite recommendations that it be routine, is not always part of the assessment for general medical problems (Balk, Dreyfus, & Harris, 1982). Therefore, primary care providers may not be skilled in identifying the specific structures that comprise the external genital examination of prepubertal children (Hornor & McCleery, 2000; Ladson, Johnson, & Doty, 1987; Lentsch & Johnson, 2000).

The physical examination of a child suspected of having been sexually abused is a unique situation owing to the specific techniques for examining the child and collecting forensic evidence. Because the examination has forensic implications, practitioners who perform these examinations must have additional training in examining the genitalia and collecting forensic evidence. The techniques for the prepubertal anogenital examination are described later in this chapter. The evidence collection techniques are described in Chapter 5, Laboratory Findings, Diagnostic Testing, and Forensic Specimens in Cases of Child Sexual Abuse.

The following sections describe general approaches to the physical examination of a child for suspected physical or sexual abuse. The specifics for the physical examination for suspected physical abuse are provided first and focus on bruises, burns, skeletal trauma, and head injury. Then, the specifics for the physical examination for suspected sexual abuse are provided. After some general information that is common to both situations, the specifics around physical and sexual abuse examination techniques are presented separately because there are unique approaches to each.

GENERAL ISSUES

STRESS AND DISTRESS REGARDING THE EVALUATION

The healthcare setting in general can be a source of stress for children, who may fear painful procedures and feel uncomfortable in the technical, adult-oriented environment (Elliott, Jay, & Woody, 1987). In cases of physical abuse, the child may be concerned and distressed about having painful injuries examined and manipulated. In child sexual abuse evaluations, the embarrassing nature of the abuse may be stressful on top of the child's anticipation of having a genital examination (Britton, 1998; Gully, Britton, Hansen, Goodwill, & Nope, 1999; Lynch & Faust, 1998).

Healthcare providers have learned a great deal about how to help children cope with the stress they may feel regarding visiting the healthcare setting. Studies determining the degree of a child's fear and feelings of distress toward medical procedures have opened the possibility of enhancing the child's coping strategies in this area (Dubowitz, 1998; Elliott et al., 1987). Efforts to decrease the child's anxiety include establishing familiarity with the setting and communicating in a child-friendly way about what to expect of the process. In considering the stress connected with a physical examination for suspected child maltreatment, the examiner should consider the following:

— The child has an injury that he or she knows will need to be examined

— The child's age and developmental level

— Previous interactions with the healthcare system

— The circumstances of the alleged maltreatment

— The child's potential concern about his or her own future safety

— The potential for further inflicted injury

— The ability and availability of a nonabusing caregiver to lend comfort and support

Strategies the examiner can use to assist the child in coping with what can be a stressful healthcare interaction include the following:

— Providing a calm and unhurried approach to the history and examination (De San Lazaro, 1995)

— Allowing the child to participate in the process as much as possible

— Talking about nonintrusive subjects with the child when possible (ask about likes and dislikes) (De San Lazaro, 1995)

— During the history from the adult who has accompanied the child, providing the child distance from the process by encouraging play in another part of the room

— Offering the child choices during the physical examination, such as what robe to wear, what position to use, what ear to first examine, and what instrument to choose first

— Distracting the child during the examination with conversation about topics of interest

— Using words that are less threatening to the child, for example, a little bump or scratch versus tears or scarring

INSPECTION OF CHILD'S GENERAL APPEARANCE

The first step in the physical examination for physical and sexual abuse is inspection of the overall appearance of the child. This is an important step that must not be overlooked. Points to consider include attention to findings that reflect the child's general well-being and findings that suggest how well the child is cared for. The examiner looks for signs indicative of caregiving that meet or fail to meet the child's basic needs and observes the child's overall appearance, especially signs of starvation, muscle wasting, or loss of weight. In short, the clinician determines if the child appears well kept or is dirty and inappropriately dressed for the climate or environmental conditions.

The overall appearance of the child tells the examiner something about the general treatment of the child. Caregiving that does not adequately deal with the child's physical condition and health needs can be a serious form of maltreatment referred to as neglect. Often the legal community only considers neglect when actual harm occurs. However, healthcare professionals and other team members often expand the definition of neglect to include the potential for harm and make every effort to refer appropriately to meet the needs of the neglected child. (See Chapter 14, Legal Issues, for further discussion.)

Specifics to look for regarding aspects of neglectful caregiving include the following:

—What is the child's height and weight?

—Are head and body circumferences age appropriate?

—Is there evidence of nutrition deficiencies? Are there subcutaneous fat deposits?

—Does the child have a diaper rash? If so, how severe is it?

—Are there any signs of skin infection?

—Are there any scars?

—Are there any insect bites?

—Does the examiner note any evidence of neglect?

—Does the child look well nourished? Clean?

—Is the clothing adequate and clean?

SPECIFIC ISSUES RELATED TO THE EXAMINATION FOR SUSPECTED PHYSICAL ABUSE

ACCIDENTAL VERSUS INFLICTED INJURY

The examiner looks for signs that indicate whether the injuries seen on physical examination appear to be accidental or inflicted on the child. Cues that help the examiner differentiate between the 2 situations are as follows:

— Location of the injury

— Prominent areas of the child's body such as forehead and shins are generally injured in accidental injuries.

— It is highly suspicious of abuse when injury is noted to padded areas such as the buttocks and relatively well-protected areas such as neck, trunk, and genitalia.

— Caregiver history and its consistency to what is observed on examination

— In cases of physical abuse, it is important to pay close attention to the caregiver's history of injuries or abuse.

— Discrepant history reported by caregivers is a key to differentiating between inflicted and accidental injury (Sirotnak & Krugman, 1994). The examiner should try to envision whether or not the injury could have occurred in a given location from the events described.

— The following are questions for the examiner to consider in formulating the diagnostic impression:

1. Is the injury location consistent with the given history of events?

2. Are injuries consistent or inconsistent with the developmental level of the child?

3. Is it developmentally possible for the child to have performed the task described and thus become injured?

— Appearance and characteristics of the injury

— Certain characteristics of injuries make them more suspicious for inflicted injuries when they are present, for example, when the child's examination or review of the medical record suggests that there have been repetitive or cumulative injuries over time.

— The appearance of the injury pattern may also raise suspicion for physical abuse, for example, cigarette burns, belt marks, and bite marks.

— Another concerning situation that should raise the suspicion for physical abuse is one in which the examination reveals a severe central nervous system injury that proves to be inconsistent with the history provided.

— The presence of defensive injuries on the arms should also raise the concern for physical abuse. These are seen in situations in which a child raises his or her arms to protect from blows.

The following are situations that should raise suspicion about physical abuse and require a complete healthcare evaluation and probably a complete investigation (Cheung, 1999):

— No reasonable explanation of injury, sometimes called the "magical injury," for which the caregiver can provide no history to how the injury occurred

— History given for injury changes over time

— History appears vague

— Injury observed is not congruent with history given

— Injury observed is incompatible with the child's developmental stage and abilities

— Caregiver appears to have an inappropriate lack of concern in the situation of a child with a severe injury

— Untimely delay in seeking medical attention for what a reasonable caregiver would have sought prompt attention

SKIN INJURIES

The skin is the largest organ in the body and the one most commonly injured in cases of physical abuse (Sirotnak & Krugman, 1994). The physical examination of a child suspected of being abused involves the careful search for findings suggestive of inflicted injury to the skin. The examiner carefully inspects the child's skin from

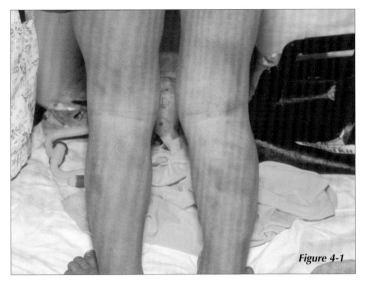

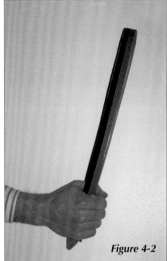

Figure 4-1

Figure 4-2

head to toe, looking for injuries requiring treatment and injuries supportive of the diagnosis of inflicted injury. The skin injuries discussed below are bruises and burns.

Bruising

A bruise injury generally results from blunt force trauma to the skin that disrupts capillaries (Richardson, 1994), with subcutaneous blood then flowing from disrupted capillaries below the intact skin. Relatively deep bruises may not appear for hours or days. Bruise injuries can develop on body areas where a child was struck or in areas where the child was held down or restrained (**Figures 4-1 to 4-6**).

Physical Examination of Bruises

Assessment of skin injuries includes examining all areas of the body where injuries are expected, such as bony prominences of the forehead, chin, and shins, as well as the atypical areas for bruises, such as the trunk, bottoms of the feet, and inside of the mouth. It is important for the validity of the investigation to carefully document the location and description of each injury. The examiner should document each identified injury in the medical record, noting the size, specific location (refer to anatomical landmarks), and appearance. The examiner notes whether the injury appears to be acute, in a healing phase, or totally healed. Ideally, each injury should be described in written form, with a hand-drawn diagram and a

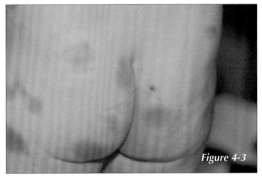

Figure 4-3

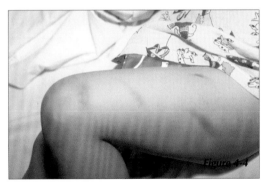

Figure 4-4

Figure 4-1. *Bruises inflicted with a belt. (Contributed by Lawrence R. Ricci, MD; Portland, Me.)*

Figure 4-2. *Belt used on child in Figure 4-1. (Contributed by Lawrence R. Ricci, MD; Portland, Me.)*

Figure 4-3. *Bruises inflicted with a wooden spoon. (Contributed by Lawrence R. Ricci, MD; Portland, Me.)*

Figure 4-4. *Bruises inflicted with a switch. (Contributed by Lawrence R. Ricci, MD; Portland, Me.)*

photograph. (See Chapter 9, Documentation of the Evaluation in Cases of Suspected Child Maltreatment, for details about documentation of findings.) See **Table 4-1** for a standard form that can useful in documenting the examination findings.

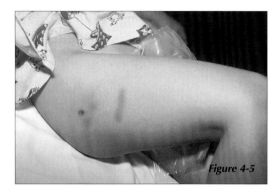

Figure 4-5

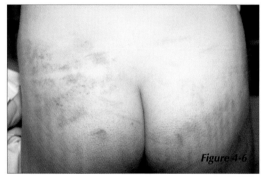

Figure 4-6

Figure 4-5.
Same child as Figure 4-4. (Contributed by Lawrence R. Ricci, MD; Portland, Me.)

Figure 4-6.
Bruises inflicted with a belt. (Contributed by Lawrence R. Ricci, MD; Portland, Me.)

Patterned Injuries

Injuries that have geometric shapes are particularly concerning and are called patterned injuries. Patterned injuries resemble the object used to physically injure the child. (See Chapter 2, Figure 2-3.) Patterned marks may be obvious or subtle in appearance. Such injuries are usually inflicted and indicate that the child was hit with something that created an impression of the object used (Richardson, 1994). Objects such as belt buckles, coiled rope, finger outlines, fists, shoes, switches, and coat hangers may form geometric patterns (Kornberg, 1992). The forensically oriented team members may be best able to assist the examiner in differentiating inflicted patterned injuries from accidental injuries. Law enforcement officials will investigate the crime scene and may be able to retrieve the exact object used to inflict injury.

Grab or pinch marks are often indicators for inflicted skin injury. Bruising in the shape of an outline of fingers or grasp marks indicates forceful holding of the child until bruising occurred. The outline of the perpetrator's fingers appears on the child's skin at the point of holding, appearing as linear bruises surrounding a clear center (Kessler & Hyden, 1991). The mechanism of injury is that during the violent holding the circulation in the child's skin is forced beyond the area where the force is applied, creating a bruise around it. Other objects can create a similar pattern, as seen when they are used to administer forceful blows (**Figures 4-7 to 4-9**).

Table 4-1. Documentation of Each Bruise

— Size of bruise

— Location (on what body part[s])

— Shape (object used)

— Color of injured area (see "Dating of Bruise Injuries" section)

— Characteristics and pattern of bruise(s)

    — Is bruise centrally located or in a protected area?

    — Do multiple bruises have different colors or different ages?

    — Is there a consistency of bruise pattern with history given?

    — Does the pattern indicate a specific mechanism of infliction?

    — Number of body surfaces injured—single or multiple episodes of trauma

— Other considerations of injury

    — Examine for other signs of organ or bone injury

    — Signs of physical neglect

Table 4-2. Progression of Bruising

BRUISES BEGIN AS REDDISH DISCOLORATIONS THAT CHANGE IN COLOR DURING THE HEALING PROCESS

Approximate age of bruise	Color range
Fresh injury	Red coloration
First day or two	Red, swollen, tender
1-5 days	Red, purple
5-7 days	Green
7-10 days	Yellow
10 or more days	Brown
14-28 days	Gone

Adapted from Farley RH, Reece RM. Recognizing When a Child's Injury or Illness is Caused by Abuse. *Portable Guides to Investigating Child Abuse. Washington, DC: US Dept of Justice; 1996. NCJ160938; Wilson E. Estimation of the age of cutaneous contusions in child abuse.* Pediatrics. *1977;60:750-752.*

Dating of Bruise Injuries

The dating of bruises based on the progression of color in the skin has received a great deal of attention over the past several decades (Schwartz & Ricci, 1996; Wilson, 1977). Bruise dating is not an exact science, and the clinician must be careful to speak in typical age ranges for various bruises rather than pronounce the specific age for a given bruise. The examiner can evaluate the potential age range of a bruise by the color of the healing bruise and document whether the given time frame between the suspected time of injury and the date of the examination is consistent or inconsistent with the estimated age. Rather than stating the exact age of a bruise injury, it is best to document that a bruise *is consistent with a given estimated age range* (Schwartz & Ricci, 1996; Wilson, 1977) because the exact age can rarely be determined.

Within the examination of the same child, it is reasonable to compare bruises that seem newer or older than other ones based on color characteristics. However, it is not accurate to compare the color of one child's bruise to the same color of a bruise in another child and say that the age of both bruises is the same. Serial or follow-up examinations for bruises are suggested so that the progression of the healing process can be documented in cases of suspected physical abuse. (See **Table 4-2** for color progression of bruises with age ranges.)

Related Injuries

Other types of skin injuries that should be looked for during the physical examination include bite marks and traumatic alopecia. A bite mark, especially a full bite mark, can help characterize the identity of the perpetrator because of its size and other dental characteristics (Mouden, 1998). This is an area where the forensically oriented members of the team can assist in documentation and evidence preservation.

Traumatic alopecia occurs when hair is pulled out of the child's head. During the physical examination the scalp should be inspected for findings indicating the loss of hair or trauma to the scalp (Monteleone & Brodeur, 1998).

Although uncommon, extragenital injury may be seen in victims of child sexual abuse. Such injury may manifest as contusions, erythema, tearing, bite marks, scratch marks, and finger pressure marks in other areas of the body, as well as the genitalia **(Figure 4-10)**.

Burns
Pathophysiology

The skin is an organ designed to function within appropriate temperatures. Extreme temperatures that come into contact with the skin cause burn injuries that produce a spectrum of injury to the affected cells. Permanent damage occurs when there is a total denaturation of proteins and enzymes and a resultant inability of cellular mechanisms to function (Robson & Heggers, 1988). The 3 layers of skin can be affected in varying degrees, depending on the temperature of the causative substance and the amount of time that the causative agent comes into contact with the skin.

After heat is applied to the skin, there are concentric zones of thermal injury. The area in most direct contact with the heat source is called the zone of coagulation and sustains irreparable damage. Outward from this is the zone of stasis, which retains some ability for repair. The most outward area is the zone of hyperemia, which has the greatest potential for repair and healing (Robson & Heggers, 1988) **(Figure 4-11)**.

There are 4 categories of burns classified according to the depth of the injury. The terms ***superficial, partial thickness*** and ***full thickness*** are used in conjunction with the 4 classifications. First-degree burns are limited to the epidermis layer. The epidermis consists of an outer layer of anucleated cornified cells, which is the stratum corneum, and an inner layer of cells that mature and differentiate into cornified

Figure 4-7.
*Handprint on leg.
(Contributed by
Lawrence R. Ricci,
MD; Portland, Me.)*

Figure 4-8.
*Handprint on face.
(Contributed by
Lawrence R. Ricci,
MD; Portland, Me.)*

Figure 4-9.
*Slap mark.
(Contributed by
Lawrence R. Ricci,
MD; Portland, Me.)*

Figure 4-10.
*Fingernail scratch.
(Contributed by
Lawrence R. Ricci,
MD; Portland, Me.)*

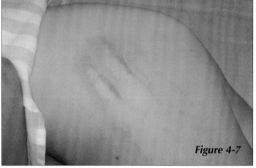

Figure 4-7

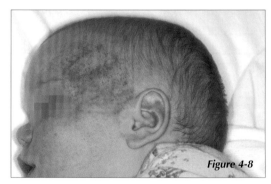

Figure 4-8

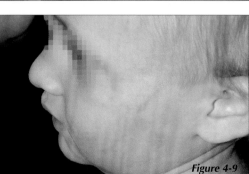

Figure 4-9

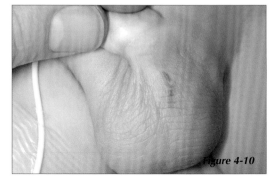

Figure 4-10

cells of the stratum corneum. The stratum corneum acts as a barrier to the entrance of microorganisms and the loss of water and electrolytes. Although painful, the superficial burn is self-limiting and rarely leads to scarring. Within a few days, the injured skin sloughs and heals as the healthy cells regenerate from the underlying skin cells. Treatment usually involves local wound care.

The second-degree burn involves injury that extends into the dermis but with some viable dermis remaining. The dermis is composed of a dense fibroelastic

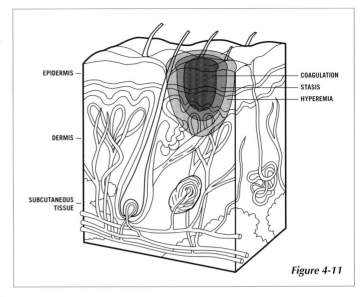

Figure 4-11

connective tissue that contains collagen, elastic fibers, and an extracellular gel, the ground substance. It has an extensive nerve and vascular network, which includes glands and appendages that communicate with the epidermis. Second-degree burns are also referred to as partial-thickness or deep partial-thickness burns. There is usually blistering of the skin, vessel disruption, and a resultant beefy red appearance of the affected area (Giardino, Christian, & Giardino, 1997a). Nerve endings are exposed, causing greater pain and discomfort during the injury and healing process. Partial-thickness burns heal in approximately 2 weeks, whereas deep partial-thickness injury may take 3 to 4 weeks (Giardino, Christian, & Giardino, 1997b).

Full-thickness burns involve destruction of the entire epidermis and dermis to the subcutaneous tissue (third degree), or the muscle, fascia, and bone (fourth degree). Fourth-degree burns are often associated with lethal injury. Full-thickness burns completely destroy blood vessels and nerve endings; they appear white because of the exposure of subcutaneous tissue. Healing occurs through means of surgical grafting or by inward growth of skin from tissues surrounding the skin.

Figure 4-11.
Diagram showing the 3 layers of skin with concentric zones of thermal injury. Adapted from Robson M, Heggers J. Pathophysiology of the burn wound. In: Carvajal H, Parks D, eds. Burns in Children: Pediatric Burn Management. St Louis, Mo: Mosby; 1988:27-32.

Relationship of History to Physical Examination of Burns

The history related to the cause of and circumstances surrounding the burn is an important part of the overall evaluation. The responses of the child (if possible) and the caregiver are carefully noted because they help to determine whether the injury was accidental or inflicted. All answers are carefully documented in the medical record. The following questions should be addressed in the history (Giardino et al., 1997a):

— How did the burn occur?

— How did the child come into contact with the burning agent?

— For how long was the burning agent in contact with the child?

— Was the skin covered with clothes or uncovered?

— Who was supervising the child?

— In what time frame was the child taken for medical care?

— If there was any delay in seeking treatment, what is the reason for the delay?

— Who brought the child to medical care?

— Did anyone other than the child witness the burn incident?

— What was the child's immediate response to the burn situation (e.g., cry, run)?

— Is the burn attributed to the actions of anyone else (sibling, playmate, child himself, adult)?

Some points to consider when evaluating burn injuries are as follows:

— What is the time of occurrence, nature, extent, and location of the burn?

— Does the burn pattern correlate with the history of the accident?

— Is the history from the caregiver plausible or implausible?

— When more than one family member is involved and questioned separately, are their stories consistent with each other and with what is seen?

— Is the history consistent with what the examiner hears from the child?

— Is the child's developmental level consistent with the actions described that precipitated the burn injury?

— Does the child have any medical conditions that mimic burning?

— Are there any other signs of abuse?

Physical Examination of Burns

The physical examination may also reveal certain burn patterns that raise a question about the possibility of inflicted injury. In cases of nonaccidental burns, the family is questioned about the cause of the burn, and in cases of inflicted injury, their answers may suggest implausible explanations. The physical examination may give clues that the history given by the caregiver or the mechanism of injury may be implausible given the developmental level of the child, as well as the depth and distribution of the burn (Hansbrough & Hansbrough, 1999).

The examiner should note all aspects of a burn injury, including:

— Location

— Size

— Appearance/severity (first-, second-, or third-degree; percentage of body surface) **(Figure 4-12)**

— Shape of the burn injury

Table 4-3 is a guideline to the physical examination of a burn injury.

Characteristics of the Burn: Accidental Versus Inflicted

The shape of the burn is important because the pattern may indicate the object used, such as an iron, radiator, or cigarette lighter **(Figure 4-13)**. Burns by forced immersion can cause sharply demarcated, circular-type injuries to the upper (glove) and lower (stocking) extremities. In forced immersion burns, characteristic patterns involving the buttocks and genitalia may result. If a child falls into a tub, the examiner would expect to find an irregular burn pattern with burns on the skin areas hit by the hot liquid. Sharp lines of demarcation would typically be absent because the child would splash around in the struggle to escape from the hot liquid. However, when held in the hot liquid, a child forcefully immersed in a sitting position with knees bent up may manifest burns on the buttocks and the legs, with sparing of the skin on the knees, hands, and arms.

An unusual pattern occurs when the child is forcefully held against the wall of a container holding the hot liquid (such as a bathtub). The central part of the child's buttock area may appear to have a milder burn than the more peripheral aspects because the solid material may be relatively cooler than the hot liquid it contains. Therefore, the point of contact where the skin touched the tub may be less burned or affected than the skin surface that was in contact with the hot liquid. This hole-in-doughnut–sparing pattern is highly associated with such a forced immersion burn (Scalzo, 1998).

Most accidental burns are related to splash or spill injuries. Splash and spill burns can either be inflicted or accidental, and there is overlap in the physical findings between the 2 mechanisms of action. The severity of the burn is related to the temperature of the burning agent, time of heat in contact with the skin, and thickness of the skin where the burn occurred. Clothing tends to keep the hot agent in contact with the skin for a longer time and, therefore, causes a more severe burn.

Accidental scalds occur in situations in which the child reaches for a container that holds hot liquid and the liquid then pours down onto the child. For example, a child who pulls down a cup of hot coffee onto himself from a table would manifest a burn pattern consistent with hot liquid falling onto the body from above. Splash marks may also appear in body areas separate from the most severe burn areas **(Figure 4-14)**.

In an inflicted burn, the perpetrator may pour a fluid onto the child or throw a liquid at a child. The history given by the caregiver is important because the story of what happened should be evaluated in relation to the pattern of the injury **(Table 4-4)**. For example, a burn on the back may indicate that liquid was thrown onto a child.

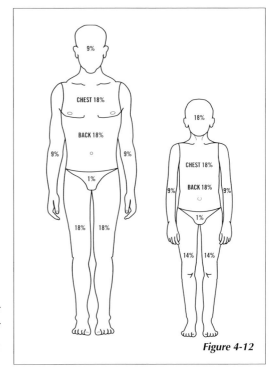

Figure 4-12

Figure 4-12. A "Rule of Nines" chart used to determine the total body surface area (TBSA) of an adult or child that has been burned. Adapted from Burn Survivor Resource Center. Medical care guide: types of burns. Available at: http://www.burnsurvivor.com/burn_types.html. Accessed March 16, 2003; Center for Pediatric Emergency Medicine. Rule of nines. Available at: http://www.cpem.org/gif/17b.gif. Accessed March 16, 2003; Scherer JC. Introductory Medical-Surgical Nursing. 4th ed. Philadelphia, Pa: Lippincott; 1986:687.

Figure 4-13.
Inflicted burn from cigarette lighter. (Contributed by Lawrence R. Ricci, MD; Portland, Me.)

Figure 4-14.
Accidental spill burn pattern.

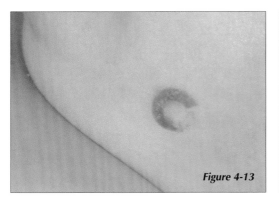

Figure 4-13

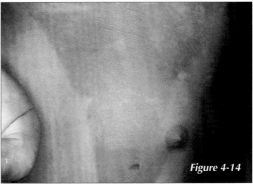

Figure 4-14

Table 4-3. Burn Examination Guidelines

DESCRIPTION OF THE BURN(S)

— Type and degree of burn(s): superficial, partial thickness (superficial or deep), full thickness

— Amount of body surface area (BSA) involved (see **Figure 4-12** for estimates for pediatric patient)

CHARACTERISTICS AND PATTERN OF BURN(S)

— Apparent age of burn (Does it appear older than given in history?)

— Consistency of burn distribution with history provided

     — Burn incompatible with described events in history

— Note signs of restraint

     — Signs of immersion in hot fluid

         — Stocking and glove demarcation on extremities

         — Sparing of flexure areas

     — Splash marks or lack of them

     — Hole-in-doughnut pattern

IDENTIFICATION OF OTHER SIGNS OF INFLICTED INJURY

— Presence of other injuries

     — Bruises, fractures, burns of differing ages

— Maltreatment evidence

     — Scars, malnourishment

— Restraint-related injuries

     — Multiple bruises resembling fingers and hands on upper extremities

---

Table 4-4. Distinguishing Accidental From Nonaccidental Burns

INDICATIONS THAT BURNS MAY NOT HAVE BEEN ACCIDENTAL

History	— The burns are attributed to siblings.
	— An unrelated adult brings the child in for medical care.
	— Accounts of the injury differ.
	— Treatment is delayed for more than 24 hours.
	— There is evidence of prior "accidents" or an absence of parental concern.
	— The lesions are incompatible with the history.

(continued)

Table 4-4. *(continued)*	
Location	— The burns are more likely to be found on the buttocks, in the anogenital region (the area between the legs, encompassing the genitals and anus), and on the ankles, wrists, palms, and soles.
Pattern	— The burns have sharply defined edges. For example, in immersion burns, the line of immersion gives the appearance of a glove or stocking on the child's hand or foot.
	— The burns are full thickness (all of the skin, and possibly muscle and bone as well, is destroyed).
	— The burns are symmetrical.
	— The burns are older than the reported history indicates.
	— The burns have been neglected or are infected.
	— There are numerous lesions of various ages.
	— The burn patterns conform to the shape of the implement used.
	— The degree of the burns is uniform (usually indicating forced contact with a hot, dry object), and they cover a large area.

INDICATIONS THAT BURNS ARE MORE LIKELY TO BE ACCIDENTAL

History	— The history of the mechanism of the burns is compatible with the observed injury.
Location	— The burns are usually found on the front of the body. They occur in locations reflecting the child's motor activity, level of development, and the exposure of the child's body to the burning agent.
Pattern	— The burns are of multiple depths interspersed with unburned areas and are usually less severe (such as splash burns).
	— The burns are of partial thickness; that is, only part of the skin has been damaged or destroyed.
	— The burns are asymmetrical.
	— Apparently only one traumatic event has occurred because the skin injuries are all of the same age.

Reprinted from Farley RH, Reece RM. Recognizing When a Child's Injury or Illness Is Caused by Abuse: Portable Guides to Investigating Child Abuse. *Washington, DC: US Dept of Justice; 1996. NCJ160938.*

Table 4-5. Classifications of Fractures

FRACTURE CLASSIFICATIONS

Fracture	Characteristics
Simple (closed fracture)	Surface of skin intact and not ruptured; bone broken in one place
Compound (open)	Fracture ruptures skin, exposing bone and causing soft tissue injury and possible infection
Greenstick (incomplete)	Bone is partly broken and partly bent; fracture occurs partly across a bone shaft, often resulting from bending or crushing mechanisms on the bone
Complete	Break is completely through the bone

CLASSIFICATION BY FRACTURE LINE

Fracture	Characteristics
Hairline	Fracture appears as a narrow crack along surface of a bone
Linear	Fracture runs parallel to the bone's axis or direction of the bone's shaft
Oblique	Angled fracture crosses bone at approximately a 45-degree angle to the bone's axis
Transverse	Fracture at a right angle to the bone's axis, at a 90-degree angle
Stellate	Fracture lines radiate from a central point
Spiral	Oblique fracture line encircles a portion of bone, crosses the bone at an oblique angle, creating a spiral pattern

CLASSIFICATION BY POSITION OF BONY FRAGMENTS

Fracture	Characteristics
Comminuted	More than one fracture line and more than 2 bone fragments; usually produced by high forces or by normal forces in a very fragile bone
Nondisplaced	Fragments of bone maintain their normal alignment after fracture
Impacted	Compression fracture, involves entire bone
Overriding	Bony fragments overlap and shorten the total length of the bone
Angulated	Fragments result in pieces of bone being at angles to each other
Displaced	Bony fragment occurs from disruption of normal bone alignment; deformity of segments separate from one another

(continued)

Table 4-5. *(continued)*

Fracture	Characteristics
Avulsed	Bone fragments pulled from normal position by forceful muscle contractions or resistance from ligaments
Segmental	Segmental alignment occurs when fractures in 2 adjacent areas happen with an isolated central segment, for example, when arm bone fractures in 2 separate places with displacement of the mid section of bone
Torus (buckle)	Impact injury specific to children; bone buckles, usually at or near the metaphysis
Depressed	Skull fracture with inward displacement of a part of the roof of the skull
Diastatic	Significant separation of bone fragments

OTHER CLASSIFICATIONS

Fracture	Characteristics
Distal	Fracture located away from center of body, usually in hands or feet
Occult	Clinical but not radiographic evidence of fracture; may also indicate a fracture seen radiographically but without manifestations of actual fracture
Pathological	Fracture occurs in area of disease-weakened bone
Proximal	Fracture located more near trunk or center of body
Supracondylar	Fracture area is above condyle, is typically of the humerus

SKELETAL INJURIES

Skeletal injury is a common indicator of child abuse because fractures are found in approximately 30% of physically abused children (Berkowitz, 1995; Kleinman, Marks, Richmond, & Blackbourne, 1995). The frequency of fractures associated with physical abuse varies from as low as 11% to as high as 55% (Kleinman et al., 1995). Physical findings in living victims of child abuse commonly include injury to the skin and bones. Fractures are the second most common manifestation of physical abuse after skin problems (Kocher & Kasser, 2000).

Fractures usually result from traumatic injury to bone, which causes the continuity of bone tissues or bony cartilage to be disrupted or broken **(Table 4-5)**. The frequency, type, location, and healing of pediatric fractures are related to the anatomical and physiological characteristics of the immature skeleton (Kleinman & Marks, 1998). The developing bones of children, which are more porous than mature bones, are a factor that affects the types of fractures that occur in children.

Relevant History

Every child suspected of physical abuse must be evaluated for bone fractures because a child may have specific signs and symptoms or none at all. The history of a child who comes for treatment of skeletal trauma should include the following details (Sirotnak & Krugman, 1994):

— Developmental stage of the child

— Supervision given by caregivers

— Child's behavior that signaled pain

— Prior history of injuries or fractures

— In cases of falls, questions regarding the height from which the child fell

— Contact surface

— Witnesses to the event

— Description of possible injury mechanisms, such as twisting, compression, traction

Patterns of Fractures in Abuse

Although no pathognomonic fracture pattern in abuse occurs, it is important to consider the child's age, stated mechanism of injury, overall injury pattern, and pertinent psychosocial factors (Kocher & Kasser, 2000). Age is an important risk factor for fractures because most fractures related to abuse are found in infants younger than age 1 year. Fractures can occur from blunt force or torsion injury (Sirotnak & Krugman, 1994). Extremities are fractured most commonly in child abuse cases, and occult fractures are also a possibility (Belfer, Klein, & Orr, 2002). Whenever skeletal injury is present, there also may be associated head and visceral trauma.

Abuse-related fractures have a variety of presentations. Therefore, the identification of an inflicted fracture depends on compiling information from a variety of factors. Relevant data include the history and description of the situation that caused the fracture, background knowledge of fracture mechanisms in children, the child's development, and physical findings of the examination. Lung or visceral damage from broken ribs may manifest as chest deformity or costochondral tenderness (Sirotnak & Krugman, 1994).

Figure 4-15.
Model for Figure 4-16. (Contributed by Lawrence R. Ricci, MD; Portland, Me.)

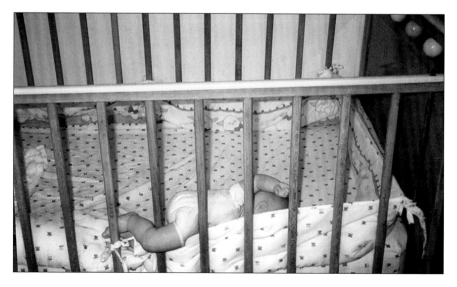

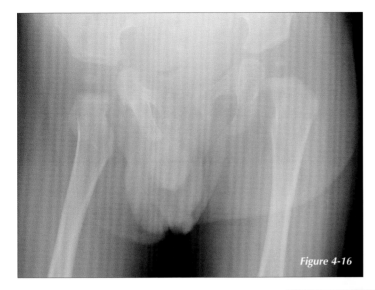

Figure 4-16

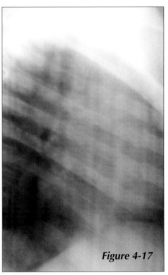

Figure 4-17

The location of a fracture may be a clue in diagnosing child abuse. Common accidental fractures that occur in the active child are often the result of falls (Berkowitz, 1995). Skeletal injury patterns that suggest inflicted injury include certain types of metaphyseal lesions in young children, multiple fractures in various stages of healing, posterior rib fractures, and long-bone fractures in children younger than 2 years of age (Kocher & Kasser, 2000) **(Figures 4-15 to 4-20)**. For example, a fractured clavicle is a common noninflicted injury,

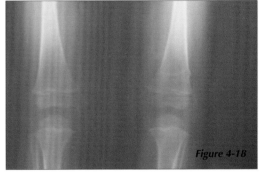

Figure 4-18

whereas fractures of the femur or ribs in a young child increase the suspicion for child abuse. Certain fractures such as rib and metaphyseal fractures in infants are so suspicious that they raise concern for abuse in the absence of a significant history. Fractures of the distal femur are a strong indicator of infant abuse and should be carefully evaluated with high-detail skeletal radiographs in all cases (Kleinman & Marks, 1998). Other uncommon and, therefore, suspicious fractures are fractures of the vertebrae, sternum, or pelvis.

Radiographic Evaluation

Radiographic imaging in child abuse cases helps identify the extent of physical injury and clarify all imaging findings that point to other diagnoses. A complete radiographic skeletal survey should be obtained of infants in whom physical abuse is suspected and in cases involving head or visceral trauma. A skeletal survey is a series of radiographs taken of the child's skeleton to identify old and new injuries. The survey identifies skeletal injuries and helps determine metabolic or genetic conditions that mimic abuse. It is also a useful screening tool for children age 2 years or younger in whom child maltreatment is being considered (American Academy of Pediatrics [AAP], 2000). The patient's age and type of suspicious injury can guide the evaluator as to the appropriateness of obtaining a skeletal survey (Belfer et al., 2002). Skeletal surveys are essential for children less than 2 years of age whose history is suspicious of abuse (AAP, 2000). For those between age 2 and 5 years, the examiner determines whether surveys are warranted based on clinical judgment. No matter what the child's age, the clinician should follow the customary radiographic protocol whenever clinical findings point to a specific site of injury (AAP, 2000).

Figure 4-16.
Femoral neck fracture from being yanked from crib in Figure 4-15. (Contributed by Lawrence R. Ricci, MD; Portland, Me.)

Figure 4-17.
Child with multiple rib fractures. (Contributed by Lawrence R. Ricci, MD; Portland, Me.)

Figure 4-18.
Buckle fracture distal femur shaft inflicted. (Contributed by Lawrence R. Ricci, MD; Portland, Me.)

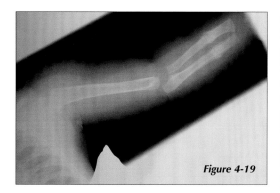

Figure 4-19

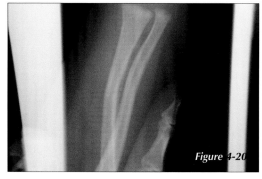

Figure 4-20

Figure 4-19.
Same child as Figure 4-9 with old radius and ulna fracture. (Contributed by Lawrence R. Ricci, MD; Portland, Me.)

Figure 4-20.
Old and new radius fracture. (Contributed by Lawrence R. Ricci, MD; Portland, Me.)

Guidelines for Imaging

Diagnosis of skeletal injury is made by the history and physical examination and then confirmed by imaging techniques. Common physical signs suggesting abusive skeletal injury include reduced range of motion, swelling, tenderness, pseudoparalysis, and limb deformity (Launius, Silberstein, Luisiri, & Graviss, 1998). Radiographs can reveal spiral fractures from twisting of the long bones, as well as old and healing fractures. In cases of suspected abuse, a radiographic skeletal survey is the method of choice for global skeletal imaging (AAP, 2000). The survey includes lateral spine views to assess vertebral fractures and dislocations and hands and feet views to identify subtle digital injuries. (See **Table 4-6** for a list of bones included in the skeletal survey.) Mandatory anteroposterior and lateral views of the skull are taken even when cranial computed tomography (CT) has been performed because a CT can miss certain skull fractures (AAP, 2000).

THORACIC AND ABDOMINAL INJURIES

In cases of child physical abuse, abdominal injuries are relatively uncommon but often serious and are the second most common cause of mortality (Berkowitz, 1995). Investigation of potential child abuse is necessary when a child sustains serious abdominal or chest injury without a known or observed mechanism.

Internal injuries usually result from blunt trauma, such as a direct blow to the abdomen. Anterior abdominal blows may cause epigastric injury, mesenteric tears, or pancreatic injury, whereas abdominal blows from the side may cause splenic, hepatic, or renal injury. It is important to inspect the abdomen carefully and examine the child for external bruises and internal injuries of underlying organs. Severe internal injuries could be present with no external signs or symptoms (Sirotnak & Krugman, 1994).

Accidental blunt trauma causes some of the same injuries as those inflicted on children. Chest injuries include pulmonary contusion, pneumothorax, pleural effusion, rib fractures, and vascular or tracheobronchial injuries (AAP, 2000). Implausible or unlikely stories should arouse suspicion of child abuse, such as falling out of bed, sibling stepping on infant, and rolling onto a child sleeping in bed (AAP, 2000). Abdominal injuries that heighten the suspicion of child abuse include blunt thoracoabdominal injury, duodenal hematomas, pancreatitis, bowel perforation, and thoracoabdominal injury associated with rib fracture.

The most common thoracic injury seen in child abuse cases is fractured ribs and underlying organ injury resulting from the fractures **(Table 4-7)**. Penetrating injuries to the chest may be seen as well and usually present as catastrophic injuries (Cooper, 1992). Significant internal injury can occur to abdominal organs without visible signs of trauma or bruising on the external skin.

Evaluation and Treatment

In abdominal injury in children, the evaluation and management of acute problems are the same for accidental and intentional injuries (AAP, 2000). The evaluation of the

Table 4-6. The Standard Skeletal Survey	
LIMBS	
Humeri	AP (anteroposterior)
Forearms	AP
Hands	Oblique PA (posteroanterior)
Femurs	AP
Lower legs	AP
Feet	AP
TRUNK AND HEAD	
Thorax	AP and lateral
Pelvis	AP; including mid and lower lumbar spine
Lumbar spine	Lateral
Cervical spine	Lateral
Skull	Frontal and lateral

Adapted from American Academy of Pediatrics. Diagnostic imaging of child abuse. Pediatrics. *2000;105:1345-1348.*

child may be determined by the stability of the patient because CT scans or ultrasounds may be more or less indicated depending on the child's physiological stability (Ludwig, 2001). Initial radiographic assessment of an injured child includes usual studies of the chest, cervical spine, and abdomen to evaluate thoracic and abdominal injuries. A CT scan should be performed when internal chest or abdominal injury is suspected and the patient's condition is stable. Ultrasonography is sometimes used, but a CT scan best reveals injuries associated with child abuse (AAP, 2000; Ludwig, 2001).

EXAMINATION OF THE HEAD
Basic Types of Head Injuries
The head and cranium of a child has multiple areas in which damage can occur. Describing injuries according to the anatomical location of the injury is common.

General Principles
The most common cause of death in child abuse cases is head injury (Berkowitz, 1995) **(Figure 4-21)**. A study of children under age 2 years admitted for head injury found that 24% of the injuries resulted from inflicted trauma (Duhaime, Christian, Rorke, & Zimmerman, 1998; Duhaime & Partington, 2002). The younger the age of the child, the more predisposed that child is to death from head injury (Berkowitz, 1995). Nonaccidental head injury is often characterized by subdural or subarachnoid hemorrhages with retinal hemorrhages but little to no external craniofacial trauma (Atwal, Rutty, Carter, & Green, 1998). Inflicted head injury accounts for a substantial number of head injuries that require hospitalization in children younger than age 6.5 years (Reece & Sege, 2000).

Table 4-7. Suspicious Thoracic and Abdominal Injuries

HISTORY

— Unsubstantiated story of how injury occurred

— Child fell out of bed

— Someone rolled onto sleeping child

— Sibling stepped on infant

SIGNS AND SYMPTOMS THE CHILD MAY MANIFEST

— Vomiting

— Abdominal pain

— Abdominal tenderness

— Hematuria

— Emesis

— Absence of bowel sounds

PHYSICAL FINDINGS ON EXAMINATION

— Blunt thoracoabdominal injury

— Duodenal hematomas

— Pancreatitis

— Bowel perforation

— Thoracoabdominal injury associated with rib fracture

Inflicted injury to the head may result from a variety of mechanisms, including shaking and the resultant rotational forces that develop, as well as impact injuries and the translational forces that develop from being slapped, hit, or punched. The head of a small child can be slammed into a hard object such as a wall (seen with and without shaking), and children can also be dropped from a height onto their heads. Children may suffer penetrating injuries to the head from firearms, knives, or glass. Penetrating injuries have a high potential for serious morbidity and mortality. Fracture of the skull (usually linear) can cause severe concussions and anoxia. Children can suffer from asphyxia as a result of choking and/or gagging.

Evaluating the child's level of consciousness is important because loss of consciousness is a common sign resulting from head injury. A study of 95 children who died from accidental head injury found that 94 had an immediate decrease in the level of consciousness (Duhaime & Partington, 2002). Another found that 2- to 3-month-old infants typically presented with a history of apnea or other breathing abnormalities and tended to have a skull fracture and subdural hemorrhage but lacked extracranial injury (Geddes, Hackshaw, Vowles, Nickols, & Whitwell, 2001). The injuries in

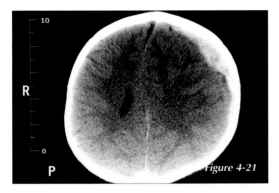

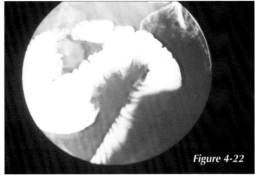

children older than 1 year were more likely to include severe extracranial injuries, particularly abdominal **(Figure 4-22)**. This age group tended to show larger subdural hemorrhages (Geddes et al., 2001). It is important to understand that a child's head and its contents are extremely vulnerable to trauma and the head should not be shaken, slapped, or struck (Felzen, 2002).

In the absence of a documented history of major trauma, subdural hematomas or retinal hemorrhages should be considered as highly suspicious for possible child abuse (Fung, Sung, Nelson, & Poon, 2002). Shaking a baby or small child can induce intracranial, ocular, and, less often, cervical spine injuries. Shaking trauma can cause subdural hematomas, subarachnoid hemorrhages, and brain contusions. It is important for the clinician to search for retinal hemorrhage as another complication of head injury because it is a common finding in shaking-related injuries. Nonspecific signs and symptoms of subdural hematomas include irritability, lethargy, or a lack of appetite. More classic signs of raised intracranial pressure are seizures, vomiting, stupor, or coma (Farley & Reece, 1996).

Subdural hematoma is a common finding in inflicted central nervous system (CNS) injury, including violent shaking of the baby with or without impact to the head, such as when a child is thrown against a stationary object like a mattress, floor, or wall (Farley & Reece, 1996).

Ophthalmological examination is essential in suspected head injury because retinal hemorrhage is found in 65% to 95% of children with inflicted head injury (Duhaime & Partington, 2002). Hemorrhages can be either unilateral or bilateral. Retinal hemorrhage is strongly associated with inflicted injury but can also be seen in accidental trauma. (See Chapter 7, Differential Diagnosis: Conditions That Mimic Child Maltreatment.) Noninflicted injuries should have a history that includes a significant trauma witnessed by others, such as a motor vehicle accident. Birth-related retinal hemorrhages heal rapidly and by 30 days are completely resolved (Anteby, Anteby, Chen, Hamvas, McAlister, & Tychsen, 2001; Emerson, Pieramici, Stoessel, Berreen, & Gariano, 2001). In infants older than 1 month, the presence of retinal hemorrhage should heighten suspicion that it may be associated with factors other than birth (Emerson et al., 2001).

Shaken Baby Syndrome

Shaken baby syndrome (SBS) accounts for a significant number of cases of head trauma in young children. The underlying cause of the damage is from vigorous manual shaking of an infant held by the chest, extremities, or shoulders, which then leads to whiplash-induced intracranial and intraocular bleeding (Wyszynski, 1999). SBS has 3 crucial components that must be present to make the diagnosis, as follows: (1) closed head

Figure 4-21.
Acute subdural with shift. (Contributed by Lawrence R. Ricci, MD; Portland, Me.)

Figure 4-22.
Duodenal hematoma. (Contributed by Lawrence R. Ricci, MD; Portland, Me.)

injury evidenced by altered level of consciousness, convulsions, coma, or death; (2) CNS injury evidenced by CNS hemorrhaging, brain contusion, laceration or concussion; and (3) retinal hemorrhages (Monteleone & Brodeur, 1998). A representative infant victim of SBS is male, younger than age 6 months, and alone with the perpetrator at the time of injury. The occurrence is unrelated to gender, race, education, or socioeconomic status (Lancon, Haines, & Parent, 1998). Characteristic injuries are subdural hemorrhage, intraocular hemorrhage, and little evidence of external trauma (Fulton, 2000; Lancon et al., 1998). SBS can go unidentified because of the absence of external injuries and no witnesses other than the perpetrator to the event. SBS can alter a child's normal developmental course by causing neuropsychological deficits (Goldberg & Goldberg, 2002; Monteleone & Brodeur, 1998).

The history often reported in the context of SBS is that the trauma the child received was of a relatively minor nature (Duhaime & Partington, 2002). As with other forms of abuse, the history may be false or misleading. Any infant or toddler with an altered level of consciousness should be considered to have head trauma until proven otherwise (Monteleone & Brodeur, 1998). The resultant uncovered damage is usually disproportionate to the type of injury described by the caregiver. The findings of SBS often involve a changing history; fractures of various ages, particularly rib fractures; subdural hematoma of the brain; and retinal hemorrhages (Kivlin, 2001).

Although retinal hemorrhages are not a necessary finding to make a diagnosis of SBS, they are the most common fundus finding. The presence of extensive bilateral retinal hemorrhages in a child less than age 3 years raises a strong likelihood of abuse. All other differential diagnoses for hemorrhages should be investigated and eliminated (Kivlin, 2001). Other clinical presentations include seizures, respiratory problems, and disturbed consciousness (Loh, Chang, Kuo, & Howng, 1998). Signs and symptoms of SBS may be nonspecific and mimic seizure disorder, infection, or metabolic abnormalities (Loh et al., 1998).

Shaking a child may also cause bruises of the upper arms and shoulders, depending on the manner in which the child is held. It is unclear whether the CNS injury from shaking is related to shaking alone or shaking followed by an impact against a solid object such as a wall or mattress. Because of this scientific debate, serious intracranial findings seen with shaking related injuries are often clinically referred to as SBS or shaking-impact syndrome.

Other head injuries include those related to the ears and the eyes. The examiner checks for tin ear syndrome, which results from blunt trauma to one ear, creating bruising of that ear, cerebral edema, and hemorrhagic retinopathy on the same side. It also involves bruising and hemorrhage in the antitragus and helix (Monteleone & Brodeur, 1998). Findings are similar to those seen in SBS or whiplash. Not all cases of tin ear syndrome are related to abuse because it can occur through trauma from sports injury. When CT, magnetic resonance imaging (MRI), or plain films of the head are needed in cases of possible head injury, consider adding chest views to look for rib fractures and old fractures.

Presenting Signs and Symptoms
The presenting signs and symptoms of head trauma are as follows:

— Caregiver is late in seeking care

— Altered level of consciousness

— Coma

— Vomiting

— Convulsions

— Opisthotonic posturing

— External injuries (may be subtle or not present at all)

— Swelling and bruising of the scalp

— Respiratory compromise

   — Apnea

   — Hypoventilation

   — Cheynes-Stokes breathing

Physical Examination

Table 4-8 is a guideline for what steps are taken to complete an examination on a child suspected of head trauma.

Table 4-8. Guidelines for Physical Examination in Head Injury

EVALUATE SKIN

— Check torso and neck for fingertip bruising

EXAMINE HEAD AND SCALP

— Examine and palpate for trauma

— Check for swelling or bruising

— Check ears

RETINAL EXAMINATION

— Direct fundoscopic evaluation

   — Look for retinal hemorrhages

— Indirect ophthalmoscopy (by ophthalmologist)

   — For specific types of hemorrhages

   — Vitreous bleeding

GLASGOW COMA SCALE

— Evaluate level of consciousness

— Difficult to apply in infants and young children

Adapted from Monteleone J, Brodeur A. Identifying, interpreting, and reporting injuries. In: Monteleone J, ed. Child Maltreatment. *2nd ed. St Louis, Mo: GW Medical Publishing; 1998:1-29.*

Radiographic Evaluation of Head Injury

Radiographic findings are important in helping to identify nonaccidental cranial trauma because the clinical presentation is often nonspecific or misleading. Initial identification and documentation of CNS injury is accomplished with a CT scan. It is superior in the acute setting over an MRI for evaluation of acute hemorrhage (AAP, 2000). MRI offers the highest sensitivity and specificity for uncovering subacute and chronic injury (AAP, 2000; Monteleone & Brodeur, 1998). The MRI can help determine whether both "old" and "new" blood are present within the hemorrhage. However, because an MRI may fail to detect acute subdural or subarachnoid hemorrhage, the AAP recommends delaying the use of MRI for up to 7 days in children who are acutely ill.

The technique of diffusion-weighted imaging (DWI) reveals nonhemorrhagic posttraumatic infarction much earlier than can be seen on conventional MRI. A study showed that DWI provided an indicator of severity that was more complete than other imaging modalities. DWI may help to guide management decisions through the identification of children at high risk for poor outcome (Suh, Davis, Hopkins, Fajman, & Mapstone, 2001).

Mouth and Teeth

The examiner should pay special attention to the mouth, gums, and mucosal lining of victims of child abuse during the physical examination. Positive findings include palatal petechiae, mucosal tears, lacerations, and abrasions or tears of the frenulum and tongue. The teeth are examined for chipping, dislocation, cleanliness, and signs of decay. In sexual abuse, the mouth is examined for signs of trauma and infection secondary to forced oral-genital contact (Botash, 1997).

There are many causes of trauma to a child's teeth and mouth structures. Caregiver frustration regarding infant feeding may result in trauma to the mouth through using excessive pressure to push the bottle nipple into the infant's mouth. This may cause contusions to the labial frenulum, the tissues of the vestibule, and the alveolar ridge (Kempe, 1975; Mouden, 1998). The most common oral injuries in child abuse include fractured teeth, avulsed teeth, oral contusions, frenulum tears, lacerations, jaw fractures, and oral burns (Mouden, 1998; Naidoo, 2000).

POISONING

Poisoning is a common medical emergency in pediatrics because children often ingest substances that are harmful. There is a high availability and accessibility to products with poisoning potential (Lifshitz & Gavrilov, 2000). Accidental poisoning is a common occurrence; in 2001, children age 3 years and younger accounted for 39% of the 2.3 million cases of reported toxin exposures, and children younger than age 6 years accounted for 51.6% of the reported cases (Litovitz et al., 2001).

Intentional poisoning is a form of child physical abuse and may be used as a type of discipline or punishment. Intentional child abuse forms a subset of poisoning incidents, with one cause of the problem being Munchausen syndrome by proxy (MSBP). The age of the child most affected by intentional poisoning is younger than age 2 years (Pray, 1997; Welliver, 1992). There are documented incidents of intentional poisoning by adults for the purpose of punishment, amusement, attempted suicide of caregiver and child for reasons decided by the adult, and quieting the child (Bays & Feldman, 2001).

Poisonous agents given to children fall into the categories of prescription and nonprescription medications and easily obtained household agents (e.g., salt, pepper, water, sugar, apple juice concentrate, sodium carbonate, vitamin A, antifreeze, naphtha, pine oil, other hydrocarbons, and lye). A wide range of substances and medications can be used to poison a child, including ipecac, laxatives, pepper, salt, water, carbon monoxide, prescription drugs, "street" drugs, household substances, and alcohol (Bays & Feldman, 2001).

The lack of detection of intentional poisoning may result from the fact that clinicians often do not consider poisoning in the differential diagnosis. Therefore, they do not obtain appropriate toxicology screens that would determine the presence of poisonous substances (Litovitz et al., 2001).

Intentional poisoning of children is often more lethal than accidental poisoning and must be considered in any case of abuse (Bays & Feldman, 2001). Ideally, the perpetrator's underlying motivation will become clearer through the history taking and physical examination. In such cases, the caregiver often does not mention the possibility of poisoning as the cause of the child's distress. When the healthcare provider mentions poisoning is a possible cause, the caregiver often denies that possibility (Welliver, 1992).

Physical Examination
The physical examination provides direction for treatment and helps to determine whether the decrease in CNS function is drug induced or from other causes of comas. The main focus of the examination is on the central and autonomic nervous systems, eye findings, changes in skin or oral and gastrointestinal mucous membranes, and odors. These areas form a collection of signs and symptoms referred to as **toxidromes**. Toxidromes include those symptoms produced by exposure to adrenergic, anticholinergic, anticholinesterase, opioid, and sedative-hypnotic agents, and certain heavy metals. Discovering the child's symptoms and physical responses to the poisoning agent may help to identify a specific toxidrome (Coulter & Scalzo, 1998).

The following are common presentation signs of a child who has been intentionally poisoned: coma, apnea, drowsiness, ataxia, lethargy, vomiting, diarrhea, dehydration, stridor, and red diapers or signs of hemorrhagic diarrhea (Bays & Feldman, 2001; Coulter & Scalzo, 1998; Welliver, 1992). For example, sympathomimetic substances cause increased pulse and pupillary dilation, and cholinergics cause bradycardia and urinary incontinence. **Table 4-9** includes recommendations for what to include in the physical examination of the child suspected of being poisoned. See also **Tables 4-10 to 4-13** (Bays & Feldman, 2001; Coulter & Scalzo, 1998; Welliver, 1992).

Laboratory data help confirm the diagnosis of poisoning. Significant tests include serum osmolality, glucose, electrolytes, creatinine, and blood urea nitrogen (BUN) (Coulter & Scalzo, 1998).

SEXUAL ABUSE EVALUATION
The physical examination of the child suspected of having been sexually abused is a fundamental component of the healthcare evaluation and is focused on the child's health status and determining whether or not there are physical findings consistent with the abuse. In most cases in which sexual abuse has occurred, the examination reveals normal or nonspecific genital or anal findings (Adams, 2001; Adams et al., 1994). Additionally, owing to the dynamics of child sexual abuse and the typical pattern of delayed disclosure, a low likelihood of finding forensic evidence occurs in the majority of cases (Christian, Lavelle, DeJong, Loiselle, Brenner, & Joffe, 2000).

Table 4-9. Criteria to Include in the Physical Examination of a Suspected Poisoning Victim

CARDIAC AND VITAL SIGNS

— Pulse

— Heart rhythm

— Temperature (normal, warm, cool): should be warm

— Capillary refill (time in seconds): 2 seconds (normal)

— Blood pressure ranges (Hogstel & Curry, 2001):

Age	Systolic/Diastolic (mm Hg)
1 month	86/54
1 year	96/65
4 years	99/65
6 years	100/60
8 years	105/60
10 years	110/60
12 years	115/60
14 years	118/60
16 years	120/65

PULMONARY FUNCTION

— Assessment of respiration

   — Normal or respiratory distress

— Respiration effort (normal, increased, decreased): normal effort

— Breath sounds (equal, asymmetric, wheezing, rales): clear, equal lung sounds bilaterally

— Excursion

   — Visible movement, depth, symmetry

   — Equal chest excursion

— Respiratory pattern

   — Apnea

— Stridor

(continued)

Table 4-9. *(continued)*

NEUROLOGICAL EXAMINATION

— Pupillary reaction

— Extremity movement (flexed, extended, tonic)

— Mental status (normal, depressed level of consciousness, unresponsive)

— Reflexes

GASTROINTESTINAL AND GENITOURINARY EXAMINATION

— Bowel activity

— Urinary retention

— Vomiting

— Diarrhea

— Hemorrhagic diarrhea

SKIN ASSESSMENT

— Facial and nasal mucosa

— Mucous membranes

— Signs of intentional poisoning

   — Restraint marks

   — Intravenous (IV) injection sites

   — Bruises or signs of physical abuse

   — Burns

   — Presence of powder on skin

ODORS

— Evaluation of odors

   — Acetone: isopropyl alcohol, phenol, and salicylates

   — Bitter almond: cyanide

   — Garlic: heavy metals, organophosphates

   — Oil of wintergreen: methylsalicylates

   — Gasoline: hydrocarbons

Adapted from Bays J, Feldman K. Child abuse by poisoning. In: Reece R, Ludwig S, eds. Child Abuse: Medical Diagnosis and Management. *2nd ed. Philadelphia, Pa: Lippincott Williams & Wilkins; 2001:405-441; Coulter K, Scalzo A. Poisoning. In: Monteleone J, ed.* Child Maltreatment: A Clinical Guide and Reference. *2nd ed. St Louis, Mo: GW Medical Publishing; 1998:315-326; Welliver J. Unusual injuries. In: Ludwig S, Kornberg A, eds.* Child Abuse: A Medical Reference. *2nd ed. New York, NY: Churchill Livingstone; 1992:213-222.*

Table 4-10. Identifying Specific Toxicological Syndrome

Poison Syndrome	Symptoms/Signs	Drugs
Sympathomimetic	Increased pulse and blood pressure, fever, pupillary dilation, sweating, agitation, psychosis	Cocaine, barbiturates, phencyclidine
Sympatholytic	Decreased pulse and blood pressure, hypothermia, small pupils, decreased peristalsis, obtundation, coma	Ethanol, barbiturates, sedative hypnotics, optiates
Cholinergic	Bradycardia, miosis, sweating, hyperperistalsis, salivation, bronchorrhea, urinary incontinence	Organophosphates, carbamates, nicotine
Anticholinergic	Tachycardia, hypertension, fever, pupillary dilation, hot dry skin, decreased peristalsis, urinary reteniton	Tricyclic antidepressants, antihistamines, phenothiazines, atropine, scopolamine

Adapted from Olsen K, Banner W. Emergency management of childhood poisoning. In: Grossman M, Dieckmann R, eds. Pediatric Emergency Medicine. *Philadelphia, Pa: JB Lippincott; 1991:332-339.*

Table 4-11. Signs Indicating That a Child Has Swallowed a Toxic Substance

— Severe throat pain

— Difficulty breathing

— Behavior changes, such as unusual sleepiness or jumpiness

— Nausea/vomiting

— Stomach cramps

— Lip or mouth burns

— Stains from the poison around lips or mouth

— Clothing stains

— Unusual drooling

— Smell of child's breath

— Unusual eye movements, such as inability to follow an object with the eyes, or eyes going around in circles

— Unconsciousness or seizures

— Open or empty container of a toxic substance found near child

Table 4-12. Physical Findings in Some Examples of Poisoning

Symptom/Sign	Agents*
Fever	Amphetamines, anticholinergics, antihistamines, aspirin, atropine, cocaine, iron, phencyclidine, phenothiazines, thyroid hormone
Hypothermia	Barbiturates, carbamazepine, ethanol, narcotics, phenothiazines
Hypertension	Amphetamines, cocaine, ephedrine, pressors, phenylpropanolamine, cyclic antidepressants (early)
Hypotension	Antihypertensive agents, arsenic, barbiturates, beta-adrenergic blockers, calcium channel blockers, carbon monoxide, clonidine, colchicine, cyanide, cyclic antidepressants (late), disulfiram, iron, nitrates, nitrites, opiates, phenothiazines, tetrahydrozoline, theophylline
Coma	Alcohols, anesthetics, anticonvulsants, barbiturates, benzodiazepines, bromide, carbon monoxide, chloral hydrate, clonidine, cyanide, cyclic antidepressants, gamma-hydroxybutyrate (GHB), hydrocarbons, hypoglycemics, inhalants, insulin, lithium, narcotics, phenothiazines, salicylates, sedative-hypnotics, tetrahydrozoline, theophylline
Seizures	Amphetamines, atropine, camphor, carbon monoxide, cocaine, gyromitra mushrooms, isoniazid, lead, lindane, lithium, meperidine, nicotine, pesticides, phencyclidine, propoxyphene, salicylates, strychnine, theophylline, cyclic antidepressants

Examples only. Not meant to be a comprehensive list.

Table 4-13. Toxidromes*

AGENT	SYMPTOMS/SIGNS
Amphetamines	Tachycardia, nausea, vomiting, hypertension, abdominal pain, diaphoresis, anorexia, tremulousness, mydriasis, tachypnea, fever, delirium, tremor, psychosis
Anticholinergic poisoning	Mydriasis, absent sweating, abdominal ileus, tachycardia, delirium, disorientation, ataxia, psychomotor agitation, hallucinations, psychosis, seizures, coma, extrapyramidal symptoms, respiratory failure, urinary retention, hyperpyrexia, dry flushed skin
Cholinergic agents (e.g., organophosphate pesticides)	Salivation, lacrimation, urination, diarrhea, gastrointestinal cramping, emesis (mnemonic: SLUDGE); also bronchorrhea, respiratory failure, seizures, miosis, bradycardia, fasciculations, profuse sweating, muscle weakness, coma
Cyclic antidepressants	Lethargy, coma, seizures, hypotension, ventricular arrhythmias, cardiac conduction disturbances (prolonged QRS duration)
Iron	Nausea, hematemesis, hemorrhagic diarrhea, shock, hypotension, coma, hyperpyrexia, metabolic acidosis, coma, arrhythmias, hepatitis, respiratory failure (late)
Narcotics	Confusion, lethargy, ataxia, coma, respiratory depression, hypotension, miosis, constipation, bradycardia, pulmonary edema, seizures (specifically meperidine, propoxyphene)
Phencyclidine	Rotatory nystagmus, dissociative delusions, aggression, coma, seizures
Salicylism	Tinnitus, tachypnea, confusion, fever, nausea, vomiting, metabolic acidosis
Theophylline	Nausea, vomiting, tremulousness, tachycardia, arrhythmias, hypotension, confusion, seizures, coma
Toxic alcohols (e.g., methanol/ethylene glycol)	Intoxication, coma, large osmolar gap, metabolic acidosis, blindness (methanol), urinary crystals, and renal failure (ethylene glycol)

*Symptoms and signs that, together, point to a clinical diagnosis.

Reprinted with permission from Pediatrics in Review, *Vol. 20, Pages 166-170, Table 3, ©1999. (Woolf AD. Poisoning by unknown agents.* Pediatr Rev. *1999;20:166-170.)*

TIME FRAME FOR FORENSIC EXAMINATION IN SEXUAL ABUSE

The nature of child sexual abuse is such that, in most cases, a child does not present as an acute assault case except with stranger rape. Generally, an urgent examination is completed if alleged contact occurred within 72 hours from the time of the evaluation. This is based on experience with adult sexual assault victims and the likelihood of finding useful forensic evidence during the examination (Finkel & DeJong, 2001). The child suspected of having been sexually abused should receive a full healthcare evaluation, which includes a complete physical examination to inspect the genitalia for suspicious findings and to determine treatment for any conditions that resulted from the sexual contact (AAP, 1999; Botash, 1997; Finkel & DeJong, 2001). If sexual contact occurred more than 72 hours before the healthcare visit and there are no immediate physical complaints such as discharge or bleeding, a physical examination can be delayed pending further investigation because forensic evidence has usually disappeared from the child by that time (Christian et al., 2000).

One of the best predictors of abnormal findings in the female genital examination is the time frame between the actual assault and the examination (Adams et al., 1994; Muram, 1989). The closer the examination is to the actual assault, the better the possibility of finding physical evidence of the assault (Christian & Giardino, 2002; Christian et al., 2000).

Examination Within 72 Hours

The purpose of the urgency to complete the physical examination within 72 hours of alleged contact is to examine the child fully and collect evidence of physical contact and sexual abuse. The examiner uses a forensic evidence collection kit, at times called a "rape kit," when there is reason to believe that evidence of trace elements and seminal products may be present (Christian & Giardino, 2002; Finkel & DeJong, 2001). It is essential that only practitioners who have experience in the collection and preservation of forensic evidence use a rape kit. Any evidence should be collected and packaged appropriately because it will be examined in a crime laboratory and possibly used as evidence in legal proceedings.

The child's body is inspected for semen and saliva using an ultraviolet light source, a Wood's lamp, or another alternate light source to help identify possible areas to sample. Any suspicious areas are swabbed, and the swabs are dried for evidence preservation. Swabs collected from the mouth, vagina or penis, and rectum are dried, packaged appropriately, and given to police, following the proper chain of evidence, for transport to the police crime laboratory. The examiner collects any debris on the child's body and sends it to the crime laboratory via the police. The child's clothing is placed into paper bags for crime laboratory analysis. (See Chapter 5, Laboratory Findings, Diagnostic Testing, and Forensic Specimens in Cases of Child Sexual Abuse.)

Anal and genital injuries are rarely found (Finkel & DeJong, 2001). Most injuries to the genital and anal tissues resulting from sexual abuse are superficial and heal quickly (Finkel, 1998). Superficial injuries in children heal in 48 to 72 hours. Injuries in sexual encounters may be fresh if less than 72 hours passed before the examination, whereas injuries older than 72 hours will be in various stages of healing.

Specific physical or emotional signs require a forensic evaluation. Signs that indicate the need for an urgent evaluation at the time of the child's presentation include the following (Botash, 1997):

— Vaginal or penile discharge

— Indications of sexually transmitted diseases (STDs) (e.g., discharge)

— Acute rectal or vaginal bleeding

— Severe emotional distress in child or caregiver

— Possible pregnancy in the pubertal child

EXAMINER EXPERTISE WITH THE SEXUAL ABUSE EXAMINATION

The question often arises as to whether a clinician who does not deal consistently with child sexual abuse evaluations has the ability to evaluate a child adequately for sexual abuse. Ideally, a child should undergo only one physical examination because the examination experience can be emotionally upsetting. To evaluate possible abuse findings appropriately, the clinician must know normal genital anatomy and variations in genital and anal tissue consistent with abuse. Inexperienced clinicians have seen normal anatomy variations and diagnosed them as abuse findings.

The clinician should refer the child to an expert examiner for further evaluation when the clinician doubts his or her ability to perform the genital examination or sees unclear findings (Adams, 1999). It is best for all involved that the examiner be someone who understands how to conduct a sexual abuse evaluation and knows how to document the findings of the assessment (Finkel & DeJong, 2001).

In cases that involve the investigation of a possible crime, a clinician who does not feel skilled to conduct such an evaluation can consult with an experienced examiner for guidance on how to proceed or defer the full examination to someone who does have expertise in forensic evaluation. The recommendation may be that the child be evaluated at a child abuse center where clinicians have expertise in performing specialized evaluations. In either case, the examiner would document that the child is being referred to a clinician or child abuse center that can provide the appropriate examination (Finkel & DeJong, 2001).

Knowledge Base of Practitioners in Child Sexual Abuse Findings

A study of pediatric nurse practitioners (PNPs) found concerning differences in the PNPs' familiarity with normal genital anatomy and in their knowledge of when to report findings significant for suspected child sexual abuse (Hornor & McCleery, 2000). Other studies examining the knowledge base of family practitioners and pediatricians regarding normal and abnormal genital findings found that physicians also had difficulty properly identifying normal prepubescent anatomy (Ladson et al., 1987; Lentsch & Johnson, 2000) **(Figure 4-23)**.

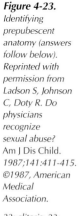

Figure 4-23. Identifying prepubescent anatomy (answers follow below). Reprinted with permission from Ladson S, Johnson C, Doty R. Do physicians recognize sexual abuse? Am J Dis Child. 1987;141:411-415. ©1987, American Medical Association.

22: clitoris, 23: labia minora, 24: urethral orifice, 25: posterior fourchette, 26: hymen, 27: labia majora.

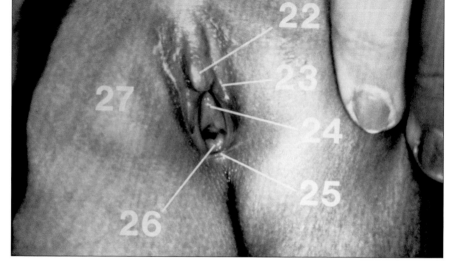

Nurse practitioners and physicians may lack the knowledge to examine effectively the prepubertal genital anatomy of a child suspected of having been sexually abused and, in such a situation, can make appropriate referrals to those more experienced with child sexual abuse evaluations. The studies discussed suggest that practitioners must reestablish their knowledge base of normal anatomy in the context of general health screening and child sexual abuse evaluations.

STRESS WITH SEXUAL ABUSE EVALUATIONS
Investigators have explored the stressful aspects of the genital examination in prepubertal children and adolescents (Hennigen, Kollar, & Rosenthal, 2000; Lazebink et al., 1994; Steward, Schmitz, Steward, Joye, & Rheinhart, 1995). The antici-pation of a genital examination is usually a stress-provoking experience for children and adolescents

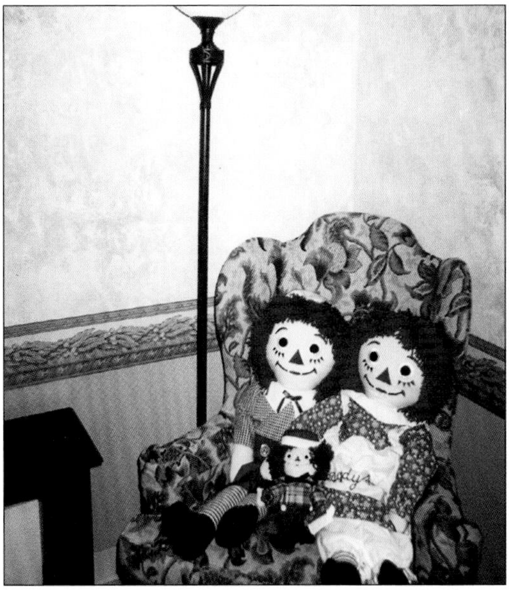

Figure 4-24.
A child abuse center provides a child-friendly setting.

undergoing a sexual abuse evaluation. Studies of children have shown that the fear associated with the examination is greater than that associated with a regular doctor visit, but the evaluation is less traumatic when performed in a controlled setting by experienced providers who support the child psychologically (Lazebink et al., 1994). (See Appendix I: Genital Evaluation Protocol Script.) Steward et al. (1995) found that children were not generally retraumatized by the colposcope examination of the genital area and the child's anxiety was lessened after completion of the examination. Few data support the examination as a form of revictimization to the child (Britton, 1998). The genital examination distress scale (GEDS) objectively measures the emotional distress of a child during the anogenital component of the sexual abuse evaluation (Fischer, 1999). The GEDS tool is used while the child undergoes the examination and may help compare different approaches to the examination. Generally, children respond well to the examination when someone talks with them about the purpose of the process and what to expect in the evaluation (Lawson, 1990). (See Appendix II: Genital Examination Distress Scale.)

SETTING
The setting for the medical examination is important. A child who requires immediate medical attention and presents to a healthcare institution is typically seen in a hospital emergency department. The examination room ideally should be dedicated to child abuse evaluations and have adequate lighting and videocolposcopy to facilitate the examination (Finkel, 2002b). Other visualization enhancement tools such as lighted magnifying glasses may be used in situations in which optimal equipment is unavailable (Finkel, 2002b).

When the sexual abuse evaluation is not urgent, practitioners can refer the child to a child abuse center. Centers provide for the needs of children and offer a friendly, comfortable environment with practitioners who are experts in evaluating and treating cases of abuse. Child abuse centers have furniture that accommodates children, child-friendly lighting, and toys available in the waiting areas **(Figure 4-24)**. Staff at child abuse referral centers, such as children's alliances, are experts in dealing with the issues of child sexual abuse and offer the child and caregiver a relaxed environment for what can be a stressful situation.

Preparing the Child for the Interview and Physical Examination

Sexual abuse, at its most basic level, is a violation of trust by an older or more powerful person toward a child (Finkel & DeJong, 2001). Perpetrators of child sexual abuse are often someone the child knows, such as family members, neighbors, people met through organized activities, or people met in school (Children's Bureau of the US Department of Health & Human Services, 2002). The abuse by a trusted person becomes a form of betrayal to the child. Therefore, the child's ability to trust other adults may be marred by the circumstances of the abuse situation (Finkelhor & Browne, 1985). The interview process is the time for the clinician to begin to establish a short-term relationship with a child who may have difficulty trusting an adult. The examiner should be open, honest, and straightforward because children respond to sincerity (Faller, 1990).

The process of building trust and rapport with the child starts by explaining the importance of the examination (De San Lazaro, 1995; Finkel, 2002b). Rapport is essential to perform a complete physical examination and collect forensic evidence. The examiner assures the child that he or she is interested in the child's health and well-being and wants to determine what has happened with the child. In cases of suspected sexual abuse, the practitioner must prepare the child for the added examination techniques that may be required to complete the forensic examination.

Children with a history of abuse need to feel like they have some control of the examination because the process involves an adult seeing and touching the child's body. Because the abuser took an element of control from the child's life, it is important to give the child as much control over the examination as possible. An approach that builds confidence and trust is essential because physically forcing or coercing a child to undergo an examination against his or her will is never appropriate. The need for the physical examination itself is not negotiable, but many aspects of the examination can be negotiated. The child should be allowed to control those aspects of the examination as much as possible. For example, the child can decide what gown or clothing to wear during the examination, where to sit, and what parts of the examination to do first. The child may keep clothes such as underwear or socks on as long as possible. Giving the child as much control as the examiner can give has the potential to reduce anxiety and help gain cooperation during the examination (Giardino, Finkel, Giardino, Seidl, & Ludwig, 1992).

The examiner should allow the child to participate in the examination as much as possible and encourage the child to become familiar with the examination instruments and room. The child should be allowed to use the stethoscope and listen to his or her heart and then palpate his or her own "belly." Children can choose the time frame for the examination unless the health of the child is in danger. Some children wish the examination to be completed as quickly as possible, while others wish to take breaks to "recover" from being touched. The clinician should give the child as many options as possible. For the genital portion of the examination, the child can choose what to hold and, within reason, who to have present in the room. Maintaining the trust of a child means never promising the child something that the examiner cannot deliver, such as rewards for behavior or control that the examiner cannot ensure.

It is helpful for the child to see how the colposcope works, and, if a videocolposcope is used, to view the picture on the screen (Mears, Heflin, Finkel, & Deblinger, 1997). The examiner can show the child how the image is viewed on the colposcope screen by first showing the image of the child's face, hands, or feet. Once the child is comfortable with the instrument and the projection process, then it is appropriate to

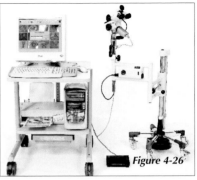

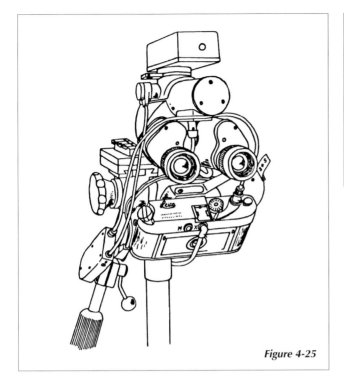

Figure 4-25. *Diagram of a coloposcope. (Contributed by Nancy D. Kellogg, MD, San Antonio, Tex.)*

Figure 4-26. *The colposcope and image documentation system. (Contributed by Nancy D. Kellogg, MD, San Antonio, Tex.)*

Figure 4-25

film the genital area and let the child also view that part of the examination. It is reassuring to the child to see, feel, and hear what the examiner is seeing, hearing, and feeling. The examiner can reassure the child by explaining health considerations whenever possible as the examination progresses.

Use of a Colposcope in the Anogenital Examination

A colposcope is a useful instrument for the detection and recording of genital injury **(Figures 4-25 and 4-26)**. It provides a noninvasive method for visualizing the anogenital structures of the male or female child (Finkel, 2002b). The child's ability to observe the genital examination via the videocolposcope screen causes a demystification of the process and a resultant sense of having more control over the situation (Finkel, 2002a). A study of children who underwent videocolposcopy found that children generally watched their evaluation and were cooperative and enthusiastic throughout the examination (Palusci & Cyrus, 2001).

Colposcopy provides magnification and an excellent light source that is helpful in identifying and capturing injury on film (Finkel, 2002a). The examiner can take still images during the examination by attaching a 35-mm camera to the colposcope. A video camera can be attached to the colposcope to document the examination through still photography or videotape. Video images have advantages over still photography because the variability of the anogenital anatomy is more easily viewed (Ricci, 2002).

Position for Genital Evaluation

For the genital examination, the child is positioned in a comfortable position that also enables the examiner to view the genitalia **(Figures 4-27 and 4-28)**. Children can be examined on a caregiver's lap or when sitting or lying on an examination table. Because the examination itself and the position required for viewing the genitalia may mimic the abuse, it is important to avoid any position or situation that reminds the child of the abuse.

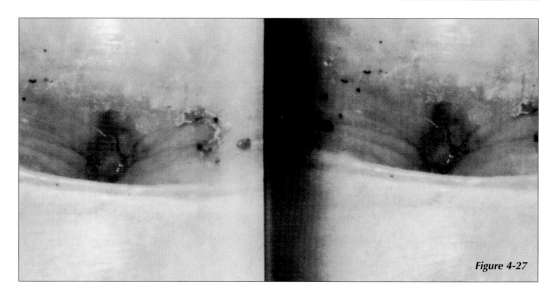

Figure 4-27

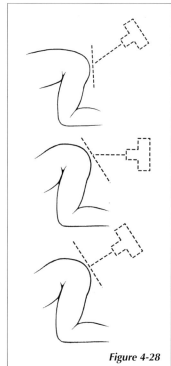

Figure 4-28

Figure 4-27. *Incorrect positioning of patient and/or photocolposcope for knee-chest position resulting in an inadequate photograph of anus. (Contributed by Nancy D. Kellogg, MD, San Antonio, Tex.)*

Figure 4-28. *Top: incorrect patient position (lower back not lordotic); Middle: incorrect photocolposcope position (colposcope not high enough); Bottom: correct position (lens is at right angle to photograph subject). (Contributed by Nancy D. Kellogg, MD, San Antonio, Tex.)*

In prepubertal and pubertal girls the most common examination positions include the supine frog-leg, frog-leg while sitting on a person's lap, and prone knee-chest position **(Figures 4-29 and 4-30)**. The lithotomy position is acceptable for pubertal girls. For boys, the genital examination may be performed in the sitting, standing, supine position, or lateral decubitus position **(Figure 4-31)** (Lahoti, McClain, Girardet, McNeese, & Cheung, 2001; McClain, Girardet, Lahoti, Cheung, Berger, & McNeese, 2000). The position in which the child is examined should be documented in the record.

Visualization of the external genitalia, including the hymen, is all that is required. It is important for the child to be as relaxed as possible to better view the hymen or anus. The supine frog-leg position and knee-chest position with the buttocks raised both allow for good visualization of the hymen **(Figures 4-32 and 33)**. The prone knee-chest position, because of the effects of gravity, is the best to achieve dilatation of the vaginal vault and hymenal orifice but is often the most uncomfortable for the child (Levitt, 1998). Lateral positions can be used if preferred by the child and are commonly used for male examinations and allow for anal examinations for boys and girls. A good light source is necessary regardless of the positions used. The examiner is better able to visualize hymenal edges and the outline of the vaginal opening on a child who is relaxed during the examination (Botash, 1997).

ANATOMY AND TERMINOLOGY IN CHILD SEXUAL ABUSE

The examination of a child who has been sexually abused requires knowledge of genital and anal anatomy. Such knowledge assists the clinician in identifying normal versus abnormal findings and variations between injuries versus anatomical variations. Knowledge of proper terminology and clinical findings also assists in documentation (American Professional Society on the Abuse of Children [APSAC], 1995). Documentation must be as specific as possible and stated in a language known and used by other examiners. Basic terms used by examiners include the following:

— ***Vulva:*** all of the components of the external genitalia—mons, labia majora and minora, clitoris, vaginal orifice

— ***Perineum:*** between the thighs; between the vulva and anus in girls, and between the scrotum and anus in boys

— ***Vestibule:*** between the labia minora, the clitoris, and the posterior fourchette

— ***Posterior fourchette:*** formed by the posterior joining of the labia minora

— ***Hymenal membrane:*** recessed in the vestibule; the internal surface of the hymenal membrane marks the beginning of the vagina

— ***Fossa navicularis:*** posterior attachment of the hymen and the fourchette

GENITAL EXAMINATION

The physical examination in the sexual abuse evaluation always occurs in the context of a complete head-to-toe examination and includes inspecting the external genitalia for normal developmental changes and findings. This requires patience, training, and experience. Injury is often subtle, and experience is needed to determine the normalcy of genitalia at various developmental stages and ages. The genital examination of males and females begins with visualization of the external genitalia. It is necessary to evaluate Tanner staging for both sexes and then document the child's stage in the record.

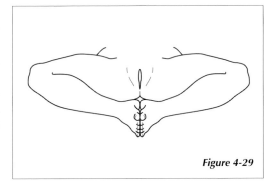

Figure 4-29

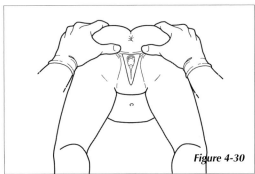

Figure 4-30

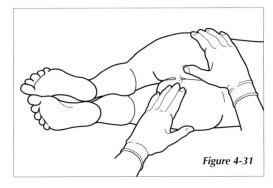

Figure 4-31

Figure 4-29. *Supine frog-leg position. (Contributed by Nancy D. Kellogg, MD, San Antonio, Tex.)*

Figure 4-30. *Prone knee-chest position. (Contributed by Nancy D. Kellogg, MD, San Antonio, Tex.)*

Figure 4-31. *Lateral decubitus position. (Contributed by Nancy D. Kellogg, MD, San Antonio, Tex.)*

(See Chapter 11, Figures 11-1 to 11-5.) For girls the Huffman staging system provides a framework from which to assess the level of estrogenization of the tissues **(Table 4-14)**.

Genitalia must be carefully observed for scarring, tears, abrasions, bruising, decreased amount or absence of hymenal tissue, and contour of the hymenal opening **(Figures 4-34 and 4-35)**. The examiner carefully documents any injury to the area. The colposcope assists with this inspection. It is uncommon to find serious physical injury in a child victim of sexual abuse. Any detected injury is usually minor and rarely requires medical intervention. It is a rare case that requires suturing. The location of

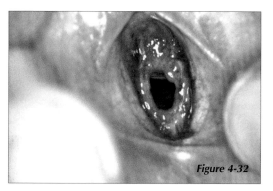

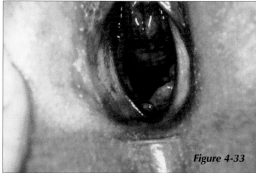

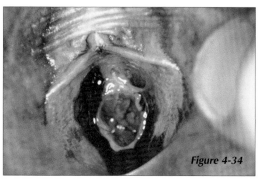

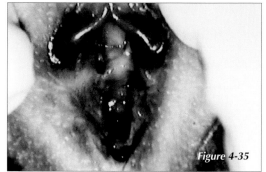

Figure 4-32. *Infant in supine frog-leg position; hymenal orifice is annular with a "bump" at 1 o'clock position and a small "notch" at 10 o'clock position. Hymenal membrane is thin, translucent, and no interruption of scarring present. (Contributed by Carol D. Berkowitz, MD; Torrance, Calif.)*

Figure 4-33. *Child examined in supine frog-leg position after genital trauma. Exam reveals suture in place at 6 o'clock position to stop bleeding from injury. Hymenal edge is irregular and asymmetric. (Contributed by Carol D. Berkowitz, MD; Torrance, Calif.)*

Figure 4-34. *Child whose genital examination reveals bruising on medial aspects of labia minora, hymenal trauma with disruption of hymenal tissue and fresh blood. (Contributed by Carol D. Berkowitz, MD; Torrance, Calif.)*

Figure 4-35. *Infant with significant bruising involving labia minora and labia majora, hymenal trauma with disruption of hymen and fresh blood. (Contributed by Carol D. Berkowitz, MD; Torrance, Calif.)*

injuries is noted in relationship to the face of a clock placed over the child in the anatomical position.

It is difficult for a child to describe sexual activity adequately. Actual penetration of a young child's vagina is unusual even when a child seems to be describing such an event. What is more common is "vulvar coitus," in which the offender rubs an erect penis between the labia for sexual stimulation. To the child, the perception may be penetration. Vulvar coitus can produce abrasions and bruising but does not usually disturb the hymen. The examination, if done immediately after the abuse, would demonstrate redness and swelling of the labia. Additionally, if the male perpetrator ejaculated during the abuse, a seminal deposit on the genitalia, the abdomen, or lower back of the child might be found if the child has not bathed. If semen or saliva is present on the external genitalia, the area should be swabbed for evidence collection.

In males, the examiner documents Tanner stage and circumcision status. (See Chapter 11, Figures 11-1 and 11-2.) The clinician inspects the penis, scrotum, testicles, and perineum for signs of trauma such as bite marks, bruising, abrasions, and suction ecchymosis. When the foreskin is intact, it is advisable to retract the foreskin and inspect the base of the glans (Botash, 1997).

Table 4-14. Huffman Rating

STAGE 1

— Birth to about 2 months of life. Maternal estrogen effects evident.

— Hymen typically appears as follows:

    — Thick

    — Pink in color

    — Moist

    — Actual secretions may be present. May see small amount of blood as the maternal estrogen effect decreases postnatally.

STAGE 2

— Low endogenous estrogen

— Occurs from about 2 months to about 6 or 7 years of age. Hymen typically appears as follows:

    — Thin

    — Translucent or whitish in color

    — Minimal secretions

    — Hymen typically appears dry

STAGE 3

— Body begins producing more estrogen. Tanner staging gives indications of estrogen effect.

— Typically, this stage occurs between the ages of 7 and 13

— Hymen appears as follows:

    — More pink in color

    — Thicker

    — Somewhat lubricated

STAGE 4

— This is the premenarcheal stage

— Genitalia more adult-like in appearance

— Hymen appears as follows:

    — Lubricated

    — Thick

    — Pink and opaque

    — Tanner staging consistent with endogenous estrogen production

Adapted from Huffman JW. The Gynecology of Childhood and Adolescence. Philadelphia, Pa: WB Saunders; 1969.

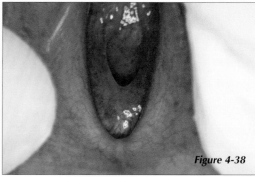

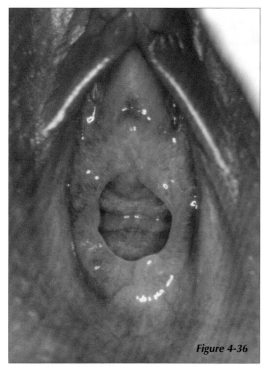

Figure 4-38

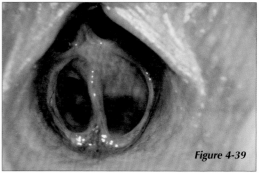

Figure 4-36

Figure 4-39

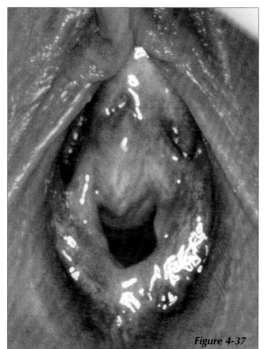

Figure 4-37

Figure 4-36. *Annular hymen, early estrogen. (Contributed by Martin A. Finkel, DO, FACOP, FAAP; Stratford, NJ.)*

Figure 4-37. *Ten-year-old with crescentic hymen. (Contributed by Martin A. Finkel, DO, FACOP, FAAP; Stratford, NJ.)*

Figure 4-38. *Crescentic hymen, translucent edge. (Contributed by Martin A. Finkel, DO, FACOP, FAAP; Stratford, NJ.)*

Figure 4-39. *Septate hymen. (Contributed by Martin A. Finkel, DO, FACOP, FAAP; Stratford, NJ.)*

Evaluation of the Hymen

The appearance of the normal hymen in prepubertal and postpubertal children varies. The range of normal variants is wide, and the examination techniques and positioning of the child can also affect what the examiner sees. Therefore, it is not always possible to determine whether sexual abuse has occurred by the examination findings (Finkel & DeJong, 2001). Studies have found normal-appearing genital tissues as well as nonspecific findings in children who have been known to be sexually abused via vaginal penetration (Finkel & DeJong, 2001).

The diameter of the hymen is easy to describe though thickness and degree of elasticity are more difficult to quantify. The prepubertal hymen has a variety of orifice configurations described as annular, crescentric, fimbriated, cribriform, or septate (Finkel & DeJong, 2001) **(Figures 4-36 to 4-39)**. The most common shapes are crescentric and annular. Estrogen affects the hymen as it does all periurethral tissue. Maternal estrogen affects the appearance of the newborn hymen by causing a thick and redundant appearance. This affect changes after 2 to 3 months and then reappears again as the child approaches puberty. Estrogen creates a thicker and paler appearance to the hymen **(Figures 4-40 and 4-41)**. The prepubertal unestrogenized hymen has an appearance of involuted tissue and tends to appear more vascular and reddened (Finkel & DeJong, 2001). Normal hymenal appearance varies between thick and elastic and thin and nonelastic (Finkel & DeJong, 2001).

Visualization of the hymen and the component parts of the vestibule in girls often requires separation and mild labial traction **(Figures 4-42 to 4-44)**. The hymen is visualized with positioning and gentle traction only. Traction is applied by grasping the labia majora between the examiner's thumb and forefinger and gently applying traction downward and lateral (Botash, 1997; Finkel, 2002b). The examiner applies gentle traction so that injury is not induced and because the more traction applied, the larger the orifice will appear. The hymenal membrane of the prepubertal child is innervated and can be sensitive to touch (Finkel & DeJong, 2001). An unestrogenized hymenal edge is tender, so too much traction or touching the hymen with items such as a cotton-tipped applicator can be uncomfortable for the child.

Warm saline solution may be applied via a catheter or syringe to "float" the hymen and allow better visualization of the hymenal edges (Botash, 1997; Finkel, 2002b).

Use of moistened cotton swabs to move the hymen may also enhance visualization. Another technique is the gentle insertion of a Foley catheter into the vagina (Finkel & DeJong, 2001). In the estrogenized hymen, improved visualization occurs by inserting a partially inflated Foley catheter into the vaginal vault behind the hymenal membrane (Levitt, 1998). This mildly retracts and stretches the tissues.

A vaginal speculum is never used with children who have not reached puberty. In prepubertal children a speculum examination, if indicated, must be done under sedation or anesthesia as required if unexplained bleeding or other unusual findings may need to be evaluated more fully (Lahoti et al., 2001). A nasal speculum is typically *not* helpful for the genital examination.

The penis can cause trauma to the clitoral hood or the fourchette. Periurethral irritation can cause dysuria. Fondling of the female child, hand placed over the mons and the index and third finger separating the labia and rubbing the vaginal vestibule, creates erythema, abrasions, scratches, and edema. Most fondling does not result in serious trauma unless a digit is introduced forcefully into the vagina. Children who are fondled complain of dysuria after the event. This symptom is related to irritation and inflammation of the urethra (Finkel, 2002b).

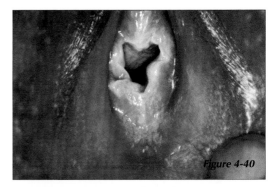

Figure 4-40

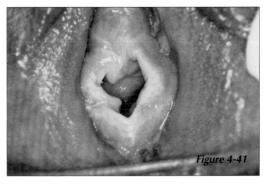

Figure 4-41

Figure 4-40. *Adolescent genital exam reveals estrogenized hymenal tissue (pink, thick, opaque); orifice appears irregular secondary to significant redundancy of tissue. (Contributed by Carol D. Berkowitz, MD; Torrance, Calif.)*

Figure 4-41. *Adolescent genital exam showing estrogenized hymenal tissue (pink, thick, opaque); orifice is irregular owing to areas of redundancy specifically at 9 o'clock position. (Contributed by Carol D. Berkowitz, MD; Torrance, Calif.)*

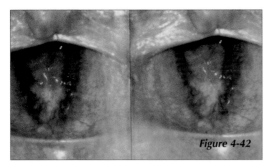

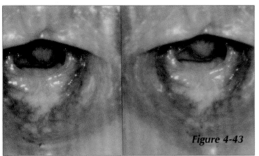

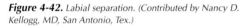

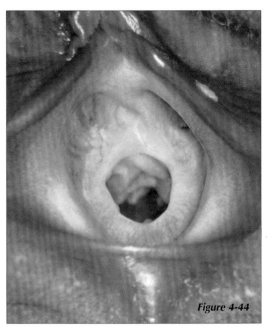

Figure 4-42. *Labial separation. (Contributed by Nancy D. Kellogg, MD, San Antonio, Tex.)*

Figure 4-43. *Labial traction (same patient as Figure 4-42). (Contributed by Nancy D. Kellogg, MD, San Antonio, Tex.)*

Figure 4-44. *Hymenal appearance with labial traction and separation. (Contributed by Martin A. Finkel, DO, FACOP, FAAP; Stratford, NJ.)*

RECTAL EXAMINATION

The anal sphincter is covered with tissue called the anal verge. Within the loose connective tissue surrounding the external orifice is the hemorrhoidal plexus. The external tissue has symmetric radiating folds known as the rugae.

The rectum is carefully inspected for injury using gentle retraction of the gluteal folds during inspection of the tissues (Lahoti et al., 2001). The anus and perianal area are evaluated with the child in a frog-leg supine, knee-chest, lithotomy with buttocks separation, or lateral decubitus position (Finkel, 2002b). The knee-chest position is more awkward for the child and may be the position in which a child was victimized. A trained examiner may need to perform an anoscopic examination if acute injury of the rectum is noted. It is typically not necessary to insert a gloved finger into the anus (Botash, 1997). As the gluteal folds are separated, the perianal muscles typically tighten reflexively; this tightening may also be stimulated by brushing the examiner's hand against the medial aspect of the child's buttock. Laxity of anal sphincter tone may be noted chronically after abuse but may be seen in normal situations such as when stool is present in the distal part of the child's rectum (Finkel, 2002b).

Abnormal findings that may be indicative of abuse include lacerations, bruising, ulcerations, external and internal scarring, bleeding, or fissures. Inflammation is seen as redness, swelling, or tenderness of perianal tissues (Muram, 1989). **Table 4-15** outlines a classification scale for anogenital findings.

Gluteal coitus occurs when the perpetrator rubs the dorsal shaft of the penis over the external anal tissues, causing pressure perceived as penetration. The penile shaft is rubbed between the gluteus and over the rectum. The anus of a child may or may not be penetrated. Such activity can cause abrasions, and seminal products may be collected if ejaculation occurs. Therefore, careful inspection for lacerations and abrasions of the anus in various stages of healing is a necessary part of the examination.

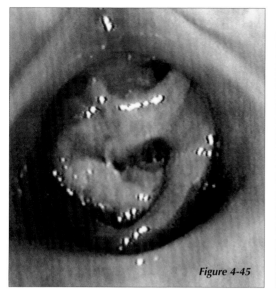

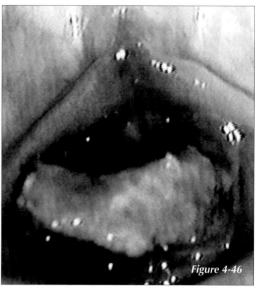

Figure 4-45. *Prepubertal child with foul-smelling, bloody discharge who, on exam, reveals the presence of a foreign body in the vagina just past the hymenal orifice. The foreign body appears to be toilet tissue that had become lodged in the vagina and colonized with bacteria. The presence of the foreign body caused a vulvovaginitis to develop. Foreign body was dislodged with gentle water flushing during exam. (Contributed by Carol D. Berkowitz, MD; Torrance, Calif.)*

Figure 4-46. *Another view of foreign body in child from Figure 4-45. (Contributed by Carol D. Berkowitz, MD; Torrance, Calif.)*

DIFFERENTIAL DIAGNOSES FOR CHILD SEXUAL ABUSE

Several conditions may create findings on physical examination that mimic the findings possible in child sexual abuse. Of course, history should support these nonabusive etiologies. Among the more common situations are the following:

— Accidental injury, for example, a fall creating bruising or abrasion on the superficial areas in the genital region such as the mons, the labia majora, the buttocks, or the penis and scrotum

— Infection creating vulvovaginitis from organisms such as *Candida albicans* or from pinworms

— Diaper dermatitis

— Foreign bodies such as toilet paper placed into the vagina **(Figures 4-45 and 4-46)**

— Labial adhesions secondary to mild inflammation often related to poor hygiene

— Anal fissures related to constipation

The differential diagnosis for genital findings is presented in more detail in Chapter 7, Differential Diagnosis: Conditions That Mimic Child Maltreatment.

PHOTOGRAPHY

Photography is an important component of evidence preservation and serves important purposes. The first is to preserve forensic evidence, and the second is to allow for expert consultation on cases of child abuse. Experts can examine photographs after the examination is complete and render opinions for courtroom purposes as well as teaching and educating other clinicians (Ricci, 2001).

Table 4-15. Revised Classification of Anogenital Findings in Suspected Sexual Abuse

CLASSIFICATION OF FINDINGS

Class 1: Normal

Found in newborns

— Periurethral or vestibular bands

— Longitudinal intravaginal ridges or columns

— Hymenal tags

— Hymenal bumps or mounds

— Hymenal clefts in the anterior (superior) half of hymenal rim, above the 3 to 9 o'clock line, with patient supine

— Estrogen changes when hymenal tissue appears thickened, redundant, and pale

— Linea vestibularis (a flat, white, midline streak in posterior vestibule)

Class 2: Nonspecific

Findings that may result from sexual abuse, depending on timing of examination with respect to abuse but that may also be normal variants or result from other causes

— Perianal skin tags

— Increased perianal skin pigmentation

— Diastasis ani, or a smooth area at 6 or 12 o'clock in perianal area, where there are no anal folds or wrinkles

— Erythema (redness) of vestibular or perianal tissues

— Increased vascularity, or dilation of existing blood vessels, in the vestibule

— Labial adhesions, or agglutination or fusion of labia minora, in midline

— Hymenal rim that appears narrow, but is 1 mm wide or less, with measurements taken from magnified photographs by means of calibrated measuring device

— Vaginal discharge (a nonspecific finding unless appropriately obtained cultures confirm the presence of a sexually transmitted infection)

— Lesions of condyloma acuminata in child less than 2 years of age

— Anal fissures

— Flattened or thickened anal folds

— Anal dilatation, or the opening of internal and external anal sphincters, which demonstrates stool in the rectal vault

— Venous congestion or venous pooling in perianal tissues causing a purple coloration, which may be localized or diffuse

(continued)

Table 4-15. *(continued)*

Class 3: Suspicious

Findings that have rarely been described in nonabused children but have been noted in children with documented abuse, and would prompt examiner to investigate carefully the possibility of abuse

— Enlarged hymenal opening, with measurements more than 2 standard deviations above mean for age and examination method

— Hymenal notch/cleft/partial transection, which appears as sudden narrowing in hymenal rim to less than 1 mm in width, located on or below 3 to 9 o'clock line (patient supine)

— Acute abrasions, lacerations, or bruising of labia or perihymenal tissue, with no history of accidental injury

— Apparent condyloma acuminata in child less than 2 years old

— Distorted anal folds, which are irregular in appearance and may have signs of edema of the tissues

— Immediate (within 30 seconds) anal dilation of 20 mm or more, with no stool visible or palpable in the rectal vault

Class 4: Suggestive of abuse or penetration

Findings, or combination of findings, that can be reasonably explained only by postulating abuse or penetrating injury of some type

— Combination of 2 or more suspicious genital findings or 2 or more suspicious anal findings

— Scar or fresh laceration of posterior fourchette, not involving the hymen

— Perianal scar

Class 5: Clear evidence of blunt force or penetrating trauma

Findings that can have no explanation other than trauma to hymen or perianal tissues

— Complete hymenal transection (healed): hymen has been torn through, to the base, so no measurable hymenal tissue remains between vaginal wall and fossa or vestibular wall

— Areas, more extensive than transections, where there is complete absence of hymenal tissue below the 3 to 9 o'clock line (patient supine)

— Acute laceration of hymen: recent tear through full thickness of hymenal tissue, which may also extend into the vagina and/or posterior fourchette

— Ecchymosis or bruising on the hymen

— Perianal lacerations extending deep to the external anal sphincter

(continued)

Table 4-15. *(continued)*

OVERALL ASSESSMENT OF LIKELIHOOD OF ABUSE

Class 1: No evidence of abuse

— Normal results of examination, no history, no behavioral changes, no witnessed abuse

— Nonspecific findings with another known or likely explanation, and no history of abuse or behavior changes

— Child considered at risk for sexual abuse, but gives no history and has only nonspecific behavior changes

— Physical findings of injury consistent with history of accidental injury, which is clear and believable

Class 2: Possible abuse

— Class 1 or 2 findings in combination with marked behavior changes, especially sexualized behaviors, but child unable to give history of abuse

— Presence of condyloma acuminata in a child less than 2 years old, or herpes type 1 genital lesions with history of abuse, and with otherwise normal results of examination

— Child has made a statement, but it is not sufficiently detailed or is not consistent

— Class 3 findings with no disclosure of abuse

Class 3: Probable cause

— Child gives a clear, consistent, and detailed description of being molested, with or without physical findings

— Class 4 findings in a child with or without a history of abuse, and with no history of accidental penetrating injury

— Positive culture (not rapid antigen test) for *Chlamydia trachomatis* from genital area in child less than 2 years old

— Positive culture for herpes simplex type 2 from genital lesions

— Confirmed condyloma acuminata, when lesions first appeared in a child 2 years old or younger

— *Trichomonas* infection, diagnosed by wet mount or culture

The technology underlying the photography of injuries and genital anatomy is extensive. There is variation in the type of camera systems that work well to meet the standards needed for use of photographs as evidence of the child's injuries (Ricci, 2001). The experience of the examiner in photographing images is another factor that affects the quality of photographic documentation of examination findings (Levitt, 1998). The examiner must take clear photographs, have adequate lighting, and include a planned composition of what parts of the body are in the picture (Ricci, 2001). The examiner documents any findings, describes them in detail, and supplements that documentation with photographs. Photographs must be taken of every injury with a scale in the frame or include anatomical landmarks to establish perspective in the photo. One overall photograph of the child is recommended to mark the beginning of the photographic set.

There are positive and negative aspects of most camera types. A forensic Polaroid camera takes clear pictures that do not fade over time. However, they also have limited ability to zoom in on an area, and the resolution is poorer than with most 35-mm cameras (Ricci, 2001). The 35-mm camera is known for taking high-quality images that are good for publication (Levitt, 1998). The fixed-focus 35-mm is problematic in focusing well at close distances. The best system is one that has close-up ability with control over aperture and shutter speed. The 35-mm SLR camera is one that provides excellent photographs taken by an examiner who is not necessarily an expert in forensic photography (Ricci, 2001). Thirty-five–millimeter photographs are standard in many healthcare practices.

Colpophotography involves photodocumentation of clinical findings using a colposcope with a camera attached to it. An advantage of using a colposcope is that the instrument magnifies and illuminates the area while allowing a photograph or video to be taken simultaneously (Finkel & DeJong, 2001; Finkel & Ricci, 1997; Ricci & Smistek, 1997). It is possible to attach a 35-mm camera or a video monitor to a colposcope for photographic documentation of anogenital findings (Finkel, 1998, 2002a).

Digital photography is an excellent way to take photographs and then transmit them to colleagues via Internet or computer-to-computer connections (Ricci, 2001). The use of digitized images should be considered after consultation with law enforcement officials and prosecutors because photographs can be manipulated more easily to alter colors or brightness of images.

Preservation of pictures must be discussed within the healthcare and forensic teams. It is important to maintain an unbroken chain of evidence and have policies in place for handling the release of photographs (Ricci, 2001; Ricci & Smistek, 1997). Many teams keep 2 sets of pictures: one in the healthcare system and one in the forensic system. When pictures are kept in the medical records department of a hospital, precautions must be taken to prevent destruction of the pictures at microfilming.

SUMMARY

The physical examination is an essential part of the evaluation and treatment of a child suspected of being abused. The examiner must consider many aspects of conducting the examination process from questioning techniques to inspecting and documenting physical examination findings. The data collected from the examination are an important component in the investigation of the allegation of child abuse. Healthcare professionals play an important role in identifying and referring possible victims of child abuse and also treating any physical injuries the child receives during an abusive episode. Therefore, evaluating children suspected of being abused requires expertise over and above that necessary for a usual examination.

Appendix I: Genital Evaluation Protocol Script

Protocol Script

Purpose: *To promote coping with the sensations and emotions felt during genital evaluation*

Outcome: *The child will actively participate in the evaluation*

Procedure Information

Nurse: My name is Ms. Lawson, and I'm going to show you everything Dr. Moore will do when she comes to examine you. Have you ever been to the doctor before?

Child: Yes, Dr. Briggs looks at my ears when they hurt. He gives me medicine that tastes like bubblegum.

Nurse: Has he ever let you look inside his ears?

Child: (Shakes her head no, looks wide-eyed, and leans toward nurse.)

Nurse: Would you like to use this light to look in mine?

Child: (Shakes her head no, pulls away.)

Nurse: Well, how about if mom looks in my ears? (Nurse positions otoscope so mother can see through.)

Child: Here! Let me see!

Nurse: What do you see?

Child: Something shiny and white.

Nurse: What's it doing now? (Nurse insufflates.)

Child: It wiggles! (Child pulls away, exclaims to her mother, and then looks again.)

Nurse: What you saw was my eardrum. And when it wiggled, it was because I put a little puff of air on it like this (nurse demonstrates insufflator on child's hand). That's what Dr. Moore will do when she looks in your ears. If your eardrum is shiny like that and it wiggles, it means you're not sick and you don't need medicine. That's the point of this whole thing: to see if what happened made you sick or hurt. If it did, we'll give you what you need to get well.

Child: But I'm not sick. At least, I don't think I am. What do you mean by, "What happened"?

Nurse: Well, remember when you told Ms. Carol about what your granddad did?

Child: She told you?

(continued)

Protocol Script *(continued)*

Nurse: Of course she did. She wants to make sure you're okay. That's why she helped your mom bring you to the doctor. We know that you've done nothing to be ashamed of. What happened is your granddad's mistake—he's the one who did something wrong.

Child: So what happens to him? Oh, I know. The cop said he'd arrest granddad if he hurt me.

Nurse: And what we want to figure out is if he hurt you. Okay?

Child: Okay. (She sits straight, uses matter-of-fact tone of voice.) What's next?

Nurse: Well, next Dr. Moore will want to look at your eyes.

Child: He didn't do anything to my eyes (scornfully).

Nurse: I know, but all your body parts are important—no one part is more important than the other. (Describes and rehearses eye examination, then proceeds through the heart and lung examination, then to the abdominal examination.)

Nurse: Once she's through listening to your lungs, Dr. Moore will check your tummy, so let's practice that part. Will you lie down with your head here?

Child: (Child lies down and looks up expectantly.)

RELAXATION EXERCISE

Nurse: Every 7-year-old girl I ever saw was ticklish. Are you?

Child: (Giggles and says yes.)

Nurse: Would you like to learn a way to not be ticklish when you don't want to be?

Child: Sure!

Nurse: Okay, then bend your knees up (demonstrates). That makes your tummy soft. Now find a spot on the ceiling and take a deep breath—in through your nose—out through your mouth (demonstrates).

Child: (Child tries several times then figures out how to regulate her breathing.)

Nurse: Now that you've figured that out, let's go to the next step. Take another deep breath in—let it out—and let all the muscles in your face get soft. Now take a deep breath in—let it out— and let the muscles in your shoulders get soft.

Child: (Child complies.)

(continued)

Protocol Script *(continued)*

Nurse: (Continues to pace child, gently touching each body part. Mentions each major body part, including her bottom. Pays particular attention to any body part that seems tense. If the child begins to giggle, gives her time to "get the giggles out." When she is completely focused and relaxed, says:) See! I touched you all over—even your tummy—and you didn't even giggle. That's because you can't feel giggly and relaxed at the same time. That will be helpful to you when Dr. Moore goes to the next part of the examination, which is to look at your "privacy" (use child's term). So to get that part done, you have to let this knee go to the wall (tap far knee) and let this muscle get soft (tap inner thigh). Then let this knee come toward me and let the muscle get soft (positions the child in frog-leg position).

Child: Ooh. Yuk (face tense).

Nurse: Sometimes children tell me that when they separate their knees like this they feel nervous or embarrassed. (Go through several words describing negative emotional responses. Stop at the one that seems to produce a reaction.)

Child: Yeah, it's like I'm doing something nasty.

Nurse: Lots of kids tell me they feel nasty when they move their legs this way, but you know what to do.

Child: (Looks puzzled.)

Nurse: Oh, you know. Take a deep breath, blow it out, then let the muscles in your legs get soft.

Child: (Child complies.)

SENSATION INFORMATION

Nurse: Next, Dr. Moore will look at your privacy. Your privacy is little and hard to see, and it's protected by skin. Dr. Moore will put on these special glasses (show optical visor) to make your privacy look bigger so she can see it. She will move the skin out of the way like this (pulls a little abdominal skin) so she can see. Then she'll touch your privacy with a Q-tip (allow the child to have one for her own). After that's done, you get to put your knees together and sit up. Dr. Moore will tap on your knees and tickle your feet, and that will be the end of that part. Do you have any questions?

Child: No, I think I'm ready.

Nurse: Okay, then you need to put on a gown. Which one do you want—the white or the blue one?

Reprinted with permission from Lawson L. Preparing sexually abused girls for genital evaluation. Issues Compr Pediatr Nurs. 1990;13:155-164. Originally published by Taylor & Francis, Ltd., PO Box 25, Abingdon, Oxfordshire OX14 3UE, UK.

APPENDIX II: GENITAL EXAMINATION DISTRESS SCALE

Genital Examination Distress Scale

Instructions: Immediately at the end of the medical examination for possible sexual abuse rate the 7 indices of behavioral distress for the child during the anogenital phase of the procedure. If the behavior was not observed, assign 1 point. Score 2 points if the behavior was somewhat displayed. A rating of 3 points should be made if the behavior was definitely displayed.

Not displayed = 1; somewhat displayed = 2; definitely displayed = 3

Rating

_____ 1. Nervous behavior (e.g., repeated nail biting, lip chewing, leg fidgeting, rocking, fingers in mouth, not listening)

_____ 2. Cry (e.g., crying sounds, tears or the onset of tears)

_____ 3. Restraint (e.g., pressure is used to hold onto the child or physical attempts to keep the child from moving)

_____ 4. Muscular dystrophy (e.g., tensing of muscles like clenched fists, facial contortions or general body tightening)

_____ 5. Verbal fear (e.g., statement of apprehension or fear such as "I'm scared" or "I'm worried")

_____ 6. Verbal pain (e.g., statement of pain in any tense such as "that hurt," "Owwwh," "You're pinching me," or "This will hurt")

_____ 7. Flail (e.g., random movement of arms, legs or body without trying to be aggressive, like pounding fists, throwing arms or kicking legs)

Reprinted with permission from Gully KJ, Britton H, Hansen K, Goodwill K, Nope J. A new measure for distress during child sexual abuse examinations: the genital examination distress scale. Child Abuse Negl. *1999;23:61-70. ©1999, with permission from Elsevier Science.*

APPENDIX III: ABUSE AND NEGLECT FORMS
(CONTRIBUTED BY THE CHILDREN'S HOSPITAL OF PHILADELPHIA AND ST. CHRISTOPHER'S HOSPITAL FOR CHILDREN)

The Children's Hospital
of Philadelphia

**CHILD PHYSICAL ABUSE
CONSULTATION FORM**

(PATIENT PLATE IMPRINT)

Patient Name:	Date of Consultation:
DOB: MR#:	Location:
CHOP SW	Attending M.D.:
Consulted by:	

HISTORY OF THE EVENTS LEADING TO THIS ADMISION

The Children's Hospital
of Philadelphia

(PATIENT PLATE IMPRINT)

**CHILD PHYSICAL ABUSE
CONSULTATION FORM**

PAGE 2

PERTINENT PAST MEDICAL HISTORY:

History of:	YES	NO	UNKNOWN	DESCRIBE
Prior significant injuries				
Prior hospitalizations				
Bleeding problems or bone disease				
Low birth weight/neonatal problems				
Developmental delay				
Prior history of child abuse				
Chronic diseases				
Medications				
Delayed Immunizations				
Allergies				

Additional pertinent past medical history:

Family/Social History:

The Children's Hospital
of Philadelphia

**CHILD PHYSICAL ABUSE
CONSULTATION FORM**

(PATIENT PLATE IMPRINT)

GENERAL PHYSICAL EXAMINATION   PAGE 3

Height: _____ Weight: _____ T _____ P _____ R _____ BP _____

PHYSICAL EXAM	NORMAL	ABNORMAL	SIGNIFICANT FINDINGS
HEAD/FACE			
EARS			
EYES			
THROAT			
NECK			
CHEST			
HEART			
ABDOMEN			
ANOGENITAL			
EXTREMITIES			
SKIN			
NEURO			

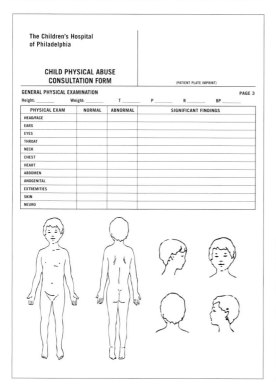

The Children's Hospital
of Philadelphia

**CHILD PHYSICAL ABUSE
CONSULTATION FORM**

(PATIENT PLATE IMPRINT)

LABORATORY/STUDIES   PAGE 4

LAB NAME	YES	NO	RESULTS	LAB NAME	YES	NO	RESULTS
CBC				Amylase/Lipase			
PT/PTT				Urine Toxicology			
LFTs				Serum Toxicology			
Bleeding Time				Urine Analysis			
Other				CPK			

STUDY NAME	RESULT
Skeletal Survey	
Bone Scan	
CT Scan	
MRI	
Ophthalmology Consult	
Other	

IMPRESSION PLAN

	YES	NO	N/A	COMMENTS
Photographs taken?				
CY 47 filed?				
Police notified?				

Attending Signature _____ Date _____
Printed Name
Fellow/Resident Signature _____ Date _____
Printed Name

Guidelines for Interviewing Children with Suspected Sexual Abuse

I. Introduction

Introduce yourself to the child; e.g., "Hi. My name is _____, and as a doctor/nurse, my job is to talk to kids about their feelings, problems and worries, and to make sure kids are doing okay. I'm going to ask you some questions, and I want you to answer them the best you can. If you don't know the answer or are not sure, I want you to tell me, 'I don't know.' I don't want you to guess. Is that okay with you?"

II. Determining Developmental Level	
Question	**Child's Answer**
1. *What's your first and last name?* *Where do you live (can they give street address?)*	
2. *Who lives with you? What are their names?*	
3. *Can you show me your nose? Eyes, etc.? Can you show me what part of your body you use to eat (i.e., mouth, etc)? Can you show me where the pee (poop) comes out (i.e., vagina, urethra, anus)? What do you call these parts?* Ask how they would refer to genitalia on person of the opposite sex?	
4. *Can you tell me what color your shirt (any object) is?*	
5. Distinguishing between lies and truth: *If I told you this shirt was blue (when it is really red), is that the truth or a lie? If I told you this pen is black (the pen is black), is that the truth or a lie?*	
6. Determining understanding of prepositions (on, in, on top of, underneath). Use a pen and a Dixie cup to illustrate. Put the pen in the Dixie cup: *Is the pen in the cup or on top of the cup?* Put the pen on top of the cup: *Is the pen on top of the cup or in the cup?* Put the pen beneath the cup: *Is the pen on top of the cup or under the cup?*	

III. Direct Questioning About Suspected Sexual Abuse	
Question	**Child's Answer**
7. *Do you know why you came to the hospital today?* If the child doesn't know, explain that as a doctor, you make sure kids' bodies are okay, and that his/her parent wanted to make sure that the child's body is okay. Explain that first, you are going to ask some more questions, and then you will take a look at his/her body.	
8. *One thing I talk to kids about is if they are hurting? Do you hurt anywhere?* If the child answers, "Yes," ask how the injury occurred and if the injury was accidental or inflicted, allowing as spontaneous a disclosure as possible. Try to get the following details, or question directly if the child doesn't spontaneously answer the question: a. If the child was hit, was s/he struck *with hand, belt, object, weapon?* b. *Who hit you?* c. *Where did you get hit? Number of times?* d. *Did it hurt? Did it leave a mark? Where?* e. *Have you been hit before? By whom?* f. Any threats to child, especially if child disclosed injury? I.e., *"I'll kill you . . , take you out . . , hurt you worse."*	
9. *Another thing I talk to kids about is if they have touching problems. Did anyone ever touch you on your body in a way that they are not supposed to?* If the child says, "Yes," ask *Can you tell me what happened?"* Allow the child to give as full and spontaneous a disclosure as possible. Try to get the following details, or if the child doesn't answer spontaneously, ask directly: a. *Who touched you?* b. *Where on your body?* c. *With what?* (Hand, penis, mouth, object?) d. *Did it go in, on top of (vaginal/rectum)?* e. *How many times?* f. *Did it hurt? Was there any blood?* g. If alleged perpetrator is male, *Did any stuff come out of his penis? Was his penis hard or soft?*	

h. *Where were you?* (during alleged incident) i. *Was anyone else there?* j. *Was it day or night? What day?* k. *Did you tell anyone?* l. Were there any threats to the child, especially if child disclosed incident? I.e., *"I'll kill you . . ,take you out . . , hurt you worse . . ."* m. *Were you told to keep this a secret?*	
10. If the child answers, "No," to Q. 10, ask: *Has anyone ever touched you on your private parts* (or child's name for genitalia)? If the child answers, "Yes," ask: *Can you tell me what happened?* Allow the child to give as full a disclosure as possible. Try to get the following details, or if the child doesn't answer spontaneously, ask directly: a. *Who touched you?* b. *Where on your body?* c. *With what?* (Hand, penis, mouth, object?) d. *Did it go in, on top of (vaginal/rectum)?* e. *How many times?* f. *Did it hurt? Was there any blood?* g. If alleged perpetrator is male, *Did any stuff come out of his penis? Was his penis hard or soft?* h. *Where were you?* (during alleged incident) i. *Was anyone else there?* j. *Was it day or night? What day?* k. *Did you tell anyone?* l. Were there any threats to the child, especially if child disclosed incident? I.e., *"I'll kill you . . ., take you out . . ., hurt you worse . . ."* m. *Were you told to keep this a secret?*	
11. *Ask about other sexual acts; use the child's own terms: Did anyone put anything in your 'pee-pee'? In your butt? In your mouth? Did anyone ask you to touch, kiss, lick their private part?*	
12. If the child refuses to answer, or appears embarrassed, offer the child a piece of paper and pencil to write down what happened, or offer to write down what happened after the child dictates it to you.	

13. *If the child denies or refuses to answer after your initial questioning, but has disclosed to someone else, question the child again, using the same terms that the child used in the original disclosure:* E.g., *Sometimes kids tell me that somebody was . . .* *ramming them in the butt or* *sexing them or* *doing the nasty or* *playing special games* *Did anyone ever do that to you?*	
14. If the child continues to deny abuse, try to determine if someone coached, threatened or bribed the child not to disclose? E.g., *Sometimes kids are afraid to tell someone when something bad happens. Did someone tell you not to tell anyone that something bad happened? Did someone ask you to keep a secret?*	
15. Determine if the child is afraid to return home.	

IV. Ending the Interview

Assure the child that whatever happened is not their fault. Commend the child for doing a good job talking to you.

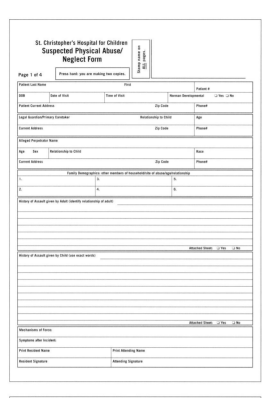

St. Christopher's Hospital for Children
Suspected Physical Abuse/ Neglect Form

Stamp name on ALL pages.

Page 1 of 4 — Press hard: you are making two copies.

Patient Last Name		First			
				Patient #	
DOB	Date of Visit	Time of Visit		Norman Developmental	❑ Yes ❑ No
Patient Current Address			Zip Code	Phone#	
Legal Guardian/Primary Caretaker		Relationship to Child		Age	
Current Address			Zip Code	Phone#	

Alleged Perpetrator Name

Age	Sex	Relationship to Child		Race	
Current Address			Zip Code	Phone#	

Family Demographics: other members of household/site of abuse/age/relationship

1.	3.	5.
2.	4.	6.

History of Assault given by Adult (identify relationship of adult)

Attached Sheet: ❑ Yes ❑ No

History of Assault given by Child (use exact words)

Attached Sheet: ❑ Yes ❑ No

Mechanisms of Force:

Symptoms after Incident:

Print Resident Name	Print Attending Name
Resident Signature	Attending Signature

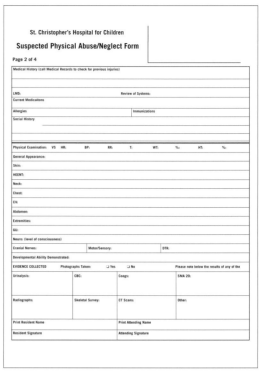

St. Christopher's Hospital for Children
Suspected Physical Abuse/Neglect Form

Page 2 of 4

Medical History (call Medical Records to check for previous injuries)

LMD: — Review of Systems:

Current Medicaitons

Allergies — Immunizations

Social History

Physical Examination: VS HR: BP: RR: T: WT: %: HT: %:

General Appearance:

Skin:

HEENT:

Neck:

Chest:

CV:

Abdomen:

Extremities:

GU:

Neuro: (level of consciousness)

Cranial Nerves: Motor/Sensory: DTR:

Developmental Ability Demonstrated:

EVIDENCE COLLECTED — Photographs Taken: ❑ Yes ❑ No — Please note below the results of any of the

Urinalysis:	CBC:	Coags:	SMA 20:
Radiographs:	Skeletal Survey:	CT Scans:	Other:

Print Resident Name	Print Attending Name
Resident Signature	Attending Signature

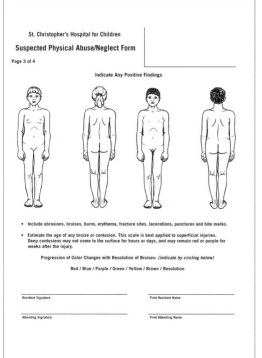

St. Christopher's Hospital for Children

Suspected Physical Abuse/Neglect Form

Page 3 of 4

Indicate Any Positive Findings

- Include abrasions, bruises, burns, erythema, fracture sites, lacerations, punctures and bite marks.
- Estimate the age of any bruise or contusion. This scale is best applied to superficial injuries. Deep contusions may not come to the surface for hours or days, and may remain red or purple for weeks after the injury.

Progression of Color Changes with Resolution of Bruises: *(indicate by circling below)*

Red / Blue / Purple / Green / Yellow / Brown / Resolution

Resident Signature	Print Resident Name
Attending Signature	Print Attending Name

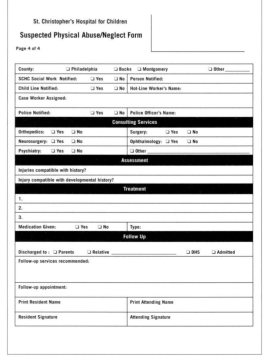

St. Christopher's Hospital for Children

Suspected Physical Abuse/Neglect Form

Page 4 of 4

County:	❑ Philadelphia	❑ Bucks ❑ Montgomery	❑ Other _____
SCHC Social Work Notified:	❑ Yes ❑ No	Person Notified:	
Child Line Notified:	❑ Yes ❑ No	Hot-Line Worker's Name:	
Case Worker Assigned:			
Police Notified:	❑ Yes ❑ No	Police Officer's Name:	

Consulting Services

Orthopedics: ❑ Yes ❑ No	Surgery: ❑ Yes ❑ No
Neurosurgery: ❑ Yes ❑ No	Ophthalmology: ❑ Yes ❑ No
Psychiatry: ❑ Yes ❑ No	❑ Other _____

Assessment

Injuries compatible with history?

Injury compatible with developmental history?

Treatment

1.

2.

3.

Medication Given: ❑ Yes ❑ No — Type:

Follow Up

Discharged to : ❑ Parents ❑ Relative _____ ❑ DHS ❑ Admitted

Follow-up services recommended:

Follow-up appointment:

Print Resident Name	Print Attending Name
Resident Signature	Attending Signature

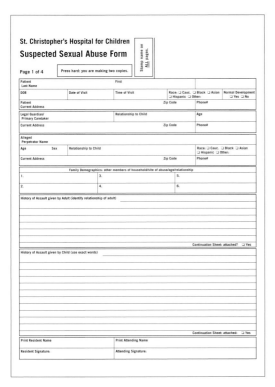

St. Christopher's Hospital for Children

Suspected Sexual Abuse Form

Stamp name on ALL pages.

Page 1 of 4 | Press hard: you are making two copies.

Patient Last Name		First		
DOB	Date of Visit	Time of Visit	Race: ❑ Cauc. ❑ Black ❑ Asian ❑ Hispanic ❑ Other:	Normal Development ❑ Yes ❑ No

Patient Current Address | Zip Code | Phone#

Legal Guardian/ Primary Caretaker | Relationship to Child | Age

Current Address | Zip Code | Phone#

Alleged Perpetrator Name

Age	Sex	Relationship to Child		Race: ❑ Cauc. ❑ Black ❑ Asian ❑ Hispanic ❑ Other:

Current Address | Zip Code | Phone#

Family Demographics: other members of household/site of abuse/age/relationship

1.   3.   5.

2.   4.   6.

History of Assault given by Adult (identify relationship of adult)

Continuation Sheet: attached? ❑ Yes

History of Assault given by Child (use exact words)

Continuation Sheet: attached: ❑ Yes

Print Resident Name | Print Attending Name

Resident Signature: | Attending Signature:

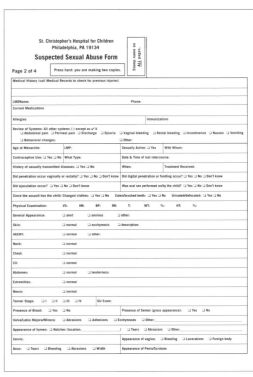

St. Christopher's Hospital for Children
Philadelphia, PA 19134

Suspected Sexual Abuse Form

Stamp name on ALL pages.

Page 2 of 4 | Press hard: you are making two copies.

Medical History (call Medical Records to check for previous injuries)

LMDName: | Phone:

Current Medicaitons

Allergies | Immunizations

Review of Systems: All other systems (-) except as ✓'d
❑ Abdominal pain ❑ Perineal pain ❑ Discharge ❑ Dysoria ❑ Vaginal bleeding ❑ Rectal bleeding ❑ Incontinence ❑ Nausea ❑ Vomiting
❑ Behavioral changes: ❑ Other:

Age at Menarche:	LMP:	Sexually Active: ❑ Yes	With Whom:

Contraceptive Use: ❑ Yes ❑ No What Type: | Date & Time of last intercourse:

History of sexually transmitted diseases: ❑ Yes ❑ No | When: | Treatment Received:

Did penetration occur vaginally or rectally? ❑ Yes ❑ No ❑ Don't know | Did digital penetration or fondling occur? ❑ Yes ❑ No ❑ Don't know

Did ejaculation occur? ❑ Yes ❑ No ❑ Don't know | Was oral sex performed on/by the child? ❑ Yes ❑ No ❑ Don't know

Since the assault has the child: Changed clothes: ❑ Yes ❑ No   Eaten/brushed teeth: ❑ Yes ❑ No   Urinated/defecated: ❑ Yes ❑ No

Physical Examination: VS: HR: BP: RR: T: WT: %: HT: %:

General Appearance: ❑ alert ❑ anxious ❑ other:

Skin: ❑ normal ❑ ecchymosis ❑ description:

HEENT: ❑ normal ❑ other:

Neck: ❑ normal

Chest: ❑ normal

CV: ❑ normal

Abdomen: ❑ normal ❑ tenderness:

Extremities: ❑ normal

Neuro: ❑ normal

Tanner Stage: ❑ I ❑ II ❑ III ❑ IV | GU Exam:

Presence of Blood: ❑ Yes ❑ No | Presence of Semen (gross appearance): ❑ Yes ❑ No

Vulva/Labia Majora/Minora: ❑ Abrasions ❑ Adhesions ❑ Ecchymoses ❑ Other:

Appearance of hymen: ❑ Notches (location:) ❑ Tears ❑ Abrasions ❑ Other:

Cervix: | Appearance of vagina: ❑ Bleeding ❑ Lacerations ❑ Foreign body

Anus: ❑ Tears ❑ Bleeding ❑ Abrasions ❑ Width | Appearance of Penis/Scrotum:

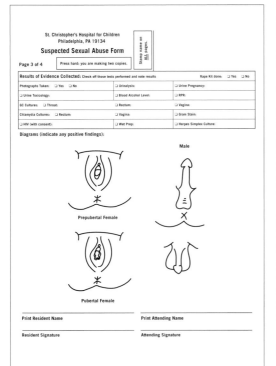

St. Christopher's Hospital for Children
Philadelphia, PA 19134

Suspected Sexual Abuse Form

Stamp name on ALL pages.

Page 3 of 4 | Press hard: you are making two copies.

Results of Evidence Collected: Check off those tests performed and note results | Rape Kit done: ❑ Yes ❑ No

Photographs Taken: ❑ Yes ❑ No	❑ Urinalysis:	❑ Urine Pregnancy:
❑ Urine Toxicology:	❑ Blood Alcohol Level:	❑ RPR:
GC Cultures: ❑ Throat:	❑ Rectum:	❑ Vagina:
Chlamydia Cultures: ❑ Rectum:	❑ Vagina:	❑ Gram Stain:
❑ HIV (with consent):	❑ Wet Prep:	❑ Herpes Simplex Culture:

Diagrams (indicate any positive findings):

Male

Prepubertal Female

Pubertal Female

Print Resident Name | Print Attending Name

Resident Signature | Attending Signature

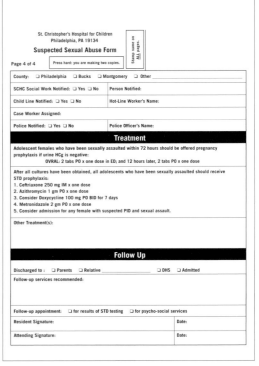

St. Christopher's Hospital for Children
Philadelphia, PA 19134

Suspected Sexual Abuse Form

Stamp name on ALL pages.

Page 4 of 4 | Press hard: you are making two copies.

County: ❑ Philadelphia ❑ Bucks ❑ Montgomery ❑ Other

SCHC Social Work Notified: ❑ Yes ❑ No | Person Notified:

Child Line Notified: ❑ Yes ❑ No | Hot-Line Worker's Name:

Case Worker Assigned:

Police Notified: ❑ Yes ❑ No | Police Officer's Name:

Treatment

Adolescent females who have been sexually assaulted within 72 hours should be offered pregnancy prophylaxis if urine HCg is negative:
    OVRAL: 2 tabs PO x one dose in ED; and 12 hours later, 2 tabs PO x one dose

After all cultures have been obtained, all adolescents who have been sexually assaulted should receive STD prophylaxis:
1. Ceftriaxone 250 mg IM x one dose
2. Azithromycin 1 gm PO x one dose
3. Consider Doxycycline 100 mg PO BID for 7 days
4. Metronidazole 2 gm PO x one dose
5. Consider admission for any female with suspected PID and sexual assault.

Other Treatment(s):

Follow Up

Discharged to : ❑ Parents ❑ Relative ❑ DHS ❑ Admitted

Follow-up services recommended:

Follow-up appointment: ❑ for results of STD testing ❑ for psycho-social services

Resident Signature:	Date:
Attending Signature:	Date:

ST. CHRISTOPHER'S HOSPITAL FOR CHILDREN

Kits of all culture materials (SCAN kits) are available in the left-hand refrigerator.

DEPARTMENT OF EMERGENCY MEDICINE
DIVISION OF PEDIATRIC EMERGENCY MEDICINE
Phone:215.427.5053
Fax:215.427.4688

Sexual Abuse Checklist

A Rape Kit should be completed in children/adolescents with a history of sexual abuse/assault in the past 72 hours. Cultures for STDs should be done in any child/adolescent with a clear disclosure of sexual abuse, a history of pain, bleeding or discharge, or an abnormal exam.

Clothing Collection for the Rape Kit:

Materials Needed: 2 bed sheets, paper bag, labels
What You Have to do: all clothing worn at the time of the attack, including shoes, must be collected as evidence. Have the child undress over 2 bed sheets placed on the floor. The top sheet is used to wrap up the clothing. If there are any stains, place a piece of paper over the stain prior to folding. Place the clothing in a labeled paper bag and seal it with staples. This stays with the Rape Kit.

Clothing collected: . . . . ❑ Yes ❑ No

Physical Examination

1. Skin

Materials Needed: Wood's lamp, red-top tube, 2 cotton-tipped swabs

For the Rape Kit: Fluoresce the skin with a Wood's lamp. Any area that fluoresces green or orange (not bright blue) may be semen. Swab the area with 2 moistened cotton swabs, air dry, and place in a labeled red-top tube, and then put in the Rape Kit.

Skin samples collected: . . . . ❑ Yes ❑ No

2. Oropharynx

Materials Needed: 2 red-top tubes, GC culture media, Chlamydia culture media (children >3 years of age), 2 cotton-tip swabs, 1 Dacron wire swab (for Chlamydia culture)

For the Rape Kit: Have the child spit into a labeled red-top tube and place in the rape kit. Swab the buccal mucosa and along the gingiva with cotton swab, air dry, place in a labeled red-top tube and then put in the Rape Kit.

For STD Cultures: Swab the tonsils and oropharynx with a cotton swab, inoculate the chocolate agar,

label and send to the St. Chris microbiology lab. Swab the tonsils and oropharynx with the Dacron wire swab, place the swab in the labeled Chlamydia culture media tube, and then send to the St. Chris lab.

Saliva sample for Rape Kit: . . . . ❑ Yes ❑ No
Oropharynx swab for Rape Kit: . . . . . . ❑ Yes ❑ No
GC throat culture for St. Chris lab: . . ❑ Yes ❑ No
Chlamydia throat culture for St. Chris lab: . . . . ❑ Yes ❑ No

3. Perineum

Materials Needed: 2 red-top tubes, GC culture media (2 for females), Chlamydia culture media (2 for females), 6 cotton swabs, 2 Dacron swabs, 2 envelopes (pubertal children), comb and scissors (pubertal children)

For the Rape Kit: Swab the vagina with 2 cotton swabs moistened with NSS, allow to air dry, place in one labeled red-top tube, and then place in the Rape Kit. Swab the rectum with 2 moistened cotton swabs, allow to air dry, place in one labeled red-top tube, and then place in the Rape Kit. If the child is pubertal, comb through the pubic hair, catching loose hairs in a paper towel. Then clip 10-15 pubic hairs with scissors, catching the hair in a folded paper towel. Place this paper towel into a labeled envelope, seal it and place in the Rape Kit.

For STD Cultures: Do GC and Chlamydia cultures (remember to use Dacron wire swab) of vagina/cervix (adolescents) and rectum (all children). Label the cultures and send to the St. Chris lab. (Please note: for males, unless there is a clear history of vaginal, anal or oral sex performed by the child, dysuria or penile discharge, penile cultures do not need to be routinely obtained.)

Vagina/cervical sample for Rape Kit: . . . . ❑ Yes ❑ No
Rectal sample for Rape Kit: . . . . ❑ Yes ❑ No
Combed pubic hair for Rape Kit: . . . ❑ Yes ❑ No

Clipped pubic hair for Rape Kit: . . . . . ❑ Yes ❑ No
GC vagina/cervical culture: . . . . ❑ Yes ❑ No
GC rectal culture: . . . . ❑ Yes ❑ No
Chlamydia vagina/cervical culture: . . . ❑ Yes ❑ No
Chlamydia rectal culture: . . . . ❑ Yes ❑ No

4. Head Hair

Materials Needed: tweezers/forceps, paper towel, envelope

For the Rape Kit: Pull 15 head hairs catching the loose hair in a paper towel. Place the paper towel into a labeled envelope, seal it and place in the Rape Kit.

Head hair collected: . . . . ❑ Yes ❑ No

5. Blood Sample Collection

Materials Needed: purple-top tube, red-top tubes (3)

For the Rape Kit: Collect 3 cc of blood, put in labeled purple-top tube, and place in the Rape Kit.

For STD Screening: In selected cases, after discussion with preceptor, blood for RPR, HIV, Hepatitis B (red tops) may be drawn. These samples go to the St. Chris lab.

Purple-top for Rape Kit collected: . . . . ❑ Yes ❑ No
Blood for RPR, HIV, Hepatitis B collected: . . . . ❑ Yes ❑ No

Paperwork:

DPH Medical Report/Sexual Assault Complaint Form: If collecting evidence for the Rape Kit, complete the Medical Report section. After examining the patient, have the parent/guardian and police officer complete the "Authorization for the Release of Information" section of form. All three copies must stay with the Rape Kit.

Evidence receipt (laboratory specimens submitted): Complete this form, and place 2 copies in the rape kit. Staple one copy to the "Suspected Sexual Abuse" ED form. (See example of how to complete this form on the inside door of the Rape Kit cabinet)

Chain of Evidence Label: complete this label and affix to front of Rape Kit. Seal Kit with red police sticker. (See example on the inside door of the Rape Kit cabinet)

CY 47: should be filed if you suspect sexual abuse/assault; and the victim is less than 18 years old; and the alleged perpetrator is a parent/guardian, person living in the same household, baby-sitter, teacher or daycare worker who is at least 14 years old.

Evidence Receipt completed, 2 copies in Rape Kit, 1 copy stapled to Suspected Sexual Abuse form: . . . . . ❑ Yes ❑ No
Chain of Evidence label completed and fixed to Rape Kit: . . . . ❑ Yes ❑ No
CY 47 completed, co-signed by preceptor, and placed in rack in chart room (not with chart): . . . . . ❑ Yes ❑ No

Phone Calls:

• Notify St. Christopher's social worker for any case of suspected sexual abuse/assault and to arrange follow-up counseling. For adolescents, Women Organized Against Rape (WOAR) is a good resource. Pamphlets are in the Rape Kit cabinet.
• Notify Sex Crimes in cases of any sexual abuse/assault that occurred within 72 hours.
• Call Childline to report CY 47.

St. Chris social worker notified: . . . . . ❑ Yes ❑ No
Name of St. Chris social worker filled in on page 4 of "Suspected Sexual Abuse" ED form: . . . . ❑ Yes ❑ No
Sex Crimes notified: . . . . ❑ Yes ❑ No
Name and badge number of officer filled in on page 4 of Suspected Sexual Abuse form: . . . . ❑ Yes ❑ No
Childline called: . . . . ❑ Yes ❑ No
Name of Childline operator filled in on page 4 of Suspected Sexual Abuse form: . . . . ❑ Yes ❑ No

What to do with the rape kit (this includes collected clothing):

• If the police take the rape kit, have the officer sign his/her name on the next line after the one you have signed (see example on door of rape kit cabinet).
• If the police do not take the kit, then place the kit in the locked refrigerator in the Walk In Clinic. The key is on the narcotics cabinet key ring.

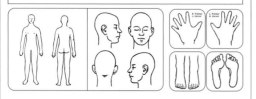

REPORT OF SUSPECTED CHILD ABUSE
(CHILD PROTECTIVE SERVICE LAW - TITLE 23 PA CSA CHAPTER 63)

PLEASE REFER TO INSTRUCTIONS ON REVERSE SIDE. EXCEPT FOR SIGNATURE, PLEASE PRINT OR TYPE

(Child abuse report form with fields for child's name, social security number, birthdate, sex, address, county, present location, biological/adoptive mother and father information, other person responsible, alleged perpetrator, family household composition, injuries/condition description, and body diagrams.)

(Second page of report form with sections: 7. ACTIONS TAKEN OR ABOUT TO BE TAKEN; 8. RISK FACTORS, CHILD; 9. RISK FACTORS, FAMILY; and instructions to mandated persons, reporting source fields.)

INSTRUCTIONS TO MANDATED PERSONS: Any persons who, in the course of their employment, occupation, or practice of their profession come into contact with children shall report or cause a report to be made to ChildLine (800-932-0313) when they have reasonable cause to suspect, on the basis of their medical, professional or other training and experience, that a child coming before them in their professional or official capacity is a victim of child abuse. Within 48 hours after making the oral report, send one copy of this report to the county children and youth agency.

NOTE: If the child has been taken into custody, you must also immediately contact the county children and youth agency where the abuse occurred. Except for confidential communications made to an ordained member of the clergy, the privileged communication between any professional person required to report and the patient or client of that person shall not apply to situations involving child abuse and shall not constitute grounds for failure to report suspected abuse.

Children's Seashore House

Abuse Referral Clinic (Safe Kids Clinic)
Abuse Evaluation Checklist

Name:		Date of Visit:
(Last)	(First)	
Birthdate:		Attending M.D.:
Address:		Referred by:
Telephone:		
Brought in by:		

History of Assault/Abuse

People present during actual interview of child (besides patient and M.D.)

Alleged perpetrator(s) (if known):

Name/nickname:	Age:	Sex:
Relationship to child:	Race:	

Time elapsed since last contact (if known):

Nature of Visit: _____

Abuse Referral Clinic (Safe Kids Clinic)
Abuse Evaluation Checklist

History of Assault/Abuse (continued)

Nature of Visit: _____

Physical Examination

Weight:			Height:	
General Description:				

General Examination: (If abnormal, please describe and include any bruising or skin injury)

PE:		Normal	Abnormal	Significant Findings
(1)	Head/Face			
(2)	Ears			
(3)	Eyes			
(4)	Throat			
(5)	Neck			
(6)	Chest			
(7)	Heart			
(8)	Abdomen			
(9)	Extremities			
(10)	Skin			
(11)	Neuro			

Genital/Pelvic Examination

Colposcope used? _____ Hand held magnifier used? _____

Position Examined: Frog Leg Supine _____ Knee Chest Prone _____
Lateral decub _____ Other _____

Female	**Male**
Tanner: Breasts _____	**Tanner:** Genitals _____
Pubic Hair _____	Pubic Hair _____
External Exam (Vulva, Hymen, Vagina)	Penis _____
	Scrotum _____
Anus _____	Anus _____
Pelvic (post pubertal):	
Cervix _____	
Adnexa _____	

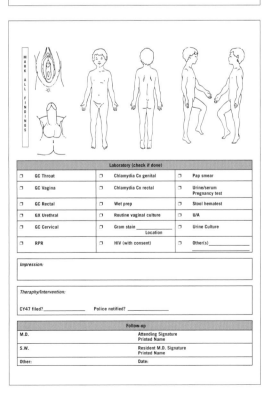

M A R K   A L L   F I N D I N G S

Laboratory (check if done)

☐ GC Throat	☐ Chlamydia Cx genital	☐ Pap smear
☐ GC Vagina	☐ Chlamydia Cx rectal	☐ Urine/serum Pregnancy test
☐ GC Rectal	☐ Wet prep	☐ Stool hematest
☐ GX Urethral	☐ Routine vaginal culture	☐ U/A
☐ GC Cervical	☐ Gram stain _____ Location	☐ Urine Culture
☐ RPR	☐ HIV (with consent)	☐ Other(s) _____

Impression:

Therapy/Intervention:

CY47 filed? _____ Police notified? _____

Follow-up

M.D.	Attending Signature
	Printed Name
S.W.	Resident M.D. Signature
	Printed Name
Other:	Date:

REFERENCES

Adams JA. Medical evaluation of suspected child sexual abuse: it's time for standardized training, referral centers, and routine peer review. *Arch Pediatr Adolesc Med.* 1999;153:1121-1122.

Adams JA. Evolution of a classification scale: medical evaluation of suspected child sexual abuse. *Child Maltreat.* 2001;6:31-36.

Adams JA, Harper K, Knudson S, Revilla J. Examination findings in legally confirmed child sexual abuse: it's normal to be normal. *Pediatrics.* 1994;94:310-317.

American Academy of Pediatrics. Diagnostic imaging of child abuse. *Pediatrics.* 2000;105:1345-1348.

American Academy of Pediatrics Committee on Child Abuse and Neglect. Guidelines for the evaluation of sexual abuse of children: subject review. *Pediatrics.* 1999;103:186-191.

American Professional Society on the Abuse of Children. *Practice Guidelines: Descriptive Terminology in Child Sexual Abuse Evaluations.* San Diego, Calif: APSAC; 1995.

Anteby II, Anteby EY, Chen B, Hamvas A, McAlister W, Tychsen L. Retinal and intraventricular cerebral hemorrhages in the preterm infant born at or before 30 weeks' gestation. *J AAPOS.* 2001;5:90-94.

Atwal GS, Rutty GN, Carter N, Green MA. Bruising in non-accidental head injured children: a retrospective study of the prevalence, distribution and pathological associations in 24 cases. *Forensic Sci Int.* 1998;96 215-230.

Balk SJ, Dreyfus NG, Harris P. Examination of genitalia in children: 'the remaining taboo'. *Pediatrics.* 1982;70:751-753.

Bays J, Feldman K. Child abuse by poisoning. In: Reece R, Ludwig S, eds. *Child Abuse: Medical Diagnosis and Management.* 2nd ed. Philadelphia, Pa: Lippincott Williams & Wilkins; 2001:405-441.

Belfer R, Klein B, Orr L. Use of the skeletal survey in the evaluation of child maltreatment. *Am J Emerg Med.* 2002;19:122-124.

Berkowitz CD. Pediatric abuse: new patterns of injury. *Emerg Med Clin North Am.* 1995;13:321-341.

Botash AS. Examination for sexual abuse in prepubertal children: an update. *Pediatr Ann.* 1997;26:312-320.

Britton H. Emotional impact of the medical examination for child sexual abuse. *Child Abuse Negl.* 1998;22:573-579.

Cheung KK. Identifying and documenting findings of physical child abuse and neglect. *J Pediatr Health Care.* 1999;13:142-143.

Children's Bureau of the US Department of Health & Human Services. *National Child Abuse and Neglect Data System (NCANDS): Summary of Key Findings From Calendar Year 2000.* Washington, DC: National Child Abuse and Neglect Data System; 2002.

Christian C, Giardino A. Forensic evidence collection. In: Finkel M, Giardino A, eds. *Medical Evaluation of Child Sexual Abuse: A Practical Guide.* 2nd ed. Thousand Oaks, Calif: Sage Publications; 2002:131-145.

Christian C, Lavelle J, DeJong A, Loiselle J, Brenner L, Joffe M. Forensic evidence findings in prepubertal victims of sexual assault. *Pediatrics.* 2000;106:100-104.

Cooper A. Thoracoabdominal trauma. In: Ludwig S, Kornberg A, eds. *Child Abuse: A Medical Reference.* 2nd ed. New York, NY: Churchill Livingstone; 1992:131-150.

Coulter K, Scalzo A. Poisoning. In: Monteleone J, ed. *Child Maltreatment: A Clinical Guide and Reference.* 2nd ed. St Louis, Mo: GW Medical Publishing; 1998:315-326.

De San Lazaro C. Making paediatric assessment in suspected sexual abuse a therapeutic experience. *Arch Dis Child.* 1995;73:174-176.

Dubowitz H. Children's responses to the medical evaluation for child sexual abuse. *Child Abuse Negl.* 1998;22:581-584.

Duhaime AC, Christian CW, Rorke LB, Zimmerman RA. Nonaccidental head injury in infants—the "shaken-baby syndrome." *N Engl J Med.* 1998;338:1822-1829.

Duhaime AC, Partington MD. Overview and clinical presentation of inflicted head injury in infants. *Neurosurg Clin North Am.* 2002;13:149-154.

Elliott C, Jay S, Woody P. An observation scale for measuring children's distress during medical procedures. *J Pediatr Psychol.* 1987;12:543-551.

Emerson MV, Pieramici DJ, Stoessel KM, Berreen JP, Gariano RF. Incidence and rate of disappearance of retinal hemorrhage in newborns. *Ophthalmology.* 2001;108:36-39.

Faller K. *Understanding Child Sexual Maltreatment.* Newbury Park, Calif: Sage Publications; 1990.

Farley RH, Reece RM. *Recognizing When a Child's Injury or Illness Is Caused by Abuse: Portable Guides to Investigating Child Abuse.* Washington, DC: US Dept of Justice; 1996. NCJ160938.

Felzen JC. Child maltreatment 2002: recognition, reporting and risk. *Pediatr Int.* 2002;44:554-560.

Finkel M. Technical conduct of the child sexual abuse medical examination. *Child Abuse Negl.* 1998;22:555-566.

Finkel M. Physical examination. In: Finkel M, Giardino A, eds. *Medical Evaluation of Child Sexual Abuse: A Practical Guide.* 2nd ed. Thousand Oaks, Calif: Sage Publications; 2002a:39-98.

Finkel M. The evaluation. In: Finkel M, Giardino A, eds. *Medical Evaluation of Child Sexual Abuse: A Practical Guide.* 2nd ed. Thousand Oaks, Calif: Sage Publications; 2002b:23-37.

Finkel M, DeJong A. Medical findings in child sexual abuse. In: Reece R, Ludwig S, eds. *Child Abuse: Medical Diagnosis and Management.* 2nd ed. Philadelphia, Pa: Lippincott Williams & Wilkins; 2001:207-286.

Finkel M, Ricci L. Documentation and preservation of visual evidence in child abuse. *Child Maltreat.* 1997;2:322-330.

Finkelhor D, Browne A. The traumatic impact of child sexual abuse: a conceptualization. *Am J Orthopsychiatry.* 1985;55:530-541.

Fischer H. The Genital Examination Distress Scale (GEDS). [Letter to the Editor.] *Child Abuse Negl.* 1999;23:1205.

Fulton DR. Shaken baby syndrome. *Crit Care Nurs Q.* 2000;23:43-50.

Fung EL, Sung RY, Nelson EA, Poon WS. Unexplained subdural hematoma in young children: is it always child abuse? *Pediatr Int.* 2002;44:37-42.

Geddes JF, Hackshaw AK, Vowles GH, Nickols CD, Whitwell HL. Neuropathology of inflicted head injury in children. I. Patterns of brain damage. *Brain.* 2001;124:1290-1298.

Giardino AP, Christian C, Giardino E. Evaluation of abuse and neglect. In: Giardino AP, Christian C, Giardino E, eds. *A Practical Guide to the Evaluation of Child Physical Abuse and Neglect.* Thousand Oaks, Calif: Sage Publications; 1997a:23-59.

Giardino AP, Christian C, Giardino E. Skin: bruises and burns. In: Giardino AP, Christian C, Giardino E, eds. *A Practical Guide to the Evaluation of Child Physical Abuse and Neglect.* Thousand Oaks, Calif: Sage Publications; 1997b:61-95.

Giardino AP, Finkel MA, Giardino ER, Seidl T, Ludwig S. *A Practical Guide to the Evaluation of Sexual Abuse in the Prepubertal Child.* Newbury Park, Calif: Sage Publications; 1992.

Giardino AP, Giardino E. Multidisciplinary teamwork issues related to child sexual abuse. In: Giardino AP, Datner E, Asher J, eds. *Sexual Assault Victimization Across the Life Span: A Clinical Guide.* St. Louis, Mo: GW Medical Publishing; 2003:173-188.

Goldberg KB, Goldberg RE. Review of shaken baby syndrome. *J Psychosoc Nurs Ment Health Serv.* 2002;40:38-41.

Gully KJ, Britton H, Hansen K, Goodwill K, Nope JL. A new measure for distress during child sexual abuse examinations: the genital examination distress scale. *Child Abuse Negl.* 1999;23:61-70.

Hansbrough J, Hansbrough W. Pediatric burns. *Pediatr Rev.* 1999;20:117-124.

Hennigen L, Kollar LM, Rosenthal SL. Methods for managing pelvic examination anxiety: individual differences and relaxation techniques. *J Pediatr Health Care.* 2000;14:9-12.

Hogstel MO, Curry LC. Body organ and system assessment. In: Hogstel MO, Curry LC, eds. *Practical Guide to Health Assessment Through the Life Span.* 3rd ed. Philadelphia, Pa: FA Davis Company; 2001:89.

Hornor G, McCleery J. Do pediatric nurse practitioners recognize sexual abuse? *J Pediatr Health Care.* 2000;14:45-49.

Huffman JW. *The Gynecology of Childhood and Adolescence.* Philadelphia, Pa: WB Saunders; 1969.

Jenny C. *Medical Evaluation of Physically and Sexually Abused Children: APSAC Study Guides, Vol. 3.* Thousand Oaks, Calif: Sage Publications; 1996.

Kempe C. Uncommon manifestations of the battered child syndrome. *Am J Dis Child.* 1975;129:1265.

Kessler D, Hyden P. Physical, sexual, and emotional abuse of children. *CIBA Found Symp.* 1991;43:1-32.

Kirschner RH, Stein RJ. The mistaken diagnosis of child abuse. A form of medical abuse? *Am J Dis Child.* 1985;139:873-875.

Kivlin JD. Manifestations of the shaken baby syndrome. *Curr Opin Ophthalmol.* 2001;12:158-163.

Kleinman PK, Marks SC. A regional approach to the classic metaphyseal lesion in abused infants: the distal femur. *AJR Am J Roentgenol.* 1998;170:43-47.

Kleinman PK, Marks SC, Richmond J, Blackbourne BD. Inflicted skeletal injury: a postmortem radiologic-histopathologic study in 31 infants. *AJR Am J Roentgenol.* 1995;165:647-650.

Kocher MS, Kasser JR. Orthopaedic aspects of child abuse. *J Am Acad Orthopaed Surg.* 2000;8:10-20.

Kornberg A. Skin and soft tissue injuries. In: Ludwig S, Kornberg A, eds. *Child Abuse: A Medical Reference.* 2nd ed. New York, NY: Churchill Livingstone; 1992:91-104.

Ladson S, Johnson C, Doty R. Do physicians recognize sexual abuse? *Am J Dis Child.* 1987;141:411-415.

Lahoti SL, McClain N, Girardet R, McNeese M, Cheung K. Evaluating the child for sexual abuse. *Am Fam Physician.* 2001;63:883-892.

Lancon JA, Haines DE, Parent AD. Anatomy of the shaken baby syndrome. *Anat Rec.* 1998;253:13-18.

Launius G, Silberstein M, Luisiri A, Graviss E. Radiology of child abuse. In: Monteleone J, ed. *Child Maltreatment.* 2nd ed. St Louis, Mo: GW Medical Publishing; 1998:31-58.

Lawson L. Preparing sexually abused girls for genital evaluation. *Issues Compr Pediatr Nurs.* 1990;13:155-164.

Lazebink R, Zimet G, Ebert J, et al. How children perceive the medical evaluation for suspected sexual abuse. *Child Abuse Negl.* 1994;18:739-745.

Lentsch K, Johnson C. Do physicians have adequate knowledge of child sexual abuse? The results of two surveys of practicing physicians, 1986 and 1996. *Child Maltreat.* 2000;5:72-78.

Levitt C. Further technical considerations regarding conducting and documenting the child sexual abuse medical examination. *Child Abuse Negl.* 1998;22:567-571.

Lifshitz M, Gavrilov V. Acute poisoning in children. *Isr Med Assoc J.* 2000;2:504-506.

Litovitz T, Klein-Schwartz W, Rodgers G, et al. 2001 annual report of the American Association of Poison Control Centers toxic exposure surveillance system. *Am J Emerg Med.* 2001;20:391-452.

Loh JK, Chang DS, Kuo TH, Howng SL. Shaken baby syndrome. *Kaohsiung J Med Sci.* 1998;14:112-116.

Ludwig S. Child abuse. In: Fleisher G, Ludwig S, eds. *Textbook of Pediatric Emergency Medicine.* 4th ed. Philadelphia, Pa: Lippincott Williams & Wilkins; 2000:1669-1704.

Ludwig S. Visceral injury manifestations of child abuse. In: Reece R, Ludwig S, eds. *Child Abuse: Medical Diagnosis and Management.* 2nd ed. Philadelphia, Pa: Lippincott Williams & Wilkins; 2001:157-175.

Lynch L, Faust J. Reduction of distress in children undergoing sexual abuse medical examination. *J Pediatr.* 1998;132:296-299.

McClain N, Girardet R, Lahoti S, Cheung K, Berger K, McNeese M. Evaluation of sexual abuse in the pediatric patient. *J Pediatr Health Care.* 2000;14:93-101.

Mears CJ, Heflin AH, Finkel M, Deblinger E. Adolescents' responses to video colposcopy and educational information provided during a sexual abuse evaluation. *J Adolesc Health.* 1997;20:128.

Monteleone J, Brodeur A. Identifying, interpreting, and reporting injuries. In: Monteleone J, ed. *Child Maltreatment.* 2nd ed. St Louis, Mo: GW Medical Publishing; 1998:1-29.

Mouden L. Oral injuries of child abuse. In: Monteleone J, ed. *Child Maltreatment.* 2nd ed. St Louis, Mo: GW Medical Publishing; 1998:59-66.

Muram D. Anal and perianal abnormalities in prepubertal victims of sexual abuse. *Am J Obstet Gynecol.* 1989;161:278-281.

Naidoo S. A profile of the oro-facial injuries in child physical abuse at a children's hospital. *Child Abuse Negl.* 2000;24:521-534.

Olsen K, Banner W. Emergency management of childhood poisoning. In: Grossman M, Dieckmann R, eds. *Pediatric Emergency Medicine.* Philadelphia, Pa: JB Lippincott; 1991:332-339.

Palusci VJ, Cyrus TA. Reaction to videocolposcopy in the assessment of child sexual abuse. *Child Abuse Negl.* 2001;25:1535-1546.

Pray W. Reversing the effects of poisoning. *US Pharmacist.* 1997;22:1-5.

Reece R, Sege R. Childhood head injuries: accidental or inflicted? *Arch Pediatr Adolesc Med.* 2000;154:11-15.

Ricci LR. Photodocumentation of the abused child. In: Reece R, Ludwig S, eds. *Child Abuse: Medical Diagnosis and Management.* 2nd ed. Philadelphia, Pa: Lippincott Williams & Wilkins; 2001:385-404.

Ricci LR. Documentation of physical evidence in child sexual abuse. In: Finkel M, Giardino A, eds. *Medical Evaluation of Child Sexual Abuse: A Practical Guide.* 2nd ed. Thousand Oaks, Calif: Sage Publications; 2002:99-110.

Ricci LR, Smistek BS. *Photodocumentation in the Investigation of Child Abuse: Portable Guides to Investigating Child Abuse.* Washington, DC: Office of Juvenile Justice and Delinquency Prevention; 1997.

Richardson A. Cutaneous manifestations of abuse. In: Reece R, ed. *Child Abuse: Medical Diagnosis and Management.* Philadelphia, Pa: Lea & Febinger; 1994:167-184.

Robson M, Heggers J. Pathophysiology of the burn wound. In: Carvajal H, Parks D, eds. *Burns in Children: Pediatric Burn Management.* St Louis, Mo: Mosby; 1988:27-32.

Scalzo A. Burns and child maltreatment. In: Monteleone J, ed. *Child Maltreatment.* 2nd ed. St Louis, Mo: GW Medical Publishing; 1998:105-128.

Scherer JC. *Introductory Medical-Surgical Nursing.* 4th ed. Philadelphia, Pa: Lippincott; 1986:687.

Schwartz A, Ricci L. How accurately can bruises be aged in abused children? Literature review and synthesis. *Pediatrics.* 1996;97:254-256.

Sirotnak A, Krugman R. Physical abuse of children: an update. *Pediatr Rev.* 1994;15:394-399.

Steward M, Schmitz M, Steward D, Joye N, Reinhart M. Children's anticipation of and response to colposcopic examination. *Child Abuse Negl.* 1995;19:997-1005.

Suh DY, Davis PC, Hopkins KL, Fajman NN, Mapstone TB. Nonaccidental pediatric head injury: diffusion-weighted imaging findings. *Neurosurgery.* 2001;49:309-318.

Welliver J. Unusual injuries. In: Ludwig S, Kornberg A, eds. *Child Abuse: A Medical Reference.* 2nd ed. New York, NY: Churchill Livingstone; 1992:213-222.

Wilson E. Estimation of the age of cutaneous contusions in child abuse. *Pediatrics.* 1977;60:750-752.

Woolf AD. Poisoning by unknown agents. *Pediatr Rev.* 1999;20:166-170.

Wyszynski ME. Shaken baby syndrome: identification, intervention, and prevention. *Clin Excell Nurse Pract.* 1999;3:262-267.

Chapter 5

Laboratory Findings, Diagnostic Testing, and Forensic Specimens in Cases of Child Sexual Abuse

Stacey Lasseter, MSN, RN, SANE-A

In evaluating a child for sexual or physical abuse, several findings help to make the diagnosis. The presence of certain sexually transmitted diseases (STDs), for example, in a prepubertal child beyond the neonatal period substantiates that sexual contact has occurred (American College of Emergency Physicians [ACEP], 1999). In child sexual abuse, the history given by the child and the caregivers often points to a specific perpetrator. Thorough evidence collection according to guidelines for forensic specimen collection and laboratory testing of possible findings is important to confirm sexual contact, identify an abuser, and ensure appropriate treatment of the child.

The Emergency Nurses Association (ENA) believes that while nurses provide physical and emotional care to victims of violence, it is also within the nursing role to evaluate the child, collect evidence, preserve the chain of evidence, and document findings in the medical record (ENA, 1998). The newly recognized specialty of forensic nursing has emerged to meet these needs. The practice of forensic nursing focuses on the forensic aspects of healthcare as related to victims, perpetrators, and families of both who experience violence, crime, and traumatic accidents (International Association of Forensic Nurses [IAFN], 1997). The ACEP supports forensic nurse programs as an excellent option for acute and chronic sexual assault evaluations, in part because of the standardized examination and evidence collection process (ACEP, 1999). When no trained forensic nurses are available to conduct the examination of a child suspected of abuse, nurses who come into contact with victims of violence must know how to interview and examine this unique population and use the methods necessary to identify, collect, and preserve evidence. The end result of the evaluation is to treat the child and gather valuable information to be used in court regarding identification of the assailant and the recentness of sexual contact (Ferris & Sandercock, 1998).

Physical evidence and injuries are not found in the majority of the child sexual abuse cases (Finkel, 2002). A recent study demonstrated that findings strongly suggestive of sexual abuse were observed in fewer than 5% of abused children in the study (Berenson et al., 2000), whereas others report abnormal findings in 1% to 14% of children (McClain et al., 2000). Reasons for this include a delay in reporting or seeking treatment, rapid healing of genital tissues, and abuse that is not physically traumatic, such as oral-genital contact or fondling (Botash, 1997). If the child comes within 72

Table 5-1. Tools Used for Evidence Collection
— Evidence collection kit
— Alternative light source (Wood's lamp or Omnichrome)
— Camera (Polaroid, 35 mm, and/or digital)
— Toluidine blue dye
— Colposcope with camera attachment
— Culture mediums (for STD testing)

hours of possible abuse, a complete physical and forensic examination is indicated. This chapter focuses on the evidence collection process, the laboratory testing involved, and the retrieval of samples for STD testing.

EVIDENCE COLLECTION

The evidence collection process is as important as the other components of the evaluation (history gathering, physical examination, and discharge process). The examiner must become competent in the procedures used to recover and preserve biological evidence. It is always imperative to check with the laboratory analyzing the forensic specimens to be sure that appropriate protocols are followed. The types of specimens collected are relatively uniform, but the techniques for testing may vary. Samples gathered may include clothing and oral, vaginal, or anal swabs. In some cases, fluids such as seminal fluid and saliva may be recovered from the skin.

The forensic examination should be conducted systematically. By beginning at the head and progressing toward the feet, each part is assessed and evidence is collected. Several tools are available to the examiner to facilitate identification and thorough collection of specimens. An evidence collection kit, an alternate light source, photography, toluidine blue dye, and a colposcope may be used for this process **(Table 5-1)**. Toluidine blue dye and the colposcope are used in the identification and documentation of genital injuries. (See Chapter 4, The Physical Examination in the Evaluation of Suspected Child Maltreatment: Physical Abuse and Sexual Abuse Examinations.)

EVIDENCE COLLECTION KITS

Many jurisdictions use a standardized kit to collect forensic evidence. These kits are designed to bring continuity to the examination so that the collection and preservation of evidence will be similar regardless of who collected it (Ferris & Sandercock, 1998). Although kits vary from state to state, they basically contain the same types of items for evidence recovery **(Table 5-2)**. A kit to collect evidence should only be used for an examination that occurs acutely; that is, if the assault occurred less than 72 hours before the evaluation of the child or if the examiner feels that biological evidence may still be present after 72 hours. The time frame for emergency evaluations is suggested from findings in adult rape victims that nonmotile and motile sperm can still be identified in the vagina 72 hours after intercourse or sexual assault. A kit should be used after 72 hours to collect evidence if the child has not bathed or changed clothes or when there is bleeding or acute injury. The applicability of the 72-hour rule for pediatric patients has been called into question. A recent study looking at forensic evidence collection based on a study of findings in children rather than in adults suggests the following (Christian et al., 2000):

— There is often little need to swab the bodies of children presenting 24 hours after the alleged event because the yield of forensic findings is extremely low after that time.

— Aggressively pursue the collection of clothing and linens of the child, particularly in cases of delayed presentation for evaluation, because there is a high yield of forensic evidence from these items.

All evidence collection kits contain detailed instructions outlining the collection and packaging of each item. Envelopes are specifically marked so the examiner knows what to put in them. The examiner seals and initials each item of evidence so that the writing is half on the seal and half on the box, envelope, or bag. Once filled, the collector returns the envelopes to the kit and then seals the kit. When evidence is received in the forensic laboratory, each sealed container is assessed for deviations in the lettering. If none, then evidence tampering has not occurred (**Appendix Figures 5-1 to 5-8**).

CLOTHING

All clothing worn by a child during an assault, particularly the underwear, may contain trace evidence and must be collected. The condition of the clothing may also assist in corroborating the child's history of the event. Clothing that is torn or has missing buttons may be evidence of force or a struggle.

Clothing that has seminal fluid or bloodstains is tested for deoxyribonucleic acid (DNA) to identify a suspect. Linens are also collected from a crime site whenever possible because they may have evidence of semen, blood, or hair on them. The examiner makes every effort to secure clothing, even if the child has already changed before the evaluation. Important physical evidence may be intact, and the opportunity for identification must not be missed. One study found forensic evidence (semen or blood) in 4 of the 5 patients who had clothing collected 24 hours after the incident (Christian et al., 2000) and recommends requesting linens and clothing for forensic evaluation.

Clothing should be carefully removed in order to protect foreign materials that are adhered to them. The child stands on a clean sheet or debris collection sheet provided in the evidence collection kit and removes each piece of clothing, so as not to shake or discard anything onto the floor (ACEP, 1999; Lynch, 1995). Any clothing that is wet or damp should be air-dried before packaging. It may be hung on a hanger or placed on butcher paper to dry while the examination continues. After drying, each clothing piece is placed separately in an individual paper bag. Next, the top of the bag is folded over, sealed with tape, and labeled with the examiner's initials (Ledray, 1999).

Table 5-2. Common Contents of Evidence Collection Kits	
— Tubes for known blood sample	— Oral samples
— Known hair samples	— Paper bags to collect clothing
— Pubic hair combings	— Paper bag to collect underwear
— Pubic hair pullings	— Swabs for suspected seminal fluid on the skin
— Vaginal swabs	— Some kits may include additional envelopes for evidence collection
— Rectal swabs	

EVIDENCE PRESENT ON THE SKIN

Biological evidence deposited on the skin should be collected so that DNA testing may be done. A nondestructive screening technique used to identify areas to be swabbed is an alternate light source called a Wood's lamp. The Wood's lamp is an ultraviolet light source used to detect potential biological substances such as semen stains on clothing or skin. The molecules of a foreign substance left on the skin or other surfaces will absorb the ultraviolet light and become excited and fluoresce, or glow. By shining the Wood's lamp over the body, the examiner can more accurately recover possible evidence. Areas of dried substances that remain on the skin may react, or glow, as a light-green to yellow-green fluorescence under the light (Finkel & DeJong, 2001). Such areas of reaction should be swabbed and placed dried in the evidence collection kit (Kini, Brady, & Lazoritz, 1996).

It is important to note that the Wood's lamp is a preliminary screening tool and a reaction does not confirm the presence of semen. Many substances, such as seminal fluid, sweat, saliva, and urine, fluoresce under this light (Auvdel, 1987, 1988); thus, one cannot determine the exact substance that fluoresces (Christian & Giardino, 2002). Other fluids, such as cosmetics, fabric cleansers with whiteners, and substances often used for children, such as Desitin, Surgilube, Balmex, and Barrier Cream also fluoresce under a Wood's lamp (Finkel & DeJong, 2001). Therefore, one can only document that a fluorescent reaction occurred and that samples were collected.

To collect samples from areas of reaction, the double swab technique is used **(Table 5-3)**. For this method, a cotton swab is immersed in sterile or distilled water and the tip is rolled over the surface of the skin, using a circular motion and moderate pressure (Sweet, Lorente, Lorente, Valunzuela, & Villaneuva, 1997). This rehydrates the dried material. A second dry swab is rolled over the surface in the same manner as the first to allow the retrieval of any additional material. The double swab technique may be used to collect any type of biological evidence left on the skin (saliva, blood, or seminal fluid). The cotton applicators are then allowed to dry and are packaged together in the same envelope. The nurse labels the envelope with the location of the area swabbed. It is then sealed and placed in the kit. This should be repeated for each area of reaction.

Table 5-3. Double Swab Technique

1. Identify area that will be swabbed.

2. Immerse one sterile cotton swab in either sterile or distilled water.

3. Roll the swab over the skin surface, using a circular motion and moderate pressure.

4. Take a second swab, which remains dry, and roll over the same surface area.

5. Apply samples to a slide (if required by a specific protocol). If not, allow them to dry and package the swabs in an envelope.

6. Seal, label, and place the envelope in the kit.

Adapted from Sweet D, Lorente M, Lorente J, Valunzuela A, Villanueva E. An improved method to recover saliva from human skin: the double swab technique. J Forensic Sci. *1997;42:320-322.*

ORAL, ANAL, AND VAGINAL SPECIMENS

Samples from each area of assault should be obtained for testing if the child comes for acute evaluation after an assault. Swabs should be specific to the body area assaulted (oral, anal, and vaginal), and 2 to 3 swabbed specimens from each area are the norm to send to the laboratory. However, if the examiner feels that all or additional orifices should be swabbed, it should be done. The swabs are tested for sperm, acid phosphatase, P30 (prostate specific protein, prostate specific antigen), and MHS-5 antigen (Finkel & DeJong, 2001). The examiner should prepare a saline wet mount of specimens from designated orifices and immediately examine for the presence of nonmotile and motile sperm (Finkel & DeJong, 2001). To minimize discomfort for the prepubertal child, the use of mini-tip culturette swabs in the vagina is recommended rather than the large cotton swabs (Finkel & DeJong, 2001). The lack of estrogenization of the hymenal membrane causes greater sensitization of that area. To decrease fears the child may have, the examiner can allow the child to see the swabs before using them.

Oral swabs are taken in cases of fellatio. The buccal pouch and along the bottom edges of the teeth and gums should be vigorously swabbed with several cotton applicators (Finkel & DeJong, 2001). Some protocols may require that an oral rinse or swabbing be collected as well. The child is allowed to rinse his or her mouth with a small amount of sterile or distilled water and then spit the contents into a sterile cup (provided in the kit). Experience has shown that only a small amount is needed to obtain an appropriate sample for laboratory evaluation.

For suspected or reported anal penetration, the nurse obtains samples from the anal/rectal area by inserting the swab one half to 1 inch beyond the anus (Finkel & DeJong, 2001). With the pull of gravity, seminal fluid may drain and pool in or around the anus. The examiner should consider obtaining anal swabs in the event of vaginal penetration. Several cotton applicators are required. Samples from the perianal area (external samples) are taken after the nurse examines the child for trauma. Then, internal swabs are retrieved. After inserting the cotton swab into the anus, the examiner rotates it several times. These applicators are then dried and packaged according to chain of evidence protocol.

The examiner collects samples from the vaginal area in the event of vaginal penetration or vulvar coitus. After inspecting for injuries, the nurse will obtain multiple swabs from the vagina or cervix. For prepubertal children, vaginal samples are required as opposed to cervical swabs. The labia is separated by using the left hand to apply traction on each buttock, and the vestibule is opened by downward and outward traction (Finkel & DeJong, 2001) **(Appendix Figures 5-9 to 5-11)**. The applicator is inserted and samples are taken. Because of the increased sensitivity of the hymenal tissue, the examiner must take care so as not to touch it while retrieving these samples (Emans, Laufer, & Goldstein, 1998). During the adolescent examination, the nurse obtains samples from the cervical os. The swabs are dried and then packaged in the envelope provided. The examiner takes care to ensure that each swab is placed in the corresponding package. The nurse seals and labels the envelope, then places it in the kit.

All swabs used must be dried before placing them in a tube or cardboard box for protection and transport to the forensic laboratory. Drying of the swabs can be time consuming; therefore, some use commercial swab dryers to aid in this process. The examiner and collector of the specimens must be careful to avoid mixing the swabs and then label each tube carefully (Christian & Giardino, 2002).

BLOOD SPECIMENS

A blood sample may be required from the child and used for comparison purposes to distinguish the child's profile from that of the suspect's (Ledray, 1997). When drawing blood samples from adolescents for pregnancy and syphilis testing, the examiner obtains an additional vial to be placed in the evidence kit. Samples may be obtained at a later date from the prepubertal child if needed, unless other laboratory studies are required. It is vital to minimize the trauma to the child. If the child was not orally assaulted, the examiner may consider obtaining buccal swabs. This is a noninvasive method for acquiring a known DNA reference sample. However, this portion of the examination may be performed at a later date if circumstances dictate.

HAIR SAMPLES

Foreign hairs recovered from the child may be used to corroborate contact and to identify an assailant. However, the significant transfer of hair (the transfer of one or more head hairs or pubic hairs between victim and assailant) has been found in only 4% of a sexually assaulted population (Ferris & Sandercock, 1998). Known hair samples collected from the child are used for comparison purposes. The scientist distinguishes head hairs from pubic hairs and animal hairs from human hairs. Because of the great variability in an individual's hair types from different sites, the examiner must collect samples from multiple sites on the child. The analysis has limited specificity, and the laboratory can conclude that the sample is consistent with, inconsistent with, or inconclusive when compared with the perpetrator's hair (Finkel & DeJong, 2001).

In the child abuse examination, hair pulling is generally no longer done. There is some controversy regarding whether or not the hair should be pulled or cut. If DNA is to be extracted, then the entire hair follicle, including the root, is needed because DNA is found in the root. It is important that local jurisdictions, forensic laboratories, and examiners take part in establishing protocols concerning hair sample collection. If protocols are in place, the examiner should confirm all practices with appropriate agencies (Ledray, 1999). It is important to establish protocols that complement the requirements of the agencies with whom the nurse works.

IDENTIFICATION OF MOTILE SPERM

The detection of motile sperm in body orifices provides strong evidence of sexual contact within a 72-hour period (Finkel & DeJong, 2001). There is a variation in survival time of sperm depending on the age of the child and the orifice in which it is found. The lack of cervical mucus in prepubertal girls causes a shortened survival time for sperm, and the action of saliva in the mouth causes a hostile environment (Finkel & DeJong, 2001). Dead or nonmotile sperm are detectable for longer periods than are motile sperm, depending on the environmental conditions of the orifice. Sperm motility decreases after ejaculation. One controlled laboratory study reveals that 50% of women tested positive for motile sperm 3 hours after consensual intercourse (Ferris & Sandercock, 1998). However, a retrospective review of 781 cases found a very low recovery rate for seminal fluid (Tucker, Ledray, & Werner, 1990). This may result from differences in the circumstances under which the intercourse occurred (Ferris & Sandercock, 1998). Therefore, any assessment for motile sperm should be done as soon as possible after an acute assault. The stability of a dry sperm specimen enables sperm to be detected on clothing for 12 months or more (Finkel & DeJong, 2001). The examiner must also remember that the lack of sperm does not discount the history.

A wet mount slide may be made for the identification of motile sperm **(Table 5-4)**. There are 2 options for the collection of fluid. The first, in the adolescent, is to swab the vaginal pool (the posterior fornix, which is the area under the cervix) while the

---

Table 5-4. Preparing a Wet Mount Slide

METHOD 1

Adolescent patient

1. During speculum insertion, place cotton-tipped applicator in the vaginal pool and collect sample (the vaginal pool is the area under the cervix). The examiner may also obtain specimens from the cervical os.

2. Place material on the slide and apply a drop of saline.

3. Take the slide and put under the microscope for viewing.

Prepubertal patient

1. Insert a Calgi swab (a very thin tipped cotton swab) into the vagina and obtain specimen.

2. Place material on the slide and apply a drop of saline.

3. Put the slide under the microscope for viewing.

METHOD 2

1. With a plastic pipette, instill several milliliters of saline into the vaginal vault.

2. Take a clean pipette to suction a sample of the fluid.

3. Place a drop of the fluid on the slide.

4. Put the slide under the microscope for viewing.

---

speculum is in place. In the prepubertal child, the cotton applicator is inserted into the vagina to capture potential samples (Emans et al., 1998). The material collected is placed on a slide and then one drop of saline solution is applied. Approximately 50% of vaginal pool specimens have no detectable sperm within 24 hours of ejaculation (Finkel & DeJong, 2001). The second method, vaginal washing, requires the examiner to instill sterile saline solution into the vaginal vault; a pipette is used to suction a small amount out, which is then placed onto a slide (Heger, Emans, & Muram, 2000). Specimens for forensic testing must be collected first to preserve any potential evidence.

Some sexual assault nurse examiners (SANEs) have found that using a light-staining microscope makes the identification of motile sperm easier **(Appendix Figure 5-12)**. This microscope enhances the image by coloring the illuminator light with filters. A yellow filter illuminates the dark field. The bright field is colored by a blue one. The result is yellow-colored sperm against a blue background (O'Brien, 1998). The examiner identifies sperm more readily with this type of microscope than with traditional microscopes. A wet mount slide is prepared and placed under the microscope for viewing.

The sperm head and tail separate quickly in an unfavorable environment such as the slide. The nurse examiner must be competent in identifying motile sperm because the possibility of misidentifying cells exists. The head resembles a white blood cell and is often mistaken for one. Such an error would be detrimental to the case. The presence of motile sperm recovered from a child confirms sexual contact and influences the investigation. Be aware that the forensic laboratory confirms the presence of sperm through enzyme and protein tests, not just visually. The scientist has the ability, through special training and experience, to distinguish between white blood cells, sperm heads, sperm tails, and other types of cells. Thus, the examiner should exercise caution when identifying sperm.

Other enzymes secreted by the prostate gland and present in sperm are indicators of sexual contact. Acid phosphatase and P30 (semen glycoprotein) are enzymes that can be detected for longer periods in certain media other than sperm (Finkel & DeJong, 2001). Acid phosphatase analysis is a complementary process to sperm identification. The length of time acid phosphatase is present may be shorter than that for sperm in some body environments, but acid phosphatase may be detected on clothing for as long as 3 years after sperm deposition (Finkel & DeJong, 2001). For P30, its detection in urine, vaginal fluid, or saliva indicates recent sexual contact within 48 hours. It is stable when dried and may be detected for up to 12 years in dried seminal stains (Finkel & DeJong, 2001).

BITE MARKS

Bite marks may be found in cases of sexual abuse as well as physical abuse. The child should be examined closely because the findings may be subtle and overlooked, especially if the wound has almost healed. Note whether the bite mark has been affected by change of position, washing of the area, and contamination (ACEP, 1999). Traditionally, bite mark evidence has been used to develop comparative evidence between the pattern and a potential suspect. The bite mark may provide biological evidence as well as physical evidence (Sweet et al., 1997). When the examiner takes the initial pictures of a bite mark, he or she should include multiple views and perspectives to show the size and shape of the bite and the texture of the mark (Ricci, 2001). Ideally, the photo should show magnified views. An expert forensic odontologist interprets the photos later. Ideally, the photos are best taken by someone who is also an expert in photographing such evidence (Barsley, West, & Fair, 1990; Finkel & DeJong, 2001; Golden, 1996), although that is not always possible.

The other technique for identification of bite mark evidence in the acute examination is to collect saliva that can be analyzed for genetic markers (Finkel & DeJong, 2001). Like other body fluids, saliva contains DNA, which is analyzed to identify perpetrators (Sweet & Pretty, 2001). The Wood's lamp is an alternative light source used to detect trace saliva evidence around the wound (ACEP, 1999). The bite mark should be swabbed as soon as possible using the double swab technique to collect saliva.

FORENSIC PHOTOGRAPHY

Photodocumentation in the forensic evaluation enables the court to see the victim through the eyes of the examiner. Photography should be considered one of the 3 necessary forms of documentation. The others are written or narrative descriptions and diagrams that pinpoint location, size, shape, and quantity of injuries. Each form of documentation builds on and supports the other. Each photograph needs to be taken so as to provide a true and accurate representation of the findings and then be properly identified as to date, time, location, case number, and magnification, to name a few of the identifying features (Ricci, 2001). Photographs must show the condition of the child's injuries as they were upon presentation to the facility. (See Chapter 2, Presentation and Overview of the Evaluation of Child Maltreatment and Chapter 9, Documentation of the Evaluation in Cases of Suspected Child Maltreatment, for further discussion.) **Table 5-5** lists equipment used in forensic photography.

Nongenital injury photographs should be taken in a series **(Appendix Figures 5-13 to 5-17)**, beginning with an overall picture of the child. This captures trauma, as well as

Table 5-5. Photography Equipment List

1. **Nylon camera bag with lots of removable sections, pockets, and a padded shoulder strap**

2. **35-mm camera body**

   — Matrix metering
   — 3-D balanced fill flash
   — TTL flash sensor
   — DX coding
   — Auto focus and manual settings
   — Date-back compatibility
   — Lens compatibility
   — Preferably uses regular AA batteries instead of lithium/nickel type batteries (less expensive and more readily available)

3. **Digital camera (a great resource to compare digital cameras is the Digital Photography Review website www.dpreview.com)**

   — Price
   — Max resolution (the more pixels the better)
   — Zoom features (telephoto and wide)
   — Digital zoom
   — Manual focus
   — White balance override (important since hospital lighting can be tricky to overcome)
   — External flash (you want the option of adding an external flash)
   — Lens compatibility
   — Storage types (compact card, disc, CD-R, memory stick)
   — Storage included
   — Uncompressed format (crucially important; the camera must have TIFF capability)
   — USB connectivity
   — Battery source or charger
   — Weight (some digital cameras can be heavy)
   — Compatible lenses to use with the 35 mm camera
   — Easy-to-use software program
   — Photo-quality printer

4. **Polaroid camera**

   — Spectra Law Enforcement Kit

5. **Camera strap**

6. **Lenses**

   — 28-80 mm
   — 105-mm Micro lens
   — 120-mm Medical lens with ringlight flash

(continued)

Table 5-5. *(continued)*

7. **Flash**

   — TTL compatibility
   — Fast recycling time
   — Removable from camera body
   — Durable, lightweight, and uses regular batteries

8. **Flash cord**

9. **Tripod**

10. **Filters**

   — UV filter
   — #15 yellow filter for UV light fluorescent photography
   — #18 A red filter for reflective UV light photography

11. **Scales and labels**

   — 6-inch scales of various colors
   — ABFO ruler
   — Color guide scale
   — Micro scales
   — 18% gray scale
   — Identification label/card

12. **Film**

   — 100 ASA
   — 200 ASA
   — 400 ASA
   — Polaroid

13. **Extra batteries of all sizes**

14. **Camera cleaning cloth/solution (soft, satiny, washable cloth works well)**

15. **Sharpie magic marker (to label film and ID card)**

Reprinted with permission from Price B. Forensic photography. Paper presented at: Sexual Assault Nurse Examiner/Forensic Nursing Training Program; September 20, 2000 (updated 2002); Richmond, Va.

---

evidence in the form of disheveled clothing and aids in identifying the patient. The next photograph is called an orientation photograph. This orients the examiner to the location of the finding. Finally, a close-up picture, showing the greatest detail, is taken of the injury itself. The examiner obtains 2 of this type of photograph—one that contains a scale or ruler comparing the size of the wound and one of the injury without a scale (Ricci, 2001). In the case of multiple wounds, orientation and close-up photos are taken of each.

Forensic Colposcopic Photography

The colposcope has become an important tool in the forensic evaluation because it provides magnification and illumination of the genital area, assisting with injury identification and documentation. Colposcopy is a noninvasive technique that has a

Table 5-6. Key Points to Consider for Colposcopic Photography

— Remember depth of field. The colposcope has a limited depth of field. The colposcope should be no more than 10-12 inches from the subject. Most 35-mm pictures should be taken at 6X and 10X for the best depth of field and field of view.

— What you see in the monitor and through the scope is not what the 35-mm camera sees. Before snapping the picture, look through the viewfinder to ensure the subject is in focus and the field of view is correct. Remember to look through the camera with your dominant eye. The dominant eye is the one in which the best focus and clarity is seen.

— The higher the magnification, the more light is needed.

— In order to prevent premature blowing of the scope bulb, allow the fan to run for approximately 10 minutes. This gives the bulb and scope time to cool.

— Keep an extra bulb for the colposcope.

— Bracket each picture to allow for overexposure and underexposure.

— Remember to document the magnification level for each picture.

— Not all film is equal. The brand name of the film may affect the quality and color balance of the photograph.

— Photographs should contain an 18% gray scale with color guide in at least one picture per roll of film. These cards may be purchased through the Lightning Powder Company, Inc., at 1-800-852-0300. A pack of 25 cards costs $6.95 and these cards also serve as an ID label.

— When examining children, let them look through the scope or take a picture with the colposcope to alleviate anxiety.

— Store your film in the refrigerator to prolong shelf life.

— Practice with multiple test rolls to perfect this type of photgraphy. Test subjects could include fruit and flowers. Raw chicken also works especially well when practicing to photograph skin characteristics and tones.

Reprinted with permission from Price B. Forensic photography. Paper presented at: Sexual Assault Nurse Examiner/Forensic Nursing Training Program; September 20, 2000 (updated 2002); Richmond, Va.

high success rate for identifying genital trauma (Ledray, 1999) and clarifying tissue findings that are difficult to see with the eye alone (Finkel & DeJong, 2001). The colposcopic examination may be assisted with a 35-mm camera attachment or a video that allows recording of the tissues throughout the entire examination (Finkel & DeJong, 2001). (See Chapter 4, The Physical Examination in the Evaluation of Suspected Child Maltreatment: Physical Abuse and Sexual Abuse Examinations, for further discussion of a colposcopic examination.) (See **Table 5-6** for key points to consider for colposcopic photography.)

The examiner must be cognizant that not all types of photodocumentation may be allowed in court. Digital cameras are used in some localities and are beneficial for the documentation of findings, peer review, and medical consultations (McClain et al., 2000). However, digital photographs may not be permitted in all courts. Protocols should be established with the assistance of the local prosecutor regarding the type of photographic documentation that can be used as evidence in court.

Becoming adept at forensic photography requires much practice; however, with practice, the examiner can perfect the ability to obtain optimal photographs. Many practice rolls taken at various camera settings should be shot and reviewed. Exploring various techniques and attending photography classes are 2 ways to increase skills in this area. There is only one opportunity to document acute injuries, and it is important not to miss that chance.

It is essential to explain to the child that the examiner will take photographs of specific parts of the medical examination. The examiner can explain to the victim that he or she is the only one who should be able to take photographs of the child without clothing (Finkel & DeJong, 2001), and then assure the child that there are trusted people present who know this is being done for the child's well-being and protection. One should always respect that a child may not want to be photographed (Finkel & DeJong, 2001).

CHAIN OF CUSTODY

Chain of custody or chain of evidence begins with the person or persons who collect any physical evidence from the child and have control or custody of evidentiary material (Lynch, 1995). It is the examiner's responsibility to document that all pieces were collected and packaged properly and that the integrity of the contents was maintained. Once the evidence is collected, the examiner must release it to the proper authorities. The next person who handles or receives it must demonstrate the same. The release of any evidence requires documentation in the medical record or on specific chain of custody forms. This includes the evidence kit and extra bags containing clothing, film, and any instant photographs. Failure to maintain chain of custody renders potentially important evidence worthless (ACEP, 1999).

To complete the chain of custody properly, the examiner and collector of the evidence documents information regarding intact evidence seals, contents of the evidence kit, and the person to whom the kit is given. The following are guidelines for what information to document in the medical record (ACEP, 1999):

— Note all personnel involved in taking the history and physical examination.

— Document any person(s) who handled specimens.

— Record the name and identity of the officer to whom the kit is given.

— Include the agency to which the officer belongs.

— Note the date the kit is transferred to the officer.

— Make a comprehensive list of evidence collected.

LABORATORY TESTING OF EVIDENCE

The forensic laboratory scientist has the ultimate authority when it comes to evidence processing. The forensic scientist receives the evidence from law enforcement, which had in turn received evidence from medical personnel or other law enforcement persons. Evidence is then dispersed to the appropriate section within the laboratory. For example, items that are to be examined for possible body fluids followed by DNA testing will be processed in the forensic biology section.

DETECTING THE PRESENCE OF SEMINAL FLUID

Because a large number of cases submitted to a forensic laboratory (forensic biology section) for evaluation involve sex crimes, probative evidence (evidence associated most closely to the crime, such as underwear or bed linens) must be examined for the presence of seminal fluid and other body secretions. Preliminary testing or screening is necessary to identify potential body fluids on evidence that is present in the evidence kit or was submitted separately. This is a 3-step process. First, the stain must be located, which may be an arduous task considering the amount of evidence (bed linens, underwear, and other articles of clothing) that may be submitted to the laboratory. Seminal fluid stains may exhibit a stiff, off-white, crusty appearance. To rely only on the identification of fluids using the naked eye is undependable (Saferstein, 1990). Depending on the item of evidence, the scientist may choose to examine the item with an alternate light source. An ultraviolet light source or Wood's lamp is recommended as an aid to detect clothing or skin stains. Semen fluorescence lasts approximately 24 hours but can then be detected by more sensitive laboratory tests (Finkel & DeJong, 2001). Once a stain is detected, it is subjected to tests that will confirm its identity as seminal fluid. The third step involves the microscopic identification of sperm cells on smears made from swabs or in extracts made from stains. After locating a suspected semen stain, the forensic scientist tests for acid phosphatase, P30, and MJS-5 (Finkel & DeJong, 2001). Acid phosphatase is an enzyme secreted by the prostate gland into seminal fluid. The scientist cuts out a tiny area of the stain or swab and places a series of 2 chemicals, sodium alpha-naphthyl acid phosphatate and Fast Blue B dye, on the cutting. The appearance of a purple color is indicative of this enzyme (Saferstein, 1990). This test allows areas to be rapidly screened and then subjected to other testing (DeForest, Gaensslen, & Lee, 1983). Other samples, however, may mimic a positive test, including some vegetable juices, fungi, bacteria, contraceptive creams, and vaginal secretions. These substances do not react to the chemicals at the rate or color typical of seminal fluid. A reaction time of less than 30 seconds strongly indicates the presence of seminal fluid (Saferstein, 1990). The ability to detect acid phosphatase in a suspected semen sample depends on various factors and deteriorates over time. Acid phosphatase may not be detected even though seminal fluid is present (DeForest et al., 1983).

The second method of identifying seminal fluid is to microscopically identify sperm cells. Spermatazoa are microscopic elongated structures that have a head, midpiece, and tail. The forensic scientist places a small amount of the stained material on a glass microscope slide. A drop of water is applied to the slide, and the material is pulled apart. The slide is either viewed as a wet mount or dried and stained. Stains may be used to highlight the presence of the spermatozoa.

Sperm are fragile and disintegrate easily, as the head and tail separate over time. Seminal fluid may be present in body orifices while sperm may not because of various reasons, such as oligospermia (an abnormally low sperm count) or aspermia (no sperm at all) in the seminal fluid (Saferstein, 1990). Frequent ejaculation, some types of cancer, and certain cancer therapies also affect the number of sperm cells found in seminal fluid (Schiermeier, 1999). Sperm can be detected in clothing stains for many months because dried semen secretions are fairly stable (Christian & Giardino, 2002).

A P30 test may be used to identify seminal fluid in the absence of sperm. The test identifies semen glycoprotein found in large concentrations in seminal fluid (Crowley, 1999; Ferris & Sandercock, 1998). P30 is of prostatic origin and can be detected in the vasectomized and nonvasectomized man. However, to perform this test, the forensic scientist requires a greater amount of the stain or swab than is needed for either the acid phosphatase test or a sperm search. With advances in DNA testing, many forensic scientists forfeit this test and proceed with DNA analysis after a positive acid phosphatase test (Finkel & DeJong, 2001).

BLOOD AND SALIVA

Blood typing and secretor status are usually determined through the testing of blood and saliva samples. These do not identify the assailant but may exclude a suspect if the evidence does not demonstrate the same typology (A, B, or O status). Approximately 80% of the population are secretors, which means that their antigen types can be detected in their saliva and semen, as well as their blood (Ferris & Sandercock, 1998). This evidence allows investigators to state if the suspect's antigen type is in the same group as that of the assailant evidence.

DNA PROFILING

DNA testing is invaluable in both identifying and eliminating suspects. It provides the most accurate identification of a perpetrator for abuse when the evidence is properly collected and preserved for testing (Finkel & DeJong, 2001). DNA is the human genetic blueprint found in the nucleus of living cells and is specific in its makeup for each individual person. Blood, hair with tissue at the root, skin cells, muscle cells, and sperm cells contain DNA. Each person receives half of his or her DNA from the biological mother and half from the biological father. It is unique to all individuals except genetically identical twins. About 99% of human DNA is the same, while the remaining 1% makes each person different.

Forensic DNA testing that has been done commonly over the past 8 years is called polymerase chain reaction (PCR) testing. PCR testing is highly sensitive and requires only small amounts of material (Dimo-Simonin, Grange, & Brand-Casadevall, 1997). Once evidence is identified and swabbed from the victim, the forensic scientist begins DNA testing. The DNA is extracted from the swabs of the unknown samples and from the known blood samples of involved individuals. Amplification of the material evidence occurs next. Finally, DNA is placed on a gel and is separated on the gel by an electrical current. The location of the DNA on the gel determines the type. The scientist then compares all samples visually and with the aid of a computer program. As a result, someone may be included as a donor of a sample or may be eliminated. In the case of an inclusion, statistics are computed to determine how rarely or commonly the particular DNA profile is found in the population.

The use of DNA typing has major implications with respect to law enforcement investigations. At state forensic laboratories throughout the United States, scientists are creating a data bank or a database of DNA profiles. These profiles are from convicted felons (criteria for inclusion varies in each state). Once there, they remain indefinitely and are compared to each subsequent case that is submitted by law enforcement. Investigators may request the scientist compare DNA profiles in cases in which the identity of the suspect is unknown to the profiles included in the databank. If the unknown profile matches one in the data bank, this is referred to as a "cold hit." This technology has allowed for cases once thought unsolvable to be reopened and the suspect possibly identified. Law enforcement agencies are finding success and have brought many perpetrators to justice.

COLLECTING SAMPLES FOR SEXUALLY TRANSMITTED DISEASE TESTING

The presence of an STD may be the only evidence that sexual contact has occurred in some cases of child sexual abuse. Observation or signs and symptoms may make positive findings of an STD indicative of transmitted diseases; serological testing may either confirm observations or identify nonsymptomatic diseases. Therefore, it is important to collect samples and then to isolate the disease. Because STDs are identified through cultures and serological tests, collecting specimens properly to identify a particular infection is essential.

When to test the prepubertal child for STDs is controversial, so guidelines are helpful concerning when to collect specimens. Specimen collection may be traumatic for the child and an unnecessary expense when testing is done indiscriminately. The clinician decides whether or not to collect specimens, along with choosing a particular site (oral, anal, vaginal, penile, or conjunctival), on an individual basis in conjunction with the facility's established protocols. Baseline testing is recommended under the following circumstances (Britton & Hansen, 1997; Ledray, 1999; McClain et al., 2000):

— The child is symptomatic.

— The suspected offender is known to have an STD or be at a high risk for one.

— The suspect has had multiple partners or a past history of an STD.

— There is a history of forced sexual assault, genital-to-genital contact, or
  possible ejaculation.

— There is evidence that suggests penetration has occurred.

— Another household member is known to have an STD.

— There is a high prevalence of STDs in the community.

GONORRHEA

A gonococcal infection in the prepubertal child typically manifests as a purulent vulvovaginitis as opposed to a cervicitis in the adolescent and adult. A Gram's stain of the discharge may show polymorphonuclear leukocytes and gram-negative intracellular diplococci. For a postpubertal, mature adolescent and adult, it is acceptable for the examiner to use either a DNA probe or a culture to screen for gonorrhea. These samples are obtained from the endocervical area. A cotton swab is inserted into the cervical os and turned several times to lift cells. The DNA probe is sent directly to the laboratory. Culture mediums must be streaked immediately after sample collection. The use of the Thayer-Martin plate requires direct transport to the bacteriology laboratory and incubation under increased carbon dioxide tension. If using the Thayer-Martin medium, the examiner inserts a carbon dioxide-generating tablet into the well of the plastic case after the sample is applied. It may be transported after an incubation of 24 to 48 hours to the laboratory (Emans et al., 1998).

In the prepubertal child, the use of Gram's stain smears alone and DNA probes is contraindicated. These nonculture techniques lack specificity and often yield false positive results (Britton & Hansen, 1997; Brodeur & Monteleone, 1994). Obtaining cervical cultures is not indicated in the prepubertal child. Vaginal samples are sufficient because gonorrhea will grow in the vaginal epithelium secondary to a neutral pH. The vaginal pH of a pubertal adolescent is acidic, and the bacteria cannot survive in this environment (Emans et al., 1998).

To gather samples from this population, the examiner gently swabs the vaginal lining. The technique of anterior labial traction is used to visualize the hymenal opening. Then a small cotton swab is passed through the opening, and vaginal samples are taken and streaked onto the culture medium. Repeat testing should occur in 2 weeks. All positive cultures must be identified by at least 2 tests that involve different principles (biochemical, enzyme substrate, or serological) to ensure specificity (Centers for Disease Control and Prevention [CDC], 1998). Only confirmed results are accepted as legal proof in court.

When collecting samples from additional sites (oral, anal, or conjunctival), the examiner must use culture media. The Food and Drug Administration (FDA) has not approved the use of DNA probes for any site other than the cervix and penis (CDC, 1998).

CHLAMYDIA

Sexual abuse must be considered in children who test positive for a chlamydial infection. However, *Chlamydia* organisms may be transmitted perinatally, which is usually manifested by neonatal conjunctivitis or pneumonia. If a child has a positive result, vertical transmission (transmission during the birth process) must be ruled out. Up to 45% of those infected with gonorrhea are also infected with chlamydia (Anderson, 1995). When testing for gonorrhea, the examiner should also collect specimens for chlamydia.

There are several detection methods for chlamydia: cultures, direct immunofluorescent smears, enzyme immunoassays (Chlamydiazyme), ligase chain reaction (LCR), PCR, and transcription-mediated amplification (TMA). Urine screening is possible with the new LCR, PCR, and TMA technologies (Emans et al., 1998). This is a non-invasive way to screen for the infection. The more invasive means includes collecting endocervical cells for adults and adolescents. The prepubertal child requires that vaginal samples be taken (by the same means as swabs taken for gonorrhea cultures) and placed immediately in the culture medium.

Even though there are many methods, nonculture tests for chlamydia in the child abuse examination are not to be used because of the possibility of false positive results. There may be a cross-reaction of test reagents with chlamydia pneumoniae, genital and anal specimens, and fecal flora (Britton & Hansen, 1997; CDC, 1998; McClain et al., 2000). However, in a study by Matthews-Greer, Sloop, Springer, McRae, LaHaye, and Jamison (1999), the detection of chlamydia by PCR testing is comparable to that of the culture. More research is needed for this type of testing to become acceptable in courts of law, and at this point, culture remains the gold standard for detecting chlamydia in child sexual abuse evaluations.

HERPES SIMPLEX

After the neonatal period, the presence of herpes lesions suggests sexual abuse. The lesions must be confirmed by culture. The best diagnostic technique is the viral culture (Emans et al., 1998). The virus grows rapidly, and a definitive diagnosis (herpes simplex type 1 or herpes simplex type 2) can be made within a few days.

Samples must be taken from an unroofed lesion. The examiner scrapes the top of the lesion. Then a cotton swab is used to obtain a good sample of the contents that have been exposed. The culture is sent directly to the laboratory for processing. (See Chapter 6, Sexually Transmitted Diseases in the Setting of Maltreatment, for more information regarding symptoms and treatment.)

SEROLOGY TESTING

In children suspected of having been sexually abused and in whom there is a risk for infection, blood samples should be obtained for syphilis, hepatitis B, and human immunodeficiency virus (HIV). While collecting blood for these tests, the examiner draws extra tubes for DNA testing in case this is an acute examination or a chronic examination conducted under anesthesia. Syphilis serology should be repeated in 6 to 8 weeks and HIV in 3 months and again in 6 months (Ledray, 1999). (See Chapter 6, Sexually Transmitted Diseases in the Setting of Maltreatment, for HIV prophylaxis.)

CONCLUSION

STD testing and evidence collection share the fact that if the samples are not collected properly, they are useless. The examiner must test for STDs when there is a suspicion or according to established protocols. Evidentiary specimens should be obtained in the event of an acute assault (less than 72 hours) or if the examiner suspects the presence of biological evidence. Competency is important in the identification, collection, and preservation of evidence so that it may undergo DNA testing to identify a perpetrator. Chain of custody issues must be addressed as well. If the chain is not maintained, potential evidence may not be admitted into the courtroom and the guilty may go free.

APPENDIX: EVIDENCE COLLECTION AND FORENSIC PHOTOGRAPHY
Diana K. Faugno, RN, BSN, CPN, FAAFS, SANE-A/A

COMPONENTS OF AN EVIDENCE COLLECTION KIT

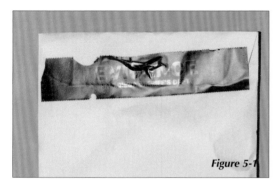

Figure 5-1.

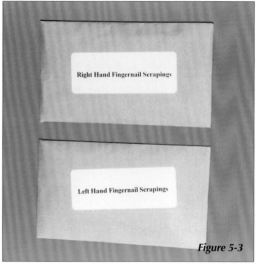

Right Hand Fingernail Scrapings

Left Hand Fingernail Scrapings

Figure 5-3

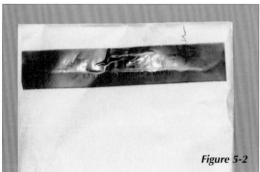

Figure 5-2

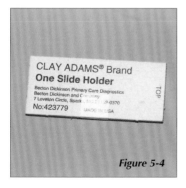

CLAY ADAMS® Brand
One Slide Holder

Becton Dickinson Primary Care Diagnostics
Becton Dickinson and Company
7 Loveton Circle, Sparks, MD 21152-0370

No:423779   MADE IN USA

TCP

Figure 5-4

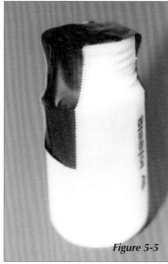

Figure 5-5

Figure 5-1. *Improperly sealed envelope (no name, date, or time).*

Figure 5-2. *Properly sealed envelope (includes name, date, and time).*

Figure 5-3. *Envelopes for fingernail scrapings.*

Figure 5-4. *Slide holder.*

Figure 5-5. *Improperly sealed urine container (no initials on the seal or bottle).*

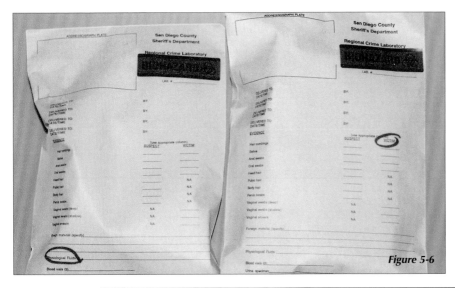

Figure 5-6.
Envelopes before use.

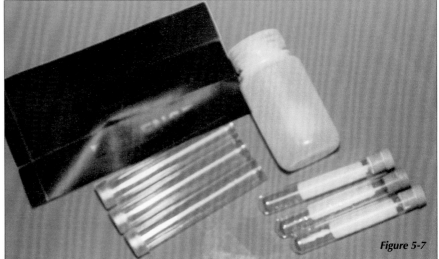

Figure 5-7.
Contents of left envelope in Figure 5-6.

Figure 5-8.
Contents of right envelope in Figure 5-6.

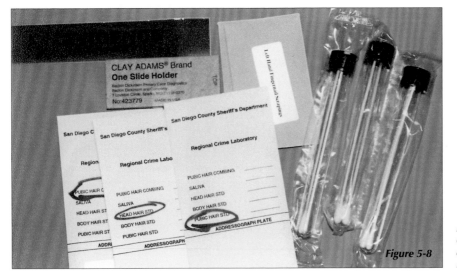

How to Separate the Labia by Applying Traction

Figure 5-9. *Separate the labia by using the left hand to apply traction on each buttock. The vestibule is opened by downward and outward traction.*

Figure 5-10. *Labial separation.*

Figure 5-11. *A closer view of labial separation.*

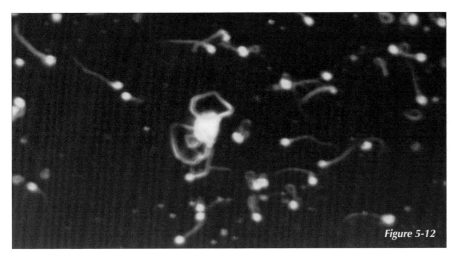

Figure 5-9

Figure 5-10

Figure 5-11

The Identification of Motile Sperm

Figure 5-12

Figure 5-12. *Identifying motile sperm by using a light-staining microscope.*

155

EXAMPLES OF FORENSIC PHOTOGRAPHY

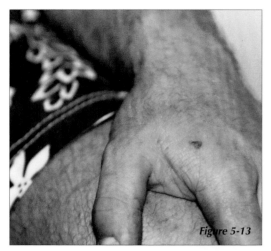

Figure 5-13.
Injury without a color scale.

Figure 5-14.
Injury with a color scale.

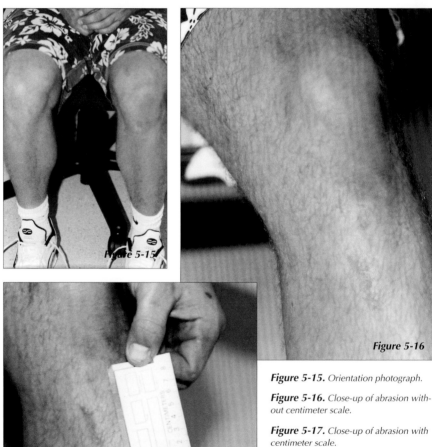

Figure 5-15. *Orientation photograph.*

Figure 5-16. *Close-up of abrasion without centimeter scale.*

Figure 5-17. *Close-up of abrasion with centimeter scale.*

REFERENCES

American College of Emergency Physicians. *Evaluation and Management of the Sexually Assaulted or Sexually Abused Patient.* Dallas, Tex: US Dept of Health & Human Services; 1999:7-8, 121.

Anderson C. Childhood sexually transmitted diseases: one consequence of sexual abuse. *Public Health Nurs.* 1995;12:41-46.

Auvdel M. Comparison of laser and ultraviolet techniques used in the detection of body secretions. *J Forensic Sci.* 1987;32:326-345.

Auvdel M. Comparison of laser and high-intensity quartz arc tubes in the detection of body secretions. *J Forensic Sci.* 1988;33:929-945.

Barsley R, West M, Fair J. Forensic photography: ultraviolet imaging of wounds on skin. *Am J Forensic Med Pathol.* 1990:11:300-308.

Berenson A, Chacko M, Wiemann C, Mishaw C, Freidrich W, Grady J. A case-control study of anatomic changes resulting from sexual abuse. *Am J Obstet Gynecol.* 2000;182:820-834.

Botash A. Examination for sexual abuse in prepubertal children: an update. *Pediatr Ann.* 1997;26:312-320.

Britton H, Hansen K. Sexual abuse. *Clin Obstet Gynecol.* 1997;40:226-240.

Brodeur A, Monteleone J. *Child Maltreatment: A Clinical Guide and Reference.* St. Louis, Mo: GW Medical Publishing; 1994.

Centers for Disease Control and Prevention. Guidelines for treatment of sexually transmitted diseases. *MMWR.* 1998;47(No RR-1):1-17.

Christian C, Giardino A. Forensic evidence collection. In: Finkel M, Giardino A, eds. *Medical Evaluation of Child Sexual Abuse: A Practical Guide.* 2nd ed. Thousand Oaks, Calif: Sage Publications; 2002:131-145.

Christian C, Lavelle J, De Jong A, Loiselle J, Brenner L, Joffe M. Forensic evidence findings in prepubertal victims of sexual assault. *Pediatrics.* 2000;106:100-104.

Crowley S. *Sexual Assault: The Medical-Legal Examination.* Stamford, Conn: Appleton and Lange; 1999:109.

DeForest P, Gaensslen R, Lee H. *Forensic Science: An Introduction to Criminalistics.* 4th ed. New York, NY: McGraw-Hill; 1983:265-277.

Dimo-Simonin N, Grange F, Brand-Casadevall C. PCR-based forensic testing of DNA from stained cytological smears. *J Forensic Sci.* 1997;42:506-509.

Emans S, Laufer M, Goldstein D. *Pediatric and Adolescent Gynecology.* 4th ed. Philadelphia, Pa: Lippincott Williams & Wilkins; 1998:16, 37, 458-460, 467-472, 761-762, 778-787.

Emergency Nurses Association. Emergency Nurses Association position statement. Forensic evidence collection. *J Emerg Nurs.* 1998;24:38A.

Ferris LE, Sandercock J. The sensitivity of forensic tests for rape. *Med Law.* 1998;17:333-350.

Finkel M. The evaluation. In: Finkel M, Giardino A, eds. *Medical Evaluation of Child Sexual Abuse: A Practical Guide.* 2nd ed. Thousand Oaks, Calif: Sage Publications; 2002:23-37.

Finkel M, DeJong A. Medical findings in child sexual abuse. In: Reece R, Ludwig S, eds. *Child Abuse: Medical Diagnosis and Management.* 2nd ed. Philadelphia, Pa: Lippincott Williams & Wilkins; 2001:207-286.

Golden G. Forensic photography: an expanding technology. *J Calif Dental Assoc.* 1996;24:50-56.

Heger A, Emans S, Muram D. *Evaluation of the Sexually Abused Child.* New York, NY: Oxford University Press; 2000:85.

International Association of Forensic Nurses. *Scope and Standards of Forensic Nursing Practice.* Washington, DC: American Nurses Association; 1997:2.

Kini N, Brady W, Lazoritz S. Evaluating child sexual abuse in the emergency department. *Acad Emerg Med.* 1996;3:966-976.

Ledray L. DNA evidence collection. *J Emerg Nurs.* 1997;23:156-158.

Ledray L. *Sexual Assault Nurse Examiner Development and Operation Guide.* Washington, DC: US Dept of Justice, Office for Victims of Crime; 1999.

Lynch V. Clinical forensic nursing: a new perspective in the management of crime victims from trauma to trial. *Crit Care Nurs Clin North Am.* 1995;7:489-507.

Matthews-Greer J, Sloop G, Springer A, McRae K, LaHaye W, Jamison R. Comparison of detection methods for *Chlamydia trachomatis* in specimens obtained from pediatric victims of suspected sexual abuse. *Pediatr Infect Dis J.* 1999;18:165-167.

McClain N, Girardet R, Lahoti S, Cheung K, Berger K, McNeese M. Evaluation of sexual abuse in the pediatric patient. *J Pediatr Health Care.* 2000;14:93-102.

O'Brien C. Light staining microscope: clinical experience in a sexual assault nurse examiner (SANE) program. *J Emerg Nurs.* 1998;24:95-97.

Price B. Forensic photography. Paper presented at: Sexual Assault Nurse Examiner/Forensic Nursing Training Program; September 20, 2000 (updated 2002); Richmond, Va.

Ricci L. Photodocumentation of the abused child. In: Reece R, Ludwig S, eds. *Child Abuse: Medical Diagnosis and Management.* 2nd ed. Philadelphia, Pa: Lippincott Williams & Wilkins; 2001:385-404.

Saferstein R. *Criminalistics: An Introduction to Forensic Science.* 4th ed. Upper Saddle River, NJ: Prentice Hall; 1990:333-339.

Schiermeier L. DNA and the PERK. Lecture handout presented at: Sexual Assault Nurse Examiner/Forensic Nursing Training Program; 1999; Richmond, Va.

Sweet D, Lorente M, Lorente J, Valunzuela A, Villanueva E. An improved method to recover saliva from human skin: the double swab technique. *J Forensic Sci.* 1997;42:320-322.

Sweet D, Pretty I. A look at forensic dentistry. Part 2: teeth as weapons of violence. *Br Dent J.* 2001;190:415-418.

Tucker S, Ledray L, Werner J. Sexual assault evidence collection. *Wis Med J.* 1990;89:407-411.

Chapter 6

SEXUALLY TRANSMITTED DISEASES IN THE SETTING OF MALTREATMENT

Marisa V. Atendido, MSN, CRNP
Angelo P. Giardino, MD, PhD, FAAP

An important component of the healthcare evaluation for suspected sexual abuse or sexual assault in the prepubertal child and the adolescent includes identifying the presence of sexually transmitted diseases (STDs) in the child or adolescent being evaluated. The American Academy of Pediatrics (AAP, 1999) and the Centers for Disease Control and Prevention (CDC, 1998, 2002) issued guidelines to assist the clinician in deciding what circumstances warrant the evaluation of children and adolescents for STDs during the suspected sexual abuse or assault evaluation. In some cases, the STD may be the presenting indicator of abuse, whereas in other cases the presence of an STD may serve to confirm the child's history of inappropriate contact. Estimates vary, but 3% to 13% of children evaluated for the presence of STDs will test positive for the organisms that cause these infections (Gardner, 1992; Ingram, Everett, Lyna, White, & Rockwell, 1992; Robinson, Watkeys, & Ridgway, 1998; White, Loda, Ingram, & Pearson, 1983). The thinking around STD screening in the setting of sexual maltreatment has evolved over the past decades as our collective professional experience has increased through working with children and adolescents being evaluated for this problem. For example, automatic screening of all prepubertal children suspected of having been sexually abused is no longer the standard of care; rather, a more thoughtful approach that considers symptomatology and level of risk for STDs in the actual clinical situation before the healthcare professional is indicated (Sirotnak, 1994). It is still important to consider screening for STDs in appropriate clinical situations, however, because the organisms responsible may be transmitted during sexually abusive contact.

This chapter provides a framework from which the nurse evaluator can consider whom to screen for which STDs in the context of a healthcare evaluation for suspected sexual abuse or assault in the prepubertal child and the adolescent. The chapter focuses on several STDs the clinician should consider when caring for those suspected of having been sexually maltreated, realizing that in this setting, legal or forensic implications exist as well. (See Chapter 5, Laboratory Findings, Diagnostic Testing, and Forensic Specimens in Cases of Child Sexual Abuse, for a description of forensic aspects of the evaluation.) The specific infections (in alphabetical order) are as follows:

— Bacterial vaginosis (BV)

— Chlamydia

— Gonorrhea

— Hepatitis B virus (HBV)

— Herpes simplex virus (HSV)

— Human immunodeficiency virus/acquired immunodeficiency syndrome (HIV/AIDS)

— Human papillomavirus (HPV, condyloma acuminata, or genital warts)

— Pediculosis pubis

— Pelvic inflammatory disease (PID)

— Syphilis

— Trichomoniasis

Each infection is discussed individually because it has its own characteristics of clinical presentation, diagnosis, and treatment. (See **Table 6-1** for the incidence of each infection in populations of sexually abused children.) The likelihood of a given infection being an indicator of sexual abuse in prepubertal children and nonsexually active adolescents varies and is addressed in the AAP (1999) guidelines on evaluating sexual abuse **(Table 6-2)**.

Other less common STDs that will not be discussed but that may need to be considered in the differential diagnosis of genital findings include chancroid, lymphogranuloma venereum (LGV), and highly contagious skin diseases, such as scabies and molluscum contagiosum **(Figures 6-1 to 6-13)**. These clinical entities should be considered when the clinical presentation is atypical and the more typical infectious diseases have been eliminated or ruled out.

Screening for STDs occurs in the context of a physical examination. Prepubertal children and adolescents may experience anxieties about the impending examination. The clinician should take time and use a gradual and sensitive approach with the patient before and during the examination, telling the patient what to expect and allowing an opportunity for questions (Sirotnak, 1994). (See Chapter 4, The Physical Examination in the Evaluation of Suspected Child Maltreatment: Physical Abuse and Sexual Abuse Examinations, for a description of the physical examination.)

There are important clinical issues to consider when evaluating the risk that a child or adolescent may have acquired an STD from sexually abusive contact. Hammerschlag (1998a, 1998b) has synthesized the clinical material in this complicated area and summarizes each issue as follows:

1. The possibility of vertical transmission (from mother to child during birth) and the extent to which vertical transmission can be used to explain an STD (e.g., prolonged colonization after perinatal acquisition)

2. The regional variation of STDs in the adult population (potential perpetrators) and the observation that variation may exist among different populations within the same region

3. Timing of examination related to time of suspected contact and the range of incubation periods and symptom presentation; *Neisseria gonorrhoeae*, for example, is several days, whereas for HPV it is several months to years

4. Controversy concerning symptomatic versus asymptomatic infection, especially in the setting of a prepubertal child

5. Inability to differentiate preexisting infections that may be related to prior sexual activity in adults and sexually active adolescents

Table 6-1. Incubation Periods, Clinical Manifestations, Transmission, and Diagnosis of STDs *

	Gonorrhea *Neisseria gonorrhoeae*	**Chlamydial infections** *Chlamydia trachomatis*
INCUBATION PERIOD	3-5 days	5-7 days
CLINICAL MANIFESTATIONS	— Vaginitis, urethritis, pharyngitis, proctitis — Rare: arthritis, conjunctivitis — Most pharyngeal (throat) and rectal infections and as many as 50% of vaginal infections in children may be asymptomatic	— Most prevalent sexually transmitted infection in the United States — In adults and adolescents: urethritis and mucopurulent cervicitis, which can lead to pelvic inflammatory disease; however, most infections in adults and children are asymptomatic
TRANSMISSION	— Through sexual contact — Exception: neonatal conjunctivitis is acquired by the infant from his/her mother at delivery — No evidence of transmission by fomites (e.g., via toilet seats, "dirty" towels)	— Sexually, in children 3 years of age or older — Perinatally acquired infection (mother-to-infant) may last in the vagina and rectum for up to 3 years or longer — No evidence of transmission by fomites
DIAGNOSIS	— Culture of *N. gonorrhoeae* using selective media with confirmation by at least 2 different methods using different principles (e.g., sugar fermentation, enzyme substances, serological or DNA hybridization) — Use of DNA probes or other nonculture methods, including Gram's stain smears or vaginal or urethral discharges, is not recommended because other bacteria may be misidentified as *N. gonorrhoeae*	— Isolation of the organism in tissue culture only with microscopic identification of the characteristic inclusions with fluorescent antibody staining — Nonculture methods, including enzyme immunoassays (EIAs), direct fluorescent antibody (DFA) tests, and DNA probes, are not approved for use in children. Use at these sites has led to many false positive tests.
PREVALENCE RANGE IN CHILDREN EVALUATED FOR SEXUAL ABUSE †	1%-2.8%	0.5%-1.3%
PREVALENCE RANGE FOR WOMEN EVALUATED FOR SEXUAL ASSAULTS ‡	0-26.3%	3.9%-17%

(continued)

Table 6-1. *(continued)*		
	Syphilis *Treponema pallidum*	**Trichomoniasis** *Trichomonas vaginalis*
INCUBATION PERIOD	— Primary infection: 10-90 days, usually 3-4 weeks — Secondary: 6 weeks-6 months after the primary lesion heals	5-28 days
CLINICAL MANIFESTATIONS	— Primary syphilis: chancre— a painless ulcer at the site of inoculation (e.g., penis, vulva, vagina, rectum). The chancre heals spontaneously after 1-2 weeks. — Secondary syphilis: diffuse rash, fever, enlarged lymph nodes, mucous patches — Latent syphilis: asymptomatic, although positive serological findings may persist for years	— Vaginitis — In males, infection appears to be asymptomatic, but *T. vaginalis* may cause some cases of nonspecific urethritis
TRANSMISSION	— Through sexual contact. The chancre and mucous patches are very infectious. — Infants may acquire congenital syphilis from their mothers. The presentation is similar to secondary syphilis.	— Through sexual contact — Has not been found in children 1 year of age or older without history of sexual contact — Infants can acquire infection from mother at delivery; can cause vaginitis — Perinatally acquired infection may persist for 6-9 months after birth — No evidence of transmission by fomites

(continued)

6. Extent to which infections in the prepubertal child and nonsexually active adolescent may be related to inadvertent nonsexual spread (if such spread is possible), sexual exploration with age-mates, and prior sexual abuse (Hammerschlag, 1998a, 1998b)

Challenging issues exist regarding adolescents suspected of having been sexually maltreated who have STDs after such contact. These are related to characteristics seen in the pubertal and postpubertal populations, such as the following:

— Determining interim consensual sexual behaviors of the affected adolescent

— Poor follow-up among sexual assault victims who are taking STD treatments (Vemillion, Holmes, & Soper, 2000)

Table 6-1. *(continued)*

	Syphilis *Treponema pallidum*	**Trichomoniasis** *Trichomonas vaginalis*
DIAGNOSIS	— Identification of *T. pallidum* in lesions by dark-field microscopy or by staining with fluorescein-conjugated monoclonal antibody — The most common methods used are serological: rapid plasma reagin (RPR) test; Venereal Disease Research Laboratory (VDRL) reaginic antibody test; and fluorescent treponemal antibody absorption (FTA-ABS) test, a test for a specific anti-*T. pallidum* antibody — Positive results on an RPR or VDRL test in a child who does not have a history of congenital syphilis — RPR and VDRL test results will be negative after effective treatment; FTA-ABS remains elevated for the lifetime of the patient	— Microscopic identification of the organism in vaginal fluid — Culture methods may be more sensitive, but not widely available — The finding of trichomonads in urine collected for another purpose is not sufficient for accurate diagnosis because the urine could be contaminated with *Trichomonas hominis*, a normal inhabitant of the bowel that is not sexually transmitted
PREVALENCE RANGE IN CHILDREN EVALUATED FOR SEXUAL ABUSE†	0.15%-1.5%	0.5%-2.5%
PREVALENCE RANGE FOR WOMEN EVALUATED FOR SEXUAL ASSAULTS‡	0-5.6%	0-19%

(continued)

Although these challenges exist, there is a clear need for the identification and treatment of sexually acquired infections, particularly those acquired as a result of abuse. The CDC (1998) recognizes this as more important for the physical and psychological well-being of the adolescent victim than for actual legal considerations. The CDC and AAP have issued guidelines for clinicians who evaluate adolescent victims of sexual abuse. These include information about the initial examination, follow-up examinations, and the need for prophylaxis **(Table 6-3)**.

The first step in clinically assessing patients for STDs is to ask questions during the history-taking process about specific symptoms that may suggest the presence of an STD. It is essential to have a direct, yet sensitive, approach to asking questions because the trauma of sexual abuse/assault can make the child, family, and adolescent uncomfortable.

Table 6-1. *(continued)*		
	Bacterial vaginosis (BV) *Gardnerella vaginalis, Bacteroides* species and other anaerobic bacteria, and *Mycoplasma hominis*	**Herpes** Herpes simplex virus (HSV), types 1 and 2
INCUBATION PERIOD	5-28 days	2-5 days
CLINICAL MANIFESTATIONS	— BV is not really an infection, but a disturbance of the normal vaginal flora, which is replaced by the organisms listed — Clinically presents as gray, foul-smelling vaginal discharge, but may be asymptomatic	— Painful vesicular lesions that become ulcers on the vulva, vagina, penis, and perirectal area — May be associated with inguinal lymphadenopathy (disease of the lymph nodes in the groin) and fever
TRANSMISSION	— Through sexual and nonsexual contact — Probably related to poor hygiene in some young children	— Through sexual contact — Primarily HSV-2, although 10% of genital herpes in adults can be due to HSV-1 — Young children with herpetic gingivostomatitis (herpetic infection of the gum tissues), a primary, nonsexually acquired infection caused by HSV-1, may autoinoculate (infect themselves) in the genital area. There should be a history of stomatitis (sores in the mouth) in the previous 2 weeks.

(continued)

WHEN TO TEST FOR STDS IN THE SETTING OF SUSPECTED MALTREATMENT

All children are not automatically tested for STDs during the sexual abuse evaluation. The likelihood of positive cultures for gonorrhea and chlamydial infection is very low in prepubertal children who have been asymptomatic before the examination, as well as in children who only report a history of fondling (AAP, 1999; Shapiro, Schubert, & Myers, 1993; Siegel, Schubert, Myers, & Shapiro, 1995). There is a relatively low incidence of STDs in children suspected of having been sexually abused, and STD testing in children is uncomfortable and costly (Siegel et al., 1995). Therefore, limiting STD testing to the most appropriate clinical scenarios is desirable.

Table 6-1. *(continued)*		
	Bacterial vaginosis (BV) *Gardnerella vaginalis, Bacteroides* species and other anaerobic bacteria, and *Mycoplasma hominis*	**Herpes** Herpes simplex virus (HSV), types 1 and 2
DIAGNOSIS	— Microscopic identification of "clue cells," which are epithelial cells studded with bacteria in vaginal secretions; a positive "whiff" or amine test, which is the release of a characteristic fishy odor when 10% potassium hydroxide (KOH) is added to the vaginal fluid; and a vaginal fluid pH of >4.5 — The latter test should only be done in adolescents, as there are no vaginal pH standards for prepubertal children — Culture of *G. vaginalis* is not indicated and is not diagnostic for BV. *G. vaginalis* can be normal vaginal flora and has been isolated in 5%-15% of normal children who have not been abused.	— Isolation of the virus from the lesions — No commercially available antibody tests will reliably differentiate between HSV-1 and HSV-2
PREVALENCE RANGE IN CHILDREN EVALUATED FOR SEXUAL ABUSE†	7%§	0.1%-0.5%
PREVALENCE RANGE FOR WOMEN EVALUATED FOR SEXUAL ASSAULTS	10%-64%‖	Not available

(continued)

The AAP (1999) recommends the following considerations to decide when to test prepubertal children for STDs:

1. The possibility of oral, genital, or rectal contact with infected secretions from the perpetrator

2. Local incidence of STDs in the adult population

3. Evidence of symptoms

The CDC (1998) advises that the decision to test prepubertal children for STDs in the sexual abuse evaluation should be made on a case-by-case basis and individualized based on risk **(Table 6-4)**. Indicators for testing according to CDC guidelines include the following:

Table 6-1. *(continued)*

	Human papillomavirus (HPV) Condyloma acuminata, venereal warts	**AIDS** Human immunodeficiency virus (HIV)
INCUBATION PERIOD	4-12 weeks, but may be clinically inapparent for up to 18 months	Seroconversion: 6 weeks after exposure; more than 90% of individuals will be HIV positive by 6 months. Development of AIDS: 5-10 years.
CLINICAL MANIFESTATIONS	— Flesh- to purple-colored papillomatous growths in the anogenital region	— Children who are HIV positive before developing AIDS are asymptomatic — Some individuals develop an acute retroviral syndrome, similar to influenza, with lymphadenopathy after infection — Has not been described in children with acquired HIV infection
TRANSMISSION	— Sexually, perinatally, and probably, but rarely, nonsexually — Major confounding variable is the long period after infection before the lesions become visible to the naked eye, which could be as long as 18 months	— Sexually, perinatally, and via blood transfusion, intravenous drug abuse (IVDA), and sharing needles — Approximately 30% of infants born to HIV-positive mothers will develop HIV infection but may not develop clinical AIDS for 5 years or longer — Acquisition by sexual abuse needs to be differentiated from perinatal infection because risk factors for maternal infection and sexual abuse are similar
DIAGNOSIS	— Clinical. HPV DNA-typing of the lesions is not generally available.	— Serological: presence of HIV antibody, detection of p24 antigen. Child being evaluated for HIV after abuse needs to be tested for 6 months. Consider HIV testing if the child is from an area of high HIV prevalence, if the abuser is in a high-risk group (e.g., IVDA, crack user), or if another STD is present.

(continued)

Table 6-1. *(continued)*

	Human papillomavirus (HPV) Condyloma acuminata, venereal warts	**AIDS** Human immunodeficiency virus (HIV)
PREVALENCE RANGE IN CHILDREN EVALUATED FOR SEXUAL ABUSE †	0.7%-1.8%	Not available
PREVALENCE RANGE FOR WOMEN EVALUATED FOR SEXUAL ASSAULTS‡	0.6%-2.3%	Not available

Reprinted from Hammerschlag MR. Sexually Transmitted Diseases and Child Abuse: Portable Guides to Investigating Child Abuse. Washington, DC: US Dept of Justice, Office of Justice Programs and Office of Juvenile Justice and Delinquency Preventions; 1996 (fourth printing, December 2002). NCJ160940.

†*Gardner JJ. Comparison of the vaginal flora in sexually abused and nonabused girls. J Pediatr. 1992;120:872-877; Robinson AJ, Watkeys JE, Ridgway GL. Sexually transmitted organisms in sexually abused children. Arch Dis Child. 1998;79:356-358; Ingram DL, Everett VD, Lyna PR, White ST, Rockwell LA. Epidemiology of adult sexually transmitted disease agents in children being evaluated for sexual abuse. Pediatr Infect Dis J. 1992;11:945-950; Schwarcz SK, Whittington WL. Sexual assault and sexually transmitted disease: detection and management in adults and children. Rev Infect Dis. 1990;12:S682-S690; White ST, Loda FA, Ingram DL, Pearson A. Sexually transmitted disease in sexually abused children. Pediatrics. 1983;72:16-21.*

‡*Reynolds MW, Peipert JF, Collins B. Epidemiologic issues of sexually transmitted diseases in sexual assault victims. Obstet Gynecol Surv. 2000;55:51-57.*

§*Difficult to quantify because the presence of G. vaginalis alone is not diagnostic of BV.*

‖*ACOG technical bulletin. Vaginitis. Number 226—July 1996 (replaces No. 221, March 1996). Committee on Technical Bulletins of the American College of Obstetricians and Gynecologists. Int J Gynaecol Obstet. 1996;54:293-302; Girardin BW, Faugno DK, Seneski PC, Slaughter L, Whelan M. Color Atlas of Sexual Assault. St. Louis, Mo: Mosby; 1997.*

— Suspected offender is known to have an STD or be at high risk for STDs

— Child has symptoms or signs of an STD

— Prevalence of STDs is high in the community

— Evidence or suspicion of anogenital or oral penetration or ejaculation

— STDs in siblings or other children (or adults) in the household

ASYMPTOMATIC VERSUS SYMPTOMATIC INFECTIONS

The prepubertal child and adolescent differ anatomically, physiologically, and with regard to the transmission, presentation, and the best means of identification of STDs (Wald, 1984). **Table 6-5** lists differences between female children and adults that affect the identification of STDs. Controversy exists as to how common asymptomatic infections are in prepubertal children versus adolescents, and some of the differences seen in frequency of asymptomatic infections between these 2 groups result from the anatomical and physiological differences that follow puberty. With regard to STDs, asymptomatic infections are more common in the adolescent than the prepubertal child.

Symptoms of STDs in the prepubertal child vary and manifest in several ways. Symptoms include vaginal or urethral discharge; genital itching and irritation, such as vulvovaginitis or urethritis; and genital lesions and growths, depending on the specific etiology. Asymptomatic genital infections have been observed to be uncommon in prepubertal children.

Table 6-2. Implications of Commonly Encountered STDs for the Diagnosis of Sexual Abuse			
	DIAGNOSTIC	HIGHLY SUSPICIOUS	SUSPICIOUS
Confirmed STD organism	Gonorrhea* Syphilis* HIV† Chlamydia*	*Trichomonas vaginalis*	Condyloma acuminata (anogenital warts) Herpes‡ (genital location)

*If not perinatally acquired.

†If not perinatally or transfusion acquired.

‡Unless there is a clear history of autoinoculation. Herpes virus types 1 and 2 are difficult to differentiate by current techniques.

Adapted from American Academy of Pediatrics Committee on Child Abuse and Neglect. Guidelines for the evaluation of sexual abuse of children: subject review (RE9819). Pediatrics. 1999;103:186-191.

In the adolescent patient, however, STDs are often asymptomatic. When symptomatic, the adolescent patient may experience vaginal discharge of varying colors and quantities, irregular bleeding, itching and/or irritation in the genital area, genital lesions or growths, a nonspecific odor, generalized urinary complaints, and mild to severe pain in the vagina or lower abdomen. Adolescent males are more likely to complain of dysuria, particularly burning on urination, urethral discharge, and genital lesions or growths. In females and males, genital lesions may be painless or extremely painful depending on the etiology.

In addition to genital complaints resulting from the presence of STDs, problems with the perianal area and rectum in prepubertal children and adolescents are possible depending on the type of sexual contact and the infecting organism involved. The presence of symptoms such as anorectal pain, tenesmus, and rectal discharge suggest the existence of proctitis (CDC, 1998).

SPECIFIC INFECTIONS

BACTERIAL VAGINOSIS

General Overview and Epidemiology

Bacterial vaginosis (BV) is a heterogeneous clinical entity marked by a disorder of vaginal flora that represents a polymicrobial syndrome in which several bacterial species interact to alter the vaginal ecosystem (Benrubi, 1999; Hammerschlag, 1998b). A shift in the ecosystem leads to a decrease in lactobacilli, usually predominant in the vagina, and an increase in anaerobes such as *Mobiluncus* species, *Gonococcus vaginalis, Bacteroides* species, peptostreptococci, and *Mycoplasma hominis* (Benrubi, 1999). BV is the most common cause of vaginitis and vaginal discharge in postpubertal women, accounting for 40% to 50% of cases, compared to vulvovaginal candidiasis, which is seen in 20% to 25% of cases, and trichomoniasis, which accounts for a discharge's presence 15% to 20% of the time (Benrubi, 1999). This nonspecific infection is probably the most common cause of vaginal discharge in female children as well (Hammerschlag, 1998b). Its prevalence and incidence are difficult to obtain, yet BV has been found in 10% to 25% of women in gynecological and obstetric clinics and in up to 64% of women seen in STD clinics. BV is not seen in adult men (American College of Obstetricians and Gynecologists [ACOG], 1996).

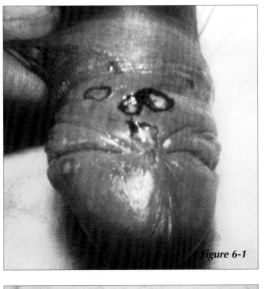

Figure 6-1

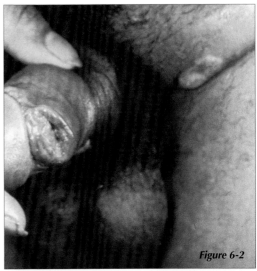

Figure 6-2

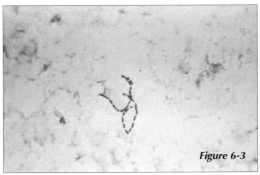

Figure 6-3

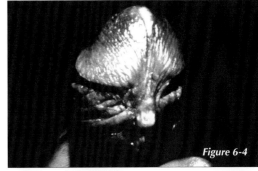

Figure 6-4

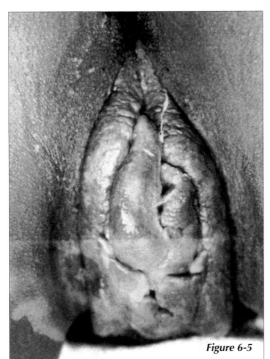

Figure 6-5

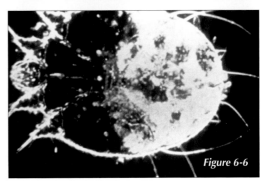

Figure 6-6

Figure 6-1. *Chancroid ulcers. (Contributed by the Centers for Disease Control and Prevention [CDC]; Atlanta, Ga.)*

Figure 6-2. *Chancroid, male. Regional adenopathy. (Contributed by the CDC; Atlanta, Ga.)*

Figure 6-3. *Chancroid; Gram's stain of* Haemophilus ducreyi. *(Contributed by the CDC; Atlanta, Ga.)*

Figure 6-4. *LGV primary lesion. (Contributed by the CDC; Atlanta, Ga.)*

Figure 6-5. *Chronic LGV in female. Genital elephantiasis. (Contributed by the CDC; Atlanta, Ga.)*

Figure 6-6. *Scabies mite. (Contributed by the CDC; Atlanta, Ga.)*

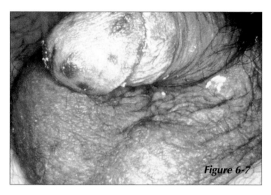

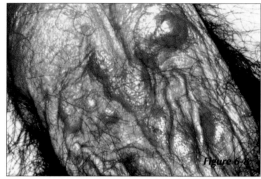

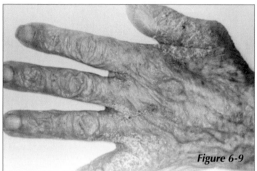

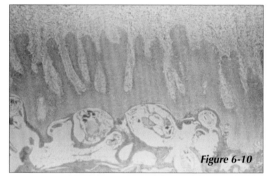

Figure 6-7.
Scabies. (Contributed by the CDC; Atlanta, Ga.)

Figure 6-8.
Scabies. (Contributed by the CDC; Atlanta, Ga.)

Figure 6-9.
Scabies causing eczema-like skin condition. (Contributed by the CDC; Atlanta, Ga.)

Figure 6-10.
Histologic section of a scabies mite burrow. (Contributed by the CDC; Atlanta, Ga.)

Although BV is not considered an STD, it is associated with sexual activity in that vaginal penetration may be the factor that alters the ecosystem, leading to an overgrowth of bacteria. BV may be present after the sexual abuse of children and in adolescents who have been sexually assaulted, but its significance as an indicator of sexual exposure is unclear (CDC, 1998; Hammerschlag, 1998b). Clinicians caring for victims of sexual assault should assess for BV and treat patients.

Clinical Findings

BV may be asymptomatic in prepubertal children and adolescents. Symptoms are present in up to 50% of adolescents and adult women with BV (American Medical Association [AMA], 1999). Common symptoms in prepubertal and postpubertal females include an unpleasant odor in the vaginal area or in the urine; a grayish white, thin, and creamy vaginal discharge; and vulvar irritation and itching. The physical examination of the adolescent female patient includes a complete pelvic examination. The patient's external genitalia may reveal the homogenous gray-white discharge either at the introitus before inserting a speculum or adherent to the vaginal walls or cervical fornices during the pelvic examination. Other clinical signs such as inflammation and erythema are not usually seen when BV exists on its own (Benrubi, 1999).

Diagnosis

Diagnosis of BV is confirmed by specific diagnostic findings because clinical signs and symptoms are not reliable on their own. In the prepubertal child, vaginal discharge is examined for the presence of "clue cells," defined as vaginal squamous epithelial cells covered with bacteria obscuring the normally well-defined edges of an epithelial cell. With adolescent patients, clinicians determine vaginal pH, perform microscopy for clue cells, and do the "whiff" test to aid in the diagnosis. Clinicians use these tests together and correlate findings with clinical symptoms and signs to diagnose BV. Clinical criteria for diagnosis in adolescents requires 3 of the 4 signs: characteristic discharge, positive whiff test, pH greater than 4.5, and presence of clue cells. Because of the polymicrobial nature of the infection, vaginal culture is of little value and Pap smears are unreliable in the diagnosis of BV (Benrubi, 1999).

In the prepubertal child, samples for the tests are obtained with a cotton swab from the vaginal discharge itself or via vaginal washings. In the adolescent, the samples may come from the vaginal sidewalls or cervical fornices, avoiding the cervix itself. For pH testing, the sample can be applied directly to the pH paper. A result greater than 4.5 is consistent with BV.

Microscopy technique involves applying the sample to a slide, adding a drop of saline solution, placing a coverslip over the sample, and visualizing 10 fields under high power (400¥). The presence of clue cells (at least 20%) indicates BV.

The whiff test involves placing the sample on a slide or in a test tube and adding a drop of 10% potassium hydroxide solution (KOH). A "fishy" odor occurs with BV and is considered a positive whiff test. The odor results from anaerobic bacteria volatized in an alkaline environment. A separate sample should be collected for the whiff test because KOH lyses the epithelial cells of a sample.

Treatment and Follow-up

The treatment guidelines for BV are summarized in **Table 6-6**. The CDC supports prophylactic treatment for BV in adolescents after a sexual assault, especially because follow-up of these patients can be difficult. (See **Table 6-3** for this regimen.) Follow-up can take place when patients come back for other reasons related to the sexual assault and involves identifying patient follow-through with prescribed medication regimens and resolution of symptoms. The treatment of male partners is not necessary (ACOG, 1996).

Figure 6-11.
Molluscum contagiosum, vulva and thighs. (Contributed by the CDC; Atlanta, Ga.)

Figure 6-12.
Molluscum contagiosum. (Contributed by the CDC; Atlanta, Ga.)

Figure 6-13.
Molluscum contagiosum, penis. (Contributed by the CDC; Atlanta, Ga.)

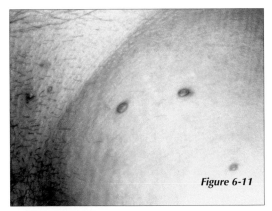

Figure 6-11

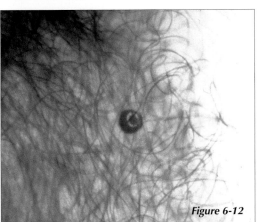

Figure 6-12

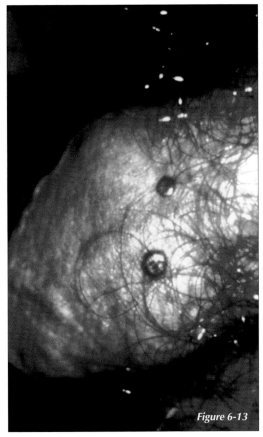

Figure 6-13

Table 6-3. Evaluation for Sexually Transmitted Infections

INITIAL EXAMINATION

An initial examination should include the following procedures:

— Cultures for *N. gonorrhoeae* and *C. trachomatis* from specimens collected from any sites of penetration or attempted penetration.

— FDA-approved nucleic acid amplification (NAA) tests (as a substitute for culture). NAA tests offer the advantage of increased sensitivity. If an NAA test is used, a positive test result should be confirmed by a second test. Confirmation tests should consist of a second FDA-licensed NAA test that targets a different sequence from the initial test. EIA, nonamplified probes, and direct fluorescent antibody tests are unacceptable alternatives for culture because false-negative test results occur more often with these nonculture tests, and false-positive test results also may occur.

— Wet mount and culture of a vaginal swab specimen for *T. vaginalis* infection. If vaginal discharge, malodor, or itching is evident, the wet mount also should be examined for evidence of BV and candidiasis.

— Collection of a serum sample for immediate evaluation for HIV, hepatitis B, and syphilis. (See **Table 6-4**.)

FOLLOW-UP EXAMINATIONS

Although it is often difficult for persons to comply with follow-up examinations weeks after an assault, such examinations are essential for the following reasons:

— To detect new infections acquired during or after the assault

— To complete hepatitis B immunization if indicated

— To complete counseling and treatment for other STDs

Examination for STDs should be repeated within 1-2 weeks of the assault. Because infectious agents acquired through assault may not have produced sufficient concentrations of organisms to result in positive test results at the initial examination, a culture (or cultures), a wet mount, and other tests should be repeated at the follow-up visit unless prophylactic treatment was provided. If treatment was provided, testing should be done only if the survivor reports having symptoms. If treatment was not provided, follow-up examination should be conducted within a week to ensure that results of positive tests can be discussed promptly with the survivor and that treatment is provided. Serologic tests for syphilis and HIV infection should be repeated 6, 12, and 24 weeks after the assault if initial test results were negative and these infections are likely to be present in the assailant.

PROPHYLAXIS

Many specialists recommend routine preventive therapy after a sexual assault because follow-up of survivors of sexual assault can be difficult and because these persons may be reassured if offered treatment or prophylaxis for possible infection. The following prophylactic regimen is suggested as preventive therapy:

(continued)

Table 6-3. *(continued)*

— Postexposure hepatitis B vaccination, without hepatitis B immunoglobulin (HBIG), should adequately protect against HBV. Hepatitis B vaccine should be administered to sexual assault victims at the time of the initial examination if they have not been previously vaccinated. Follow-up doses of vaccine should be administered 1-2 and 4-6 months after the first dose.

— An empiric antimicrobial regimen for chlamydia, gonorrhea, trichomonas, and BV may be administered.

RECOMMENDED REGIMEN

Ceftriaxone 125 mg IM* in a single dose
       PLUS
Metronidazole 2 g PO in a single dose
       PLUS
Azithromycin 1 g PO in a single dose
       OR
Doxycycline 100 mg PO twice daily for 7 days

Note: **For patients requiring alternative treatments, see the sections in the CDC report that specifically address those agents.**

The efficacy of these regimens in preventing gonorrhea, trichomoniasis, BV, and *C. trachomatis* genitourinary infections after sexual assault has not been evaluated. Clinicians should counsel patients regarding the possible benefits, as well as the possible toxicity, associated with these treatment regimens; gastrointestinal side effects can occur with this combination. Providers may also consider antiemetic medications if prophylaxis is administered, particularly if emergency contraception is also provided.

OTHER MANAGEMENT CONSIDERATIONS

At the initial examination and, if indicated, at follow-up examinations, patients should be counseled regarding the following:

— Symptoms of STDs and the need for immediate examination if symptoms occur

— Abstinence from sexual intercourse until STD prophylactic treatment is completed

---

For this and all future tables in this chapter, IM=intramuscularly, PO=orally, and IV=intravenously.

Reprinted from Centers for Disease Control and Prevention. Sexually transmitted disease treatment guidelines 2002. MMWR Morb Mortal Wkly Rep. 2002;51(No. RR-6):1-84. Available at: http://www.cdc.gov/STD/treatment/rr5106.pdf. Accessed February 28, 2003.

Drug dosage recommendations listed herein are those of the authors and are not endorsed by the US Public Health Service or the US Department of Health & Human Services.

Table 6-4. General Guide for STD Testing in Prepubertal Children Suspected of Having Been Sexually Abused

Decision to test must be made on an individual basis, based on suspected risk. Single examination may be sufficient if:

— Abuse occurred over an extended period, and

— Last suspected episode of abuse occurred well before the medical evaluation.

For appropriate high-risk cases, the following multivisit-testing scheme is suggested.

INITIAL VISIT AND 2-WEEK FOLLOW-UP EXAMINATIONS

Visual inspection of genital, perianal, and oral areas for:

— Genital discharge

— Odor

— Bleeding

— Irritation

— Warts

— Ulcerative lesions

Cultures for *N. gonorrhoeae*

— Vagina

— Urethra in boys (meatal specimen is adequate if urethral discharge is present)

— Pharynx in girls and boys

— Anus in girls and boys

Cultures for *C. trachomatis*

— Vagina

— Anus in girls and boys

— If urethral specimen should be collected, obtain a meatal specimen if urethral discharge is present

— Pharyngeal specimens not recommended in either girls or boys

Cultures and wet prep for *T. vaginalis*

— Vagina

— Bacterial vaginosis suggested by presence of clue cells and/or positive whiff test

Serum sample for *T. pallidum*, HIV, and hepatitis B surface antigen (HBsAg)

— Decision made on case-by-case basis

— Evaluate immediately and preserve for subsequent analysis

(continued)

Table 6-4. *(continued)*

RECOMMENDATIONS FOR POSTEXPOSURE ASSESSMENT OF CHILDREN WITHIN 72
HOURS OF SEXUAL ASSAULT

— Review HIV/AIDS local epidemiology and assess risk for HIV infection in the
assailant.

— Evaluate circumstances of assault that may affect risk for HIV transmission.

— Consult with a specialist in treating HIV-infected children if postexposure
prophylaxis is considered.

— If the child appears to be at risk for HIV transmission from the assault, discuss
postexposure prophylaxis with the caregiver(s), including its toxicity and its
unknown efficacy.

— If caregivers choose for the child to receive antiretroviral postexposure
prophylaxis, provide enough medication until the return visit at 3-7 days after
initial assessment to reevaluate the child and to assess tolerance of medication.
Dosages should not exceed those for adults.

— Perform HIV antibody test at original assessment, 6 weeks, 3 months, and
6 months.

12 WEEKS AFTER LAST SUSPECTED SEXUAL EXPOSURE

— Recommended to allow for antibodies to infectious agents to develop if
baseline tests are negative

— Interpret results of HBsAg carefully because HBV can be transmitted
nonsexually

— Presumptive treatment for STDs

    — Not recommended in prepubertal children

        — Prevalence of most STDs is low following abuse/assault

        — Lower risk for ascending infection in girls before puberty

        — Regular follow-up can be better ensured with children

    — Patient or caregiver concerns must be considered, however, and may be
an indication for treatment

*Adapted from Centers for Disease Control and Prevention. Sexually transmitted disease treatment
guidelines 2002. MMWR Morb Mortal Wkly Rep. 2002;51(No. RR-6):1-84. Available at:
http://www.cdc.gov/STD/treatment/rr5106.pdf. Accessed February 28, 2003.*

Table 6-5. Difference Between Female Adults and Female Children Affecting the Diagnosis of Sexually Transmitted Diseases

CHARACTERISTICS	ADULTS	CHILDREN	EFFECT ON DIAGNOSIS/TREATMENT
Vaginal pH	< 4.5 (acidic)	6.6-7.5 (alkaline)	Vagina supports a different flora. Example: alkaline pH is hostile to yeast. Vaginal yeast infections are rare in children.
Vaginal mucosa	Stratified squamous	Columnar epithelium	Pathogens such as *N. gonorrhoeae* and *C. trachomatis* infect columnar epithelium and cause vaginitis in children instead of cervicitis.
Vaginal mucous glands	Present	Absent	Child's vagina is probably a more "hostile" environment to some pathogens such as *T. vaginalis* because of lack of vaginal mucus.
Normal vaginal flora	Lactobacilli	Gram-positive cocci and anaerobic gram-negatives more common; flora resembles that of postmenopausal women.	Gram-positive cocci and gram-negative anaerobes can "cross-react" with immunofluorescent stains for *C. trachomatis*. Gram-negative enteric pathogens are more likely to cause vaginitis in prepubertal children.
Vaginal length	11-12 cm	4-5 cm	Cuboidal mucosa closer to external genitalia might increase the likelihood of STD microorganisms entering the vagina without actual penile penetration.
Vaginal anatomy	Thick protective labia; elastic distensible vaginal structure	Comparatively thin labia; rigid, non-elastic, thin-walled vagina	Sexual activity is probably more likely to cause bleeding and mucosal disruption in children, possibly increasing the likelihood of infection with HIV after exposure.

Reprinted with permission from Jenny C. Sexually transmitted diseases and child abuse. Pediatr Ann. 1992;21:497-503.

Table 6-6. Bacterial Vaginosis Treatment Guidelines

PREPUBERTAL

Metronidazole 15-30 mg/kg/day in 3 divided doses for 7 days

ADOLESCENT

Recommended regimens

Metronidazole 500 mg PO twice daily for 7 days
     OR
Metronidazole gel 0.75%, one full applicator (5 g) intravaginally once daily for 5 days
     OR
Clindamycin cream 2%, one full applicator (5 g) intravaginally at bedtime for 7 days

Alternative regimens

Metronidazole 2 g PO in a single dose
     OR
Clindamycin 300 mg PO twice daily for 7 days
     OR
Clindamycin ovules 100 g intravaginally once at bedtime for 3 days

---

Reprinted from Centers for Disease Control and Prevention. Sexually transmitted disease treatment guidelines 2002. MMWR Morb Mortal Wkly Rep. 2002;51(No. RR-6):1-84. Available at: http://www.cdc.gov/ STD/treatment/rr5106.pdf. Accessed February 28, 2003.

Drug dosage recommendations listed herein are those of the authors and are not endorsed by the US Public Health Service or the US Department of Health & Human Services.

CHLAMYDIA

General Overview and Epidemiology

Chlamydia organisms are obligate intracellular bacterial parasites (Darville, 1998). Three species exist: *C. psittasi* (causes human infection from infected birds), *C. pneumoniae* (causes pneumonia, pharyngitis, and bronchitis), and *C. trachomatis*, which in the United States is most often associated with genital tract infections. Infection with *C. trachomatis* does not confer immunity from subsequent infection (CDC, 1996). Acute and chronic inflammatory responses are seen with chlamydial infection. From 2% to 30% of pregnant women have a cervical chlamydial infection. Infants born through an infected birth canal can acquire interstitial pneumonia and inclusion conjunctivitis and may manifest urogenital tract and rectal infection (Hammerschlag, 1994). The organism may persist for nearly 2 1/2 years after birth in the child's nasopharynx and oropharynx and for approximately 1 year in the vagina and rectum (Jenny, 1992). The AAP (1999) considers nonvertically transmitted chlamydial infection in prepubertal children to be diagnostic of sexual abuse and recommends reporting such cases to child protective services (CPS) for complete investigation.

Chlamydial infection is the most common STD in the United States, with an estimated 3 to 4 million new cases occurring each year. It is thought that more than 2 million people are currently infected with this disease, with the highest infection rate among adolescents (CDC, 2000). Although it is difficult to determine the prevalence of STDs in victims of sexual assault, one study estimated that chlamydial infection occurred in 4% to 17% of cases; prevalence estimates vary widely depending on the population studied and known risk factors for STDs (Reynolds, Peipert, & Collins, 2000).

Approximately 75% of postpubertal females and 50% of postpubertal males infected with chlamydia are symptom free (Cates, 1999). This accounts for the high incidence and prevalence of this infection. Rectal and vaginal infection in prepubertal children suspected of having been sexually abused is relatively infrequent, with a prevalence of less than 5% (Hammerschlag, 1998b). When chlamydial infection is diagnosed in adolescents, clinicians should be alert to the possibility of transmission through sexual assault while keeping in mind that the infection could also have been acquired through consensual intercourse.

Symptoms
Prepubertal Children
Symptoms in the prepubertal child differ from those in the adolescent and adult. Perinatally acquired chlamydia typically expresses itself as congenital pneumonia, and the organism may persist for several years. There is debate concerning symptomatology in older children infected with *C. trachomatis*, specifically around the prevalence of asymptomatic infection. Asymptomatic infection with chlamydia may occur in prepubertal children although it appears that chlamydial infections in prepubertal children suspected of sexual abuse present either symptomatic or with a history of symptoms before the evaluation (Siegel et al., 1995).

Symptomatic chlamydial infection in female children may be associated with a history of vaginal discharge, a chief complaint of vaginitis, a discharge on examination, and/or a history of exposure to sexual abuse (Siegel et al., 1995). Symptomatic ascending infections of the prepubertal girl's uterus and fallopian tubes have not been reported (Jenny, 1992). When symptomatic, a chlamydial infection in a prepubertal child who has been sexually abused may present as a vulvovaginitis in females, with inflammation and vaginal discharge, and as a urethritis in both males and females (Jenny, 1992). It has not been definitively determined whether these structures can be asymptomatically infected. Little information exists concerning boys who are suspected of having been abused that are infected with chlamydia.

Adolescents
Adolescent patients infected with chlamydia may be asymptomatic or minimally symptomatic, which is consistent with patterns seen in 70% of adult women. Diagnosis often occurs when screening at-risk populations or because a sexual contact develops symptoms (Darville, 1998). Common symptoms of chlamydial infection in postpubertal women include the following:

— Abnormal vaginal discharge

— Irregular bleeding

— Dysuria

— Vaginal pain

— Lower abdominal pain

Symptomatic adolescent males usually complain of urethral discharge and dysuria. *C. trachomatis* is the most common organism identified in nongonorrheal urethritis in males and also in 20% of men diagnosed with gonococcal urethritis.

Chlamydial infections in the adolescent female genital tract may develop into an ascending infection spreading to the uterus (endometritis) and fallopian tubes (salpingitis). (See the section on pelvic inflammatory disease for further discussion of this complication.)

Clinical Findings
Prepubertal Children

The examination of the prepubertal child includes inspection of the external genitalia for signs of inflammation and discharge (ACOG, 1995). An internal examination is unnecessary. Vulvitis or vulvovaginitis may be present in which mucous membranes appear inflamed and may be friable. Prepubertal children suspected of having been sexually abused and found to have a chlamydial infection may be asymptomatic upon presentation but often have a history of a vaginal discharge or a concurrent gonococcccal infection in addition to the chlamydial infection (Shapiro, Schubert, & Myers, 1993).

Adolescents

Examination of the adolescent female includes inspection of the external genitalia for the presence of discharge or inflammation. A grayish-yellow discharge may suggest chlamydial or other infections. On initial visualization the discharge may come from the vagina, the urethra, or the Skene's glands. Bartholinitis (Bartholin's gland inflammation) may also suggest chlamydial infection **(Figure 6-14)**.

For the internal examination, symptomatic adolescents may experience pain in specific genital areas, externally and internally. Clinicians examine the entire cervix for abnormal discharge and bleeding. A cervix that appears edematous and bloody, even when touched lightly with an application swab, is highly suspicious for chlamydial infection or other STDs. Samples for microscopic viewing should come from the posterior or lateral fornices of the cervix or other places where the discharge is free from obscuring blood. In the presence of abnormal discharge, microscopy may show a few to too-numerous-to-count white blood cells (WBCs) per high power field.

Chlamydial infection is always considered in an adolescent male patient who has a urethral discharge. Typically, the discharge color ranges from clear to white to grayish-yellow or green. Less common findings include penile and/or scrotal edema and/or tenderness.

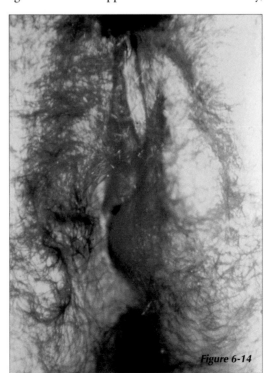

Figure 6-14.
Bartholin's abscess. (Contributed by the CDC; Atlanta, Ga.)

Figure 6-14

Diagnosis

A cell culture is the gold standard for testing to confirm the diagnosis of chlamydial infection (Hammerschlag, Ajl, & Laraque, 1999). This is essential in the context of sexual victimization because of the forensic nature of the examination. Rapid tests are not adequate from a forensic standpoint, especially for prepubertal children. The technique to obtain the culture involves the use of nonwooden, synthetic swabs because cotton swabs with wooden shafts may contain substances that are toxic to *Chlamydia* organisms. The timing of the sexual assault or contact is significant when testing for the presence of *Chlamydia* organisms because it may take up to 2 weeks from the time of contact to produce sufficient concentrations of the organism to result in a positive test. Testing may need to be repeated in a subsequent visit if the assault was a recent one and prophylactic treatment was not provided during the initial evaluation (CDC, 1998).

Prepubertal Children

For the prepubertal child, microswabs are ideal because typically adult-sized swabs are not easily introduced into the smaller prepubertal genital structures. The swab is moistened and rubbed against the mucosa to collect a sample with mucosal cells. The swab is inserted into the urethral meatus for the prepubertal boy.

Adolescents

A culture can be obtained from the endocervical canal after excess cervical discharge is removed from the area. The swab should be placed 1 to 2 cm into the endocervix, rotated several times for 15 to 30 seconds, then removed from the vagina and placed in the appropriate culture media for immediate transport.

To obtain a culture from a male adolescent, the clinician removes excess discharge from the meatus, inserts the swab 2 to 4 cm into the urethra, and rotates the swab in one direction for at least one revolution for 5 seconds. The swab is then removed and placed in the same type of culture media for transport. The CDC recommends obtaining specimens from other sites of penetration or attempted penetration to test for chlamydial infection (CDC, 1998).

Treatment and Follow-up

The treatment recommendations for chlamydial infection are the same for female and male patients, as summarized in **Table 6-7**. There is a CDC-recommended regimen for chlamydia prophylaxis after an assault **(Table 6-3)**. Follow-up includes assessing patients for symptom resolution and compliance with prescribed medication regimens. Patients with incomplete treatment should be retreated. When treating postpubertal patients, single-dose therapy increases the rate of treatment success over multidose regimens primarily because of compliance issues for adolescent patients, and makes repeat testing unnecessary. If repeat testing is done for any reason, it should be delayed until 4 to 6 weeks after initial treatment to avoid false-positive results.

GONORRHEA

General Overview and Epidemiology

Gonorrhea is caused by *N. gonorrhoeae*, a gram-negative bacterium infecting mucous membranes, with a preference for the columnar epithelium of the genitourinary tract (Darville, 1999b; Sung & MacDonald, 1998a) **(Figures 6-15 to 6-20)**. *N. gonorrhoeae* has antigenic diversity that allows it to survive host defenses and develop resistance to various antibiotics as well. Sexual contact is the most common means of transmission, including the mucous membranes of the genitalia, rectum, and oropharynx (AAP, 1998). Infants born through an infected birth canal may contract the infection from their mothers and present with a purulent exudative acute conjunctivitis within 1 week of birth.

Table 6-7. Treatment of *Chlamydia trachomatis* Infection

UNCOMPLICATED GENITAL INFECTION IN CHILDREN AGE 8 YEARS OR OLDER, ADOLESCENTS, ADULT MEN, AND ADULT NONPREGNANT WOMEN

Recommended regimens

Azithromycin 1 g PO in a single dose
     OR
Doxycycline 100 mg PO twice daily for 7 days

Alternative regimens

Erythromycin base 500 mg PO 4 times daily for 7 days
     OR
Erythromycin ethylsuccinate 800 mg PO 4 times daily for 7 days
     OR
Ofloxacin* 300 mg PO twice daily for 7 days
     OR
Levofloxacin 500 mg PO for 7 days

RECOMMENDED REGIMEN FOR CHILDREN WHO WEIGH LESS THAN 45 KG

Erythromycin base or ethylsuccinate 50 mg/kg/day PO divided into 4 doses daily for 14 days

RECOMMENDED REGIMEN FOR CHILDREN WHO WEIGH MORE THAN 45 KG BUT ARE YOUNGER THAN AGE 8 YEARS

Azithromycin 1 g PO in a single dose

UNCOMPLICATED GENITAL INFECTION IN PREGNANT WOMEN

Recommended regimens

Erythromycin base 500 mg PO 4 times daily for 7 days
     OR
Amoxicillin 500 mg PO 3 times daily for 7 days

Alternative regimens

Erythromycin base 250 mg PO 4 times daily for 14 days
     OR
Erythromycin ethylsuccinate 800 mg PO 4 times daily for 7 days
     OR
Erythromycin ethylsuccinate 400 mg PO 4 times daily for 14 days
     OR
Azithromycin 1 g PO in a single dose

(continued)

Table 6-7. *(continued)*

INFANTS WHO HAVE CONJUNCTIVITIS

Erythromycin base or ethylsuccinate 50 mg/kg/day (maximum dose, 500 mg) PO divided into 4 doses daily for 14 days†

INFANTS WHO HAVE PNEUMONIA

Erythromycin base or ethylsuccinate 50 mg/kg/day (maximum dose, 500 mg) PO in 4 divided doses for 14 days

*Ofloxacin and other quinolone antibiotics are contraindicated for pregnant and lactating women and for children and adolescents younger than age 18 years.

†An association between oral erythromycin and infantile hypertrophic pyloric stenosis (IHPS) has been reported in infants aged <6 weeks who were treated with this drug. Infants treated with erythromycin should be followed for signs and symptoms of IHPS. Data on use of other macrolides (e.g., azithromycin, clarithromycin) for the treatment of neonatal chlamydia infection are limited. The results of one study involving a limited number of patients suggests that a short course of azithromycin, 20 mg/kg/day PO, one dose daily for 3 days, may be effective.

Reprinted from Centers for Disease Control and Prevention. Sexually transmitted disease treatment guidelines 2002. MMWR Morb Mortal Wkly Rep. 2002;51(No. RR-6):1-84. Available at: http://www.cdc.gov/STD/treatment/rr5106.pdf. Accessed February 28, 2003.

Drug dosage recommendations listed herein are those of the authors and are not endorsed by the US Public Health Service or the US Department of Health & Human Services.

Infection with *N. gonorrhoeae* does not confer immunity. Most cases are symptomatic although asymptomatic infections may occur. Infants born to *N. gonorrhoeae*-positive women rarely have the organism isolated when they are age 1 to 6 months because of the rarity of asymptomatic infection (Sung & MacDonald, 1998a). Thus, outside of the perinatal period, gonorrhea in a prepubertal child should lead to investigation of sexual abuse. In peer-reviewed medical literature, there is no credible evidence outside of the neonatal period for nonsexual transmission of *N. gonorrhoeae* to children. Gonorrhea is spread by direct contact of infected secretions with the genital, anal, or pharyngeal mucous membranes. *N. gonorrhoeae* is very sensitive to dry and cool temperatures, so transmission by inanimate objects is unlikely. Gonorrhea is the most common STD in children who have been sexually abused (Darville, 1999b).

An estimated 650 000 people are infected annually with gonorrhea (AMA, 1999). Although the number of reported cases of this disease has decreased from approximately 20 years ago, trends show a disproportionate number of certain populations that continue to have a higher incidence of the infection, with the highest incidence in urban areas among persons under age 24 years who have multiple sex partners and who engage in unprotected sexual intercourse (Division of STD Prevention, 1998). The CDC lists gonorrhea as second to chlamydia as the most reported infection (Division of STD Prevention, 1998). The reported rates increased between 1997 and 1999 (CDC, 2000).

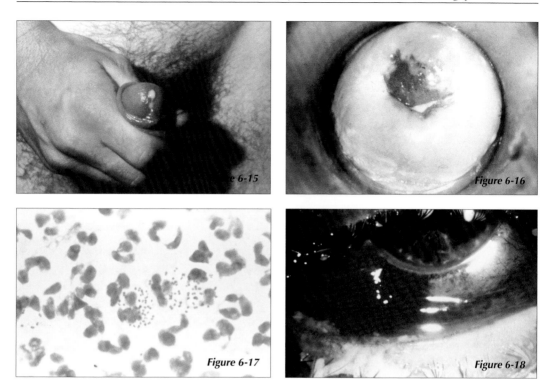

Adolescents and young adults between ages 15 and 24 years have the highest incidence of gonorrhea infection (Sung & MacDonald, 1998a). Approximately 50% of adolescent and adult females and a similar percentage of adolescent and adult males are thought to remain asymptomatic for a varied period of time, when infected with gonorrhea. *N. gonorrhoeae* infection frequently occurs together with *C. trachomatis* infection.

An estimated 3% prevalence of gonorrhea infection is noted among abused children (Hammerschlag, 1998b; Siegel et al., 1995). There are selective criteria for collecting vaginal cultures because of the low incidence of gonorrhea in prepubertal children who have asymptomatic vaginal infection. Rectal and pharyngeal infections are more likely to be asymptomatic. Definitive advice on genital infections in boys is not available because of few case reports. Asymptomatic gonococcal urethritis in prepubertal boys is believed to be uncommon (Hammerschlag, 1998b). The AAP (1999) considers nonvertically transmitted gonorrhea infection in prepubertal children to be diagnostic of sexual abuse and recommends reporting such cases to CPS for complete investigation.

Symptoms and Clinical Findings
Prepubertal Children
In prepubertal girls, the alkaline pH of the vagina and the lack of estrogenization allow vaginal infection to occur and appear as a purulent vulvovaginitis. Prepubertal boys may have a purulent urethral discharge and dysuria. The perianal tissues and oropharynx also may be involved.

Adolescents
Estrogenization of the adolescent protects the vaginal area from *N. gonorrhoeae* (Wald, 1984), but the organism ascends further to infect the cervix and cause a purulent cervicitis. Adolescent females may complain of symptoms similar to those with chlamydia, including abnormal vaginal discharge, vaginal irritation and/or itching, irregular bleeding, dysuria, vaginal pain, and lower abdominal pain. Adolescent males may have moderate to large amounts of urethral discharge and dysuria. The acute

Figure 6-15.
Gonococcal urethritis. (Contributed by the CDC; Atlanta, Ga.)

Figure 6-16.
Gonococcal cervicitis. (Contributed by the CDC; Atlanta, Ga.)

Figure 6-17.
N. gonorrhoeae: Gram's stain of urethral discharge. (Contributed by the CDC; Atlanta, Ga.)

Figure 6-18.
Gonococcal ophthalmia. (Contributed by the CDC; Atlanta, Ga.)

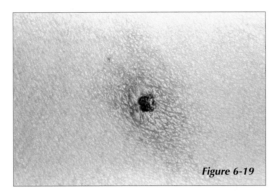

Figure 6-19

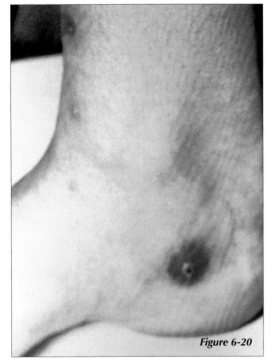

Figure 6-20

epididymitis that may develop is characterized by pain, tenderness, and testicular swelling. If perianal and rectal tissues are infected and symptomatic, painless mucopulent anorectal discharge or, rarely, an acute proctitis with pain on stooling (tenesmus), itching, and bleeding may develop. The pharynx is infrequently infected, but when it is, swollen, exudative tonsils and cervical adenopathy are present.

Adolescent female patients may have visible discharge from the vagina, urethra, or Skene's glands. Discharge is typically a purulent yellowish-green color. Bartholinitis may also be present. Cervical discharge is the same color, and microscopic evaluation may reveal several to too-numerous-to-count WBCs per high power field. When bleeding is seen, particularly bleeding of the cervical body itself, the clinician should have a high index of suspicion for gonorrhea. As with symptomatic chlamydial infections, gonorrhea infection may also cause pain during the speculum and bimanual examinations.

A purulent urethral discharge with a yellowish-green color seen in adolescent males is suspicious for gonorrhea. Generalized penile and scrotal edema is uncommon but is more likely in gonorrhea than with chlamydial infection.

Diagnosis
The gold standard for the diagnosis of *N. gonorrhoeae* is a culture (AAP, 1998; Hammerschlag, 1998b). Rapid tests are not adequate for forensic purposes, especially in prepubertal children. They are used for the sexual abuse evaluation in pubertal girls and boys. The examiner takes samples for culture from the endocervical canal in adolescent females and from the urethra in adolescent males. This is done in the same way as when testing for chlamydial infection. The media used to test for gonorrhea vary from modified Thayer-Martin medium, used for urethral samples, to selective Thayer-Martin medium, used for endocervical samples. The media differ from the cell culture media used to test for *C. trachomatis*. Nonselective chocolate agar plates are also used when culturing for gonorrhea. Samples are obtained for microscopy in the same way they are for *C. trachomatis*. It is possible that blood may be seen in the culture area and should be avoided when sampling.

Treatment and Follow-up
Table 6-8 summarizes treatment guidelines for gonorrhea infection. **Table 6-3** presents the prophylaxis regimen for adolescent patients after an assault. Retesting is unnecessary if symptoms resolve and treatment regimens are completed. Any follow-up testing should also be delayed for 4 to 6 weeks to avoid false-positive results. Clinicians should again consider the timing of the assault as it relates to testing for gonorrhea when deciding on initial and follow-up testing.

PELVIC INFLAMMATORY DISEASE
General Overview and Epidemiology
Pelvic inflammatory disease (PID) **(Figure 6-21)**, an infectious disease complication, affects adolescent females and can result from chlamydial infection, gonorrhea, or both. PID may ascend into the upper genital tract of adolescent females but is not known to occur in prepubertal girls. Adolescents and young adult women seem to be at particularly high risk for this condition. Pubertal females may be at higher risk because of a lack of local immunity and immaturity of the epithelial lining of the cervix.

PID is a polymicrobal infection that produces an inflammation of the female upper genital tract, which may involve the uterus (endometritis, parametritis), fallopian tubes (salpingitis), ovaries (oophoritis), and peritoneum (peritonitis and perihepatitis). PID may lead to the formation of a tubo-ovarian abscess (TOA) (Pletcher & Slap, 1998). Infections with organisms such as *N. gonorrhoeae*, BV, and *C. trachomatis* are often involved, either alone or together, and other vaginal and gastrointestinal (GI) flora may also be involved. Specifically, the transitional zone between the columnar and squamous epithelium of the vagina is more distal, thus creating a biological susceptibility (Pletcher & Slap, 1998).

Approximately 1 million women in the United States contract PID annually (AMA, 1999). Adolescent women account for about one quarter of all cases, and they have a tenfold-higher risk compared with adult women. From 20% to 40% of pubertal females with chlamydial infection and 10% to 40% of those with gonorrhea develop PID if these infections are not treated effectively (National Institute of Allergy and Infectious Diseases [NIAID], 1998). In the context of sexual abuse of pubertal females, PID is a particularly important complication because of the serious long-term consequences, including chronic pelvic pain (18%), infertility (20%), and increased risk of ectopic pregnancy (9%) (Benaim, Pulaski, & Coupey, 1998; NIAID, 1998).

Clinical Findings
Females with PID may have all of the symptoms seen with chlamydial infection and gonorrhea, along with more extensive symptoms of fever, chills, generalized fatigue, anorexia, abdominal pain, nausea, and vomiting. A distinguishing feature found on bimanual pelvic examination is the presence of cervical motion tenderness. Patients may also have fullness or masses on palpation of the fallopian tubes and ovaries, especially if a TOA develops. Uterine tenderness is also possible. Other signs include a guarding-like posture by patients who are trying to minimize movement of the pelvic region.

Diagnosis
PID is diagnosed by looking at the entire clinical picture. No single factor confirms the diagnosis. Minimal diagnostic criteria include lower abdominal tenderness, bilateral or unilateral adnexal tenderness, and cervical motion tenderness (CDC, 1998). Fever, elevated WBC counts, and sedimentation rates are consistent with PID, as are positive chlamydia and gonorrhea tests. Clinicians should be aware that mild cases of PID or those seen early in the disease process could be subtle with minimal signs and symptoms.

Treatment and Follow-up
Treatment for PID involves combination antibiotic therapy to include aerobic and anaerobic bacterial coverage. Patients may be treated on an outpatient or inpatient basis depending on the severity, but inpatient management is strongly recommended for cases occurring in pubertal females. Close follow-up is needed for any patient diagnosed and treated for PID, whether managed as an inpatient or outpatient. **Table 6-9** contains treatment guidelines for PID.

Table 6-8. Treatment of Gonococcal Infection*

UNCOMPLICATED GENITAL INFECTION IN ADOLESCENT OR ADULT

Cefixime 400 mg PO in a single dose
> OR

Ceftriaxone 125 mg IM in a single dose
> OR

Ciprofloxacin 500 mg PO in a single dose†
> OR

Ofloxacin 400 mg PO in a single dose†
> OR

Levofloxacin 250 mg PO in a single dose†
> PLUS,

IF CHLAMYDIAL INFECTION IS NOT RULED OUT

Azithromycin 1 g PO in a single dose
> OR

Doxycycline 100 mg PO twice daily for 7 days

DISSEMINATED GONOCOCCAL INFECTION IN ADOLESCENT OR ADULT

Recommended regimen

Ceftriaxone 1 g IM or IV every 24 hours

Alternative regimens

Cefotaxime 1 g IV every 8 hours
> OR

Ceftizoxime 1 g IV every 8 hours
> OR

Ciprofloxacin 400 mg IV every 12 hours†
> OR

Ofloxacin 400 mg IV every 12 hours†
> OR

Levofloxacin 250 mg IV daily†
> OR

Spectinomycin 2 g IM every 12 hours

All of the preceding regimens should be continued for 24-48 hours after improvement begins, at which time therapy may be switched to one of the following regimens to complete at least 1 week of antimicrobial therapy.

Cefixime 400 mg PO twice daily
> OR

Ciprofloxacin 500 mg PO twice daily†
> OR

Ofloxacin 400 mg PO twice daily†
> OR

Levofloxacin 500 mg PO once daily†

(continued)

Table 6-8. *(continued)*

MENINGITIS IN ADOLESCENT OR ADULT

Ceftriaxone 1-2 g IV every 12 hours for 10-14 days

ENDOCARDITIS IN ADOLESCENT OR ADULT

Ceftriaxone 1-2 g IV every 12 hours for a minimum of 28 days

UNCOMPLICATED GENITAL INFECTION IN CHILDREN

Ceftriaxone 125 mg IM in a single dose
     OR
Spectinomycin 40 mg/kg (maximum dose, 2 g) IM in a single dose

DISSEMINATED GONOCOCCAL INFECTION IN CHILDREN WITHOUT COMPLICATIONS

Ceftriaxone 50 mg/kg/day (maximum 1 g/day) IV or IM once daily for 7 days

MENINGITIS IN CHILDREN

Ceftriaxone 50 mg/kg/day twice daily for 10-14 days

ENDOCARDITIS IN CHILDREN

Ceftriaxone 50 mg/kg/day twice daily for a minimum of 28 days

NEONATAL GONOCOCCAL OPHTHALMIA

Ceftriaxone 25-50 mg/kg (maximum 125 mg) IV or IM in a single dose

*Concomitant treatment for C. trachomatis *should be administered to all patients outside the neonatal period. Children may be treated with erythromycin 40/mg/kg/day PO (maximum 2 g/d) in 4 divided doses for 7 days or azithromycin 10 mg/kg PO (maximum 1 g) in a single dose. Neonates should have tests performed for* C. trachomatis *infection.*

†Quinolones should not be used for infections acquired in Asia or the Pacific, including Hawaii. In addition, use of quinolones is probably inadvisable for treating infections acquired in California and in other areas with increased prevalence of quinolone resistance.

Adapted from Centers for Disease Control and Prevention. Sexually transmitted disease treatment guidelines 2002. MMWR Morb Mortal Wkly Rep. *2002;51(No. RR-6):1-84. Available at: http://www.cdc.gov/STD/treatment/rr5106.pdf. Accessed February 28, 2003.*

Drug dosage recommendations listed herein are those of the authors and are not endorsed by the US Public Health Service or the US Department of Health & Human Services.

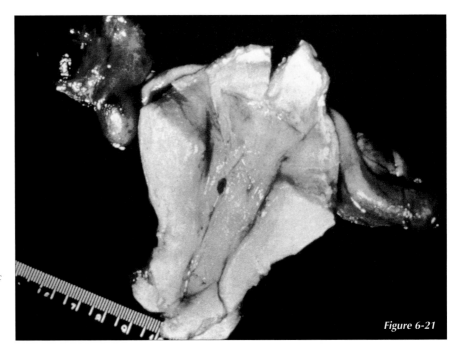

Figure 6-21.
Pathology specimen from patient with pelvic inflammatory disease. (Contributed by the CDC; Atlanta, Ga.)

Figure 6-21

HUMAN PAPILLOMAVIRUS
General Overview and Epidemiology

Human papillomavirus (HPV) is the most common viral STD in the United States (ACOG, 1994). It is a double-stranded DNA virus that presents a challenging dilemma to the healthcare professional evaluating cases of suspected sexual abuse. A large number of people with HPV are asymptomatic and believed to be shedding the viral pathogen. Further complicating the clinical picture are the many subtypes of HPV and the growing recognition that several of these subtypes are associated with the onset of cervical cancer in affected women.

Infants born to HPV-infected women through an infected birth canal can acquire the viral infection as well. The HPV virus in such perinatal cases may have a prolonged incubation period of up to 3 years, thus making the possibility of perinatal transmission an important consideration (Cohen, Honig, & Androphy, 1990; DeJong, Weiss, & Brent, 1982). Perinatal HPV-exposed infants may have transient mucosal colonization that clears by age 6 weeks (Hammerschlag, 1998b). Other infants may harbor the viruses and develop anal or genital warts and, uncommonly, juvenile-onset laryngeal papillomatosis months to years after birth (Puranen, Yliskoski, Saarikoski, Syrjanen, & Syrjanen, 1996).

Numerous HPV types are identified and continue to be closely studied (Koutsky, 1997). Statistics from epidemiological studies demonstrate that over 20 million people in the United States are infected with HPV, with more than 5 million new cases occurring annually, reaching epidemic proportions (Cates, 1999). Certain HPV types are the etiological agents that can lead to condyloma acuminata, or genital warts.

Between 18% and 33% of sexually active female adolescents have tested positive in various clinical studies of STDs (ACOG, 1990). It is difficult to estimate the number of HPV infections in adolescents that occur as a result of sexual assault. The time from initial viral exposure to detection of the infection by the patient or clinician varies widely, making it almost impossible to identify the original source of the infection in adolescents with interim sexual contact. The prevalence of HPV infections in one study in assault victims was 0.6% to 2.3%, yet no direct evidence showed those infections were the result of the assault (Reynolds et al., 2000).

HPV infection or condyloma acuminata is present in 1% to 2% of children who have been evaluated for suspected sexual abuse (Hammerschlag, 1998b). Children less than age 3 years are generally unable to give clear histories of sexual contact, thus making the assumption of perinatal transmission problematic (Cohen et al., 1990). The most prudent clinical approach is to always consider the possibility of sexual abuse in children who have signs and symptoms of HPV infection, realizing that younger children may acquire the virus perinatally. The AAP (1999) considers nonvertically transmitted HPV infection as suspicious for sexual abuse and recommends reporting the infection to child protective services (CPS) for full investigation.

Clinical Findings
Prepubertal Children
Genital warts associated with HPV infection, condyloma acuminata, have a predilection for warm, moist areas and appear as flesh- to gray-colored papillomatous growths. Warts can be as small as 1 mm to several square centimeters if several lesions condense and may form clusters of multidigitated, papillomatous fibroepitheliomas

---

Table 6-9. Recommendations for the Treatment of Pelvic Inflammatory Disease

PARENTERAL TREATMENT

Regimen A

Cefotetan 2 g IV every 12 hours
    OR
Cefoxitin 2 g IV every 6 hours
    PLUS
Doxycycline 100 mg PO or IV every 12 hours

Regimen B

Clindamycin 900 mg IV every 8 hours
    PLUS
Gentamicin loading dose IV or IM (2 mg/kg of body weight) followed by a maintenance dose (1.5 mg/kg) every 8 hours. Single daily dosing may be substituted.

Alternative regimens

Ofloxacin 400 mg IV every 12 hours
    OR
Levofloxacin 500 mg IV once daily
    WITH OR WITHOUT
Metronidazole 500 mg IV every 8 hours
    OR
Ampicillin/Sulbactam 3 g IV every 6 hours
    PLUS
Doxycycline 100 mg PO or IV every 12 hours

(continued)

Table 6-9. *(continued)*

ORAL TREATMENT

Regimen A

Ofloxacin 400 mg PO twice daily for 14 days
　　　OR
Levofloxacin 500 mg PO once daily for 14 days
　　　WITH OR WITHOUT
Metronidazole 500 mg PO twice daily for 14 days

Regimen B

Ceftriaxone 250 mg IM once
　　　OR
Cefoxitin 2 g IM once and Probenecid 1 g PO administered concurrently in a single dose
　　　OR
Other parenteral third-generation cephalosporin (e.g., ceftizoxime or cefotaxime)
　　　PLUS
Doxycyline 100 mg PO twice daily for 14 days
　　　WITH OR WITHOUT
Metronidazole 500 mg PO twice daily for 14 days

Reprinted from Centers for Disease Control and Prevention. Sexually transmitted disease treatment guidelines 2002. MMWR Morb Mortal Wkly Rep. 2002;51(No. RR-6):1-84. Available at: http://www.cdc.gov/STD/treatment/rr5106.pdf. Accessed February 28, 2003.

Drug dosage recommendations listed herein are those of the authors and are not endorsed by the US Public Health Service or the US Department of Health & Human Services.

(Darville, 1999a). Genital warts have various descriptions. **Figures 6-22 to 6-26** represent the varied shapes, sizes, and locations of exophytic warts, including the classic "cauliflower-like" growths, the "finger-like" projections, and the smooth papular growths. Flat genital warts are usually subclinical and can be detected by applying acetic acid to the wart, which opacifies the growths and makes them more distinct (Handsfield, 1997).

The appearance of HPV on the vulvar mucous membranes may be subtle and resemble a stippled area on the hymen or medial aspect of the labia minora. In addition to the anogenital area, genital warts may be found on the umbilicus, axilla, mouth, conjunctiva, and webbing between the toes. When HPV infection is subclinical, there may be no obvious warts or signs of infection.

In prepubertal females, the most common areas are on the vulva; in prepubertal males, the most likely area is the perianus.

Adolescents

In adolescent females, HPV growths can be located on the vulva, perianal area, vagina, and cervix. Common sites in adolescent males include the prepuce, glans, and urethra as well as the penile shaft, scrotum, and perianal area (Handsfield, 1997). Adolescent females and males may report the presence of growths or "bumps" anywhere on the external genitalia and perianal region (Handsfield, 1997). These growths are usually painless and do not involve bleeding unless manipulation of those growths has taken place. External lesions may coexist in the adolescent female with flat condyloma of the cervix and in the adolescent male on the urethra. Subclinical infection is also possible.

Diagnosis

The diagnosis of HPV is largely based on clinical inspection of the female and male genitalia. Biopsy can be used to confirm the diagnosis in cases that are unclear but is usually unnecessary. In adolescent females, HPV may be initially found on Pap smear and colposcopic examination (Trofatter, 1997). Although HPV typing is being studied for use in detecting of cervical neoplasia, it is not routinely recommended (Rohan, Burk, & Franco, 2001). Syphilis should be considered in the differential diagnosis because condylomata lata, a clinical manifestation of secondary syphilis infection, can mimic the appearance of condyloma acuminata, in which the etiology is HPV.

Condylomata lata, the wartlike lesions from secondary syphilis, are generally flattened, broad-based lesions with less surface irregularity than the condyloma acuminata. Of course, the serological tests for syphilis are positive in cases of condylomata lata. Serological testing for syphilis is recommended in the context of evaluating patients after sexual assault (CDC, 1998).

Treatment and Follow-up

Several options are available for treatment of genital warts. The goal of therapy is to remove the external warts, keeping in mind that the viral infection with HPV cannot be eradicated. Treatment choice for external warts depends on the location and severity of the growths and ranges from patient- and provider-applied topical agents to cryotherapy and surgical removal (Beutner & Ferenczy, 1997). **Table 6-10** contains HPV treatment suggestions.

Prepubertal and pubertal female and male patients may need regular weekly or monthly follow-up depending on the treatment regimen used. It may take several weeks or months to eradicate the warts. A regrowth of external warts may occur, at which time treatment must start over. Adolescent females need close cytological evaluation with Pap smears and possibly colposcopy, because cervical cancer is directly linked to HPV infection. Close evaluation is required for women with subclinical infection (detected on Pap smear or colposcopy) because their risk for cervical neoplasia is also increased and possibly at an even higher rate (Koutsky, 1997).

Figure 6-22.
Condyloma acuminata, penile. (Contributed by the CDC; Atlanta, Ga.)

Figure 6-23.
Condyloma acuminata, anal. (Contributed by the CDC; Atlanta, Ga.)

Figure 6-24.
Condyloma acuminata, meatal. (Contributed by the CDC; Atlanta, Ga.)

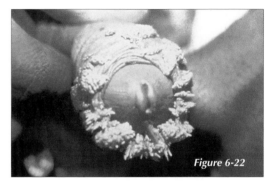

Figure 6-22

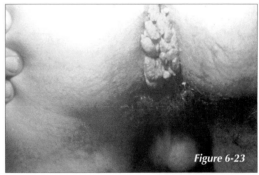

Figure 6-23

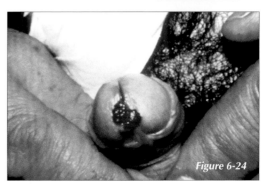

Figure 6-24

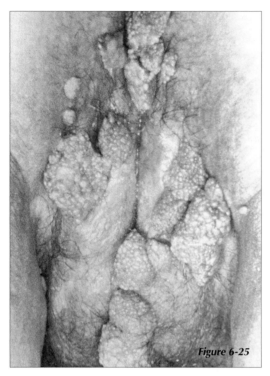

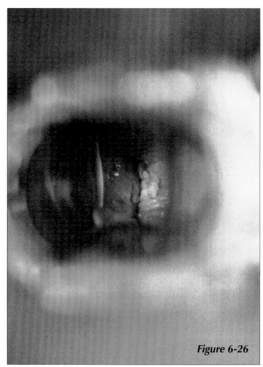

Figure 6-25

Figure 6-26

Figure 6-25.
Condyloma
acuminata, vulva.
(Contributed
by the CDC;
Atlanta, Ga.)

Figure 6-26.
Condyloma
acuminata, vaginal
wall. (Contributed
by the CDC;
Atlanta, Ga.)

HERPES SIMPLEX VIRUS
General Overview and Epidemiology

Herpes simplex virus (HSV) is a large DNA virus with 2 major subtypes. Type 1 HSV commonly infects the oral area, causing stomatitis, and type 2 HSV more often infects the genitalia. These predilections for infection sites are not absolute, however, and type 1 HSV can infect the genitals and type 2 can infect the mouth. HSV 2 is the etiological agent in 85% to 90% of cases of genital herpes, while type 1 HSV is implicated in the other cases (Schack & Neinstein, 1996).

In children, a type 1 HSV infection can be spread to the genitals by autoinoculation; however, a genital herpes infection in children should be evaluated for the possibility of it having been acquired from sexual abuse. An HSV-positive mother may transmit the virus to the infant born through the infected birth canal. This may lead to a catastrophic, disseminated HSV infection of the neonate.

The prevalence of HSV 2 in the adult population is increasing, and asymptomatic shedding in adults is frequent. One in 5 people age 12 years and older in the United States (approximately 45 million individuals) are infected with genital herpes (Fleming et al., 1997). It is estimated that 1 million new cases are diagnosed each year (CDC, 1998). Children are known to contract HSV 2 outside of the perinatal period by sexually abusive contact, and they may present with recurring skin ulcers and vesicles. Infections that may be confused with HSV infections include varicella, herpes zoster, erythema multiforme, impetigo, and syphilis. The AAP (1999) considers herpes infections involving the genital areas as suspicious for sexual abuse and recommends reporting these cases to CPS for complete investigation.

Clinical Findings

Prepubertal and postpubertal female and male children with genital herpes complain of painful lesions or "sores" located anywhere on the external genitalia. They often report that pain occurs during urination. Other symptoms include a

Table 6-10. Treatment of Human Papillomavirus Infection

EXTERNAL GENITAL WARTS

Recommended treatments

Patient-applied:

Podofilox 0.5% solution or gel
         OR
Imiquimod 5% cream

Provider-administered:

Cryotherapy with liquid nitrogen or cryoprobe. Repeat applications every 1-2 weeks.
         OR
Podophyllin resin 10%-25% in a compound tincture of benzoin. A small amount should be applied to each wart and allowed to air dry. The treatment can be repeated weekly, if necessary. To avoid the possibility of complications associated with systemic absorption and toxicity, some specialists recommend that application be limited to <0.5 mL of podophyllin or an area of <10 cm^2 of warts per session. Some specialists suggest that the preparation should be thoroughly washed off 1-4 hours after application to reduce local irritation. *The safety of podophyllin during pregnancy has not been established.*
         OR
Trichloroacetic acid (TCA) or bichloroacetic acid (BCA) 80%-90%. A small amount should be applied only to warts and allowed to dry, at which time a white "frosting" develops. If an excess amount of acid is applied, the treated area should be powdered with talc, sodium bicarbonate (i.e., baking soda), or liquid soap preparations to remove unreacted acid. This treatment can be repeated weekly, if necessary.
         OR
Surgical removal either by tangential scissors excision, tangential shave excision, curettage, or electrosurgery.

Alternative treatments

Intralesional interferon
         OR
Laser surgery

CERVICAL WARTS

For women who have exophytic cervical warts, high-grade squamous intraepithelial lesions (SIL) must be excluded before treatment is initiated. Management of exophytic cervical warts should include consultation with a specialist.

VAGINAL WARTS

Cryotherapy with liquid nitrogen. The use of a cryoprobe in the vagina is not recommended because of the risk for vaginal perforation and fistula formation.
         OR
TCA or BCA 80%-90% applied to warts. A small amount should be applied only to warts and allowed to dry, at which time a white "frosting" develops. If an excess amount of acid is applied, the treated area should be powdered with talc, sodium bicarbonate (i.e., baking soda), or liquid soap preparations to remove unreacted acid. This treatment can be repeated weekly, if necessary.

(continued)

Table 6-10. *(continued)*

ANAL WARTS

Cryotherapy with liquid nitrogen
    OR
TCA or BCA 80%-90% applied to warts. A small amount should be applied only to warts and allowed to dry, at which time a white "frosting" develops. If an excess amount of acid is applied, the treated area should be powdered with talc, sodium bicarbonate (i.e., baking soda), or liquid soap preparations to remove unreacted acid. This treatment can be repeated weekly, if necessary.
    OR
Surgical removal

ORAL WARTS

Cryotherapy with liquid nitrogen
    OR
Surgical removal

Reprinted from Centers for Disease Control and Prevention. Sexually transmitted disease treatment guidelines 2002. MMWR Morb Mortal Wkly Rep. *2002;51(No. RR-6):1-84. Available at: http://www.cdc.gov/STD/treatment/rr5106.pdf. Accessed February 28, 2003.*

Drug dosage recommendations listed herein are those of the authors and are not endorsed by the US Public Health Service or the US Department of Health & Human Services.

burning or tingling sensation, and the lesions appear as blisters, "bumps," or a rash. Anal and genital lesions typically progress from maculopapular lesions to vesicles, ulcers, and finally to lesions that may crust. Lesions tend to heal completely without leaving scars. Approximately 70% of adolescent female patients and 40% of adolescent males have systemic complaints in a primary infection. Symptoms may include fever, malaise, myalgias, headache, neck pain, and photophobia (Schack & Neinstein, 1996). Genital herpes may be resolved by the time patients come in for a physical examination; therefore, clinicians should assess them for a history of these symptoms. HSV-infected adults and adolescents may shed virus intermittently from their cervix or urethra when no visible lesions are seen. It is currently not known if prepubertal children also shed virus between recurrences.

Prepubertal Children
In prepubertal children the clinical manifestation of genital herpes is the presence of vesicles or ulcers in the genital or perianal area (Hammerschlag, 1998b).

Adolescents
For female patients, the evaluation for genital herpes begins with inspection of the external genitalia and continues with the speculum examination when internal structures are examined. The examination of males involves thorough inspection of the external genitalia, taking into consideration that herpes lesions may be found in the perinanal region in both male and female adolescents (CDC, 1997b).

Primary infections **(Figures 6-27 to 6-29)** are usually severe, with the presence of multiple vesicles or lesions and tender, enlarged inguinal lymph nodes, especially in type 2 HSV, while type 1 HSV may be less severe even with a primary infection. Therefore, clinicians should attempt to culture all suspicious lesions. Most recurrent infections are less severe in both female and male patients (Schack & Neinstein, 1996) **(Figure 6-30)**.

The course of a genital herpes infection varies among individual patients in terms of the length of time of each stage and the severity of the infection. In females and males, systemic symptoms precede the presence of vesicles, followed by lesions that eventually end with crusting and reepithelialization (Schack & Neinstein, 1996).

Diagnosis

The diagnosis of genital herpes is largely based on patient history and clinical findings. At this time, viral culture remains the gold standard when testing for HSV. Serological values have not proved especially helpful. The ideal culture is obtained directly from an intact vesicle that is gently ruptured, using a cotton or Dacron swab. When an ulcer is present, samples are obtained by swabbing the base of the lesion, being sure to remove any crusting before sampling and limiting the amount of blood present in the sample. A moderate amount of friction is necessary when culturing these ulcers, to obtain an adequate sample (Schack & Neinstein, 1996). Samples are then placed in the appropriate viral media for transport. From a forensic perspective, commercially available serological assays have difficulty differentiating HSV 1 from 2; therefore, in children, viral cultures are the test of choice when sexual abuse is being considered.

Treatment and Follow-up

The treatment of genital herpes in female and male patients, prepubertal and pubertal, should emphasize pain management as the first priority. This includes the use of topical anesthetics, nonsteroidal anti-inflammatory drugs (NSAIDs), and possibly narcotics if severe pain is present. Other palliative measures can also be used, including sitz baths, light application of petroleum jelly, and keeping lesions clean and dry (Schack & Neinstein, 1996). The goal of antiviral agents is to accelerate the healing process of an acute infection and to decrease the overall number of recurrent infections. See **Table 6-11** for genital herpes treatment options.

Figure 6-27.
Primary herpes, male. (Contributed by the CDC; Atlanta, Ga.)

Figure 6-28.
Primary herpes, female. (Contributed by the CDC; Atlanta, Ga.)

Figure 6-29.
Same patient as Figure 6-28, 4 days later. (Contributed by the CDC; Atlanta, Ga.)

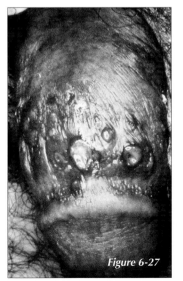

Figure 6-27

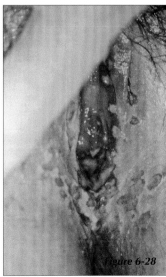

Figure 6-28

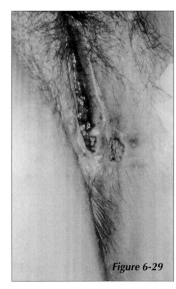

Figure 6-29

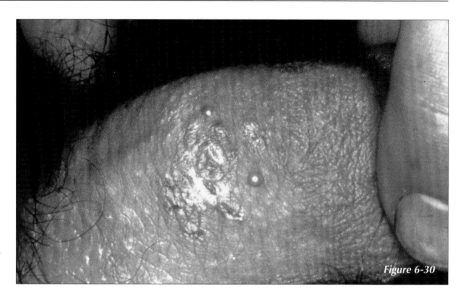

Figure 6-30

Figure 6-30.
Recurrent herpes, male. (Contributed by the CDC; Atlanta, Ga.)

Regular follow-up is necessary to ensure that primary herpes infections heal appropriately without complications. Clinicians should evaluate the effectiveness of antiviral treatments and adjust dosages as needed. Patients with a history suspicious for herpes who could not previously be cultured should be advised to return if lesions recur. Sampling recurrent lesions helps to confirm the diagnosis. It is possible to determine whether a herpes outbreak is primary by testing for antiviral serologies in the blood. If the outbreak is primary, the blood sample will be negative because the body has not had enough time to build up antiviral markers (CDC, 1997b).

Ongoing counseling and education are essential for all patients who are diagnosed with herpes because it is a lifelong infection requiring ongoing management and social lifestyle modifications. Counseling provides children and their families with needed support and allows clinicians to identify patients who may require referral for further therapy.

TRICHOMONIASIS
General Overview and Epidemiology
Trichomonas vaginalis is a flagellated protozoon that is a common cause of vaginitis in adult women (Hammerschlag, 1998b). Adult and adolescent females and nearly all males infected with *T. vaginalis* may be asymptomatic. The extent to which prepubertal children may be asymptomatic is not known. Infants born to *T. vaginalis*-positive women may become colonized or infected for up to 1 year if not treated (Hammerschlag, 1998b). After infancy, it is appropriate to assume a child acquired *T. vaginalis* in a sexually abusive manner (Ross, Scott, & Busuttil, 1993). It is important to differentiate the protozoa from *T. hominis*, a common species that inhabits the human bowel (Garcia, 2001). Distinction may be made by appearance under the microscope based on the length of the undulating membrane. *T. hominis* is often differentiated from *T. vaginalis* by the expert laboratory microscopists looking at a fresh wet prep (Garcia, 2001).

Trichomoniasis affects approximately 5 million people annually in the United States (Cates, 1999). The World Health Organization (WHO, 1998) estimated that 170 million people globally were infected with this parasite in 1997. The AAP (1999) considers *T. vaginalis* infection outside of infancy to be highly suspicious for sexual abuse and recommends reporting to CPS for complete investigation.

Table 6-11. Treatment of Genital Herpes

PREPUBERTAL

Acyclovir 80 mg/kg PO divided in 3-5 doses for 7-10 days (maximum dose = 80 mg/kg/day)

ADOLESCENTS

Recommended regimens for first clinical episode

Acyclovir 400 mg PO 3 times daily for 7-10 days
        OR
Acyclovir 200 mg PO 5 times daily for 7-10 days
        OR
Famciclovir 250 mg PO 3 times daily for 7-10 days
        OR
Valacyclovir 1 g PO twice daily for 7-10 days

Recommended regimens for episodic recurrent infection

Acyclovir 400 mg PO 3 times daily for 5 days
        OR
Acyclovir 200 mg PO 5 times daily for 5 days
        OR
Acyclovir 800 mg PO twice daily for 5 days
        OR
Famciclovir 125 mg PO twice daily for 5 days
        OR
Valacyclovir 500 mg PO twice daily for 3-5 days
        OR
Valacyclovir 1 g PO once daily for 5 days

Recommended regimens for daily suppressive therapy

Acyclovir 400 mg PO twice daily
        OR
Famciclovir 250 mg PO twice daily
        OR
Valacyclovir 500 mg PO once daily
        OR
Valacyclovir 1 g PO once daily

Reprinted from Centers for Disease Control and Prevention. Sexually transmitted disease treatment guidelines 2002. MMWR Morb Mortal Wkly Rep. 2002;51(No. RR-6):1-84. Available at: http://www.cdc.gov/STD/treatment/rr5106.pdf. Accessed February 28, 2003; Jew R. Pharmacy Handbook and Formulary. The Children's Hospital of Philadelphia, Department of Pharmacy Services. Hudson, Ohio: Lexi-Comp; 2000.

Drug dosage recommendations listed herin are those of the authors and are not endorsed by the US Public Health Service or the US Department of Health & Human Services.

Table 6-12. Trichomoniasis Treatment Guidelines

PREPUBERTAL

Metronidazole 30 mg/kg/day in divided doses PO every 8 hours for 7 days

ADOLESCENTS

Recommended regimen

Metronidazole 2 g PO in a single dose

Alternative regimen

Metronidazole 500 mg twice daily for 7 days

Adapted from Centers for Disease Control and Prevention. Sexually transmitted disease treatment guidelines 2002. MMWR Morb Mortal Wkly Rep. *2002;51(No. RR-6):1-84. Available at: http://www.cdc.gov/ STD/treatment/rr5106.pdf. Accessed February 28, 2003.*

Drug dosage recommendations listed herein are those of the authors and are not endorsed by the US Public Health Service or the US Department of Health & Human Services.

Clinical Findings
Prepubertal Children
In the context of the sexual abuse examination, all vaginal discharges should be examined for *T. vaginalis*, which causes vaginitis (Jones, Yamauchi, & Lambert, 1985). Very little information is available for symptomatology in prepubertal boys.

Adolescents
Approximately 25% to 50% of adolescent and adult females and up to 90% of adolescent and adult males infected with *T. vaginalis* are asymptomatic. Those adult and adolescent females who have symptoms complain primarily of vaginal irritation and/or itching and a "bubbly" cream-colored or greenish discharge. Initial presentation may include irregular bleeding, dysuria, vaginal odor, or lower abdominal pain, but these symptoms are less common. The relatively low number of males who have symptoms include the same type of discharge and urethral irritation as experienced by females.

The external and internal genitalia of females who have trichomoniasis may reveal slight inflammation and erythema. The presence of a frothy, cream-colored, or greenish discharge coming from the vagina or cervix or petechiae of the cervix ("strawberry cervix") should cause suspicion for trichomoniasis. This same discharge may be seen coming from the urethra in males and should be sampled for microscopic evaluation. A male with this discharge may also have some urethral inflammation and erythema although this is uncommon.

Diagnosis
The discharge of a prepubertal child should be prepared and examined under the microscope using wet prep technique. The sample is combined with a small amount of saline solution, spread gently on a slide, and topped with a cover slide.

Clinicians should microscopically evaluate samples from any discharge seen in any area from the posterior or lateral fornices in adolescent female patients and from the urethra in adolescent male patients.

The diagnosis of trichomoniasis is made when the oval-shaped, motile protozoa are visualized on high power field microscopy. These protozoa usually have an undulating membrane with visible flagella and are slightly larger than WBCs. There may be a few to multiple protozoa seen microscopically, and WBCs may be an additional finding (ACOG, 1996).

Treatment and Follow-up

Trichomoniasis treatment guidelines are discussed in **Table 6-12**. Follow-up includes the assessment for completion of prescribed treatment regimens and resolution of symptoms. Repeating treatment is appropriate if clinicians suspect failure with initially prescribed regimens. Repeat microscopical testing is only needed if symptoms persist or recur after several months.

PEDICULOSIS PUBIS
General Overview and Epidemiology

Pediculosis pubis is a parasite that may be sexually transmitted through close contact. It is caused by the pubic crab louse, *Pthirus pubis*, which is an oval-shaped insect approximately 1 to 4 mm in length. The parasite lives on the skin, usually where hair is present, and feeds on host blood. The female pubic louse **(Figure 6-31)** lays about 3 eggs per day, which attach to the shaft of the hair as nits and hatch within 8 to 10 days (Nelson & Neinstein, 1996).

Clinical Findings

Pediculosis pubis is an infection primarily seen in adolescent and adult males and females and typically not in children because of the absence of pubic hair in the prepubertal child. Symptoms usually occur in females and males, approximately 1 to 2 weeks after initial contact. Patients primarily complain of itching throughout all areas of the external genitalia particularly in areas where there is hair growth. They or a family member may also have seen an actual crab louse in the genital area. Infestation on eyelashes and eyebrows occurs in prepubertal children and adolescents.

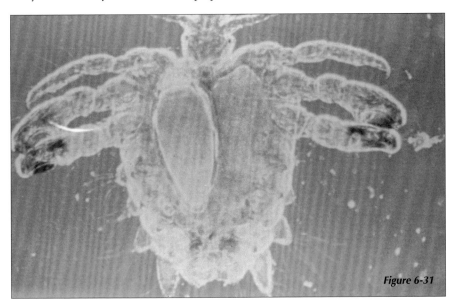

Figure 6-31.
Female crab louse.
(Contributed
by the CDC;
Atlanta, Ga.)

Figure 6-31

Diagnosis

During inspection of the external genitalia of female and male patients, clinicians may first notice small yellowish-white nits attached to the base of the pubic hair shafts. If these are seen, they should be collected as evidence and sent to the laboratory. It may be possible to type the DNA from the louse and, if the alleged perpetrator is also infected, attempt to match the louse DNA from the child or adolescent with the comparable louse DNA from the perpetrator. The eyelashes and eyebrows are also inspected, looking for nits and the crab louse. The diagnosis of *P. pubis* infestation is made by a combination of the clinical history and clinical findings.

Treatment and Follow-up

Treatment guidelines are summarized in **Table 6-13**, and follow-up is required to determine if the infestation was adequately treated. Retreatment may be indicated in 7 to 10 days if nits are still visible. Pediculosis of eyelashes is treated differently with ophthalmic ointment to the eyelid margins twice daily for 10 days (Nelson & Neinstein, 1996). Clinicians should advise patients to remove all residual nits with a fine-toothed comb. In the context of sexual abuse, all clothing and linen that has come in close contact with the patient and alleged perpetrator should be turned over to the police for forensic evaluation. Articles of clothing and linen should be washed in hot soapy water on their return.

SYPHILIS

General Overview and Epidemiology

Syphilis is caused by *Treponema pallidum*, a unicellular spirochete that cannot be cultivated in vitro (Sung & MacDonald, 1998b). Congenital infection **(Figures 6-32 to 6-35)** may be acquired in utero or at the time of delivery. Congenital syphilis infection may cause miscarriage or stillbirth in up to one fifth of cases.

Table 6-13. Pediculosis Pubis Treatment Guidelines

Permethrin 1% creme rinse applied to affected areas and washed off after 10 minutes.

OR

Lindane 1% shampoo applied for 4 minutes to the affected area and then thoroughly washed off. This regimen is not recommended for pregnant or lactating women or for children under 2 years of age.

OR

Pyrethrins with piperonyl butoxide applied to the affected area and washed off after 10 minutes.

Reprinted from Centers for Disease Control and Prevention. Sexually transmitted disease treatment guidelines 2002. MMWR Morb Mortal Wkly Rep. 2002;51(No. RR-6):1-84. Available at: http://www.cdc.gov/ STD/treatment/rr5106.pdf. Accessed February 28, 2003.

Drug dosage recommendations listed herein are those of the authors and are not endorsed by the US Public Health Service or the US Department of Health & Human Services.

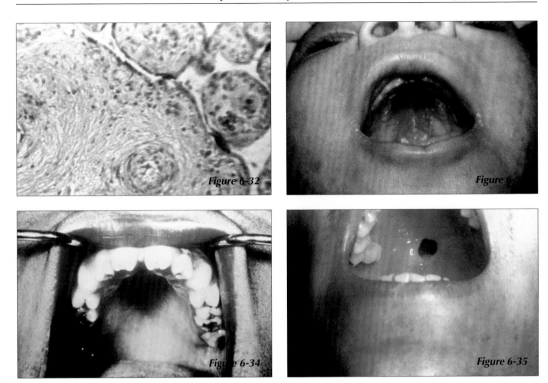

Figure 6-32

Figure 6-33

Figure 6-34

Figure 6-35

Infected infants are categorized into 2 groups: early (symptoms before and up to 3 months of age) and late (symptomatic period followed by symptoms after age 2 years). Early congenital signs and symptoms include mucocutaneous abnormalities, bone findings, and involvement of various organ systems, such as the hematological, hepatic, and renal systems. Late congenital syphilis presents with serious central nervous system, musculoskeletal, and sensory involvement.

The overall rate of syphilis has decreased dramatically in the United States over the last decade, and efforts are under way to eliminate this disease from the United States by 2005 (CDC, 1997a; NCHSTP, 1999). Despite this remarkable decline there are populations in the United States and internationally in which the prevalence of syphilis remains quite high and has even increased (CDC, 2000). The infecting agent, *T. pallidum*, enters the body through small skin abrasions and during exposure to mucocutaneous lesions **(Figures 6-36 to 6-38)**. Syphilis is then spread through the blood vessels and lymphatics (Neinstein & Himebaugh, 1996). Estimates vary based on study, but 0% to 1.8% of children evaluated for suspected sexual abuse are found to have positive serological tests for syphilis (Hammerschlag, 1998b). The AAP (1999) considers syphilis that is not vertically transmitted to be diagnostic of sexual abuse and recommends reporting all cases to CPS for complete investigation.

Clinical Findings

Females and males with primary syphilis are usually asymptomatic (CDC, 1997a). Their primary complaint may be a sore (chancre) **(Figures 6-39 to 6-43)** anywhere on the external genitalia, yet this ulcer can often go unnoticed. Chancres may heal over a 4- to 6-week period and are often accompanied by regional lymphadenopathy. Nodes are usually firm and nontender (Neinstein & Himebaugh, 1996).

Figure 6-32.
Congenital syphilis; increased size of villi secondary to vasculitis and increased connective tissue. (Contributed by the CDC; Atlanta, Ga.)

Figure 6-33.
Congenital syphilis; mucous patches. (Contributed by the CDC; Atlanta, Ga.)

Figure 6-34.
Congenital syphilis; Hutchinson's teeth. (Contributed by the CDC; Atlanta, Ga.)

Figure 6-35.
Congenital syphilis; perforation of palate. (Contributed by the CDC; Atlanta, Ga.)

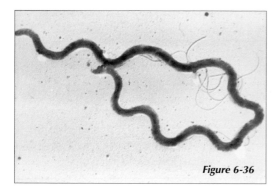

Figure 6-36

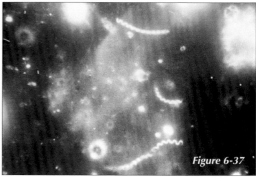

Figure 6-37

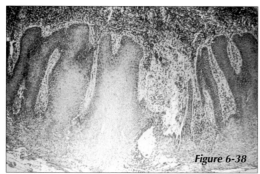

Figure 6-38

Figure 6-36. Syphilis; Treponema pallidum. *(Contributed by the CDC; Atlanta, Ga.)*

Figure 6-37. Syphilis; T. pallidum *on darkfield. (Contributed by the CDC; Atlanta, Ga.)*

Figure 6-38. Syphilis; migration of polys through epidermis, acanthosis (prickle cell layer), elongation of rete ridges, and edema of rete cells. (Contributed by the CDC; Atlanta, Ga.)

Between 6 and 8 weeks after initial exposure to syphilis, female and male patients may have the clinical symptoms of secondary syphilis **(Figures 6-44 to 6-49)**. The primary complaint is a rash on the skin, particularly on the palms of the hands and soles of the feet, and in the mucous membranes. Condylomata lata **(Figure 6-50)**, which are hypertrophic granulomatous lesions whose appearance may be confused with that of the condyloma accuminata of HPV, may also occur near the site of the original chancre. Therefore, both females and males may complain of genital growths. Although classic rashes are seen with syphilis, clinicians should be aware that the complaint of any rash could be indicative of secondary syphilis, especially in the context of a history of sexual maltreatment. Children may also have flulike symptoms and regional or general lymphadenopathy on physical examination (Neinstein & Himebaugh, 1996).

Patients with early latent syphilis, occurring within the first year of the infection, and those with late latent syphilis, referring to the period after the first year, are usually asymptomatic. Female and male patients who develop neurosyphilis **(Figures 6-51 and 6-52)**, which can occur at any time during a syphilis infection, may remain asymptomatic or have neurological symptoms; those with tertiary or late syphilis may have the symptoms of cardiac involvement and/or granulomatous lesions of the skin, soft tissue, and bone **(Figures 6-53 and 6-54)**. Tertiary syphilis is uncommon today but can occur 2 to 10 years after initial exposure (Neinstein & Himebaugh, 1996).

Diagnosis
The diagnosis of syphilis includes an index of suspicion, careful history taking, physical examination, and serological testing. Nontreponemal antibody tests such as the rapid plasma reagin (RPR) and Venereal Disease Research Laboratory (VDRL) tests are used for screening purposes of patients at risk for syphilis. If screening tests are positive, a quantitative VDRL test should be done to obtain titers. This test is used to follow the

course of syphilis and to ensure adequate treatment. A specific treponemal antibody test such as MHA-TP or FTA-ABS should also be done after a positive screening test to confirm the diagnosis. Clinicians should be aware that false positive screening tests may occur and specific tests can be used to clear up any confusion.

Treatment and Follow-up

Treatment involves the use of benzathine penicillin G given intramuscularly and in a single dose for primary, secondary, and early latent syphilis. Multiple treatment regimens are used when the infection has been present for a year or more or when treatment failure occurs. All infected individuals should be examined and repeat serological testing (VDRL) completed at 3 and 6 months. Patients with confirmed syphilis should be considered for HIV virus testing as well.

Children with a history of sexual maltreatment and who are clinically judged to be at risk for syphilis infection should have an initial screening test for syphilis with a follow-up test at 3 and 6 months. Minimum criteria have been suggested for the selective testing for syphilis in children suspected of having been sexually abused and include the following (Bays & Chadwick, 1991, 1993):

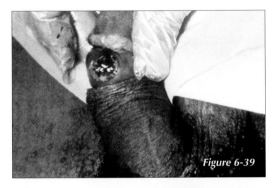
Figure 6-39

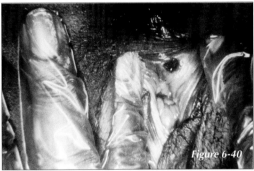
Figure 6-40

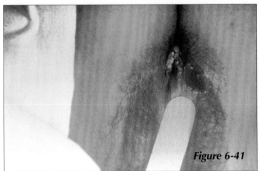
Figure 6-41

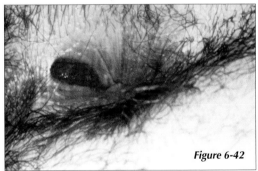
Figure 6-42

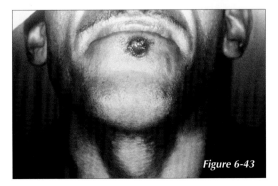
Figure 6-43

Figure 6-39. *Primary syphilis chancre. (Contributed by the CDC; Atlanta, Ga.)*

Figure 6-40. *Primary syphilis chancre. (Contributed by the CDC; Atlanta, Ga.)*

Figure 6-41. *Primary syphilis chancre. (Contributed by the CDC; Atlanta, Ga.)*

Figure 6-42. *Primary syphilis chancre of anus. (Contributed by the CDC; Atlanta, Ga.)*

Figure 6-43. *Primary syphilis chancre. (Contributed by the CDC; Atlanta, Ga.)*

Figure 6-44. *Secondary syphilis; papulosquamous rash. (Contributed by the CDC; Atlanta, Ga.)*

Figure 6-45. *Secondary syphilis; papulopustular rash. (Contributed by the CDC; Atlanta, Ga.)*

Figure 6-46. *Secondary syphilis. (Contributed by the CDC; Atlanta, Ga.)*

Figure 6-47. *Secondary syphilis. (Contributed by the CDC; Atlanta, Ga.)*

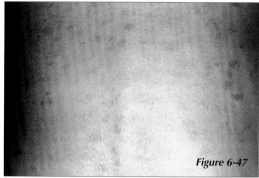

Figure 6-47

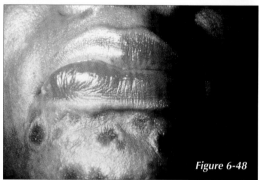

Figure 6-48

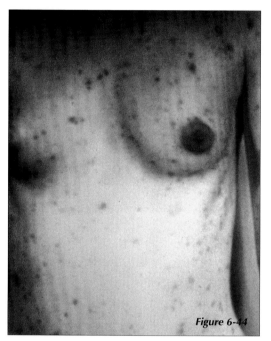

Figure 6-44

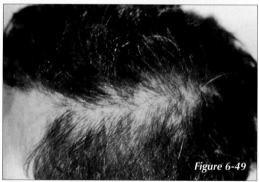

Figure 6-49

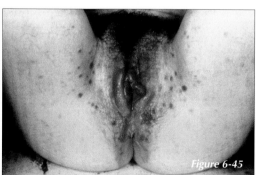

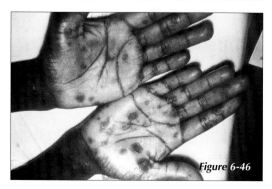

Figure 6-45

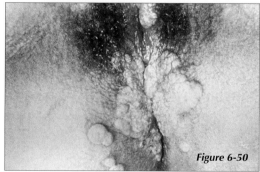

Figure 6-50

Figure 6-46

Figure 6-48. *Secondary syphilis. (Contributed by the CDC; Atlanta, Ga.)*

Figure 6-49. *Secondary syphilis; alopecia. (Contributed by the CDC; Atlanta, Ga.)*

Figure 6-50. *Secondary syphilis; condylomata lata. (Contributed by the CDC; Atlanta, Ga.)*

— Evidence of an STD

— Adolescent age range

— Children from endemic areas/nations

— Parent, family member, or alleged perpetrator with syphilis

— High incidence of syphilis in child's community

If screening for syphilis is initiated, follow-up serological testing for syphilis should be repeated 6, 12, and 24 weeks after a sexual assault when initial testing was negative (CDC, 1998). Repeat testing should be done at any time after the initial 6 months if clinicians are suspicious of syphilis. See **Table 6-14** for syphilis treatment guidelines.

HUMAN IMMUNODEFICIENCY VIRUS/ACQUIRED IMMUNODEFICIENCY SYNDROME
General Overview and Epidemiology
Human immunodeficiency virus (HIV) is a retroviral infection that provides a challenging dilemma to health professionals working with children and adolescents suspected of sexual abuse (Gutman et al., 1991). Although one can acquire an HIV infection via sexual abuse and sexual assault, the risk is low (CDC, 1998). However, the seriousness of acquiring HIV makes the risk of this STD a particular concern in the context of the healthcare evaluation for sexual maltreatment. Issues that arise for the healthcare provider are whether or not to perform screening tests for the infection and whether or not to initiate postexposure medications (Lindegren, Hanson, Hammett, Beil, Fleming, & Ward, 1998). The majority of information about what to do in the clinical context of sexual abuse and sexual assault does not come from research in this specific area but instead from extrapolations on data from occupational exposures, which is a less than ideal situation (CDC, 1998; Moe & Grau, 2001). What is known at this point is that the majority of cases of HIV infection in children have been

Figure 6-51.
Neurosyphilis; spirochetes in neural tissue. (Contributed by the CDC; Atlanta, Ga.)

Figure 6-52.
Neurosyphilis; tabes dorsalis, demyelinization of posterior columns and degeneration of dorsal roots. (Contributed by the CDC; Atlanta, Ga.)

Figure 6-53.
Late syphilis; serpiginous gummata of forearm. (Contributed by the CDC; Atlanta, Ga.)

Figure 6-54.
Late syphilis; ulcerating gumma. (Contributed by the CDC; Atlanta, Ga.)

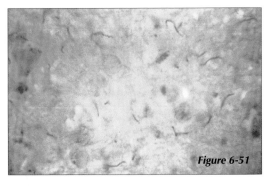

Figure 6-51

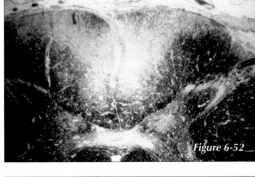

Figure 6-52

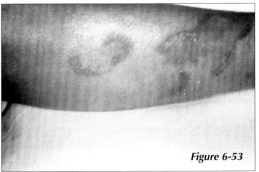

Figure 6-53

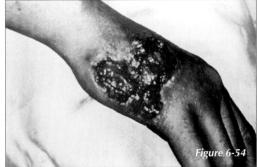

Figure 6-54

Table 6-14. Guidelines for the Treatment of Syphilis

CONGENITAL SYPHILIS IN INFANTS YOUNGER THAN AGE 4 WEEKS

Crystalline penicillin G 50 000 U/kg per dose twice daily for 7 days, then 3 times daily to complete a 10 day course

CONGENITAL SYPHILIS IN INFANTS OLDER THAN AGE 4 WEEKS

With no neurological involvement

Benzathine penicillin G* 50 000 U/kg IM once weekly for 3 weeks

With neurological involvement

Crystalline penicillin G* 50 000 U/kg per dose IV 4 times daily for 10 days followed by benzathine penicillin G* 50 000 U/kg IM once weekly for 3 weeks

PRIMARY, SECONDARY, OR LATENT SYPHILIS WITH LESS THAN 1-YEAR DURATION

Benzathine penicillin G*† 50 000 U/kg IM single dose

LATENT SYPHILIS GREATER THAN 1 YEAR OR TERTIARY SYPHILIS, EXCLUDING NEUROSYPHILIS

Benzathine penicillin G* 50 000 U/kg IM once weekly for 3 weeks

NEUROSYPHILIS

Crystalline penicillin G* 50 000 U/kg IM once weekly for 3 weeks

FOR PENICILLIN-ALLERGIC PATIENTS

Uncomplicated early syphilis

Doxycycline 100 mg PO twice daily for 14 days (for children older than age 8 years)
　　　　OR
Erythromycin 10 mg/kg per dose 4 times daily for 14 days

Uncomplicated late syphilis

Doxycycline 100 mg PO twice daily for 28 days (for children older than age 8 years)
　　　　OR
Erythromycin 10 mg/kg per dose PO 4 times daily for 28 days

(continued)

Table 6-14. *(continued)*

FOR PREGNANT WOMEN

If penicillin-allergic

Undergo testing and desensitization followed by penicillin treatment.
If treated with nonpenicillin regimens, infants should be evaluated for possible congenital syphilis and treated with penicillin.

*Maximum doses: Benzathine penicillin G, 2.4 million U per dose; crystalline penicillin G, 3.4 million U per dose.

†If patient is pregnant, some recommend 2 doses of benzathine penicillin 2.4 million U 1 week apart.

Adapted from Centers for Disease Control and Prevention. Guidelines for treatment of sexually transmitted diseases. MMWR Morb Mortal Wkly Rep. 1998;47(RR-1):1-118.

Drug dosage recommendations listed herein are those of the authors and are not endorsed by the US Public Health Service or the US Department of Health & Human Services.

acquired perinatally. Several reports in the pediatric literature indicate a very small number of cases of HIV infection acquired with the sole risk factor of sexual abuse (CDC, 1999, 2001a; Gellert, Durfee, Berkowitz, Higgins, & Tubiolo, 1993; Gutman et al., 1991; Lindegren et al., 1998; Siegel, Christie, Myers, Duma, & Green, 1992). The risk for an adolescent or adult woman acquiring HIV from a sexual assault is also believed to be low and dependent on related factors such as the following: type of intercourse (oral, vaginal, or anal); presence of oral, vaginal, or anal trauma; ejaculate exposure site; viral load in ejaculate; the presence of other STDs (e.g., syphilis) (CDC, 1998). Although the risk is difficult to determine precisely, a given clinical situation may warrant needing to make a decision about testing and the initiation of antiretroviral agents relatively urgent. Therefore, the CDC recommends a case-by-case approach regarding HIV prophylaxis in cases of sexual abuse and sexual assault. The following selective screening criteria for HIV are suggested because the risk to the prepubertal child of acquiring HIV from sexual abuse is low (Hammerschlag, 1998b):

— Presence of STD

— Perpetrator is a member of a high-risk group (e.g., homosexual, intravenous drug abuser, known to be infected with HIV)

— Perpetrator is unknown to have:

— Multiple partners

— Symptoms suggesting immunodeficiency

— Parents have requested HIV screening

The CDC (1998) suggests that for adolescents and adults who are being evaluated for sexual assault, clinicians consider the following:

— Likelihood of exposure to HIV

— Potential benefits and risks of antiretroviral therapy

— Interval between exposure and initiation of treatment

— HIV status of assailant and, if not known, local epidemiology of HIV/AIDS

If antiviral postexposure prophylactic medications are offered/initiated, the CDC (1998) recommends a discussion with the patient that covers the following:

— Efficacy and toxicity of antiretrovirals

— Need for frequent dosing of medications

— Need for close follow-up

— Importance of strict compliance

— Need for immediate initiation for maximal effectiveness

The number of children and adolescents who acquired HIV infection from sexual abuse is very low, and the number who become HIV positive from a sexual assault is not known but also believed to be low (Hammerschlag, 1998b). No universally accepted standard protocols exist at the present time related to testing or initiation of postexposure antiretroviral therapy. **Table 6-15** contains the HIV protocol recommended by the CDC. The information related to HIV will increase as more study is done, so clinicians will need to pay close attention and consult with regional experts on this important issue. The AAP (1999) considers the presence of HIV

Table 6-15. Recommendations for HIV Postexposure Assessment

RECOMMENDATIONS FOR POSTEXPOSURE ASSESSMENT OF CHILDREN WITHIN 72 HOURS OF SEXUAL ASSAULT

— Review HIV/AIDS local epidemiology and assess risk for HIV infection in the assailant.

— Evaluate circumstances of assault that may affect risk for HIV transmission.

— Consult with a specialist in treating HIV-infected children if postexposure prophylaxis is considered.

— If the child appears to be at risk for HIV transmission from the assault, discuss postexposure prophylaxis with the caregiver(s), including its toxicity and its unknown efficacy.

RECOMMENDATIONS FOR POSTEXPOSURE ASSESSMENT OF ADOLESCENT AND ADULT SURVIVORS WITHIN 72 HOURS OF SEXUAL ASSAULT*

— Review HIV/AIDS local epidemiology and assess risk for HIV infection in the assailant.

— Evaluate circumstances of assault that may affect risk for HIV transmission.

— Consult with a specialist in HIV treatment if postexposure prophylaxis is considered.

— If the survivor chooses to receive antiretroviral postexposure prophylaxis, provide enough medication to last until the next return visit; reevaluate survivor 3-7 days after initial assessment and assess tolerance of medications.

— Perform HIV antibody test at original assessment; repeat at 6 weeks, 3 months, and 6 months.

Assistance with postexposure prophylaxis decisions can be obtained by calling the National HIV Telephone Consultation Service (tel: 800-933-3413).

Adapted from Centers for Disease Control and Prevention. Sexually transmitted diseases treatment guidelines 2002. MMWR Morb Mortal Wkly Rep. *2002;51(No. RR-6):1-84.*

infection that is nonvertically transmitted in the prepubertal child to be indicative of sexual abuse and recommends reporting to CPS.

Clinical Findings

The incubation period for HIV infections varies and may be quite long before symptoms appear. Males and females infected with the HIV virus can have a wide range of signs and symptoms. Many are asymptomatic, whereas others may initially have mild and vague complaints. Clinicians are referred to major pediatric and adolescent textbooks for a complete discussion of the presentation of HIV/AIDS.

Diagnosis

HIV infection is diagnosed by serological testing after obtaining informed consent. Initial screening, if it is to be done, should take place after the identification of child sexual maltreatment with repeat testing as described below. Repeat testing is important because negative antibody tests cannot exclude infection that occurred less than 6 months before the test (Belzer & Neinstein, 1996). The CDC (1998) recommends repeat HIV testing 6, 12, and 24 weeks after initial testing in sexual assault cases, along with syphilis testing. A positive antibody test is followed by a more specific test, such as the Western blot or the immunofluorescence assay to confirm HIV infection.

Treatment and Follow-up

Many medications are used to slow the progression of HIV infection. Patients who are HIV positive require comprehensive medical care to manage this, as well as extensive psychosocial support. At the present time a case-by-case approach is to be followed and routine prophylaxis is not recommended for child victims of sexual maltreatment but may be necessary in individual cases based on the clinical situation of the abuse (Vermillion et al., 2000). A similar case-by-case approach is to be followed for adolescents and adult women who have been sexually assaulted. In the pediatric setting, the patient and family's input is highly valued and serves as a factor in the clinical decision making. Because of the rapidly changing recommendations for HIV care, consultation with an infectious disease specialist is recommended to have access to the most current recommendations for therapy.

HEPATITIS B VIRUS

General Overview and Epidemiology

The hepatitis B virus (HBV) is a DNA virus considered a blood-borne pathogen and an STD. It is estimated that 250 000 new cases of HBV are diagnosed each year, with 30% to 60% acquired through sexual transmission (Vermillion et al., 2000). Some of these acute infections progress to chronic infections, with approximately 6% of children infected after age 6 years developing chronic infections (CDC, 2001b). Approximately 6000 deaths each year are attributable to HBV infection (CDC, 1998). The number of cases has steadily declined since the HBV vaccine became available in the early 1980s. HBV vaccination is highly effective, with protective levels of antibody present in approximately 50% of recipients after the first dose, 85% after 2 doses, and greater than 90% after 3 doses (CDC, 1998). Passive immunization with hepatitis B immune globulin (HBIG) prevents up to 75% of infections after sexual contact with individuals who have acute HBV infections, and HBV vaccine without HBIG is effective in preventing infections after sexual contact with individuals with chronic infection (CDC, 1998).

In pediatrics, the majority of infections of prepubertal children occur via perinatal infection and via person-to-person contact with chronically infected household members over the first 5 years of life (CDC, 1998). In adolescents, sexual transmission is most common. Because of the potential long-term consequences of HBV, clinicians should consider its possibility in the context of sexual maltreatment.

Symptoms and Clinical Findings

Those infected with the HBV have a wide range of signs and symptoms, and approximately 30% of individuals are asymptomatic. Acutely symptomatic children and adolescents may complain of fatigue, anorexia, nausea, fever, right upper quadrant pain, myalgias, and arthralgias (CDC, 2001b). Clinical findings include liver or spleen tenderness, icteric sclera, arthritis, and skin rash (Mason & Neinstein, 1996).

Diagnosis

Several serological tests are available to assess for HBV. A hepatitis B surface antigen (HBsAg) becomes positive during the incubation period and in most cases becomes negative during the clinical disease phase. A positive result suggests acute hepatitis B infection, except in cases in which the person is a chronic carrier of the disease, when this test will remain positive for life (Mason & Neinstein, 1996). The anti-hepatitis B core antigen (anti-HBc) becomes positive after the incubation period, when the HBsAg is decreasing. This test can be divided into immunoglobulin M (IgM) and immunoglobulin G (IgG), which is helpful when trying to identify an acute versus older infection. The IgM and IgG will both be present when an acute infection is present, while the presence of IgG alone indicates an infection that is at least 6 months old (Mason & Neinstein, 1996). These are the baseline tests used when initially evaluating someone for hepatitis B. Others are available for use when an initial diagnosis is made, and further information is needed to understand the disease phase.

Clinicians caring for victims of sexual maltreatment should keep in mind that patients may have been immunized against hepatitis B. A history of completing the vaccination series may eliminate the need for testing and should be a reassurance. The hepatitis Bs antibody (HBsAb) is the serological test that will be positive when a person has been successfully immunized.

Treatment and Follow-up

Patients who are diagnosed with hepatitis B require long-term care with a gastrointestinal specialist. Much of the care for an acute infection is supportive and palliative, while follow-up is necessary. There is currently no curative treatment for hepatitis B, yet medical regimens using alpha interferon and lamivudine are being investigated (CDC, 1998, 2001b). Unless the perpetrator is known to be acutely infected with HBV, the initiation of the HBV vaccination series in an unimmunized child or adolescent should be adequate protection. In the unlikely scenario of a perpetrator with a known acute HBV infection, HBIG along with the initiation of the active vaccination series would be indicated.

SUMMARY

The healthcare evaluation of a child or adolescent in the context of possible sexual abuse or sexual assault requires careful attention to risk for exposure to STDs. In prepubertal children and nonsexually active adolescents, outside of perinatal transmission, the presence of an STD warrants investigation for sexual maltreatment. The CDC guidelines offer a reasonable approach to testing for possible STDs and treatment. Prepubertal children and adolescents differ anatomically and physiologically, and because of this, their presentation with STDs may differ. Prepubertal children are most often symptomatic with the majority of STDs; asymptomatic infections in adolescents are not uncommon, especially in males. Clinicians must also be aware of the forensic issues that arise in evaluating for STDs in the context of sexual abuse evaluations.

REFERENCES

ACOG technical bulletin. Vaginitis. Number 226—July 1996 (replaces No. 221, March 1996). Committee on Technical Bulletins of the American College of Obstetricians and Gynecologists. *Int J Gynaecol Obstet.* 1996;54:293-302.

American Academy of Pediatrics Committee on Child Abuse and Neglect. Gonorrhea in prepubertal children: subject review (RE9803). *Pediatrics.* 1998;101:1324-1135.

American Academy of Pediatrics Committee on Child Abuse and Neglect. Guidelines for the evaluation of sexual abuse of children: subject review (RE9819). *Pediatrics.* 1999;103:186-191.

American College of Obstetricians and Gynecologists. The adolescent obstetric-gynecologic patient. *ACOG Tech Bull 145.* Washington DC; 1990.

American College of Obstetricians and Gynecologists. Genital human papillomavirus infections. *ACOG Tech Bull 193.* Washington, DC; 1994.

American College of Obstetricians and Gynecologists. Pediatric gynecologic disorders. *ACOG Tech Bull 201.* Washington DC; 1995.

American College of Obstetricians and Gynecologists. Vaginitis. *ACOG Tech Bull 226.* Washington, DC; 1996.

American Medical Association. Sexually transmitted diseases statistics. *JAMA.* 1999. Available at: http://www.ama-assn.org//special/std/support/stdstat.htm. Accessed April 8, 2000.

Bays J, Chadwick D. The serologic test for syphilis in sexually abused children and adolescents. *Adolesc Pediatr Gynecol.* 1991;4:148-152.

Bays J, Chadwick D. Medical diagnosis of the sexually abused child. *Child Abuse Negl.* 1993;17:91-110.

Belzer M, Neinstein L. HIV infections and AIDS. In: Neinstein L, ed. *Adolescent Health Care: A Practical Guide.* Baltimore, Md: Williams & Wilkins; 1996:513-544.

Benaim J, Pulaski M, Coupey S. Adolescent girls and pelvic inflammatory disease: experience and practices of emergency department pediatricians. *Arch Pediatr Adolesc Med.* 1998;152:449-454.

Benrubi G. Bacterial vaginosis: diagnosing and treating the most common vaginal infection. *Female Patient.* August 1999;(Suppl):S4-S8.

Beutner K, Ferenczy A. Therapeutic approaches to genital warts. *Am J Med.* 1997;102:28-37.

Cates W. Estimates of the incidence and prevalence of sexually transmitted diseases in the United States. *Sex Transm Dis.* 1999;26(suppl):S2-S7.

Centers for Disease Control and Prevention. *Some Facts About Chlamydia: What Is Chlamydia?* 1996. Available at: http://www.cdc.gov/nchstp/dstd. Accessed January 14, 1999.

Centers for Disease Control and Prevention. *Syphilis Facts.* 1997a. Available at: http://www.cdc.gov/nchstp/dstd. Accessed January 14, 1999.

Centers for Disease Control and Prevention. *Genital Herpes.* 1997b. Available at: http://www.cdc.gov/nchstp/dstd. Accessed January 14, 1999.

Centers for Disease Control and Prevention. Guidelines for treatment of sexually transmitted diseases. *MMWR Morb Mortal Wkly Rep.* 1998;47(RR-1):1-118.

Centers for Disease Control and Prevention. *HIV/AIDS Statistics: Semi-Annual HIV/AIDS Surveillance Report.* 1999. Accessed telephone information June, 2000.

Centers for Disease Control and Prevention. *Tracking the Hidden Epidemics: Trends in STDs in the United States.* 2000. Available at: http://www.cdc.gov/nchstp/ dstd/stats_Trends/Trends2000.pdf. Accessed July 26, 2001.

Centers for Disease Control and Prevention. *HIV/AIDS Update: A Glance at the HIV Epidemic.* 2001a. Available at: http://www.cdc.gov/nchstp/od/new/At-a-Glance. Accessed July 26, 2001.

Centers for Disease Control and Prevention. *Viral Hepatitis B.* 2001b. Available at: http://www.cdc.gov/ncidod/diseases/hepatiti/b/fact.htm. Accessed January 15, 2002.

Centers for Disease Control and Prevention. Sexually transmitted disease treatment guidelines 2002. *MMWR Morb Mortal Wkly Rep.* 2002;51(No. RR-6):1-84. Available at: http://www.cdc.gov/STD/treatment/rr5106.pdf. Accessed February 28, 2003.

Cohen BA, Honig P, Androphy E. Anogenital warts in children. Clinical and virologic evaluation for sexual abuse. *Arch Dermatol.* 1990;126:1575-1580.

Darville T. Chlamydia. *Pediatr Rev.* 1998;19:85-91.

Darville T. Genital warts. *Pediatr Rev.* 1999a;20:271-272.

Darville T. Gonorrhea. *Pediatr Rev.* 1999b;20:125-128.

DeJong AR, Weiss JC, Brent RL. Condyloma acuminata in children. *Am J Dis Child.* 1982;136:704-706.

Division of STD Prevention. *Sexually Transmitted Disease Surveillance.* Atlanta, Ga: US Dept of Health & Human Services, Public Health Service, Centers for Disease Control; 1998.

Fleming D, McQuillian G, Johnson R, et al. Herpes simplex virus type 2 in the United States, 1976 to 1994. *N Engl J Med.* 1997;337:1105-1111.

Garcia LS, ed. Protozoa from other body sites. In: *Diagnostic Medical Parasitology.* 4th ed. Washington, DC: ASM Press; 2001:106-131.

Gardner JJ. Comparison of the vaginal flora in sexually abused and nonabused girls. *J Pediatr.* 1992;120:872-877.

Gellert GA, Durfee MJ, Berkowitz CD, Higgins KV, Tubiolo VC. AIDS and child sexual abuse. *Hosp Community Psychiatry.* 1993;44:186.

Girardin BW, Faugno DK, Seneski PC, Slaughter L, Whelan M. *Color Atlas of Sexual Assault.* St. Louis, Mo: Mosby; 1997.

Gutman LT, St Claire KK, Weedy C, et al. Human immunodeficiency virus transmission by child sexual abuse. *Am J Dis Child.* 1991;145:137-141.

Hammerschlag MR. *Chlamydia trachomatis* in children. *Pediatr Ann.* 1994;23:349-353.

Hammerschlag MR. *Sexually Transmitted Diseases and Child Abuse: Portable Guides to Investigating Child Abuse.* Washington, DC: US Dept of Justice, Office of Justice Programs and Office of Juvenile Justice and Delinquency Preventions; 1996 (fourth printing, December 2002). NCJ160940.

Hammerschlag MR. Sexually transmitted disease in sexually abused children: medical and legal implications. *Sex Transm Infect.* 1998a;74:167-174.

Hammerschlag MR. The transmissibility of sexually transmitted diseases in sexually abused children. *Child Abuse Negl.* 1998b;22:623-626.

Hammerschlag MR, Ajl S, Laraque D. Inappropriate use of nonculture tests for the detection of *Chlamydia trachomatis* in suspected victims of child sexual abuse: a continuing problem. *Pediatrics.* 1999;104:1137-1139.

Handsfield H. Clinical presentation and natural course of anogenital warts. *Am J Med.* 1997;102:16-20.

Ingram DL, Everett VD, Lyna PR, White ST, Rockwell LA. Epidemiology of adult sexually transmitted disease agents in children being evaluated for sexual abuse. *Pediatr Infect Dis J.* 1992;11:945-950.

Jenny C. Sexually transmitted disease and child abuse. *Pediatr Ann.* 1992;21:497-503.

Jew R. *Pharmacy Handbook and Formulary.* The Children's Hospital of Philadelphia, Department of Pharmacy Services. Hudson, Ohio: Lexi-Comp; 2000.

Jones JG, Yamauchi T, Lambert B. *Trichomonas vaginalis* infestation in sexually abused girls. *Am J Dis Child.* 1985;139:846-847.

Koutsky L. Epidemiology of genital human papillomavirus infection. *Am J Med.* 1997;102:3-8.

Lindegren ML, Hanson IC, Hammett TA, Beil J, Fleming PL, Ward JW. Sexual abuse of children: intersection with the HIV epidemic. *Pediatrics.* 1998;102:e46.

Mason W, Neinstein L. Hepatitis. In: Neinstein L, ed. *Adolescent Health Care: A Practical Guide.* Baltimore, Md: Williams & Wilkins; 1996:493-512.

Moe K, Grau A. HIV prophylaxis within a treatment protocol for sexual assault victims: rationale for the decision. *J Emerg Nurs.* 2001;27:511-515.

National Institute of Allergy and Infectious Diseases. *Sexually Transmitted Diseases Statistics.* 1998. Available at: http://www.niaid.nih.gov/factsheets/stdstats.htm. Accessed June 19, 2001.

NCHSTP News & Notes. *Efforts to Eliminate Syphilis in the United States by 2005.* 1999. Available at: http://www.gov/nchstp/od/cccwg/syphelimination1.pdf. Accessed January 15, 2002.

Neinstein L, Himebaugh K. Syphilis. In: Neinstein L, ed. *Adolescent Health Care: A Practical Guide.* Baltimore, Md: Williams & Wilkins; 1996:924-941.

Nelson A, Neinstein L. Pediculosis pubis and scabies. In: Neinstein L, ed. *Adolescent Health Care: A Practical Guide.* Baltimore, Md: Williams & Wilkins; 1996: 969-973.

Pletcher JR, Slap GB. Pelvic inflammatory disease. *Pediatr Rev.* 1998;19:363-367.

Puranen M, Yliskoski M, Saarikoski S, Syrjanen K, Syrjanen S. Vertical transmission of human papillomavirus from infected mothers to their newborn babies and persistence of the virus in childhood. *Am J Obstet Gynecol.* 1996;174:694-699.

Reynolds M, Peipert J, Collins B. Epidemiologic issues of sexually transmitted diseases in sexual assault victims. *Obstet Gynecol Surv.* 2000;55:51-57.

Robinson AJ, Watkeys JEM, Ridgway GL. Sexually transmitted organisms in sexually abused children. *Arch Dis Child.* 1998;79:356-358.

Rohan T, Burk R, Franco E. Toward a reduction of the global burden of cervical cancer. *Clin J Women's Health.* 2001;1:103-106.

Ross JD, Scott GR, Busuttil A. *Trichomonas vaginalis* infection in prepubertal girls. *Med Sci Law.* 1993;33:82-85.

Schack L, Neinstein L. Herpes genitalis. In: Neinstein L, ed. *Adolescent Health Care: A Practical Guide.* Baltimore, Md: Williams & Wilkins; 1996:942-953.

Schwarcz SK, Whittington WL. Sexual assault and sexually transmitted disease: detection and management in adults and children. *Rev Infect Dis.* 1990;12:S682-S690.

Shapiro RA, Schubert CJ, Myers PA. Vaginal discharge as an indicator of gonorrhea and chlamydia infection in girls under 12 years old. *Pediatr Emerg Care.* 1993;9:341-345.

Siegel R, Christie C, Myers M, Duma E, Green L. Incest and Pneumocystis carinii pneumonia in a twelve-year-old girl: a case for early human immunodeficiency virus testing in sexually abused children. *Pediatr Infect Dis J.* 1992;11:681-682.

Siegel RM, Schubert CJ, Myers PA, Shapiro RA. The prevalence of sexually transmitted diseases in children and adolescents evaluated for sexual abuse in Cincinnati: rationale for limited STD testing in prepubertal girls. *Pediatrics.* 1995;96:1090-1094.

Sirotnak AP. Testing sexually abused children for sexually transmitted diseases: who to test, when to test, and why? *Pediatr Ann.* 1994;23:370-374.

Sung L, MacDonald NE. Gonorrhea: a pediatric perspective. *Pediatr Rev.* 1998a;19:13-16.

Sung L, MacDonald NE. Syphilis: a pediatric perspective. *Pediatr Rev.* 1998b;19:17-22.

Trofatter K. Diagnosis of human papillomavirus genital tract infection. *Am J Med.* 1997;102:21-27.

Vermillion S, Holmes M, Soper D. Adolescents and sexually transmitted diseases. *Obstet Gynecol Clin North Am.* 2000;27:163-179.

Wald ER. Gynecologic infections in the pediatric age group. *Pediatr Infect Dis.* 1984; 3:S10-S13.

White ST, Loda FA, Ingram DL, Pearson A. Sexually transmitted diseases in sexually abused children. *Pediatrics.* 1983;72:16-21.

World Health Organization. *World Health Report.* Geneva: WHO; 1998.

DIFFERENTIAL DIAGNOSIS: CONDITIONS THAT MIMIC CHILD MALTREATMENT

Frances M. Nadel, MD
Angelo P. Giardino, MD, PhD, FAAP

This chapter outlines the differential diagnosis for various signs and symptoms to be considered when the healthcare professional evaluates a child suspected of having been maltreated. Conditions whose presentation mimic physical abuse and neglect manifesting as failure to thrive (FTT) and sexual abuse are discussed. The differential diagnostic process is a form of clinical reasoning and decision making that requires the clinician to obtain a thorough history, complete physical examination, and appropriate laboratory and diagnostic studies. With this information in hand, the clinician considers the various diagnostic possibilities to determine which findings support the diagnostic possibility and which do not. Further information may be required to rule a diagnosis "in" or "out"; then a diagnostic impression is formed, with the most likely diagnosis or diagnoses given as the probable cause for the child's signs and symptoms.

For the purpose of this discussion, differential diagnoses will be considered for the following possibilities:

— Physical abuse in children with injury patterns including bruising, burns, fractures, and eye injuries

— Neglect in children with a growth pattern that fails to meet expectations for given age (so-called FTT)

— Sexual abuse in children with signs and symptoms of vulvitis, vulvovaginitis, and vaginitis

Discussing the various diagnostic possibilities that mimic findings in cases of child maltreatment is in no way meant to diminish the need to consider child maltreatment as a possibility. Instead, considering all possibilities highlights the clinical imperative to consider anything relevant to a given clinical situation before arriving at the final diagnosis. Misdiagnosis can have catastrophic consequences for a child who is left with caregivers who have failed to protect the child from injury. However, misdiagnosing child maltreatment in a child and family where it is not present can also have a devastating impact (Kirschner & Stein, 1985). Differentiating conditions that appear similar to those found in cases of child abuse requires practice and experience. Therefore, clinicians may find that consultation with the multidisciplinary team at a local or regional center may help during the clinician's evaluation, especially in complicated or unusual cases (Hibbard, 1998).

Physical Abuse

Many diagnostic possibilities must be considered when looking for causes of bruises, burns, fractures, and eye injuries in children, including physical maltreatment. The clinician must pay careful attention to the history given, the child's developmental ability, the plausibility of the mechanism of injury described by the caregivers, the pattern of injury observed on examination, and the result of any laboratory and diagnostic testing.

The evaluation of cases of suspected child abuse and neglect is often complex and typically not straightforward. At times, the presentation of children who are physically abused is so clear-cut that other diagnostic possibilities are limited, but many cases of physical abuse present in a less obvious manner, with a confusing history and without pathognomonic signs of child maltreatment. A more extensive evaluation in these cases is necessary, and an extensive differential diagnosis may be warranted.

Bruising

Bruises that are extensive, multiple, patterned, in unusual locations, or not consistent with the caregiver's reported history raise suspicions for abuse (Altemeier, 2001; Kini & Lazoritz, 1998; Mayer & Burns, 2000). However, accidental trauma, cultural practices, and hematological, vasculitic, and inherited disorders may result in findings similar to those seen in cases of child maltreatment (Jenny, 2001; Richardson, 1994). Additionally, birthmarks, dermatological conditions, and exposure to skin irritants or even fabric dyes that tattoo the skin may be confused with bruising and child maltreatment (Tunnessen, 1988). **Table 7-1** lists commonly mistaken etiologies and helpful distinguishing characteristics for bruises.

Actual Bruising
Accidental Bruising

Ambulatory children and those learning to walk often have multiple bruises of different ages on their body. The location of bruises and the developmental stage and age of the child help distinguish inflicted from accidental bruising. Two recent studies described bruising in young children who came for a well-child care visit and in whom physical abuse was not suspected. In both studies, bruising increased in children who were older and more ambulatory (Carpenter, 1999; Sugar, Taylor, & Feldman, 1999). In fact, bruising was extremely rare in children younger than age 6 months (0.6%) and in preambulatory infants (2.2%) (Sugar et al., 1999). Bruises in ambulatory children were found on the front of the body and over bony prominences, especially the pretibial region, upper leg, and forehead.

Folk Remedies

Some folk remedies (Stewart & Rosenberg, 1996b) intended to treat medical ailments may lead to a distinctive pattern of bruising or burns that arouse suspicion of abuse to a naive observer. For example, coining *(cao gio)* is an Asian practice often used to treat fever or pain (Yeatman & Dang, 1980) **(Figure 7-1)**. A hot coin or spoon is rubbed on a child's back and results in linear bruising. Cupping may be used in some Eastern European and South American cultures to treat various ailments (Sandler & Haynes, 1978). In this practice, a cup is dipped in alcohol and then ignited. The hot cup is then placed on the child multiple times, creating suction between the skin and cup. After the cup is removed, a circular ecchymosis or superficial burn may appear. Other folk remedies include biting the child, shaking infants who are dehydrated *(mollera caida)*, or placing burning incense and yarn on sites of pain (moxibustion). These are established practices of a culture, and thus they are not considered abusive. However, some of these practices, such as *mollera caida*, can cause significant harm, and public

Table 7-1. Factors That May Be Helpful in Distinguishing Bruising Mimics

MIMIC	HISTORY	PHYSICAL EXAMINATION FINDINGS	LABORATORY ABNORMALITIES
Accidental bruising	Child is ambulatory	Bruising over bony prominences	None
Coining	Family is Asian, practices alternative medicine	Linear ecchymosis, usually in a Christmas tree pattern on the back	May have myoglobinuria if extensive bruising
Idiopathic thrombocytopenic purpura	Often preceded by viral illness	Petechiae with minimal trauma (e.g., with blood pressure cuff inflation)	Low platelet count with the rest of the complete blood count normal
Hemophilia	Family history of hemophilia Excessive bleeding at circumcision or cord separation	Bruises in unusual locations Hemarthrosis after minimal trauma	Prolonged partial thromboplastin time (PTT), abnormal factor assay
Ehlers-Danlos (ED) syndrome	Family history of Ehlers-Danlos syndrome	Fragile skin with poor wound healing Joint hyperextensibility Elastic skin	Not applicable
Leukemia	May have weight loss, prolonged fever, night sweats, fatigue	Pallor Hepatosplenomegaly Adenopathy Cachexia	Abnormal cells on smear Many other laboratory abnormalities, which may include prolonged prothrombin time (PT)/PTT

(continued)

Table 7-1. *(continued)*

MIMIC	HISTORY	PHYSICAL EXAM-INATION FINDINGS	LABORATORY ABNORMALITIES
Henoch-Schönlein purpura	Acute onset of a rash that initially may have been urticarial Patient may complain of abdominal and joint pain	Purpura, often predom-inately on the buttocks and exterior surfaces of the extremities Swollen joints Scrotal edema or bruising Tender abdomen	May have eosinophilia, leukocytosis, hematuria
Tattooing	Recent new clothes (especially jeans)	Marks wash off	Not applicable
Mongolian spots	Present since birth	Not tender, uniform gray-blue color, no swelling, takes months to resolve	Not applicable

Adapted from Tunnessen WW Jr. Signs & Symptoms in Pediatrics. 2nd ed. Philadelphia, Pa: JB Lippincott; 1988.

health education at the community level may be helpful in preventing future injuries (Monteleone & Brodeur, 1998).

Disorders of the Hemopoietic System

Extensive bruises in unusual places or without a consistent mechanism may occur in children because of coagulation abnormalities. For example, hemophiliacs may have joint and soft tissue bleeding after minimal trauma. This X-linked disorder is caused by a deficiency in one of the factors responsible for normal clotting (**Figure 7-2**). A history of prolonged bleeding with circumcision or cord separation may be elicited in children with unsuspected hemophilia (Montgomery & Scott, 2000).

Thrombocytopenia or platelet dysfunction may cause generalized petechiae and purpura without a corresponding history of trauma. The most common platelet abnormality in children is idiopathic thrombocytopenic purpura (ITP) (**Figures 7-3 and 7-4**). ITP is caused by an immune-mediated destruction of platelets and is usually self-limited. Von Willebrand's factor is necessary for normal platelet adherence and function. Platelet dysfunction with prolonged bleeding and easy bruisability may result if this factor is abnormal in number or function (Monteleone & Brodeur, 1998). Children with leukemia or bone marrow failure from any etiology may also have easy bruisability and bleeding because they lack many of the components needed for normal coagulation. A complete blood count, prothrombin time/partial thromboplastin time (PT/PTT), and consultation with a pediatric hematologist should be considered in children with unexplained bruising.

Deficiencies or dysfunction of vitamin K can cause easy bruisability because of abnormal clotting. Newborn babies who did not receive the usual intramuscular injection of vitamin K are at risk for the classic form of hemorrhagic disease of the newborn (Wetzel, Slater, & Dover, 1995). These babies are often breastfed (a poor source of vitamin K) and usually present at age 2 to 7 days with nasal, gastrointestinal, and even central nervous system bleeding. Children with gut malabsorption secondary to cystic fibrosis or short bowel syndrome may be deficient in vitamin K. Vitamin K activity also may be inhibited in curious toddlers who ingest rat poisons that contain anticoagulant substances (Johnson & Coury, 1988). Treatment for these circumstances is vitamin K administration.

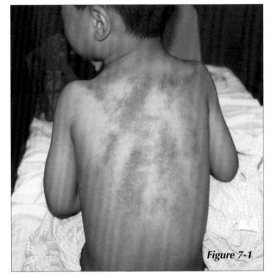

Figure 7-1

Vasculitis

Vasculitic processes causing extensive purpuric lesions may initially be confused with bruising from abuse. A complete history and physical examination are usually sufficient in distinguishing Henoch-Schönlein purpura (HSP), meningococcemia, rickettsial infection, and other causes of palpable purpura from an abusive etiology (Jenny, 2001). Often, more systemic findings, such as fever and general malaise, will predominate. In HSP, the typical petechial and purpuric rash occurs on bilateral extensor surfaces, often limited to below the waist. Arthralgias, arthritis, and abdominal pain are also common findings in HSP.

Inherited defects in collagen synthesis such as Ehlers-Danlos (ED) syndrome or osteogenesis imperfecta (OI) may result in easy bruisability and poor wound healing (Bays, 2001) **(Figure 7-5)**. There are many types of ED, but the common features in all patients are joint hyperextensibility, skin fragility, and skin elasticity. A complete family history and thorough physical examination are usually sufficient to make these diagnoses.

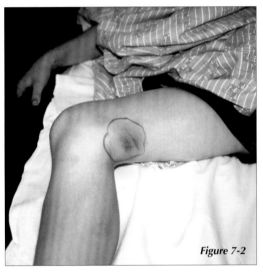

Figure 7-2

Figure 7-1.
Coining. To treat his fever, this child's family practices cao gio. A coin is rubbed up and down his back, usually in a pine tree pattern.

Figure 7-2.
Factor VIII deficiency. This patient did not recall a specific trauma to his leg.

Pseudobruising
Birthmarks
Mongolian spots have been mistaken for an abusive injury (Richardson, 1994). The typical location of these birthmarks over the sacrum and back or an uncommon location such as the face or legs in a baby may make one suspicious for abuse. However, unlike bruises, Mongolian spots are not tender, are often more uniform in color, and, most importantly, have been present since birth. Mongolian spots fade slowly over months to years, unlike bruises, which usually resolve in days to weeks.

For another example of pseudobruising, see **Figures 7-6 and 7-7**.

Dermatological Conditions
The sudden appearance of the typical target lesions found in erythema multiforme (EM) may be confused with bruising (Giardino, Christian, & Giardino, 1997a).

These lesions are characterized by an erythematous, irregular border and a dusky or ecchymotic center. EM may result from many causes, including infections with herpes simplex virus and mycoplasma and exposure to drugs such as sulfonamides or phenytoin. The tendency of more lesions to appear and for plaques to coalesce helps distinguish EM from abuse.

Figure 7-8 gives an example of another dermatological disorder.

Toxins

The rash caused by phytophotodermatitis may be easily confused with an inflicted bruise or burn. Often parents cannot offer an explanation for this "injury." However, further questioning may elicit a history of exposure to the juice of limes, figs, celery, or parsnips, all of which contain plant psoralens. The child's skin comes in contact with the psoralen-containing juice and, on exposure to sunlight, the psoralens undergo a photoreaction and irritate the skin. A rash results that is initially erythematous and then may progress to vesicles or even bullae (Leopold & Tunnessen, 1993). Dye from clothing such as a pair of new jeans or from ink pens may "tattoo" the skin and be confused with a bruise (Tunnessen, 1988).

BURNS

Just as with bruising, children may sustain burns from abusive and nonabusive mechanisms. It is often difficult to distinguish accidental from intentional burns (Kini & Lazoritz, 1998; Mayer & Burns, 2000). However, most children quickly withdraw from a heat source hot enough to burn. Therefore, burns that are extensive, deep, or

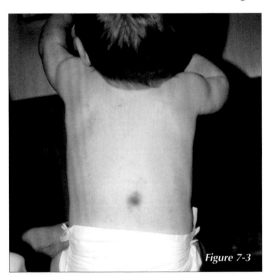

Figure 7-3

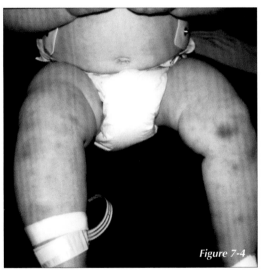

Figure 7-4

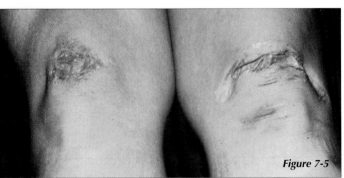

Figure 7-5

Figure 7-3. *Idiopathic thrombocytopenic purpura (ITP). This patient had petechiae and easy bruisablity. His platelet count was less than 13 000.*

Figure 7-4. *The ITP patient in Figure 7-3 (front view of the legs).*

Figure 7-5. *Scars from Ehlers-Danlos syndrome. (Contributed by Paul J. Honig, MD; Philadelphia, Pa.)*

uniform in severity; that have well-demarcated borders; or that show a distinctive pattern should arouse suspicions for abuse (Ayoub & Pfeiffer, 1979; Lenoski & Hunter, 1977).

Accidental Burns
Scalds

It is not uncommon for a curious preschooler to pull a cup of hot liquid from the table above him or her. The resulting burn from the hot liquid is usually located on the face and chest and is triangular with a narrower distal apex. The burn is less severe at the distal aspect because the liquid cools during its descent. There are irregular borders and a surrounding splatter appearance of smaller "droplets" of burns (Giardino et al., 1997a). However, it is difficult to distinguish an accidental scald burn from an inflicted one. For children who have repeated "accidental" burns or injuries, a home evaluation may assist in identifying and modifying unsafe environments or parenting practices.

Patterned Burns

When hot objects come in contact with the skin they may leave a patterned burn resembling the actual object because the object essentially brands the skin (Johnson, 1990). Such patterned burns may be accidental or inflicted on the child. For example, a curious toddler may touch, pick up, or run into a hot iron, leaving the distinctive burn of the iron grid. However, one should be concerned about the level of supervision of the child when a hot iron is being used and certainly be more suspicious of abuse if the burn is deep, multiple, or not consistent with the child's developmental abilities when compared with the history offered.

Pseudoburns

Infections, chemical irritants, and inherited skin disorders can cause erythema or blistering that may be confused with an inflicted burn **(Figure 7-9)**.

Infections

The circular lesions of impetigo caused by staphylococcal and streptococcal infections may be confused with a cigarette burn. The lesions are often more superficial, appear less uniform in shape, and heal more quickly and with less scarring than an inflicted cigarette burn. In addition, the bacterial-caused lesions often occur in crops in various stages of formation from blister to ulcers (Stewart & Rosenburg, 1996b).

The craterlike erosions seen in eczema herpeticum may also be confused with inflicted cigarette burns. Children with this condition often appear ill, with multiple vesiculated lesions in areas of eczematous involvement because of a disseminated herpes simplex infection. A scraping of a fresh lesion can be sent for diagnosis.

Bullous impetigo is a localized form of staphylococcal skin infection in infants and young children. The bullae commonly appear in the diaper area and rupture easily, causing an area of moist denuded skin. Extensive areas of infection have been confused with an immersion burn (Scales, Fleischer, & Krowchuk, 1997).

Chemical Irritants

A local contact dermatitis may be confused with an inflicted immersion burn. Diaper dermatitis **(Figure 7-10)** may result from a new diaper cream that is allergenic, the ingestion of an irritant (Leventhal, Griffin, Duncan, Starling, Christian, & Kutz, 2001), or the prolonged exposure to urine from an unchanged diaper.

A child with epidermolysis bullosa may raise concern for inflicted burns because of extensive unexplained blistering. Epidermolysis bullosa is an inherited disorder characterized by blistering with minimal trauma. Disease severity and age of presentation vary greatly among the disorder's different forms (Darmstadt, 2000).

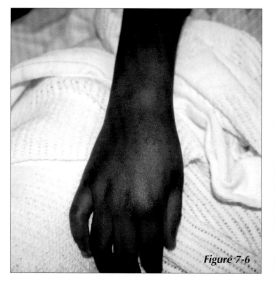

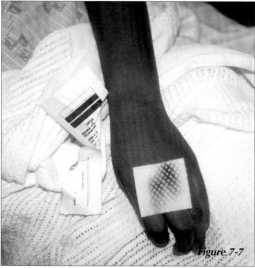

Figure 7-6

Figure 7-7

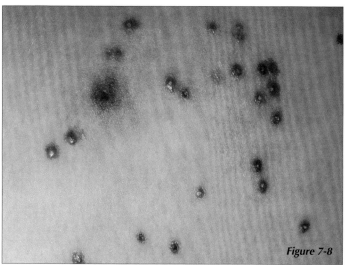

Figure 7-6. *Pseudobruise. This patient had recently dyed her hair red.*

Figure 7-7. *The "bruise" came off easily with alcohol.*

Figure 7-8

Figure 7-8. *Crop of molluscum contagiosum lesions with several demonstrating inflammation surrounding the base of the classic core-filled pearly lesions. (Contributed by Paul J. Honig, MD; Philadelphia, Pa.)*

Figure 7-9. *Ecthyma. This patient has a history of bug bites. Notice the smaller red papule on her left lower quadrant, which may evolve into a similar lesion. The lesion is bigger than expected from a cigarette burn. (Contributed by Martha Stevens, MD, MSCE; Milwaukee, Wisc.)*

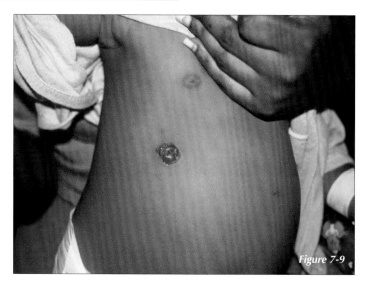

Figure 7-9

FRACTURES

Broken bones may arouse suspicions for child abuse if they are found in a very young, preambulatory child, if there are multiple fractures at different stages of healing, or if the fracture is not consistent with the reported mechanism and/or the child's developmental abilities (Kini & Lazoritz, 1998; Mayer & Burns, 2000). Certain fracture types are also very concerning for abuse because they are highly associated with abusive causes, such as metaphyseal bucket handle or rib fractures (Kleinman, 1998). When evaluating skeletal fractures in children it is important to consider accidental and abusive etiologies because both may be possible. In addition, birth-related fractures and inherited, metabolic, and infectious disorders may cause some of the same findings found with inflicted trauma (Giardino, Christian, & Giardino, 1997b). **Table 7-2** describes some mimics of abusive fractures and their distinguishing characteristics.

Accidental Injury

Ambulatory children may have signs and symptoms of a broken bone, and the history provided by the caregiver may point to everyday activities of play and exploration (Rivara, Parrish, & Mueller, 1986). If the child is older and involved in sport activities, he or she may even have multiple fractures over time. Although there is no magical number of fractures that should be considered "too many," each child who presents with a fracture should have a complete evaluation that considers abuse as a possible etiology. In addition, the clinician must always make sure the history fits the injury and the child's developmental level.

Birth-Related Fractures

In a recent study of over 30 000 births, the incidence of fractures attributed to labor and delivery was 0.1% (Bhat, Kumar, & Oumachigui, 1994). Macrosomia, shoulder dystocia, difficult or prolonged delivery, and prematurity have been implicated as risk factors for antenatal fractures (Nadas & Reinberg, 1992; Roberts et al., 1995). The clavicle is by far the most commonly fractured bone, followed by the humerus, femur, and skull (Bhat et al., 1994; Strait, Siegel, & Shapiro, 1995; Thomas, Rosenfield, Leventhal, & Markowitz, 1991; Turnpenny & Nimmo, 1993). Rib fractures are extremely rare birth injuries (Bulloch, Schubert, Brophy, Johnson, Reed, & Shapiro, 2000; Rubin, 1964). An important distinguishing characteristic of a birth fracture is that there should be signs of healing by age 2 weeks (Cumming, 1979).

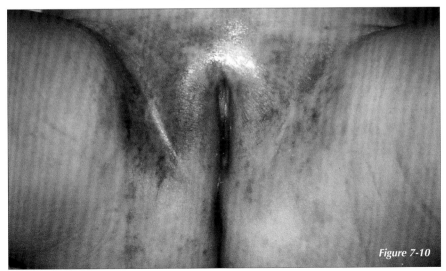

Figure 7-10.
Dermatitis in perineal area, secondary to use of super absorbent diapers. (Contributed by Paul J. Honig, MD; Philadelphia, Pa.)

Figure 7-10

Table 7-2. Disorders That Mimic Fractures Occuring From Abuse

DISORDER	HISTORY	PHYSICAL EXAM-INATION FINDINGS	LABORATORY ABNORMALITIES	X-RAY FINDINGS
Congenital syphilis*	Two thirds of patients may be asymptomatic at birth. Symptoms may include profuse rhinitis, erythematous rash with subsequent desquamation of hands and feet, or decreased use of limb secondary to pain from perio-steal or bone inflammation.	Infants may have snuffles, saddle nose deformity, or extramedullary hematopoiesis. Hepatospleno-megaly, failure to thrive (FTT).	CBC: anemia, thrombocytopenia UA: hematuria, proteinuria Elevated liver funtion tests CSF pleocytosis Serological testing is diagnostic	Diffuse periostitis of long bones Osteochondritis of joints
Fracture from birth trauma	A prolonged or difficult delivery, forceps use, and macrosomia have been associated with fracture from birth.†‡	The usual findings of swelling or extremity disuse may not be found on the newborn screening examination. Callus formation over a healing clavicle fracture may be palpable.		Evidence healing fracture within 11-14 days from birth. Rest of skeletal survey is without fractures. The clavicle is most commonly fractured, followed by humerus, femur, and skull fractures. Rib fractures are rarely a result of birth trauma.†‡§

(continued)

Table 7-2. *(continued)*

DISORDER	HISTORY	PHYSICAL EXAM-INATION FINDINGS	LABORATORY ABNORMALITIES	X-RAY FINDINGS
Osteogenesis imperfecta (OI)	Inherited in auto-somal dominant fashion History of early deafness, frequent fractures, easy bruisability	Patient may have evidence of poor wound healing, blue sclera, abnormal dentition, joint hypermobility, and hearing impairment.	Collagen bio-chemical studies of skin biopsy confirm diagnosis and type of OI.	Multiple fractures at different stages of healing. Osteopenia is a late finding secondary to lack of weight bearing. Fracture severity will vary with the different types of OI.
Rickets	Patients at risk include pre-mature infants, breastfed babies not receiving vitamin supple-ments, and children with liver or kidney disease. Patients may present with seizures or with complaints related to etiology of rickets.‖	Prominent costochondral junctions. Findings will be primarily related to the underlying etiology.	Normocalcemia Hypocalcemia Hypopho-sphatemia Elevated alkaline phosphatase	Fraying of metaphysical and costochondral junctions Epiphyseal widening Periosteal evaluation Osteopenia

*Azimi P. Syphilis. In: Behrman RE, Kleigman RM, Jensen HB, eds. Nelson Textbook of Pediatrics. 16th ed. Philadelphia, Pa: WB Saunders; 2000:903-907.

†Bhat BV, Kumar A, Oumachigui A. Bone injuries during delivery. Indian J Pediatr. 1994;61:401-405.

‡Harmann RW. Radiologic case of the month. Arch Pediatr Adolesc Med. 1997;151:947-948.

§Cumming WA. Neonatal skeletal fractures: birth trauma or abuse? J Assoc Can Radiol. 1979;30:30-33.

‖Giardino AP, Christian CW, Giardino ER. Evaluation of fractures and skeletal injuries. In: Giardino AP, Christian CW, Giardino ER, eds. A Practical Guide to the Evaluation of Child Abuse and Neglect. Thousand Oaks, Calif: Sage Publications; 1997b:97-126.

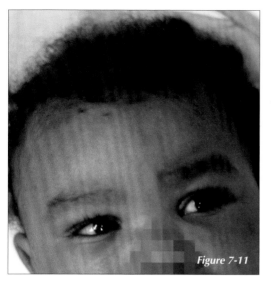

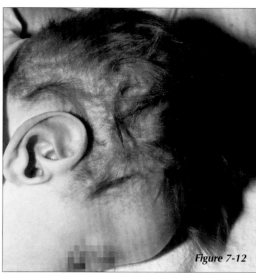

Figure 7-11

Figure 7-12

Figure 7-11.
This patient has osteogenesis imperfecta (OI) with blue sclera.

Figure 7-12.
Menkes' kinky hair syndrome. (Contributed by Paul J. Honig, MD; Philadelphia, Pa.)

Inherited/Metabolic Disorders

Osteogenesis imperfecta (OI) is a rare inherited disorder caused by a defect in collagen synthesis (Paterson & McAllion, 1989). Children with OI may suffer multiple fractures with minimal trauma because of brittle bones. The 4 major types of OI vary in clinical expression. A thorough history and physical examination are usually sufficient in differentiating types I, II, and III from abuse. These patients have additional findings that suggest OI, including blue sclera **(Figure 7-11)**, abnormal dentition, short stature, wormian bones of the skull, joint laxity, easy bruisability, perinatal fractures, and/or a positive family history of OI (Giardino et al., 1997b). Type IV, a rare form of OI, may not have any of these distinguishing features, which has led to misdiagnosis of abuse. A helpful clue to type IV is continued fractures despite different caretakers (Giardino et al., 1997b). However, children with OI might also be abused. In addition, OI is much rarer than child abuse. Therefore, abuse is much more likely in a young child with a history of multiple unexplained fractures and no other suggestion of OI (Stewart & Rosenberg, 1996a).

Deficiencies in copper and in vitamins A, D, and C may cause skeletal changes that mimic abusive injuries. In Menkes' syndrome **(Figure 7-12)**, copper malabsorption leads to characteristic hematological, neurological, and dermatological derangements, as well as metaphyseal bone spurs and diffuse periostitis. These skeletal anomalies may be confused with a metaphyseal fracture or evidence of an old healing fracture.

Nutritional rickets is the most common form of vitamin D deficiency. Breastfed babies with little sun exposure are particularly susceptible. The periosteal bone formation and metaphyseal changes that occur during the healing phase have been confused with fractures from abuse. The fraying that occurs at the costochondral junctions, the so-called rachitic rosary, should not be mistaken for rib fractures (Stewart & Rosenberg, 1996a). Regarding laboratory values, calcium levels will be low to normal, phosphate levels low, and alkaline phosphatase levels high. Vitamin C deficiency, or scurvy, may result in metaphyseal fractures that could be confused with abuse. A complete dietary history and additional typical radiographic changes seen in scurvy help discriminate between the 2 diagnoses (Stewart & Rosenberg, 1996a).

Osteopenia, for many reasons, such as prematurity or prolonged immobilization, will make bones more susceptible to fractures with minor trauma. For example, an increase in range-of-motion exercises during physical therapy can result in a long bone fracture in a nonambulatory child with spina bifida. Plain radiographs should demonstrate generalized osteopenia.

Blount's disease is a rare disorder that causes bilateral metaphyseal abnormalities of the proximal tibia because of asymmetric growth of the medial aspect. Untreated, this disease can lead to length discrepancy or bowing of the lower extremities (Thompson & Scoles, 2000).

Hereditary sensory neuropathy is a rare inherited disorder in which the child does not feel pain or extremes of temperature. Because these children do not sense painful stimuli they may not seek treatment until a deformity of a healed fracture is apparent. They may also have extensive bruises, old abrasions, and burns because of their insensitivity to pain (Spencer & Grieve, 1990; Stewart & Rosenberg, 1996a).

Infections

Congenital syphilis may lead to radiographic findings that raise the suspicion for inflicted injury. Metaphysitis, diffuse periostitis, and pathological fractures associated with congenital syphilis may be confused with abuse (Stewart & Rosenberg, 1996a). Most children with congenital syphilis are seen within the first 6 months of life and will have serological results that indicate infection with *Treponema pallidum* **(Figure 7-13).**

EYE INJURIES
Retinal Hemorrhages

Although the vast majority of infants and young children with retinal hemorrhages are victims of abuse, this injury is not pathognomonic for abuse. Retinal hemorrhages have been described in children related to birth, major trauma, infections, blood dyscrasias, metabolic disorders, and intracranial lesions (Gayle, Kissoon, Hered, & Harwood-Nuss, 1995). Most children who have retinal hemorrhages because of abuse are younger than age 1 year (Ophthalmology Child Abuse Working Party, 1999). The shearing and sudden deceleration forces that cause many of the findings in shaken baby syndrome (SBS) **(Figures 7-14 to 7-20)** play an important role in the development of retinal hemorrhages. A baby's relatively large head size, weak neck musculature, and immature myelination puts him/her at higher risk for such an injury (Duhaime et al., 1992).

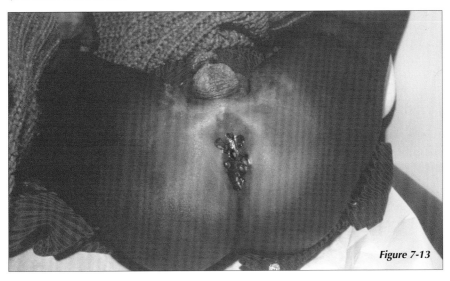

Figure 7-13.
Perineum of a prepubertal child who has perinatally acquired syphilis. Condylomata lata surround the perianal area. (Contributed by Paul J. Honig, MD; Philadelphia, Pa.)

Figure 7-13

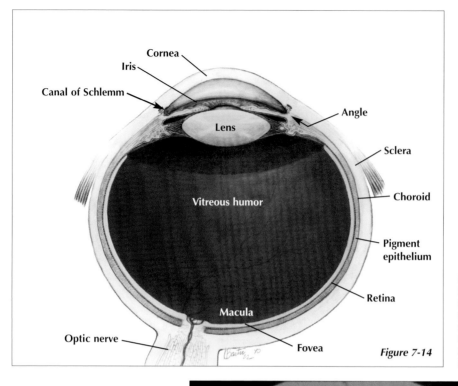

Figure 7-14.
Illustration of the normal eye. (Contributed by the National Eye Institute, National Institutes of Health; Bethesda, Md.)

Figure 7-15. *Color fundoscopic photo showing a normal retina and optic nerve. (Contributed by Brian J. Forbes, MD, PhD; Philadelphia, Pa.)*

Figure 7-16. *Color fundoscopic photo showing marked retinal hemorrhages at all layers of the retina in the eye of an SBS victim. (Contributed by Brian J. Forbes, MD, PhD; Philadelphia, Pa.)*

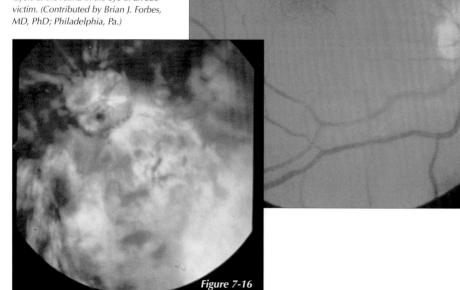

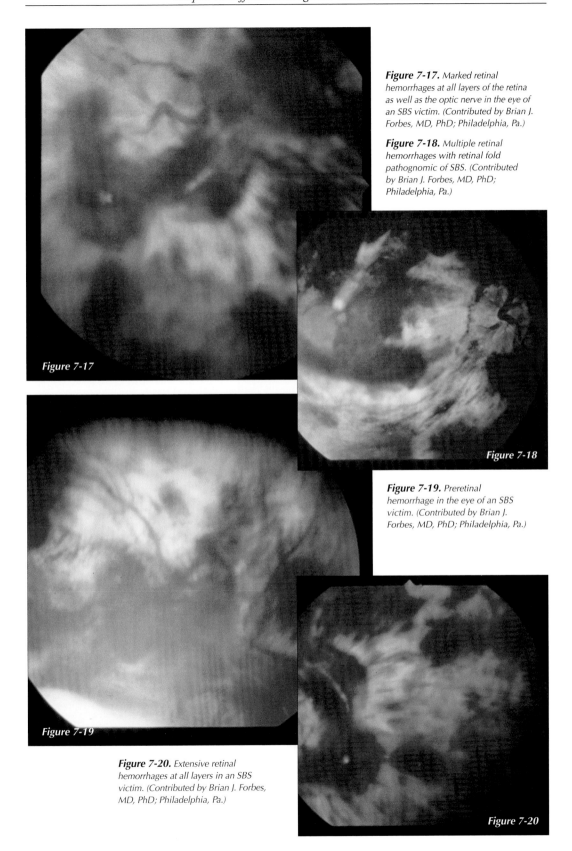

Figure 7-17. *Marked retinal hemorrhages at all layers of the retina as well as the optic nerve in the eye of an SBS victim. (Contributed by Brian J. Forbes, MD, PhD; Philadelphia, Pa.)*

Figure 7-18. *Multiple retinal hemorrhages with retinal fold pathognomic of SBS. (Contributed by Brian J. Forbes, MD, PhD; Philadelphia, Pa.)*

Figure 7-19. *Preretinal hemorrhage in the eye of an SBS victim. (Contributed by Brian J. Forbes, MD, PhD; Philadelphia, Pa.)*

Figure 7-20. *Extensive retinal hemorrhages at all layers in an SBS victim. (Contributed by Brian J. Forbes, MD, PhD; Philadelphia, Pa.)*

Figure 7-17

Figure 7-18

Figure 7-19

Figure 7-20

Retinal Hemorrhage From Birth Trauma

Approximately 11% to 30% of newborns are found to have retinal hemorrhages after delivery (Baum & Bulpitt, 1970; Jain, Singh, Grupta, & Gupta, 1980). The exact mechanism is not completely understood, and hemorrhages have been found in children after a cesarean section. Retinal hemorrhages from birth resolve relatively quickly with no visual deficits, most by age 2 weeks, though some may take longer. All of these are gone by 4 to 6 weeks after birth (Levin, 2001; Ophthalmology Child Abuse Working Party, 1999).

Trauma

Retinal hemorrhages have been described after major polytrauma, such as a motor vehicle collision (Johnson, Braun, & Friendly, 1993). Although retinal hemorrhages in infants have been described after "household trauma," the mechanisms were not trivial, and the possibility of child abuse must fully be explored in such cases (Christian, Taylor, Hertle, & Duhaime, 1999).

Infections

Retinal hemorrhages have been reportedly associated with malaria, rickettsia, cytomegalovirus, and human immunodeficiency virus (HIV) (Gayle et al., 1995). Any infection that causes disseminated vascular coagulopathy or septic emboli may also cause retinal hemorrhage.

Hematological Disorders

Retinal hemorrhages may be associated with many of the inherited or acquired hematological disorders, including leukemia, aplastic anemia, and sickle cell disease (Gayle et al., 1995).

Metabolic Disorders

Retinal hemorrhages have been associated with galactosemia (Levy, Brown, Williams, & de Juan, 1996) and glutaric aciduria (Morris et al., 1999). Distinguishing glutaric aciduria from abuse may be particularly troublesome because children with this disorder have many of the same features as those with SBS, specifically subdural hematomas, irritability, and FTT. Findings on imaging studies and laboratory evaluation are helpful in establishing the diagnosis of glutaric aciduria. However, the 2 conditions of disease and abuse can coexist, especially because these babies are often irritable and difficult to feed (Morris et al., 1999).

Intracranial Lesions

Retinal hemorrhages are also associated with subdural hematomas, arteriovenous malformations, and subarachnoid hemorrhages (Gayle et al., 1995). The role cardiopulmonary resuscitation (CPR) plays in causing retinal hemorrhages is controversial. Autopsy and animal model data do not support CPR as the sole mechanism of retinal hemorrhages (Gayle et al., 1995). In addition, one recent prospective study of 43 children found only one child who had small punctate retinal hemorrhages after receiving CPR (Odom et al., 1997).

Retinal hemorrhages have been seen in association with severe hypertension, HSP, postoperative ocular and cardiac surgery, and extracorporeal membrane oxygenation (Ophthalmology Child Abuse Working Party, 1999).

Subconjunctival Hemorrhages

Although bruising anywhere in a newborn is concerning for abuse, up to one third of newborns may have subconjunctival hemorrhages after delivery that resolve quickly (Baum & Bulpitt, 1970; Jain et al., 1980; Katzman, 1992). Subconjunctival hemorrhages may also occur if the patient has had particularly forceful coughing episodes, as may occur in pertussis. In addition, any coagulation disorder may lead to subconjunctival hemorrhages.

Periorbital Bruising

Parents may seek care because their child has periorbital bruising without a history of trauma. However, on further questioning, many of these children have had some minor head trauma in the preceding 1 to 2 weeks or a bruise may be on the forehead. These "raccoon eyes" can result from the pooling of blood in the more dependent interorbital region.

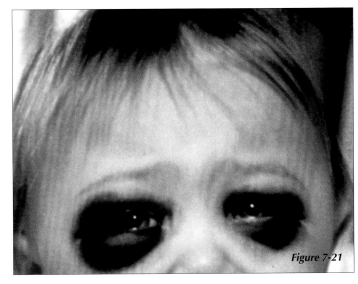

Figure 7-21

An unusual cause of "spontaneous" periorbital bruising with proptosis is neuroblastoma that has metastasized to the orbits **(Figure 7-21)**. Such "bruising" is probably the result of venous congestion (Caron & Pearson, 1998).

Figure 7-21.
Orbital neuroblastoma can invade the orbits and cause "magical" periorbital bruising. (Contributed by Marc Gorelick, MD; Milwaukee, Wisc.)

FAILURE TO THRIVE AND GROWTH FAILURE

Many situations uncovered in clinical practice may indicate neglect as a possible etiology, including a child who fails to grow as expected, one who lacks routine primary care, a situation in which the caregiver or child seeks medical attention later than would be normally expected, and a child who has poor hygiene. The healthcare provider should carefully consider the child's basic needs and determine whether or not these are being met (Dubowitz, Giardino, & Gustavson, 2000).

Children who do not grow according to expected parameters raise concerns about several possible medical conditions and are often said to be experiencing growth failure or FTT (Zenel, 1997). In general, FTT is a nonspecific term that may be synonymous with growth failure, undernutrition, and growth retardation, depending on a given set of clinical circumstances (Wilcox, Nieburg, & Miller, 1989). Alexander (1992) conceptualizes the fundamental nutritional issues that lie at the root of all FTT cases as being too few calories going into the child, too many calories going out of the child, or too many calories being used up by the child. Children are said to suffer from FTT when their growth pattern becomes problematic and their growth parameters demonstrate the following:

— Weight and/or weight for height measurements follow a curve less than 3%, essentially more than 2 standard deviations from the mean for their age.

— Weight measurements (less commonly height and head circumference) drop across at least 2 formal growth curves (i.e., 95th, 90th, 75th, 50th, 25th, 10th, 5th).

— Fluctuating growth pattern of near normal periods of growth followed by abnormal delayed periods, producing what has been described as a "sawtooth pattern."

Early thinking about FTT categorized the etiologies for this syndrome into organic (or medical) and nonorganic (or psychosocial) causes (Cantwell, 1997; Helfer, 1990). Organic etiologies represented bona fide medical conditions as the cause for the growth failure, whereas nonorganic causes were psychosocially related and revolved around neglectful parenting styles and significant environmental stressors in the child's life. Over time, the overlap between these categories was understood, and mixed cases were identified that represented combinations of organic and nonorganic causes in which a medical problem, nutrition issue, or feeding style expressed itself in an environment that was unable to meet the challenges of the child's needs (Homer & Ludwig, 1981). (See Chapter 8, Clinical Aspects of Child Neglect, for a further discussion of FTT.)

Many medical causes can lead to FTT, and extensive workups may be needed to rule out various suspected medical conditions (Berwick, Levy, & Kleinerman, 1982). As with any differential diagnostic process, the workup must be tailored to the clinical circumstances of the case. Knowing that many FTT cases are in fact mixed, and understanding that the adequacy of the caregiving environment around nutritional issues must be assessed, adds to the information the clinician should collect and factor into the differential diagnostic process.

Central to the workup for FTT are a history, physical examination, and laboratory assessment. The history should focus on signs and symptoms of the various medical conditions and explore the child's nutritional intake (Gahagan & Holmes, 1998). The physical examination focuses on growth parameters, patterns of growth, and findings consistent with various congenital or acquired medical conditions. The physical examination also evaluates other findings that may suggest a neglectful environment, such as poor grooming and hygiene, excessive diaper rash, or improper dress for the climate. The laboratory workup focuses on diagnostic possibilities suggested by the history and physical examination and should not be composed of an automatic extensive set of laboratory tests not indicated by the history or physical examination because such "fishing expeditions" rarely yield new or useful information (Berwick et al., 1982; Homer & Ludwig, 1981). However, once the clinician completes the basic history and physical examination and considers reasonable diagnoses, he or she considers possible screening laboratory tests. Evaluations that are reasonable as a first step and that may be indicated in the preliminary evaluation of FTT include the following:

— Complete blood count to include hemoglobin, hematocrit, platelet count, white blood count, and standard red cell indices

— Basic electrolyte panel to include sodium, potassium, chloride, bicarbonate, blood urea nitrogen, and creatinine

— Erythrocyte sedimentation rate (ESR)

— Urinalysis

— Bone age radiographs

Other tests and diagnostic studies should be considered based on the clinical situation and diagnostic factors being considered.

Medical conditions to be considered include growth variations, congenital anatomical anomalies, congenital and chromosomal disorders, and organ system disorders.

GROWTH VARIATIONS

Constitutional short stature may be seen in a well-nourished child whose height and weight are at a similar percentile and in whom a weight-for-height curve is normal. Normal leanness is seen in an adequately nourished healthy child whose family members demonstrate a propensity for a slender body habitus. Shifting linear growth may be seen in some children as they establish their appropriate formal growth curves, but the FTT workup should be pursued in situations before crossing the 5th percentile (Bithoney, Dubowitz, & Egan, 1992). Prematurity affects the child's birth measurements, and adequate assessment requires correction for the child's gestational age for approximately 2 years for weight and 3 years for length or height (Brandt, 1979). Finally, intrauterine growth restriction (IUGR) also affects the child's growth. Symmetric IUGR, in which head circumference, weight, and length are all affected, may arise for various reasons, including prenatal drug and alcohol exposure, congenital infections, and several chromosomal syndromes. Asymmetric or head-sparing IUGR is seen when the weight measurement is decreased out of proportion to the head circumference and often results from insufficient nutrition reaching the growing fetus. Asymmetric IUGR has the best prognosis for postnatal growth provided that adequate nutrition is provided.

CONGENITAL ANATOMICAL ANOMALIES

Congenital anomalies may be associated with growth problems for various reasons, depending on the impact of the anomaly on the child's growth potential and ability to feed. Cleft lip and cleft palate are among the clearest examples of how a congenital anomaly can affect growth and the child's ability to thrive. Cleft lip and cleft palate are midline craniofacial defects that make proper nutritional intake difficult because the baby cannot create an adequate seal for sucking. Feeding techniques for children with cleft lip and cleft palate have been developed but are challenging. These children also experience frequent otitis media infections that adversely affect their growth.

CONGENITAL AND CHROMOSOMAL DISORDERS

A large number of identified congenital syndromes have growth failure as a component. Some syndromes have a clearly defined genetic basis. One of the better understood syndromes is Turner syndrome (Ulrich-Turner syndrome), which is caused by the complete or partial absence of the X chromosome in females (Wiedemann, Kunze, & Grosse, 1997). In this syndrome, affected children fail to grow as expected, manifest short stature, and fail to undergo pubertal development. Growth failure, however, is rarely the only finding indicating a genetic syndrome. In Turner syndrome, the growth failure is also associated with other findings, such as neck webbing, various skeletal anomalies (hand, shield chest), and retarded bone age. For the well-recognized syndromes, chromosomal analysis is diagnostic.

ORGAN SYSTEM DISORDERS

Cardiovascular System

In congenital heart disease (CHD), poor cardiovascular function does not provide adequate oxygen and other nutrients to the body's tissues, nor are metabolic waste products adequately removed. Over time this leads to a clinical situation marked by acidosis, polycythemia, and increased caloric requirements. Growth is impaired secondary to the inability to provide adequate nutrition. Children who develop congestive heart failure as part of their clinical picture experience poor cardiac pumping function that also impairs oxygen delivery capacity and other normal metabolic functions, such as removal of waste products. In the setting of impaired cardiac function, the exertion of feeding leads to increased caloric consumption, which only further worsens the growth failure.

Endocrine System

Some endocrinological disorders may affect growth, especially those affecting growth hormone and thyroid hormone. Growth hormone deficiency leads to impaired growth and short stature. Thyroid disorders are among the most common endocrinological disorders that may cause a child to not grow according to expectations. Hyperthyroidism may present as congenital hyperthyroidism in the neonate or, more commonly, can present as an autoimmune thyroid disease or Graves' disease, with tachycardia, nervousness, and weight loss in the face of increased appetite. Hypothyroidism, if present at birth, is usually diagnosed by newborn screening and includes decreased tone, lethargy, poor feeding, and diminished growth. After the neonatal period, hypothyroidism in the child presents primarily as a slowing of linear growth with delayed bone age and often delayed puberty. Serum thyroid function tests are abnormal.

Gastrointestinal System

Children may be born at normal weight but during the first few weeks to months of life may experience feeding problems. Such problems may be related to incorrect formula preparation, breastfeeding problems, difficulties with mother-infant attachment, and anatomical problems of the airway and/or esophagus. Gastroesophageal reflux, present to some degree in almost all neonates, may become problematic. The movement of stomach contents into the esophagus may occur with or without vomiting and can interfere with adequate caloric intake. Inflammatory bowel disease may manifest itself as a pattern of remitting and relapsing signs and symptoms including cramping, abdominal pain, diarrhea, blood in the stool, fever, anorexia, weight loss, and growth failure. Severe growth restriction may precede the onset of gastrointestinal symptoms.

Malabsorption of nutrients may lead to growth failure and conditions such as celiac disease with intolerance to gluten, carbohydrate malabsorption with intolerance to sugars such as lactose, cow's milk allergy, soybean allergy, and pancreatic enzyme deficiency (Shwachman-Diamond syndrome). The presentation for malabsorption syndromes includes diarrhea, flatulence, bloating, unintended weight loss, and poor growth pattern over time.

Hematological and Oncological Disorders

Malignancies in children can result in abnormal growth patterns based on a number of possible etiologies. These include the direct effects of the neoplasm, a poor metabolic state, loss of appetite secondary to the disease or the treatment of recurrent infections resulting from immunosuppression, chronic diarrhea secondary to the effects of chemotherapy/radiation, and central nervous system disorders secondary to the disease or the treatment that have an impact on the hypothalamic-pituitary axis, such as irradiation.

Immunological System

Immunodeficiency may be a component of many congenital syndromes. Congenital growth failure may result from recurrent infections that develop and lead to increased work of breathing associated with chronic pneumonia, painful swallowing with chronic candidiasis, and chronic diarrhea with related malabsorption. Children with HIV/AIDS may manifest growth failure for various reasons, including esophagitis; diarrhea from parasitic, viral, or bacterial infections; and malabsorption. Constitutional symptoms such as malaise lead to decreased appetite, and a variety of recurrent infections may lead to weight loss.

Autoimmune-type disorders such as juvenile rheumatoid arthritis (JRA), systemic lupus erythematosus (SLE), and dermatomyositis may be associated with growth failure secondary to the presence of malaise, decreased appetite, chronic inflammation, weight loss, gastrointestinal involvement, and chronic steroid use.

Metabolic Disorders

Metabolic disorders typically present with recurring episodes of lethargy, poor feeding, vomiting, and seizures. The laboratory evaluation necessary depends on the clinical situation and the suspected defect. Galactosemia is a well-studied defect that manifests itself in the neonatal period after the initiation of routine feedings that contain the sugar galactose. The child's signs and symptoms include vomiting, diarrhea, jaundice (elevated conjugated bilirubin level), poor feeding, abdominal distention with ascites and hepatosplenomegaly, poor weight gain, hypoglycemia, and aminoaciduria.

Renal System

Renal tubular acidosis (RTA) occurs as several types with various causes and results in a metabolic acidosis associated with poor growth. The urine pH has excess base present, and the serum bicarbonate level is low. Bacterial urinary tract infection (UTI), if chronic, may lead to kidney damage that significantly affects growth. Renal failure leads to metabolic abnormalities and nutritional restrictions that affect growth. The treatments for these problems may also affect growth.

Respiratory System

Cystic fibrosis is a multisystem exocrine dysfunction that leads to serious respiratory and gastrointestinal manifestations associated with growth failure. Respiratory involvement includes wheezing, recurrent pneumonia, and sinusitis, while gastrointestinal involvement is seen with pancreatic insufficiency and associated malabsorption. Growth failure results from the combined effects of the increased caloric needs from the respiratory effort and infections, as well as decreased nutrition secondary to poor absorption. Chronic lung disease is associated with growth failure because of chronic hypoxia, recurrent pneumonia, and the increased caloric requirement from the work of breathing.

SEXUAL ABUSE

GENITAL AND ANAL FINDINGS

The differential diagnosis for anogenital signs and symptoms, such as erythema, excoriation, pruritus, bruising, bleeding, genital discharge, and unusual anogenital appearance, includes physical and sexual abuse (Emans & Goldstein, 1990; Wilson, 1992; Woodruff, 1992). Several conditions affecting the anogenital area may have physical findings similar to those seen in sexual maltreatment and consequently could be confused with this type of abuse. As with most differential diagnoses, the diagnostic process begins with careful attention to the history provided by the child and caregivers. This is especially true with regard to suspected sexual abuse because the presenting complaint often includes various nonspecific behavioral changes. Next, the diagnostic process collects information from the physical examination. The physical examination in potential sexual maltreatment cases frequently does not uncover definitive findings for abuse, and findings that are present are often nonspecific (Adams, 2001; Kellogg, Parra, & Menard, 1998). The laboratory evaluation in sexual abuse cases is often not diagnostic unless seminal products or a noncongenitally acquired sexually transmitted disease (STD) is found (American Academy of Pediatrics, 1999). Because possible sexual abuse cases are rarely straightforward, consultation with a multidisciplinary team at a regional center may be necessary to sort out the evaluation findings and to work through the differential diagnoses of the child with anogenital complaints (Kini & Lazoritz, 1998).

Vaginitis, vulvitis, and vulvovaginitis cause a wide range of signs and symptoms referable to the anogenital area (Emans & Goldstein, 1990; Jaquiery, Stylianopoulos, Hogg, & Grover, 1999; Koumantakis, Hassan, Deligeoroglou, & Creatsas, 1997). Vulvitis occurs when the vulvar structures (labia majora, labia minora, clitoris, and components of the vestibule) become inflamed and friable. Vaginitis occurs when the vaginal mucosa becomes inflamed, is friable, may bleed, and produces a discharge. Vulvovaginitis is a combination of both entities, and one frequently leads to the other

(Paradise, Campos, Friedman, & Frishmuth, 1982). Males may also have genital inflammation, but this is seen less frequently than in girls. In boys, comparable inflammatory conditions affecting the most distal portion of the penis include phimosis, paraphimosis in the uncircumcised male, and urethritis in circumcised and uncircumcised males. Male and female children have perianal signs and symptoms that result from inflammation.

This chapter addresses the differential diagnosis for the following anogenital signs and symptoms in the prepubertal child:

— Anogenital erythema, excoriation, and pruritus

— Anogenital bruising

— Anogenital bleeding and/or bloody vaginal discharge

— Nonbloody vaginal discharge

— Unusual anogenital appearance, congenital and acquired

Anogenital Erythema, Excoriation, and Pruritus

Redness in the anogenital tissues and structures may arise from several causes related to inflammation **(Figure 7-22)**. A vicious cycle may ensue in which inflammation, irritation, and pruritus lead to repeated scratching of the affected area, increased scratching leads to a worsening in the inflammatory process, and the cycle continues (O'Brien, 1995; Wilson, 1992; Woodruff, 1992). Causes of this situation that should be considered include various local conditions, systemic disease, inappropriate genital manipulation, and STDs. Depending on the history and clinical index of suspicion, other diagnostic possibilities include local irritation, dermatological disorders, infections, and, uncommonly, systemic conditions such as Crohn's disease, Kawasaki disease, and Stevens-Johnson syndrome.

Local Irritation

Poor hygienic practices such as wiping the anogenital area from back to front (instead of the hygienic front to back) lead to possible fecal contamination of the vagina and the development of vaginitis and its accompanying irritation and pruritus (Paradise et al., 1982). Retained urine in the skin folds of obese children, urinary reflux, and poor drainage of urine into the vagina may lead to inflammation and irritation (Tunnessen,

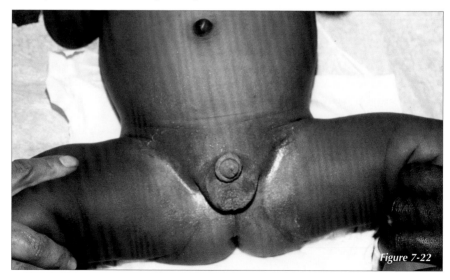

Figure 7-22.
Male infant with perineal erythema and fever raising concern about bacterial superinfection. (Contributed by Paul J. Honig, MD; Philadelphia, Pa.)

Figure 7-22

1988). Any type of restrictive or poorly ventilated clothing, whether underwear, pants, or tights, may lead to friction and increased heat that can result in inflammation, irritation, pruritus, and erythema (Altchek, 1985). Chemical irritants including soaps, fragrances, colored toilet tissue, and bubble baths commonly lead to inflammation in the anogenital area as well. Sandbox vulvitis deserves special mention because it is caused by the entrapment of particles of dirt or sand in the child's vulvar area (Tunnessen, 1988). In the prepubertal child, the labia majora do not fully surround the vulvar structures, and the child may come into contact with contaminating material while sitting on the ground during play outdoors.

Dermatological Disorders

Contact dermatitis is a skin irritation that results after contact with substances to which the skin is sensitive, typically on an allergic basis (Woodruff, 1992). Seborrhea in the genital area is common in infancy, although it may occur at any age. It involves the folds of the diaper area between the labia minora and labia majora. Seborrheic rashes may be pruritic and frequently become secondarily infected from scratching as a result of breaks in the skin's protective barriers. Seborrheic lesions in the genital area appear elevated and erythematous. The yellow, greasy scales of seborrhea are also commonly observed in extragenital areas (Gordon, 1983; Williams, Callen, & Owen, 1986). Psoriasis is a dermatological condition that affects children at any age. The diagnostic lesions vary in size and location and are sharply demarcated, pruritic, erythematous plaques with silvery scales on a flat surface (Altchek, 1996; Quint & Smith, 1999).

Lichen sclerosis is an uncommon dermatological condition of unknown etiology that is often seen in the anogenital area. In females, it presents as irregular ivory macules or papules that coalesce to form atrophic hypopigmented plaques in an hourglass or figure-eight pattern (Albers, Taylor, Huyer, Oliver, & Krafchik, 2000; Berth-Jones, Graham-Brown, & Burns, 1989; Loening-Baucke, 1991). In males, lichen sclerosis, known as balanitis xerotica obliterans, presents as a chronic, progressive, atrophic, sclerosing process of the glans and foreskin (Laymon & Freeman, 1944; Rickwood, Hemalatha, Batcup, & Spitz, 1980). The skin in both the male and female becomes thin and fissured, may appear reddened and edematous, and is easily traumatized by minimal pressure (**Figure 7-23**).

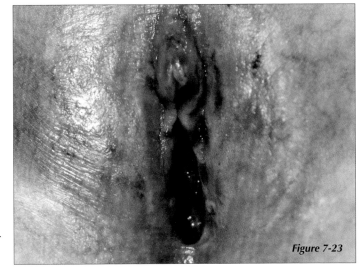

Figure 7-23

Figure 7-23. Prepubertal female child's external genitalia demonstrating the friable skin findings seen in lichen sclerosis. (Contributed by Paul J. Honig, MD; Philadelphia, Pa.)

Infections

Infection caused by STDs may lead to local irritation and redness. (See Chapter 6, Sexually Transmitted Diseases in the Setting of Maltreatment for further discussion.) Therefore, such findings need to be assessed for possible STDs. Nonspecific vaginitis is a mixed bacterial infection caused by a combination of coliforms, streptococci, *Haemophilus vaginalis*, and other bacteria (Preminger & Pokorny, 1998). Vaginitis frequently leads to a secondary vulvitis with local irritation, inflammation, erythema, and pruritus (Wilson, 1992). Infestation with pinworms may cause vulvovaginitis as well. The female pinworm *(Enterobius vermicularis)* resides in the child's intestinal tract and migrates to the perianal area to deposit eggs. This causes pruritus, scratching, and irritation. Pinworms may move from the rectum to the vagina and can introduce fecal flora into the vagina, resulting in a bacterial vulvovaginitis (Altchek, 1972).

Scabies, caused by a parasitic mite *(Sarcoptes scabiei)*, results in the development of pruritic erythematous papules with wavy burrows. Candidal overgrowth in the anogenital area may occur after a course of antibiotics, with diabetes mellitus, when the child is in diapers, or as a result of other risk factors, such as immunodeficiency (Emans & Goldstein, 1990). Exposure to antibiotics may change the makeup of the vaginal flora, which keeps the yeast in check.

Finally, perianal streptococcal cellulitis is recognized as an etiology leading to a perianal rash that has an intense confluent erythematous area surrounding the anus (Mogielnicki, Schwartzman, & Elliott, 2000). The rash is irregular but well demarcated. The condition may cause painful defecation, blood-streaked stools, and perianal inflammation and irritation **(Figure 7-24)**.

Systemic Conditions

Crohn's disease, an inflammatory bowel disease, may have vulvar or perianal involvement and may be confused with sexual abuse (Clayden, 1987; Quint & Smith, 1999). The skin findings associated with Kawasaki disease may involve the anogenital area and present with a perineal rash that is painful, erythematous, and macular and that eventually desquamates (Fink, 1983). Stevens-Johnson syndrome, with its characteristic mucositis, may lead to findings consistent with vulvovaginitis (Emans, 1986). These serious systemic disorders have other associated findings, so a careful history and physical examination are required to rule them either in or out.

Anogenital Bruising

Anogenital trauma may cause genital or anal bruising. The differential diagnoses for anogenital bruises include both sexual abuse and nonsexually sustained blunt and/or impaling injuries. Accidental injury should present with a plausible history that details an appropriate mechanism of injury. Additionally, bruising in the genital area may also be seen in a variety of hematological, connective tissue, and dermatological conditions (Bays & Jenny, 1990).

Local Injury

A straddle injury occurs when a child falls on a hard object, crushing the soft tissues of the genitalia between the object and the pubic bone. Straddle injuries tend to be anterior **(Figure 7-25)**. In girls, the hymen, an internal structure, would not be expected to be affected by this mechanism of injury because of its relatively recessed position. Impaling or penetrating injuries **(Figure 7-26)**, however, such as a fall onto an exposed stick or broom handle, may conceivably injure the hymen. Boys may also suffer impaling or penetrating injuries **(Figure 7-27)** and injure their genitalia if an object such as a toilet seat falls on the penis. In addition, zipper injuries to the penis may be seen.

Dermatological Disorders

Mongolian spots are slate blue, well-demarcated areas of hyperpigmentation that may be confused with bruising in infants and toddlers. Over half of African American children have Mongolian spots (Behrman & Kliegman, 1983). The most common locations for Mongolian spots are the back and buttocks.

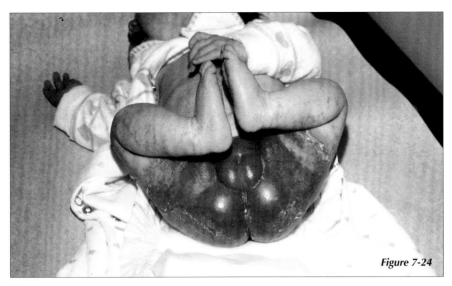

Figure 7-24

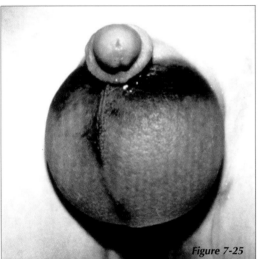

Figure 7-25

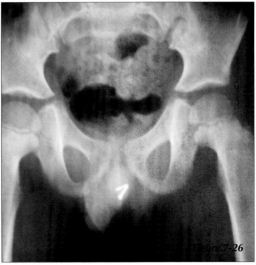

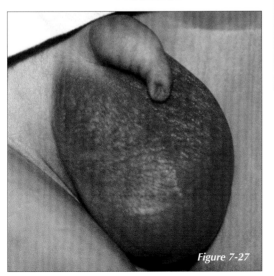

Figure 7-27

Figure 7-24. *An infant's perineum revealing diffuse erythema and swelling consistent with perianal streptococcal cellulites. (Contributed by Paul J. Honig, MD; Philadelphia, Pa.)*

Figure 7-25. *Scrotal hematoma from a straddle bicycle injury. (Contributed by Douglas A. Canning, MD; Philadelphia, Pa.)*

Figure 7-26. *Straight pin in female child's bladder caused bladder trauma and urethral injuries. Pin was removed endoscopically from urethra. (Contributed by Douglas A. Canning, MD; Philadelphia, Pa.)*

Figure 7-27. *Swollen scrotum from a ten-penny nail injury. (Contributed by Douglas A. Canning, MD; Philadelphia, Pa.)*

Lichen sclerosis, a dermatological condition, is easily traumatized from minimal pressure and may become blue and discolored as a result. Vascular nevi may give the appearance of bruising secondary to the visible accentuation of the capillary bed. Phytodermatitis mimics bruising and burns on the child's skin and has been confused with child physical abuse (Coffman, Boyce, & Hansen, 1985; Dannaker, Glover, & Goltz, 1988). This photosensitivity reaction occurs when the child's skin comes in contact with plant psoralens (e.g., lemon juice) and then is exposed to sunlight, leaving a discoloration. If this is offered as a reason for anogenital bruising, the history must account for contact with the psoralen and exposure of the anogenital skin to sunlight.

Systemic Conditions

Some hematological conditions, including bleeding disorders such as hemophilia, von Willebrand's disease, and ITP may cause anogenital bruising. Bruising in extragenital sites would also be expected and is typical. Appropriate laboratory studies should rule these bleeding disorder causes in or out. In addition, disorders with a vasculitis component may also cause bruising in the anogenital area and would be expected to have other characteristic findings associated with the specific vasculitis, such as generalized lower extremity petechiae with HSP.

Anogenital Bleeding and/or Bloody Vaginal Discharge

Bleeding in the anogenital area may represent a medical emergency and requires identification and management of the source of the bleeding (Altchek, 1996). Bloody or blood-tinged urethral discharge is a separate clinical entity that may initially be difficult to differentiate from anogenital bleeding. A bloody vaginal discharge, including frank bleeding, requires prompt diagnosis and treatment.

Local Irritation

Bleeding in the anogenital region may result from inappropriate anogenital manipulation from sexually abusive contact. Although nonaccidental trauma should be considered to be caused by sexual abuse, the differential diagnosis of localized injury and bleeding includes accidental trauma, superficial abrasions, and friability of the mucosa from a vulvovaginitis. A foul-smelling vaginal discharge raises the possibility of a foreign body, especially if the discharge is bloody (Paradise & Willis, 1985). Toilet tissue is the most frequently described foreign body found in a young girl's vagina and causes a foul-smelling bloody discharge.

Dermatological Disorders

Bleeding may also arise from the effects of pruritic dermatological conditions such as atopic, contact, and seborrheic dermatitis; psoriasis; and lichen sclerosis (Koumantakis et al., 1997; Quint & Smith, 1999; Wilson, 1992). The inflammation leads to pruritus and irritation and ultimately to local trauma and bleeding.

Infection

Infections may lead to friable vulvar and vaginal tissues that bleed. A vulvovaginitis-like picture may be seen with STDs contracted during sexual abuse and may present with a characteristic discharge. Less common genital infections may lead to vulvovaginitis as well, including group A beta-hemolytic streptococcus, which may cause vaginitis, especially following pharyngitis, and *Shigella* and *Yersinia*, which cause similar findings and should be considered if diarrhea is present (Altchek, 1996; Emans & Goldstein, 1990; Murphy & Nelson, 1979; Watkins & Quan, 1984).

Endocrinological Disorders

What appears to be bleeding from the vagina may actually be menstrual flow from precocious pubertal development in a child. If this is suspected, hormone-producing

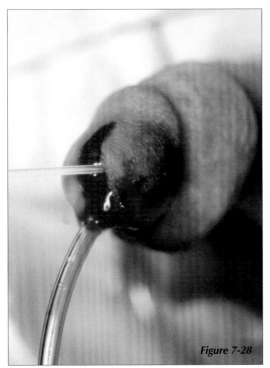

Figure 7-28. *Laceration of glans penis. (Contributed by Douglas A. Canning, MD; Philadelphia, Pa.)*

Figure 7-29. *Postoperative appearance of laceration of glans penis. (Contributed by Douglas A. Canning, MD; Philadelphia, Pa.)*

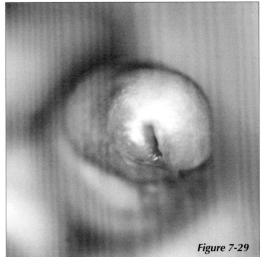

Figure 7-29

Figure 7-28

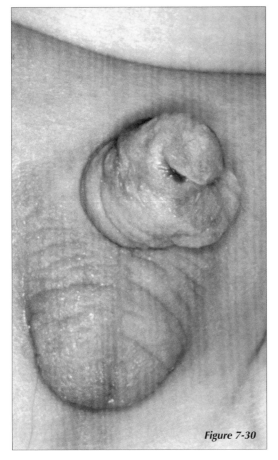

Figure 7-30

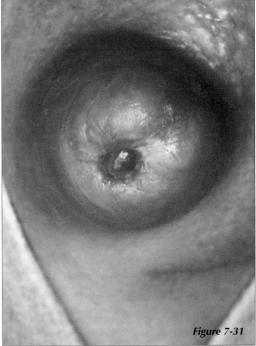

Figure 7-31

Figure 7-30. *Circumcision injury. Child had part of glans removed with the Mogen clamp. (Contributed by Douglas A. Canning, MD; Philadelphia, Pa.)*

Figure 7-31. *Circumcision injury. Shows postcircumcision cicatrix. (Contributed by Douglas A. Canning, MD; Philadelphia, Pa.)*

tumors should be excluded and endocrinological evaluation will be necessary (Breen & Maxson, 1977). Endocrinological reasons for bleeding would be expected to have no signs of genital trauma. In female neonates, a well-described bloody discharge may be transiently observed during the first weeks of life as a result of maternal estrogen withdrawal.

Structural/Neoplastic Disorders

Anatomical structures, such as vaginal polyps and benign growths, may erode and bleed. Vulvar hemangiomas are prone to ulceration and bleeding (Levin & Selbst, 1988). Neoplastic conditions such as sarcoma botryoides may present as vaginal bleeding. Sarcoma botryoides is a grapelike malignant tumor that typically arises from the anterior vaginal wall near the cervix and may involve the vagina, uterus, bladder, and urethra (Emans & Goldstein, 1990; Imai, Horibe, & Tamaya, 1995). Its peak incidence is in the first 2 years of life, with most cases presenting before age 5 years. Prognosis is poor unless found early, so all suspicious lesions should be fully evaluated.

Nonbloody Vaginal Discharge

Vaginal discharge is a genital complaint that requires thorough evaluation in the prepubertal child. Nonpathological leukorrhea, a physiological clear, white, mucoid discharge, may be considered a normal variant in prepubertal girls, and the skilled examiner should not confuse it with pathological discharges associated with vulvitis, vaginitis, and vulvovaginitis (Emans & Goldstein, 1990). Infections are often associated with vaginal discharges, and sexually and nonsexually acquired infections and certain systemic infections may lead to discharges, including varicella, measles, scarlet fever, and typhoid (Woodruff, 1992).

Genitourinary tract anomalies may lead to persistent wetness and can be initially misdiagnosed as a vaginal discharge. Additionally, such anatomical anomalies may lead to inflammation in the anogenital area, also causing a vulvovaginitis and subsequent discharge. For example, an ectopic ureter may drain into the vagina, cervix, uterus, or urethra, cause wetness, and produce a purulent perineal discharge, especially if a kidney infection is present (Emans & Goldstein, 1990). Other examples include rectovaginal fistula or an acquired draining pelvic abscess, which may also lead to similar findings.

Unusual Anogenital Appearance, Acquired and Congenital

At times various genital structures may appear abnormal and may simulate the chronic changes observed in anogenital appearance after sexual abuse. Both congenital and acquired anomalies of the genitourinary tract may alter the expected appearance of the genital structures (Woodruff, 1992) **(Figures 7-28 to 7-31)**.

Acquired Conditions

Acquired conditions may cause abnormalities in anogenital appearance, including labial agglutination, urethral prolapse, labial abscess, paraphimosis, phimosis, and hair-thread tourniquet syndrome. Some of these acquired conditions may arise from either sexual or nonsexual etiologies. Labial agglutination or adhesions occur when the labia minora join in the midline as a result of inflamed surfaces adhering and then fusing. This fusion may be near total and may cause poor drainage of vaginal secretions and diversion of urinary flow. Labial adhesions are believed to be secondary to the combined effects of vulvar irritation, poor hygiene, and low estrogen levels that make the mucosa more friable. Labial adhesions are believed to be acquired typically in a nonsexual fashion; however, genital fondling or vulvar coitus may result in irritation of the medial aspects of the labia minora and predispose it to agglutination (Berkowitz, Elvik, & Logan, 1987; McCann, Voris, & Simon, 1988). Urethral prolapse occurs when the distal portion of the female urethral mucosa becomes everted and edematous, creating the appearance of a doughnut-shaped structure surrounding the urethral meatus (Johnson, 1991; Lowe, Hill, Jeffs, & Brendler, 1986). Most common in prepubescent African American girls, it may be related to an antecedent episode of increased intraabdominal pressure.

Phimosis and paraphimosis are conditions affecting the foreskin of uncircumcised males. Phimosis is a congenital or acquired inflammatory condition of the foreskin resulting in pathological nonretractability that is not consistent with the developmentally normal state of nonretractability seen in most young boys under age 3 years (Rickwood et al., 1980). If left untreated, phimosis results in inadequate hygiene, severe inflammation, and ulceration of the glans and undersurface of the prepuce (Dodson, 1970).

Alternatively, paraphimosis is an acquired inflammatory condition that results when a retracted foreskin is left retracted, which causes venous and lymphatic obstruction. The distal penis becomes swollen and inflamed.

Finally, the uncommon hair-thread tourniquet syndrome affects various appendages and may involve the genitalia. In this situation, fibers of hair or thread become tightly wrapped around external genitalia structures such as the penis, labia minora, and clitoris (Barton, Sloan, Nichter, & Reinisch, 1988; Bays, 2001; Press, Schachner, & Paul, 1980; Singh, Kim, & Wax, 1978). The tourniquet effect leads to various degrees of lymphatic, venous, and arterial obstruction, with subsequent swelling, discoloration, ischemia, and eventually necrosis. Both accidental and intentional cases have been described (Barton et al., 1988).

Congenital Conditions

Normal anatomical landmarks may be altered by congenital abnormalities, including imperforate hymen, vaginal septum, distal vaginal agenesis, phimosis, and ambiguous genitalia. Imperforate hymen is a congenital condition in which no hymenal orifice is present. If the imperforate hymen is left untreated, mucocolpos (retention of vaginal secretions) may develop, and eventually, with the onset of menses, hematocolpos (retention of menstrual flow) will develop at puberty (Emans & Goldstein, 1990; Wilson, 1992).

Other congenital anomalies that may alter the appearance of the genitalia include paraurethral cysts, urethral diverticulum, ectopic ureterocele, hymenal or vaginal cysts, vulvar hemangioma, congenital pit, and congenital failure of midline genital fusion (Adams & Horton, 1989; Bays & Jenny, 1990; Emans & Goldstein, 1990; Levin & Selbst, 1988).

REFERENCES

Adams JA. Evolution of a classification scale: medical evaluation of suspected child sexual abuse. *Child Maltreat.* 2001;6:31-36.

Adams JA, Horton M. Clinical experiences: is it sexual abuse? *Clin Pediatr.* 1989;28:146-148.

Albers SE, Taylor G, Huyer D, Oliver G, Krafchik BR. Vulvitis circumscripta plasmacellularis mimicking child abuse. *J Am Acad Dermatol.* 2000;42:1078-1080.

Alexander R. Failure to thrive. *The Advisor.* 1992;5:1, 11-12.

Altchek A. Pediatric vulvovaginitis. *Pediatr Clin North Am.* 1972;19:559-580.

Altchek A. Recognizing and controlling vulvovaginitis in children. *Contemp Pediatr.* 1985;2:59-70.

Altchek A. Finding a cause of genital bleeding in prepubertal girls. *Contemp Pediatr.* 1996;3:80-92.

Altemeier WA III. Interpreting bruises in children. *Pediatr Ann.* 2001;30:517-520.

American Academy of Pediatrics Committee on Child Abuse and Neglect. Guidelines for the evaluation of sexual abuse of children: subject review (RE9819). *Pediatrics.* 1999;103:186-191.

Ayoub C, Pfeiffer D. Burns as a manifestation of child abuse and neglect. *Am J Dis Child.* 1979;133:910-914.

Azimi P. Syphilis. In: Behrman RE, Kliegman RM, Jenson HB, eds. *Nelson Textbook of Pediatrics.* 16th ed. Philadelphia, Pa: WB Saunders; 2000:903-907.

Barton DJ, Sloan GM, Nichter LS, Reinisch JF. Hair-thread tourniquet syndrome. *Pediatrics.* 1988;82:925-928.

Baum JD, Bulpitt CJ. Retinal and conjunctival haemorrhage in the newborn. *Arch Dis Child.* 1970;45:344-349.

Bays J. Conditions mistaken for child physical abuse. In: Reece RM, Ludwig S, eds. *Child Abuse: Medical Diagnosis and Management.* Philadelphia, Pa: Lippincott Williams & Wilkins; 2001:177-206.

Bays J, Jenny C. Genital and anal conditions confused with child sexual abuse trauma. *Am J Dis Child.* 1990;144:1319-1322.

Behrman RE, Kliegman RM. The fetus and the neonatal infant: physical examination of the newborn infant. In: Behrman RE, Vaughan VC, eds. *Nelson Textbook of Pediatrics.* 12th ed. Philadelphia, Pa: WB Saunders; 1983:322-416.

Berkowitz CD, Elvik SL, Logan MK. Labial fusion in prepubescent girls: a marker for sexual abuse? *Am J Obstet Gynecol.* 1987;156:16.

Berth-Jones J, Graham-Brown RA, Burns DA. Lichen sclerosus. *Arch Dis Child.* 1989;64:1204-1206.

Berwick DM, Levy JC, Kleinerman R. Failure to thrive: diagnostic yield of hospitalisation. *Arch Dis Child.* 1982;57:347-351.

Bhat BV, Kumar A, Oumachigui A. Bone injuries during delivery. *Indian J Pediatr.* 1994;61:401-405.

Bithoney WG, Dubowitz H, Egan H. Failure to thrive/growth deficiency. *Pediatr Rev.* 1992;13:453-459.

Brandt L. Growth dynamics of low birthweight infants with emphasis on the perinatal period. In: Falkner F, Tanner J, eds. *Human Growth: Neurobiology and Nutrition.* New York, NY: Plenum; 1979.

Breen JL, Maxson WS. Ovarian tumors in children and adolescents. *Clin Obstet Gynecol.* 1977;20:607-623.

Bulloch B, Schubert CJ, Brophy PD, Johnson N, Reed MH, Shapiro RA. Cause and clinical characteristics of rib fractures in infants. *Pediatrics.* 2000;105:E48.

Cantwell HB. The neglect of child neglect. In: Helfer ME, Kempe RS, Krugman RD, eds. *The Battered Child.* 5th ed. Chicago, Ill: University of Chicago Press; 1997:347-373.

Caron H, Pearson A. Neuroblastoma. In: Voute PA, Kalifa C, Barrett A, eds. *Cancer in Children: Clinical Management.* Oxford: Oxford University Press; 1998:279-280.

Carpenter RF. The prevalence and distribution of bruising in babies. *Arch Dis Child*. 1999;80:363-366.

Christian CW, Taylor AA, Hertle RW, Duhaime AC. Retinal hemorrhages caused by accidental household trauma. *J Pediatr*. 1999;135:125-127.

Clayden G. Anal appearances and child sex abuse. *Lancet*. 1987;1:620-621.

Coffman KB, Boyce WT, Hansen RC. Phytodermatitis simulating child abuse. *Am J Dis Child*. 1985;139:229-240.

Cumming WA. Neonatal skeletal fractures: birth trauma or child abuse? *J Assoc Can Radiol*. 1979;30:30-33.

Dannaker CJ, Glover RA, Goltz RW. Phytodermatitis: a mystery case report. *Clin Pediatr*. 1988;27:289-290.

Darmstadt GL. The skin. In: Behrman RE, Kliegman RM, Jenson HB, eds. *Nelson Textbook of Pediatrics*. 16th ed. Philadelphia, Pa: WB Saunders; 2000:1965-2054.

Dodson AI. *Urological Surgery*. St. Louis, Mo: CV Mosby; 1970.

Dubowitz H, Giardino AP, Gustavson E. Child neglect: guidance for pediatricians. *Pediatr Rev*. 2000;21:111-116.

Duhaime AC, Alario AJ, Lewander WJ, et al. Head injury in very young children: mechanisms, injury types, and ophthalmologic findings in 100 hospitalized patients younger than 2 years of age. *Pediatrics*. 1992;90:179-185.

Emans SJ. Vulvovaginitis in the child and adolescent. *Pediatr Rev*. 1986;8:12-19.

Emans SJH, Goldstein DP. *Pediatrics and Adolescent Gynecology*. 3rd ed. Boston, Mass: Little, Brown; 1990.

Fink CW. A perianal rash in Kawasaki disease. *Pediatr Infect Dis*. 1983;2:140-141.

Gahagan S, Holmes R. A stepwise approach to evaluation of undernutrition and failure to thrive. *Pediatr Clin North Am*. 1998;45:169-187.

Gayle MO, Kissoon N, Hered RW, Harwood-Nuss A. Retinal hemorrhage in the young child: a review of etiology, predisposed conditions, and clinical implications. *J Emerg Med*. 1995;13:233-239.

Giardino AP, Christian CW, Giardino ER. Skin: bruises and burns. In: Giardino AP, Christian CW, Giardino ER, eds. *A Practical Guide to the Evaluation of Child Abuse and Neglect*. Thousand Oaks, Calif: Sage Publications; 1997a:61-95.

Giardino AP, Christian CW, Giardino ER. Evaluation of fractures and skeletal injuries. In: Giardino AP, Christian CW, Giardino ER, eds. *A Practical Guide to the Evaluation of Child Abuse and Neglect*. Thousand Oaks, Calif: Sage Publications; 1997b:97-126.

Gordon IB. Pediatric gynecology and adolescent issues: infections and skin disorders of the genitalia. In: Behrman RE, Vaughan VC, eds. *Nelson Textbook of Pediatrics*. 12th ed. Philadelphia, Pa: WB Saunders; 1983:1515-1530.

Harmann RW. Radiologic case of the month. *Arch Pediatr Adolesc Med*. 1997;151:947-948.

Helfer RE. The neglect of our children. *Pediatr Clin North Am*. 1990;37:923-942.

Hibbard RA. Triage and referrals for child sexual abuse medical examinations from the sociolegal system. *Child Abuse Negl*. 1998;22:503-513.

Homer C, Ludwig S. Categorization of etiology of failure to thrive. *Am J Dis Child.* 1981;135:848-851.

Imai A, Horibe S, Tamaya T. Genital bleeding in premenarcheal children. *Int J Gynaecol Obstet.* 1995;49:41-45.

Jain IS, Singh YP, Grupta SL, Gupta A. Ocular hazards during birth. *J Pediatr Ophthalmol Strabismus.* 1980;17:14-16.

Jaquiery A, Stylianopoulos A, Hogg G, Grover S. Vulvovaginitis: clinical features, aetiology, and microbiology of the genital tract. *Arch Dis Child.* 1999;81:64-67.

Jenny C. Cutaneous manifestations of child abuse. In: Reece RM, Ludwig S, eds. *Child Abuse: Medical Diagnosis and Management.* Philadelphia, Pa: Lippincott Williams & Wilkins; 2001:23-45.

Johnson CF. Inflicted injury versus accidental injury. *Pediatr Clin North Am.* 1990;37:791-814.

Johnson CF. Prolapse of urethra: confusion of clinical and anatomic traits with sexual abuse. *Pediatrics.* 1991;87:722-725.

Johnson CF, Coury DL. Bruising and hemophilia: accident or child abuse? *Child Abuse Negl.* 1988;12:409-415.

Johnson DL, Braun D, Friendly D. Accidental head trauma and retinal hemorrhage. *Neurosurgery.* 1993;33:231-234.

Katzman GH. Pathophysiology of neonatal subconjunctival hemorrhage. *Clin Pediatr.* 1992;31:149-152.

Kellogg ND, Parra JM, Menard S. Children with anogenital symptoms and signs referred for sexual abuse evaluations. *Arch Pediatr Adolesc Med.* 1998;152:634-641.

Kini N, Lazoritz S. Evaluation for possible physical or sexual abuse. *Pediatr Clin North Am.* 1998;45:205-219.

Kirschner RH, Stein RJ. The mistaken diagnosis of child abuse: a form of medical abuse? *Am J Dis Child.* 1985;139:873-875.

Kleinman PK. *Diagnostic Imaging of Child Abuse.* 2nd ed. St. Louis, Mo: Mosby; 1998.

Koumantakis EE, Hassan EA, Deligeoroglou EK, Creatsas GK. Vulvovaginitis during childhood and adolescence. *J Pediatr Adolesc Gynecol.* 1997;10:39-43.

Laymon CW, Freeman C. Relationship of balantis xerotica obliterans to lichen sclerosus et atrophicus. *Arch Dermatol.* 1944;49:57-59.

Lenoski EF, Hunter KA. Specific patterns of inflicted burn injuries. *J Trauma.* 1977;17:842-846.

Leopold JC, Tunnessen WW Jr. Picture of the month. Phytophotodermatitis. *Am J Dis Child.* 1993;147:311-312.

Leventhal JM, Griffin D, Duncan KO, Starling S, Christian CW, Kutz T. Laxative-induced dermatitis of the buttocks incorrectly suspected to be abusive burns. *Pediatrics.* 2001;107:178-179.

Levin AV. Ocular manifestations of child abuse. In: Reece RM, Ludwig S, eds. *Child Abuse: Medical Diagnosis and Management.* Philadelphia, Pa: Lippincott Williams & Wilkins; 2001:97-107.

Levin AV, Selbst SM. Vulvar hemangioma simulating child abuse. *Clin Pediatr.* 1988;27:213-215.

Levy HL, Brown AE, Williams SE, de Juan E Jr. Vitreous hemorrhage as an ophthalmic complication of galactosemia. *J Pediatr.* 1996;129:922-925.

Loening-Baucke V. Lichen sclerosus et atrophicus in children. *Am J Dis Child.* 1991;145:1058-1061.

Lowe FC, Hill GS, Jeffs RD, Brendler CB. Urethral prolapse in children: insights into etiology and management. *J Urol.* 1986;135:100-103.

Mayer BW, Burns P. Differential diagnosis of abuse injuries in infants and young children. *Nurse Pract.* 2000;25:15-18.

McCann J, Voris J, Simon MA. Labial adhesions and posterior fourchette injuries in childhood sexual abuse. *Am J Dis Child.* 1988;142:659-663.

Mogielnicki NP, Schwartzman JD, Elliott JA. Perineal group A streptococcal disease in pediatric practice. *Pediatrics.* 2000;106:276-281.

Monteleone JA, Brodeur AE. *Child Maltreatment: A Clinical Guide and Reference.* Vol. 1. 2nd ed. St. Louis, Mo: GW Medical Publishing; 1998.

Montgomery RR, Scott JP. Hereditary clotting factor deficiencies. In: Behrman RE, Kliegman RM, Jenson HB, eds. *Nelson Textbook of Pediatrics.* 16th ed. Philadelphia, Pa: WB Saunders; 2000:1508-1513.

Morris AA, Hoffmann GF, Naughten ER, et al. Glutaric aciduria and suspected child abuse. *Arch Dis Child.* 1999;80:404-405.

Murphy TV, Nelson JD. Shigella vaginitis: results of 38 patients and review of the literature. *Pediatrics.* 1979;63:511-516.

Nadas S, Reinberg O. Obstetric fractures. *Eur J Pediatr Surg.* 1992;2:165-168.

O'Brien TJ. Paediatric vulvovaginitis. *Aust J Dermatol.* 1995;36:216-218.

Odom A, Christ E, Kerr N, et al. Prevalence of retinal hemorrhages in pediatric patients after in-hospital cardiopulmonary resuscitation: a prospective study. *Pediatrics.* 1997;99:E3.

Ophthalmology Child Abuse Working Party. Child abuse and the eye. *Eye.* 1999;13:3-10.

Paradise JE, Campos JM, Friedman HM, Frishmuth G. Vulvovaginitis in premenarcheal girls: clinical features and diagnostic evaluation. *Pediatrics.* 1982;70:193-198.

Paradise JE, Willis ED. Probability of vaginal foreign body in girls with genital complaints. *Am J Dis Child.* 1985;139:472.

Paterson CR, McAllion SJ. Osteogenesis imperfecta in the differential diagnosis of child abuse. *BMJ.* 1989;299:1451-1454.

Preminger MK, Pokorny SF. Vaginal discharge: a common pediatric complaint. *Contemp Pediatr.* 1998;15:115-122.

Press S, Schachner L, Paul P. Clitoris tourniquet syndrome. *Pediatrics.* 1980;66:781.

Quint EH, Smith YR. Vulvar disorders in adolescent patients. *Pediatr Clin North Am.* 1999;46:593-606.

Richardson AC. Cutaneous manifestations of abuse. In: Reece RM, ed. *Child Abuse: Medical Diagnosis and Management.* Philadelphia, Pa: Lea & Febiger; 1994:167-184.

Rickwood AMK, Hemalatha V, Batcup G, Spitz L. Phimosis in boys. *Br J Urol*. 1980;52:147-150.

Rivara FP, Parrish RA, Mueller BA. Extremity injuries in children: predictive value of clinical findings. *Pediatrics*. 1986;78:803-807.

Roberts SW, Hernandez C, Mayberry MC, et al. Obstetric clavicular fracture: the enigma of normal birth. *Obstet Gynecol*. 1995;86:978-981.

Rubin A. Birth injuries: incidence, mechanisms, and end results. *Obstet Gynecol*. 1964;23:218.

Sandler AP, Haynes V. Nonaccidental trauma and medical folk belief: a case of cupping. *Pediatrics*. 1978;61:921-922.

Scales JW, Fleischer AB Jr, Krowchuk DP. Bullous impetigo. *Arch Pediatr Adolesc Med*. 1997;151:1168-1169.

Singh B, Kim H, Wax SH. Strangulation of glans penis by hair. *Urology*. 1978;11:170-173.

Spencer JA, Grieve DK. Congenital indifference to pain mistaken for non-accidental injury. *Br J Radiol*. 1990;63:308-310.

Stewart GM, Rosenberg NM. Conditions mistaken for child abuse: Part I. *Pediatr Emerg Care*. 1996a;12:116-121.

Stewart GM, Rosenberg NM. Conditions mistaken for child abuse: Part II. *Pediatr Emerg Care*. 1996b;12:217-221.

Strait RT, Siegel RM, Shapiro RA. Humeral fractures without obvious etiologies in children less than three years of age: when is it abuse? *Pediatrics*. 1995;96:667-671.

Sugar NF, Taylor JA, Feldman KW. Bruises in infants and toddlers: those who don't cruise rarely bruise. Puget Sound Pediatric Research Network. *Arch Pediatr Adolesc Med*. 1999;153:399-403.

Thomas SA, Rosenfield NS, Leventhal JM, Markowitz RI. Long-bone fractures in young children: distinguishing accidental injuries from child abuse. *Pediatrics*. 1991;88:471-476.

Thompson GH, Scoles PV. Torsional and angular deformities. In: Behrman RE, Kleigman RM, Jenson HB, eds. *Nelson Textbook of Pediatrics*. 16th ed. Philadelphia, Pa: WB Saunders; 2000:2069-2070.

Tunnessen WW Jr. *Signs & Symptoms in Pediatrics*. 2nd ed. Philadelphia, Pa: JB Lippincott; 1988.

Turnpenny PD, Nimmo A. Fractured clavicle of the newborn in a population with a high prevalence of grand-multiparity: analysis of 78 consecutive cases. *Br J Obstet Gynaecol*. 1993;100:338-341.

Watkins S, Quan L. Vulvovaginitis caused by Yersinia enterocolitica. *Pediatr Infect Dis*. 1984;3:444-445.

Wetzel RC, Slater AJ, Dover GJ. Fatal intramuscular bleeding misdiagnosed as suspected nonaccidental injury. *Pediatrics*. 1995;95:771-773.

Wiedemann HR, Kunze J, Grosse FR. *Clinical Syndromes*. 3rd ed. London: Times Mirror International Publishers; 1997:214-215.

Wilcox WD, Nieburg P, Miller DS. Failure to thrive: a continuing problem of definition. *Clin Pediatr*. 1989;28:391-394.

Williams TS, Callen JP, Owen LG. Vulvar disorder in the prepubertal females. *Pediatr Ann.* 1986;15:588-605.

Wilson MD. Vaginal discharge and vaginal bleeding in childhood. In: Carpenter SE, Rock JA, eds. *Pediatric and Adolescent Gynecology.* Philadelphia, Pa: Lippincott-Raven; 1992:139-151.

Woodruff JD. Vulvar disease in the prepubertal child. In: Carpenter SE, Rock JA, eds. *Pediatric and Adolescent Gynecology.* Philadelphia, Pa: Lippincott-Raven; 1992:123-137.

Yeatman GW, Dang VV. Cao gio (coin rubbing): Vietnamese attitudes toward health care. *JAMA.* 1980;244:2748.

Zenel JA. Failure to thrive: a general pediatrician's perspective. *Pediatr Rev.* 1997;18:371-379.

Chapter 8

Clinical Aspects of Child Neglect

Ann L. O'Sullivan, PhD, CPNP, FAAN

Angelo P. Giardino, MD, PhD, FAAP

Neglect is the most common form of child maltreatment and is a major threat to the health and well-being of children in our society. Neglect as a clinical entity spans a wide continuum of caregiving from slightly less than adequate parenting, when measured against a generally accepted community standard, to severely dangerous omissions in care that are likely to cause death (Dubowitz, Black, Starr, & Zuravin, 1993). Neglect is a heterogeneous collection of various situations and typologies that have been formulated to help professionals categorize the various forms of neglect. Schmitt (1981) described 5 types of child neglect: medical, physical, safety, educational, and emotional. Zuravin (1999) identified at least 12 types of neglect:

1. Refusal or delay in providing physical healthcare

2. Refusal or delay in providing mental healthcare

3. Supervisory neglect

4. Custody refusal

5. Custody-related neglect

6. Abandonment/desertion

7. Failure to provide a stable home

8. Neglect of personal hygiene

9. Housing hazards

10. Inadequate housing sanitation

11. Nutritional neglect

12. Educational neglect

Table 8-1 lists the federal government's categorization scheme for the various forms of child neglect that it recognizes (Gaudin, 1993). The unifying principle underlying each of these categories is that a child's basic needs are not being met (Dubowitz, Giardino, & Gustavson, 2000).

Despite year-to-year variation, the number of cases of neglect per year is approximately twice the number for physical abuse and approximately 4 times the number for sexual abuse. Data from 2000 show 53.5% of maltreatment cases were for neglect, 22.7% for physical abuse, and 11.5% for sexual abuse (National Clearinghouse on Child Abuse and Neglect Information [NCCANI], 2000). Neglect generally receives less attention in professional literature and the public policy arena compared to physical and sexual abuse. This prompts some to criticize the "neglect of neglect" (Cantwell, 1997; Wolock

Table 8-1. Types of Neglect	
PHYSICAL NEGLECT	
Safety	Conspicuous inattention to avoidable hazards in the home; inadequate nutrition, clothing, or hygiene; and other forms of reckless disregard of the child's safety and welfare, such as driving with the child while intoxicated and leaving a young child unattended in a motor vehicle.
MEDICAL NEGLECT	
Refusal of healthcare	Failure to provide or allow needed care in accordance with recommendations of a competent healthcare professional for a physical injury, illness, medical condition, or impairment.
Delay in healthcare	Failure to seek timely and appropriate medical care for a serious health problem that any reasonable layman would have recognized as needing professional medical attention.
CUSTODY-RELATED NEGLECT	
Abandonment	Desertion of a child without arranging for reasonable care and supervision. This category includes cases in which children were not claimed within 2 days and when children were left by parents/substitutes who gave no (or false) information about their whereabouts.
Expulsion	Other blatant refusals of custody, such as permanent or indefinite expulsion of a child from the home without adequate arrangements for care by others, or refusal to accept custody of a returned runaway.
Inadequate supervision	Child left unsupervised or inadequately supervised for extended periods or allowed to remain away from home overnight without the parent/substitute knowing (or attempting to determine) the child's whereabouts.
Other custody issues	Custody-related forms of inattention to the child's needs other than those covered by abandonment or expulsion. For example, repeated shuttling of a child from one household to another because of apparent unwillingness to maintain custody, or chronically and repeatedly leaving a child with others for days/weeks at a time.
EMOTIONAL NEGLECT	
Inadequate nurturance/affection	Marked inattention to the child's needs for affection, emotional support, attention, or competence.

(continued)

Table 8-1. *(continued)*

Chronic/extreme abuse or domestic violence	Chronic or extreme spousal abuse or other domestic violence in the child's presence.
Permitted drug/ alcohol abuse	Encouraging or permitting drug or alcohol use by the child; cases of the child's drug/alcohol use are included if it appears that the parent/guardian had been informed of the problem and had not attempted to intervene.
Permitted other maladaptive behavior	Encouragement or permittance of other maladaptive behavior (e.g., severe assaultiveness, chronic delinquency) in circumstances in which the parent/guardian has reason to be aware of the existence and seriousness of the problem but does attempt to intervene.
Refusal of psychological care	Refusal to allow needed and available treatment for a child's emotional or behavioral impairment or problem in accordance with competent professional recommendation.
Delay in psychological care	Failure to seek or provide needed treatment for a child's emotional or behavioral impairment or problem that any reasonable layman would have recognized as needing professional psychological attention (e.g., severe depression, suicide attempt).
Other emotional neglect	Other inattention to the child's developmental/emotional needs not classifiable under any of the above forms of emotional neglect (e.g., markedly overprotective restrictions that foster immaturity or emotional overdependence, chronically applying expectations clearly inappropriate in relation to the child's age or level of development).

EDUCATIONAL NEGLECT

Permitted chronic truancy	Habitual truancy averaging at least 5 days a month is classifiable under this form of maltreatment if the parent/guardian has been informed of the problem and has not attempted to intervene.
Failure to enroll/ other truancy	Failure to register or enroll a child of mandatory school age, causing the school-age child to remain at home for nonlegitimate reasons (e.g., to work, to care for siblings) an average of at least 3 days a month.
Inattention to special education need	Refusal to allow or failure to obtain recommended remedial educational services, or neglect in obtaining or following through with treatment for a child's diagnosed learning disorder or other special education need without reasonable cause.

Reprinted from Gaudin JM Jr. Child Neglect: A Guide for Intervention. *Washington, DC: US Dept of Health & Human Services, Administration for Children and Families, Westover Consultants (Contract No. HHS-105-89-1730); 1993.*

& Horowitz, 1984). Despite its prevalence, political and medical leaders over past decades have paid less attention to neglect than physical and sexual abuse. This is true even though neglect affects more children. The neglect of neglect may result from its relationship to poverty, its indolent and insidious nature, its generally "low-tech" management, and its relationship to a host of other associated social problems (Oates, 1996; Reece & Ludwig, 2000; Wolock & Horowitz, 1984).

The professional view of neglect has evolved over time, and the field has moved from psychopathological models focused on blaming deficient parents to ecological models, which focus more on the contributing factors that cause those in a given environment to inadequately meet a child's basic needs (Crittenden, 1999; Dubowitz, 1999). In the ecological approach, parents in specific communities and the larger community in general each have a role to play in making sure that the child's basic needs are met. (Ecological perspectives are discussed below and in further detail in Chapter 1, The Problem of Child Abuse and Neglect.) Rather than absolving parents from the responsibility to nurture and protect their children, ecologically based models seek to define a shared responsibility that identifies social factors that influence caregiver ability to provide care (Dubowitz et al., 1993).

Intervention strategies are best designed with attention to the shared contributions the individual caregiver, family, community, and society can each make toward the solution (Runyan et al., 1997). This takes into account that parents and other caregivers remain ultimately responsible, and they are accountable for the well-being of their children despite challenging environmental conditions (Dubowitz et al., 1993). Over time, approaches that merely blame parents have proven to be clinically ineffective and do not seem to have produced much improvement for the children involved (Polansky, 1981).

Neglect has far-reaching effects on children, influencing physical health and psychological adjustment, as well as intellectual, social, behavioral, and affective development (Crouch & Milner, 1993). The impact of neglect on an individual child depends on many factors, including developmental level at the time of the neglect and type, severity, and chronicity of the neglectful behavior (Gaudin, 1999). One can conceptualize the consequences of neglect as having acute, short-term, and long-term effects in the realms of physical and psychological functioning, depending on specific clinical circumstances present. Additionally, neglect has societal effects, especially when one considers the impact on child health and well-being and social programs needed to deal with later effects. Other social impacts are seen in law enforcement, in the courts, and within the juvenile and adult criminal justice systems. The overall impact of neglect on a child's life is immeasurable, and financial costs are estimated to be in the billions of dollars each year (Daro, 1988; NCCANI, 1998).

Nurses have the opportunity to participate in the multidisciplinary efforts directed at prevention, identification, evaluation, and management of the healthcare-related aspects of neglect. This chapter defines neglect, describes its presentation, and discusses how nurses can identify a longitudinal pattern of caregiving that meets the diagnostic criteria for neglect. The prevention of neglect requires establishing a relationship with the caregivers to facilitate a fair degree of parental education and close clinical follow-up (Wolfe, 1993). Nurses are ideal participants on the team that provides such a comprehensive, longitudinal approach to intervention.

A particular focus of this chapter is on the healthcare evaluation and management of forms of neglect that are likely to be identified in the healthcare setting, namely, physical neglect (form of neglect related to safety and avoidance of obvious environmental dangers), medical neglect (form of neglect related to failure to access or provide reasonable medical care), and failure to thrive (FTT) (form of neglect that manifests itself in the child as inadequate growth when compared to peers).

DEFINITION AND CONCEPTUAL MODELS

No theory fully explains or predicts neglectful behavior, but research has identified associated risks for neglect. A specific predictive model has not been developed (Garbarino, 1977a), but related literature addresses neglect as a heterogeneous clinical entity with variation in the definitions used to describe it (Garbarino & Collins, 1999; Zuravin, 1999). Some definitions that focus exclusively on the parent's deficits have proven to be of little value in designing interventions and have been criticized for reinforcing negative images of some societal groups such as the poor or young parents (Burke, Chandy, Dannerbeck, & Watt, 1998). Despite this criticism, most researchers and clinicians would agree that for neglect to occur, the caregiving inadequacy or omission must result in some observable disruption in the general well-being of the child (Dubowitz, 1999; Gaudin, 1993; Ludwig & Rostain, 1992). In clinical practice, disruption spans a wide continuum of observations ranging from minor disruptions in the child's care to cases so severe that a lack of provision for the child's basic needs leads to disability and/or death (Johnson & Coury, 1992; Ludwig, 1992b).

Neglect may have an associated risk for mortality as evidenced by the observation that each year more children die from neglect than from physical abuse (Brown, Cohen, Johnson, & Salzinger, 1998). Of approximately 1100 deaths in 1999 known to have occurred from child maltreatment, 38.2% were due to neglect alone, 26.1% to physical abuse, and an additional 22.7% to a combination of physical abuse and neglect (US Department of Health & Human Services [USDHHS], 2001).

Professionals working in the child maltreatment area rely on legal definitions of what constitutes neglect to guide practice and intervention decisions (Ludwig, 1992a). Law enforcement and prosecution use legal definitions to determine if they should become involved in a case. Criminal justice system involvement usually requires a level of seriousness that places the child at significant risk for severe bodily harm. The less severe forms of maltreatment tend to be handled by child protective services (CPS) agencies without police or prosecutor involvement (Pence & Wilson, 1994). The healthcare provider may see a pattern of neglect emerge early on in the care of the child and report the situation to CPS. Identified patterns of neglect may include a failure to meet the child's basic needs despite reasonable healthcare interventions such as parent education, more frequent office-based health supervision visits, or the use of home nursing (English, 1999).

States define neglect in various ways, ranging from statutes that contain detailed listings of what constitutes neglect to broad, inclusive language to describe neglectful caregiving **(Table 8-2)**.

Most state statutes and research literature, however, agree on 9 components of neglect that revolve around a conceptualization of what comprises a child's basic needs. Neglect exists when these basic needs are not met and may be seen in cases that demonstrate the following (Rose & Meezan, 1996):

1. Inadequate food

2. Inadequate clothing

3. Inadequate shelter

Table 8-2. Variations in State Definitions of Neglect	
STATE	DEFINITION
Arkansas (detailed description)	***Neglect*** means those acts or omissions of a parent, guardian, custodian, foster parent, or any person who is entrusted with the juvenile's care by a parent, custodian, guardian, or foster parent, including, but not limited to, an agent or employee of a public or private residential home, child care facility, public or private school, or any person legally responsible under state law for the juvenile's welfare, which constitute the following: — Failure or refusal to prevent the abuse of the juvenile when such person knows or has reasonable cause to know the juvenile is or has been abused; — Failure or refusal to provide the necessary food, clothing, shelter, education required by law, and medical treatment necessary for the juvenile's well-being except when the failure or refusal is caused primarily by the financial inability of the person legally responsible and no services for relief have been offered or rejected; — Failure to take reasonable action to protect the juvenile from abandonment, abuse, sexual abuse, sexual exploitation, neglect, or parental unfitness where the existence of such condition was known or should have been known; — Failure or irremediable inability to provide for the essential and necessary physical, mental, or emotional needs of the juvenile; — Failure to provide for the juvenile's care and maintenance, proper or necessary support, or medical, surgical, or other necessary care; — Failure, although able, to assume responsibility for the care and custody of the juvenile or participate in a plan to assume such responsibility; or — Failure to supervise the juvenile appropriately, which results in the juvenile's being left alone at an inappropriate age or in inappropriate circumstances, which puts the juvenile in danger.
Colorado (detailed description)	***Neglected*** or ***dependent***—a child is neglected or dependent if: — A parent, guardian, or legal custodian has abandoned the child or has subjected him or her to mistreatment or abuse or a parent, guardian, or legal custodian has suffered or allowed another to mistreat or abuse the child without taking lawful means to stop such mistreatment or abuse and prevent it from recurring; — The child lacks proper parental care through the actions or omissions of the parent, guardian, or legal custodian; — The child's environment is injurious to his or her welfare;

(continued)

Table 8-2. *(continued)*	
STATE	DEFINITION

— A parent, guardian, or legal custodian fails or refuses to provide the child with proper or necessary subsistence, education, medical care, or any other care necessary for his or her health, guidance, or well-being;

— The child is homeless, without proper care, or not domiciled with his or her parent, guardian, or legal custodian through no fault of such parent, guardian, or legal custodian;

— The child has run away from home or is otherwise beyond the control of his or her parent, guardian, or legal custodian;

— A parent, guardian, or legal custodian has subjected another child or children to an identifiable pattern of habitual abuse; and

— Such parent, guardian, or legal custodian has been the respondent in another proceeding under this article in which a court has adjudicated another child to be neglected or dependent based upon allegations of sexual or physical abuse, or a court of competent jurisdiction has determined that such parent's, guardian's, or legal custodian's abuse or neglect has caused the death of another child; and

— The pattern of habitual abuse described above and the type of abuse pose a current threat to the child.

EXCEPTIONS
Colo. Rev. Stat. Ann. § 19-1-103(1)(b) (West Supp. 1998)
In all cases, those investigating reports of child abuse shall take into account accepted child-rearing practices of the **culture** in which the child participates.

Nothing in this subsection shall refer to acts that could be construed to be **a reasonable exercise of parental discipline** or to acts reasonably necessary to subdue a child being taken into custody that are performed by a peace officer acting in good faith performance of the officer's duties.

Colo. Rev. Stat. Ann. § 19-3-103 (West Supp. 1998)
No child who in lieu of medical treatment is under treatment solely by spiritual means through prayer in accordance with a **recognized method of religious healing** shall, for that reason alone, be considered to have been neglected or dependent within the purview of this article. However, the religious rights of a parent, guardian, or legal custodian shall not limit the access of a child to medical care in a life-threatening situation or when the condition will result in serious disability. In order to make a determination as to whether the child is in a life-threatening situation or that the child's condition will result in serious disability, the court may order a medical evaluation of the child. If the court

(continued)

Table 8-2. *(continued)*	

STATE	DEFINITION
	determines, on the basis of any relevant evidence before the court, including the medical evaluation ordered pursuant to this section, that the child is in a life-threatening situation or that the child's condition will result in serious disability, the court may order that medical treatment be provided for the child. A child whose parent, guardian, or legal custodian inhibits or interferes with the provision of medical treatment in accordance with a court order shall be considered to have been neglected or dependent for the purposes of this article and injured or endangered for the purposes of section 18-6-401, C.R.S. A method of religious healing shall be presumed to be a recognized method of religious healing if: — Fees and expenses incurred in connection with such treatment are permitted to be deducted from taxable income as medical expenses pursuant to regulations or rules promulgated by the United States Internal Revenue Service; and — Fees and expenses incurred in connection with such treatment are generally recognized as reimbursable healthcare expenses under medical policies of insurance issued by insurers licensed by this state; or — Such treatment provides a rate of success in maintaining health and treating disease or injury that is equivalent to that of medical treatment.
New York **(detailed description)**	***Neglected child*** means a child less than 18 years of age: — Whose physical, mental, or emotional condition has been impaired or is in imminent danger of becoming impaired as a result of the failure of his parent or other person legally responsible for his care to exercise a minimum degree of care—In supplying the child with adequate food, clothing, shelter or education in accordance with the education law, or medical, dental, optometrical or surgical care, though financially able to do so or offered financial or other reasonable means to do so; or—In providing the child with proper supervision or guardianship, by unreasonably inflicting or allowing to be inflicted harm, or a substantial risk thereof, including the infliction of excessive corporal punishment; or by misusing a drug or drugs; or by misusing alcoholic beverages to the extent that he loses self-control of his actions; or by any other acts of a similarly serious nature requiring the aid of the court provided, however, that where the respondent is voluntarily and regularly participating in a rehabilitative program, evidence that the respondent has repeatedly misused a drug or drugs or alcoholic beverages to the extent that he loses self-control of his actions shall not establish that the child is

(continued)

Table 8-2. *(continued)*

STATE	DEFINITION
	a neglected child in the absence of evidence establishing that the child's physical, mental or emotional condition has been impaired or is in imminent danger of becoming impaired; or
	— Who has been abandoned, in accordance with the definition and other criteria set forth in the social services law, by his parents or other person legally responsible for his care.
West Virginia **(moderate description)**	*Neglected child* means a child: — Whose physical or mental health is harmed or threatened by a present refusal, failure, or inability of the child's parent, guardian or custodian to supply the child with necessary food, clothing, shelter, supervision, medical care or education, when such refusal, failure or inability is not due primarily to a lack of financial means on the part of the parent, guardian or custodian; or — Who is presently without necessary food, clothing, shelter, medical care, education or supervision because of the disappearance or absence of the child's parent or custodian.
Idaho **(moderate description)**	*Neglected* means a child: — Who is without proper parental care and control, or subsistence, education, medical or other care or control necessary for his well-being because of the conduct or omission of his parents, guardian or other custodian or their neglect or refusal to provide them; or — Whose parents, guardian or other custodian are unable to discharge their responsibilities to and for the child because of incarceration, hospitalization, or other physical or mental incapacity; or — Who has been placed for care or adoption in violation of law. **EXCEPTION** **Idaho Code § 16-1602(t)(1) (Supp. 1998)** However, no child whose parent or guardian chooses for such child **treatment by prayers through spiritual means** alone in lieu of medical treatment shall be deemed for that reason alone to be neglected or lack parental care necessary for his health and well-being, but further provided this subsection shall not prevent the court from acting pursuant to statute.
Iowa **(minimal description)**	*Child abuse* or *abuse* means: — The failure on the part of a person responsible for the care of a child to provide for the adequate food, shelter, clothing or other care necessary for the child's health and welfare when financially able to do so or when offered financial or other reasonable means to do so.

(continued)

Table 8-2. *(continued)*	

STATE	DEFINITION
Kansas (minimal description)	***Physical, mental*** or ***emotional abuse*** means the infliction of physical, mental or emotional injury or the causing of a deterioration of a child and may include, but shall not be limited to maltreatment or exploiting a child to the extent that the child's health or emotional well-being is endangered.
Montana (minimal description)	***Child abuse*** or ***neglect*** means: — Actual harm to a child's health or welfare; or — Substantial risk of harm to a child's health or welfare. The term includes actual harm or substantial risk of harm by the acts or omissions of a person responsible for the child's welfare. The term does not include self-defense, defense of others, or action taken to prevent the child from self-harm that does not constitute harm to a child's health or welfare.
Vermont (minimal description)	***Abused*** or ***neglected child*** means a child whose physical health, psychological growth and development or welfare is harmed or is at substantial risk of harm by the acts or omissions of his or her parent or other person responsible for the child's welfare. An "abused or neglected child" also means a child who is sexually abused or at substantial risk of sexual abuse by any person.
Washington (minimal description)	***Negligent treatment*** or ***maltreatment*** means an act or omission which evidences a serious disregard of consequences of such magnitude as to constitute a clear and present danger to the child's health, welfare, and safety. The fact that siblings share a bedroom is not, in and of itself, negligent treatment or maltreatment.
California (minimal description)	***Neglect*** means the negligent treatment or the maltreatment of a child by a person responsible for the child's welfare under circumstances indicating harm or threatened harm to the child's health or welfare. The term includes acts and omissions on the part of the responsible person.
Georgia (minimal description)	***Child abuse*** means: — Neglect or exploitation of a child by a parent or caretaker thereof.

Adapted from US Department of Health & Human Services. Child Abuse and Neglect State Statutes Elements: Reporting Laws: Number 1: Definitions of Child Abuse and Neglect. *National Clearinghouse on Child Abuse and Neglect Information; 1999. Available at:* http://www.calib.com/nccanch/pubs/stats02/define/index.cfm. *Accessed February 27, 2003.*

4. Inadequate supervision

5. Inadequate medical care

6. Inadequate emotional care

7. Inadequate education

8. Exploitation

9. Exposure to unwholesome circumstances

Ludwig and Rostain (1992) developed a useful description based on family functioning and dysfunction that contrasts too much and too little attention to a child's basic needs. **Table 8-3** juxtaposes the excess and inadequate provision of the child's needs.

The basic needs of children vary at different ages and developmental levels, for example, a 2-month-old infant's total dependence on the responses of caregivers for all needs contrasts with an 8-year-old child in second grade. Another clinical viewpoint addresses the positive needs of children and includes the following (Hobbs, Hanks, & Wynne, 1993b):

— Food

— Warmth

— Clothing

— Shelter and protection

— Grooming and hygiene

— Fresh air and sunlight

— Activity and rest

— Prevention from illness and accidents

— Affection

— Continuity of care

— Security of belonging

— Self-esteem

— Opportunity to learn

— Opportunity to achieve independence and success

To determine the extent to which a caregiver fails to meet a child's basic needs requires consideration of legal definitions of neglect and discussions with multidisciplinary professionals who each bring a variety of perspectives to the discussion and to the diagnostic process.

Organizations serving children, and the professionals operating within these organizations, must then work on legal definitions and mandates to determine acceptable practice (Ludwig, 1992a). Professionals should familiarize themselves with policies and procedures in place within the organization in which one is practicing. Finally, professionals and lay people within a community need to interpret what constitutes adequate caregiving or parenting. A person's own definition of neglect is the most prone to variation, because many factors influence an individual's view of providing care to children. These include the person's upbringing, training, knowledge, and other life experiences over time (Ludwig, 1992a).

Table 8-3. Family Dysfunction

TASK	DYSFUNCTIONAL INADEQUACY	DYSFUNCTIONAL EXCESS
Providing for physical needs		
— Protection	— Failure to protect — Child abuse	— Overprotection and overanxiety
— Food	— Underfeeding	— Overfeeding, obesity
— Housing	— Homelessness	— Multiple residences — "Yo-yo"/vagabond children
— Healthcare	— Medical neglect	— Excessive medical care — Munchausen syndrome by proxy
Providing for developmental, behavioral, and emotional needs		
Stimulation	*Understimulation*	*Overstimulation*
— Developmental and cognitive	— Neglect	— "Hothousing" — Parental perfectionism
— Guidance: approval and discipline	— Inadequate approval — Overcriticism — Psychological abuse	— Overindulgence — Spoiled child
— Affection: acceptance, intimacy	— Inadequate affection — Emotional neglect — Rejection — Hostility	— Sexual abuse — Incest
Socialization		
— Intrafamilial relationship	— Attenuated family relationships — Distanced parents	— Parenting enmeshment — Overinvolved relationships
— Extrafamilial, community relationships	— Boundaryless families — Deficiency in training in extrafamilial relationships	— Insular families — Excessive restriction from extrafamilial relationships

Reprinted with permission from Ludwig S, Rostain A. Family function and dysfunction. In: Levine MD, Carey WB, Crocker AC, eds. Developmental-Behavioral Pediatrics. *2nd ed. Philadelphia, Pa: WB Saunders; 1992:147-159.*

The results of studies comparing the perceptions of parents and professionals around the presence or absence of child neglect vary but suggest that differences do exist between professional and lay people's views of neglect (Magura & Moses, 1986; Rose, 1999; Rose & Meezan, 1996). In general, child protection professionals tended to be less concerned than mothers regarding physical and psychological care. CPS workers differed amongst themselves, with investigative workers more likely to see most types of neglect as more serious than service-providing CPS workers (Rose & Meezan, 1996). Depending on responsibilities and experience, CPS workers may be raising the threshold of what constitutes neglect so as not to overwhelm their child welfare system with unfounded reports. However, parents and their children are less able to benefit from helpful community resources when the threshold for determining neglect is set too high.

There are perceived differences among ethnic and racial groups concerning physical care of a child and neglect as well (Dubowitz, Klockner, Starr, & Black, 1998; Rose, 1999; Rose & Meezan, 1996). For example, African American and Latino mothers generally perceived some types of neglect as more serious than their white mother counterparts, as identified in neglect ratings (Rose, 1999). In a different study that used vignettes of an imaginary 18-month-old child, lower- and middle-class African American parents were more concerned than their middle-class white counterparts about the physical care described (Dubowitz et al., 1998). In the coming years, more scholarly work in the area of ethnic and cultural expectations will be necessary to characterize the trends in this area, as well as to understand their implications fully with regard to intervention and management strategies.

Garbarino (1977a) applied ecological concepts initially developed by Hawley (1950) and Bonfenbrenner (1977) to the problem of child maltreatment and neglect. In the ecological model (see Chapter 1, The Problem of Child Abuse and Neglect), neglect arises from a mismatch between child and family, as well as a mismatch between family and neighborhood and/or community. This ecological "asynchrony" manifests itself in that neglectful families are consistently unable to access basic family support systems within their environments. The notion of neglectful families being essentially isolated has given rise to the conceptualization of social impoverishment as a risk factor for child neglect. An impoverished environment often lacks consistent supportive relationships that are a source of nurturance and feedback to the family and that provide a protective barrier against neglectful behavior (Garbarino & Crouter, 1978; Garbarino & Sherman, 1980). There is also a relationship between socially impoverished neighborhoods and neglectful parents. These parents do not seem to have the social/interpersonal connections with others generally characterized among nonneglectful parents, who experience and describe a healthier and more supportive environment (Burke et al., 1998; Polansky, Gaudin, Ammons, & Davis, 1985).

Research studies have shown that neglectful parents tend to perceive their neighborhoods and communities as more socially cold and isolated than do nonneglectful parents (Garbarino, 1977b; Garbarino & Crouter, 1978; Garbarino & Sherman, 1980). Neglectful parents may manifest a self-fulfilling prophecy of sorts in that their perception of a socially impoverished environment leads to behavioral patterns that further isolate them. This self-fulfilling prophecy may be realized because the neglectful parents' neighbors perceive that neglectful parents will not appreciate or reciprocate positive interchanges when extended in social situations. What develops is a vicious cycle in which one's perceptions of isolation lead to further isolation. The etiology of child neglect depends on several complex factors and interactions. However, in the neglect scenario, there seems to be a fairly consistent component of social isolation or impoverishment, whether actual or perceived (Garbarino, 1977b).

The preceding discussion of the ecological approaches to the issue of neglect demonstrates the systemic nature of this model and makes clear the interrelatedness of the participants and their social and physical environments (Belsky, 1993; Dubowitz, 1999; Garbarino & Barry, 1997; Kaplan, 1999; Lutzker, Bigelow, Doctor, Gershater, & Greene, 1998). The "eco-" in each of these approaches comes from the belief that maltreatment/neglect is the end result of complex interactions among potential risk factors within the abuser (e.g., depression), his/her family (e.g., single-parent family), and the environment (e.g., social isolation). To understand the prevention and treatment of neglect, ecological theorists focus on interactions between a large number of risk and resilience factors present among the child, the parents, and the sociocultural environment. The ecological model ensures a broad approach to the study of neglect and is concordant with the health promotion role that underpins the role and function of nurses and nursing in the healthcare setting.

Burke et al. (1998) define neglect as a characteristic pattern of parental behavior sustained by problematic parent capacities to use knowledge, support, and resources in carrying out the parental role. This definition describes a general pattern of parenting performance that would be amenable to nursing approaches to health promotion discussed by various nursing theorists, including that by Henderson. Viewing this in the context of a shared-responsibility paradigm as advocated by Dubowitz et al. (1993) ideally speaks to the strengths the nursing profession brings to dealing with child neglect.

INCIDENCE STATISTICS

The Third National Incidence Study (NIS-3) attempted to assess the overall national incidence of child maltreatment going beyond cases known to the official CPS system (Sedlak & Broadhurst, 1996). The NIS-3 used 2 standards known as the Harm Standard and the Endangerment Standard to categorize available data. The Harm Standard considered children as maltreated if they had already experienced harm. The Endangerment Standard included children at risk for harm and those who were already harmed. Looking specifically at physical neglect, the NIS-3 reported cases involving inadequate nutrition, clothing, and personal hygiene; disregard for safety; medical neglect; abandonment; and other custody-related and supervision issues (Sedlak & Broadhurst, 1996). To be included in the Harm Standard for physical neglect, a parent or parent substitute must have been responsible for demonstrable injury or impairment in the child that was serious or fatal. Those counted under the Endangerment Standard included any adult caregiver who failed to provide appropriate care (thus, not meeting the child's basic needs) or who demonstrated disregard for the child's safety.

Using 1993 statistics, 338 900 children experienced physical neglect under the Harm Standard, for an incidence rate of 5.0 children per 1000. Using the more inclusive Endangerment Standard, 1 961 300 children were neglected, yielding a more staggering rate of 29.2 children per 1000. Boys and girls were equally as likely to be physically neglected under either standard. The child's age did not differ under the Harm Standard, but the Endangerment Standard found a higher incidence of children 0 to 11 years old than children in the older age groups. This reflects that younger children have greater needs for physical care and supervision than do older children (Sedlak & Broadhurst, 1996). No differences in rates of physical neglect could be attributed to racial differences.

Finally, marked differences existed in the rate of physical neglect for various family income levels using both standards. The highest rates were for children in families earning less than $15 000 per year, followed by those in families earning between $15 000 and $29 999 per year. The lowest rate of physical neglect was in families earning $30 000 or more (Sedlak & Broadhurst, 1996). The professional literature debates whether or not the income relationship is real or merely an artifact of how the data are reported and collected.

Using 1999 data reporting on cases of child maltreatment known to CPS agencies, almost three fifths (58.4%) of the 826 000 children known to have been maltreated after CPS investigation were victims of neglect (USDHHS, 2001). An estimated 1100 children were known to have died from maltreatment, with the largest proportion, 38.2%, attributed to neglect alone as the cause of death (Bonner, Crow, & Logue, 1999; USDHHS, 2001).

NURSING AS A BASIS FOR CLINICAL PRACTICE WITH CHILD NEGLECT

Healthcare providers usually have a definition of their role, whether nurse, physician, physical therapist, or social worker, that guides their clinical practice. In 1958, Virginia Henderson was asked by the Nursing Service Committee of the International Council of Nurses to prepare a pamphlet on nursing. Her 1961 definition continues to guide nursing clinical practice and is particularly relevant to nurses' work with children and families in regard to neglect. The definition states:

The unique function of the nurse is to assist the individual, sick or well, in the performance of those activities contributing to health or its recovery (or to a peaceful death) that he/she would perform unaided if he/she had the necessary strength, will, or knowledge. (p. 15.)

This definition reinforces the conclusion that the most effective nursing involves continuous observation and interpretation of client behavior, validation by the client of the nurse's interpretation of his or her need for help, and action based on this validated inference (Dumas, 1963; Henderson, 1966). In addition to a definition of the nursing role, nursing often adds a model or theory to practice for a particular issue.

With the amount of documented neglect, nurses must respond to neglect and identify factors indicative of child neglect in the nursing assessment. For example, the utility of an ecological framework might suggest adding questions to the family history during the initial newborn visit, such as the following:

— Were you (mother or father) abused or neglected as a child?

— Do you have a supportive, close relationship with someone?

— Have you ever been in therapy or used social support services and had a positive experience with them?

Obtaining additional information from parents gives the nurse a place to begin to assist them in performing the parental role, which will contribute to the infant's health.

Nurses have varied roles in the pediatric healthcare setting ranging from health promotion to direct patient care. With advanced practice nursing, nurse practitioners take on even more complex responsibilities. Nurses in both traditional and nontraditional roles may play a significant part in dealing with child neglect, especially its prevention, evaluation, and ongoing management, as follows:

— ***Prevention:*** nurses have played significant roles in various prevention efforts regarding child maltreatment, including the prevention of neglect (Olds, Hill, Mihalic, & O'Brien, 1998). Nurse home visiting programs have been shown to be effective in preventing child abuse and neglect for at least 15 years after the intervention (Olds et al., 1997). Research findings on these programs show that the nurse's intervention contributes to changing the mother's life course (Olds &

Kitzman, 1993). In other words, the ability of nursing intervention to persuade mothers to make better decisions for their children and themselves in terms of education, job choices, and health relationships, to name a few, has been validated. (Chapter 17, Prevention of Child Abuse and Neglect: Approaches and Issues, contains a full discussion of nurse-related prevention efforts.)

— ***Evaluation:*** nurses participate on multidisciplinary teams in a variety of ways in evaluating neglect (Bridges, 1978; McCleery & Pinyerd, 1988). Participation ranges from the office-based nursing professional who collects growth parameters and performs a nursing assessment to the advanced practice nurse who delivers a full range of primary care services. Regardless of the role, nursing's focus on the assessment and evaluation of the child and the adult caregivers and on restoration of their health and well-being makes the nurse ideally suited for detection and prevention of abuse.

— ***Management:*** once neglect is identified, nurses play various roles in the management of neglect (McCleery & Pinyerd, 1988). By building strong relationships with families, nurses may provide ongoing education concerning child development and the basic needs of the child. Nurses may teach the family skills in caring for children and provide a variety of educational experiences in which the family may learn necessary skills. Additionally, the nurse may be the service provider who monitors the child's progress (either in the office or in the child's home) and may be part of a support team that encourages the family to meet the challenges they face. This type of ongoing intervention is essential and contributes to secondary and tertiary prevention efforts while providing treatment to the involved child.

NEGLECT IN THE HEALTHCARE SETTING

The nurse may identify many forms of neglect, but some forms are more likely to come to the healthcare provider's attention than others. This is a result of healthcare settings' focus on anticipatory guidance concerning environmental safety and child development, physical assessment, and medical treatment for acute and chronic disease.

PRESENTATION
Physical Neglect

Physical neglect may come to light either from single episodes that point to a serious breach in acceptable parenting or from multiple episodes that represent patterns of signs and symptoms suggesting a lack of reasonable supervision or little attention to creating and maintaining a safe environment. In addition, poor hygiene and little attention to appropriate grooming may be obvious during the visit. Custody-related forms of physical neglect may or may not be apparent to the healthcare provider. At times, the child may be brought in for care by a responsible caregiver who reports the child as abandoned; this is an obvious case of neglect. The more subtle forms of custody-related neglect may elude the healthcare provider, especially if the parent does not provide accurate information about the child's caregiving and living situation.

Possible indicators for physical neglect in the healthcare setting might be the following:

— Multiple bruises or scabs on old injuries from falls

— Unresolved tinea infections on the scalp

— Very hungry children at each visit who have not eaten yet that day

— Improper clothing for seasonal or environmental conditions

— Unkempt appearance with dirty, excessively soiled clothing and/or filth in skin creases

Medical Neglect

Medical neglect may present variably as well. A pattern over time of apparent disregard for the importance of routine healthcare may be manifested as a failure to immunize the child according to generally accepted schedules. Delay in seeking healthcare assistance at a reasonable point in an acute illness may also be a sign of medical neglect. This may be seen when illness is recognized long after symptoms that would normally prompt a reasonable parent to bring the child in for assessment. In medical neglect, the child is brought in only after the clinical situation is well beyond what would be considered reasonable or when the child has deteriorated to the point of being seriously ill or perhaps near death. Additionally, medical neglect may be seen in families with a child who has a chronic illness where medical therapies are not followed as prescribed, with serious consequences to the child's health. Not seeking assistance for obvious developmental delays also qualifies for medical neglect. Finally, refusing appropriate medical care for treatable illness that places the child at risk for serious complications is also a form of medical neglect (Hobbs, Hanks, & Wynne, 1993b).

Possible indicators for medical neglect in the healthcare setting are as follows:

— Infected burns that have not been seen by a primary care provider

— Many school days missed for lack of appropriate treatment of asthma or diabetes

— Medications not being taken as prescribed or prescriptions not filled at all

In discussing medical neglect, the clinician must keep in mind that there is a baseline level of noncompliance or nonadherence with medical regimens in adults and pediatric patients (LaGreca, 1990). Therefore, all nonadherence is not automatically medical neglect. It is widely reported that in pediatrics, compliance rates vary from 7% to 89% for short-term medical regimens and 11% to 83% for long-term regimens (Matsui, 1997). Specifically, in treating acute otitis media, approximately 7% of children completed the entire therapy and 53% took less than half the prescribed antibiotics. The compliance figures are not much better for chronic conditions such as asthma and cystic fibrosis (Matsui, 1997). A variety of reasons have been offered by caregivers to account for the noncompliance with medication administration, including forgetting, stopping the medication because of symptom improvement, misunderstanding the instructions, child resistance, perceived ineffectiveness, and onset of side effects. Assessing the impact of the noncompliance on the child as well as the pattern of adherence to prescribed medical regimens by the caregivers is paramount in distinguishing noncompliance from medical neglect.

FAILURE TO THRIVE

A child who fails to grow as expected, compared to peers of the same age and ethnicity, is traditionally referred to as having failure to thrive (FTT). FTT is a symptom rather than a diagnosis (Oates & Kempe, 1997). Although some suggest more appropriate terms, such as growth failure, these have not taken root in the healthcare setting and FTT remains entrenched in the lexicon of most pediatric clinicians (Haecker, Cockerill, Giardino, Christian, & Giardino, 1997; Wilcox, Nieburg, & Miller, 1989). FTT typically is identified when a recognized pattern of growth can be classified as organic or nonorganic.

Early on, FTT was described as either organic or nonorganic. Organic FTT was initially seen as a failure to grow adequately based on the presence of an underlying medical condition that could be evaluated and diagnosed. Nonorganic FTT, on the other hand, was seen as a failure to grow according to expectations secondary to underlying psychosocial dysfunction, which unfavorably affected the parenting received by the child. The polarity between organic and nonorganic FTT was eventually seen to be less than complete, and a great deal of overlap existed. Taking a more holistic approach, Homer and Ludwig (1981) described many cases of FTT as "mixed FTT." Several medical conditions may be associated with FTT, and Chapter 7, Differential Diagnosis: Conditions That Mimic Child Maltreatment, discusses the differential diagnosis for a child who has symptoms and signs of growth failure.

Indicators for FTT in the healthcare setting are as follows:

— Either height or weight dropping below the 5th or 3rd percentile curves

— Either height or weight crossing at least 2 curves (usually falling)

— No weight gain after addressing feeding and provision of appropriate calories issues with the caregivers

EVALUATION

In conceptualizing the evaluation of possible neglect in the healthcare setting, because of neglect's heterogeneous definition and its many forms and types, the healthcare provider should consider generic and specific screens. Generic screens are broadly applicable and seek to find any pattern of caregiving or symptoms and/or signs that suggest the need to explore further for possible neglect. Building on the generic screens, a set of specific screens can then be done for particular forms of neglect that may be suspected. Thus, every child assessed by a healthcare provider should be screened for general appearance, hygiene and grooming, height and weight (**Figures 8-1 to 8-4**), and, if under age 2 years, head circumference.

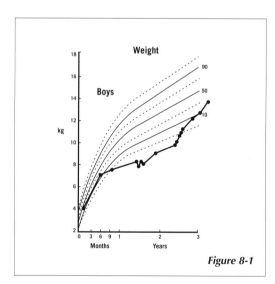

Figure 8-1.

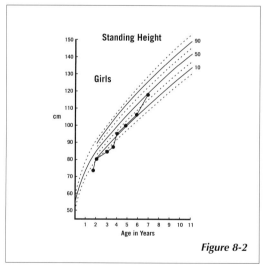

Figure 8-2.

Figure 8-1. Weight chart showing catch-up growth from age 2½ years when a diagnosis of neglect was made and conveyed to the parents. The child remained at home showing that his normal growth potential could be reached. Reprinted from Hobbs CJ, Hanks HGI, Wynne JM. Failure to thrive. In: Hobbs CJ, Hanks HGI, Wynne JM, eds. Child Abuse and Neglect: A Clinician's Handbook. New York, NY: Churchill Livingstone; 1993a:25-28. ©1993, with permission from Elsevier.

Figure 8-2. Height chart demonstrating gradual catch-up of height to 50th centile at age 7 years in an emotionally abused child (same case as Figure 8-4). Reprinted from Hobbs CJ, Hanks HGI, Wynne JM. Failure to thrive. In: Hobbs CJ, Hanks HGI, Wynne JM, eds. Child Abuse and Neglect: A Clinician's Handbook. New York, NY: Churchill Livingstone; 1993a:25-28. ©1993, with permission from Elsevier.

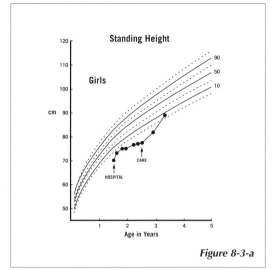

Figure 8-3-a

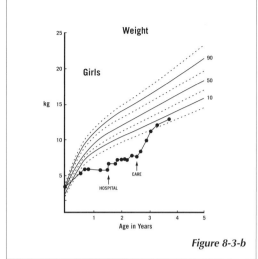

Figure 8-3-b

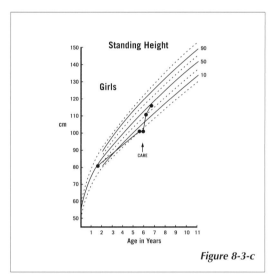

Figure 8-3-c

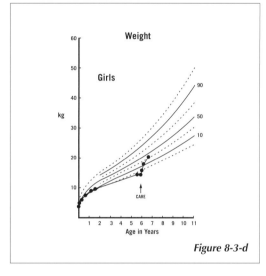

Figure 8-3-d

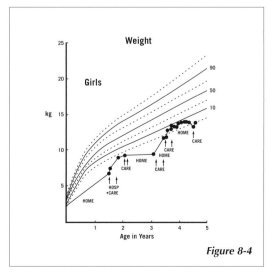

Figure 8-4

Figure 8-3. *(a)* and *(b)*: *Height and weight charts of index child failing to thrive who shows 2 episodes of catch-up growth. (c) and (d): Height and weight charts of older sibling whose FTT was unrecognized prior to admission to foster care but recognized only retrospectively when she showed accelerated growth. Reprinted from Hobbs CJ, Hanks HGI, Wynne JM. Failure to thrive. In: Hobbs CJ, Hanks HGI, Wynne JM, eds.* Child Abuse and Neglect: A Clinician's Handbook. *New York, NY: Churchill Livingstone; 1993a:25-28. ©1993, with permission from Elsevier.*

Figure 8-4. *Weight chart demonstrating the use of weights and life events to chart progress in a child with severe emotional abuse and FTT. Prolonged efforts of rehabilitation to parents' care have failed while the child repeatedly shows catch-up growth in substitute care. Reprinted from Hobbs CJ, Hanks HGI, Wynne JM. Failure to thrive. In: Hobbs CJ, Hanks HGI, Wynne JM, eds.* Child Abuse and Neglect: A Clinician's Handbook. *New York, NY: Churchill Livingstone; 1993a:25-28. ©1993, with permission from Elsevier.*

During primary care visits, nurses should generically ask screening questions about child safety at home, car restraints, and immunizations status. More probing may need to be done if more focused questions or concerns arise. A specific screen related to the possible form of neglect should be undertaken when the generic screen or clinical situation causes one to suspect a particular form of neglect.

Generic Screening

Generic screening includes attention to what Dubowitz et al. (2000) term "core issues" in assessing neglect. The core issues that globally apply to any child suspected of any type of neglect include attention to the following 6 areas:

1. Indications that basic needs are not being met (general appearance, signs of actual harm, risk of harm based on clinical situations, and child's past medical history)

2. Pattern of caregiving that suggests the presence of neglect (lack of adherence to routine healthcare recommendations, past episodes of neglect, previous CPS involvement)

3. Assessment of potential contributing factors (parental coping strategies, presence of domestic violence in family)

4. Assessment of strengths and possible resources available to the child and family (parental interest in child's well-being, other involved family members who are genuinely helpful, access to community-based family support programs)

5. Past successes and failures with previous interventions (what did and did not work before, who was involved, reasons for success or failure)

6. Prognostic information related to family motivation, capacity to change, and access to resources (Does the family have a track record of accepting help and achieving goals? Is there a record of resistance to recommendations? Are resources available with the family and community?)

After the generic assessment of the core issues described, the healthcare provider can move into a more specific, direct assessment of issues that need attention based on the type or form of neglect suspect (**Table 8-4**).

Specific Screening

Specific screening for particular forms of neglect such as physical neglect, medical neglect, and FTT is discussed in terms of the healthcare evaluation. The evaluation includes a medical history, physical examination, possible laboratory and diagnostic studies, and careful observation of the parent-child interaction during the office visit. It is also important to incorporate reports by other disciplines, especially professionals who visit the child at home. More specific evaluations would be for physical neglect, medical neglect, and FTT.

Physical Neglect

The types of physical neglect that may come to light in the healthcare setting revolve around patterns of care that demonstrate an inattention to avoidable risks to the child. Additionally, poor hygiene and inappropriate dress may become apparent. Depending on the setting, custody-related issues may or may not come to light. This often depends on the history provided by the caregiver and the presence of other responsible adults in the child's environment who may fill in the gaps for the child.

In assessing for physical neglect, the healthcare provider looks for any indication of exposure to avoidable and well-known environmental hazards. Examples include the following:

— Exposure to poisons left within the child's reach

— Failure to child-proof the house in which the child lives, with resultant risk of injury (e.g., turning the water heater down to the lowest setting)

— Installation and use of smoke detectors

— Appropriate use of child restraints in motor vehicles

— Use of bicycle helmets

— Presence of unsecured firearms in the home

— Presence of illicit drugs in household (the child or siblings may present with injuries or ingestion resulting form these exposures)

Additionally, the healthcare provider may use potential screening questions to identify the following situations that could present a risk:

— Hygiene: frequency of bathing, laundering, and toileting behaviors

— Clothing/shelter: types of clothing available, resources to acquire the clothing, how seasonal clothing is selected (if the child is in summer clothing and without a coat during a mid-winter visit, then the nurse must explore who made the decision and whether a winter coat is available)

— Questions about housing and its state of repair, as well as safety regarding electrical, heat, and cooking issues

— Custody/supervision: determine who besides the caregiver watches the child and what caregivers do when they need a break from childcare responsibilities

Observation. It is important to assess the physical appearance of the child. The nurse should note general appearance, including appropriateness of dress for climate and weather conditions, cleanliness, and infestations with parasites such as scabies and pediculosis capitis. Additionally, the nurse looks for evidence of acute or healed injuries and checks records to determine the history that the caregiver provided for each. If clothing is inappropriate for climate, the nurse should look for any evidence of environmental exposure, for example, frostbite on the fingers or toes. Lack of gloves or inappropriate foot coverings in cold weather should be noted.

Laboratory. The clinician orders laboratory assessments according to diagnostic considerations suggested by the clinical information. For example, a toxicology screen may be indicated if there is concern about ingestion, or a serum protein and albumin level is required if the clinician is concerned about long-standing calorie deprivation (Owen & Coant, 1992).

Caregiver-Child Interaction. In observing the caregiver-child interaction, the nurse should note whether the caregiver responds to the child's natural curiosity about the environment in a supportive manner but one that also redirects the child to safer activities. For example, if the child fingers the electric receptacle, does the caregiver redirect to a more appropriate activity? If the child climbs on a chair, does the caregiver move into a position to offer assistance and protection or does it appear that the child is ignored?

Medical Neglect

Medical neglect is a broad term that, at times, is included under physical neglect (Johnson & Coury, 1992). However, it is best to separate medical from physical neglect to highlight the unique expertise that healthcare providers have in identifying this form of neglect and fashioning specific interventions. The following discussion outlines guidelines to determine medical neglect.

Table 8-4. US Department of Health & Human Services Assessment of Neglect

TYPE OF NEGLECT

— Specific indicators of neglect

— Chronicity

PROBLEMS

— Identified by referral source

— Identified by parent

— Identified by helper

FACTORS AFFECTING PROVISION OF ADEQUATE CARE

— Individual personality

  — Strengths

  — Mental status/intelligence

  — Parenting knowledge and skills

  — Interpersonal skills

  — Physical health

  — Cooperation, motivation

— Family system

  — Strengths

  — Family size and composition

  — Income

  — Marital relationship

  — Special needs of children

  — Stability of family composition/membership

  — Structure, organization and communication/interaction patterns

  — Family boundaries

(continued)

Table 8-4. *(continued)*

ENVIRONMENTAL/COMMUNITY-BASED STRESSORS AND RESOURCES

— Housing

— Job/employment

— Neighborhood

— Informal social networks

— Cultural factors

— Availability and responsiveness of formally organized services

SETTING PRIORITIES

— Break goals into manageable, achievable subgoals

STRUCTURED ASSESSMENT MEASURES

— Learn about neglect characteristics

— Provide focus for interventions

— Provide a means for assessing intervention outcomes

Adapted from Gaudin JM Jr. Child Neglect: A Guide for Intervention. *Washington, DC: US Dept of Health & Human Services, Administration for Children and Families, Westover Consultants (Contract No. HHS-105-89-1730); 1993.*

History. First, the provider should determine appropriateness of the caregiver's response to the child, given the illness present. This involves the following aspects:

1. Timeliness for routine care

2. Response to presence of symptoms and signs

3. Reported adherence to medical regimens (supplemented by pharmacy records of filling prescriptions and, if appropriate, refill frequency)

4. Whether the caregiver expresses concern and seems interested in the evaluation

5. Whether caregiver asks appropriate questions about possible causes of the problem and treatments

Physical Examination. Evaluation of the child's condition is guided by the presenting symptoms and history provided and information gleaned from the medical record. The following are assessed:

1. Observe the general appearance, looking for signs of neglect. For specific clinical conditions, the physical examination will be directed by what is present.

2. Evaluate any delay in seeking treatment for new or acute symptoms:

   — What are the findings?

— How obvious are they?

— How severe do they appear?

3. For ongoing care of chronic conditions, assess the state of control of the disease, especially compared to expectations relative to prescribed treatment if followed as planned.

4. For routine care, evaluate:

— How well does the child appear in general?

— Is the child's development concordant with chronological age?

Laboratory Findings. The laboratory studies requested usually depend on the child's present condition. If there was delay in the caregiver seeking treatment for care, some laboratory tests may give information on diagnostic possibilities. In dehydration, the severity or chronicity of the situation can be revealed by an electrolyte panel. For certain chronic conditions, laboratory tests help determine the child's current clinical state. For example, the hemoglobin A1c test for diabetes management may indicate blood glucose control in the past. Finally, wide-ranging laboratory panels are generally not useful for routine care issues (Berwick, Levy, & Kleinerman, 1982).

Failure to Thrive

FTT is diagnosed when a child fails to grow as expected, compared to appropriate peers. The evaluation of a child's growth pattern involves a history, physical examination, and laboratory evaluations, as well as observations of parent-child interactions, especially regarding feeding.

History. The history in an FTT evaluation focuses on several key issues, including the following:

1. Child's dietary intake, preferences, and growth pattern over time

2. General health and well-being beginning with birth and up until the present time

3. Any known food intolerances or allergies

4. Presence of symptoms and signs such as vomiting, diarrhea, discomfort after feeding, or rashes with specific foods, which may suggest malabsorption or the presence of a disorder

5. Any recent or intercurrent illnesses since the last visit

6. Family dietary practices and process for food preparation

7. The family's ability to obtain appropriate foods for the child

8. Previous medical workups and results of previous interventions

9. Whether the caregiver seems concerned; if not, why not?

Physical Examination. When considering FTT, the accurate measurement of growth parameters and trends over time are essential. General appearance should be assessed for symptoms and signs of other forms of neglect or maltreatment, for example, severe diaper rash that has not been cared for. The examiner completes a head-to-toe physical examination, focusing on any findings that suggest a primary pathophysiological condition of the various systems examined. For example, wheezing and decreased breath sounds on lung examination suggest pulmonary disease, whereas a noninnocent murmur on heart examination suggests cardiac disease. It is important to assess skin integrity and evaluate muscle mass to determine the child's general nutritional status. The neurological examination also helps to assess coordination and developmental level. (See Chapter 7, Differential Diagnosis: Conditions That Mimic Child Maltreatment.)

Laboratory Assessment. The laboratory assessment in the FTT workup is focused and directed by the history and physical examination (Zenel, 1997). Large-scale "fishing expeditions" are rarely useful and tend to identify what would have been indicated in a more focused examination (Berwick et al., 1982; Homer & Ludwig, 1981). In general, a basic screening set of laboratory tests should be sufficient initially, followed by more involved or invasive laboratory or diagnostic studies as suggested by the clinical data. A bone age test may be helpful in considering primary growth disorders. A screening chemistry panel may help rule out basic metabolic, hepatic, and renal aberrations. A complete blood count can assist in evaluating basic hematological pathology, and a screening urinalysis can help in excluding urinary pathology, such as a urinary tract infection, as a possible etiology.

Caregiver-Child Interaction. As with any evaluation for child neglect, careful observation of how the caregiver interacts with the child is quite valuable. In the FTT evaluation, special attention is given to how the parent addresses the child's hunger and thirst, how food is provided, and the observable care given in responding to the child's cues (Chatoor, Schaefer, Dickson, & Egan, 1984). Additionally, the response of the child to the caregiver is important to note, looking at problems or ease with feeding. Does the child or parent appear frustrated or satisfied? Are the perceptions that are verbalized consistent with what is being observed?

Case Study of Neglect

The following case study presents a neglect situation, noting possible findings and outlining guidance for evaluation.

Sara is an 18-month-old female infant in your office today, Friday, for a sick visit. Her mother is concerned about her pulling on her right ear and her increased crying during the night. Sara has a history of one previous ear infection that started the same way, according to her mother. Sara lives with her mother Susan, age 16 years, her maternal grandmother, Sally, age 34 years, who has just started to work as part of a new state initiative, her aunt Shelly, age 18 years, and her 2 cousins, Joseph, age 2 years, and Jasmine, age 3 years. Susan is a junior in the neighborhood high school, and Shelly provides day care for the 3 children. The ear pulling started 2 nights ago and was slightly relieved with 2 droppersful of Tylenol Infant Drops every 4 hours. Susan wants an antibiotic for the ear pain.

A history reveals bowel and bladder function, sleep, and nutrition are within normal limits. Immunizations are not up to date; the child is missing booster DtaP. There are no allergies, emergency room visits, hospitalizations, or other illnesses since the last visit at age 12 months.

On doing the physical examination you see a bright red, bulging tympanic membrane, with a diffuse light reflex and no mobility. Her nose has boggy red turbinates and a yellow mucous discharge comes from both nostrils. Her throat is normal.

You also notice on the left side of the forehead a healing scab 3 cm by 0.5 cm, and on her right thigh 2 additional healing scabs. When asked about these, Susan tells you that Sara got burned with her curling iron that was left on the floor of her room while she was getting ready for school on Monday. She describes how the blisters formed and how after they broke she applied some medicine her sister used on her children for minor burns.

You finish the physical assessment and sit down to talk to Susan about leaving "small appliances that get hot, like a curling iron, plugged in and within a child's reach." You also ask about a safe place for the toddler to play while she is getting ready for school. Currently, there is no playpen or gate to keep any of the children confined to a safe space while an adult prepares for school or work or answers a ringing phone or doorbell.

Questions you must ask yourself at this time relate to the injury, the lack of seeking medical care, and using someone else's medicine.

— Is this a case of neglect?

— Should it be reported to CPS in your state?

A practical definition of neglect looks at the role of responsibility and intent of the child's care-taker (Johnson & Coury, 1992).

— Was Susan extraordinarily inattentive?

— What was the degree of avoidable suffering or actual harm—the burns?

— Did Susan respond in a reasonable way?

— How serious is it that Sara is not up to date on her immunizations and was not brought for medical care?

— If this were the second or third occurrence of burns, how would you change your plan of care?

Now for concerns based on community resources:

— What role does the primary care setting play, since the last appointment for immunizations is 3 pm and there are no evening or Saturday hours?

— Can no one other than a parent sign permission for the immunizations?

— Does her high school have a school-based clinic?

— Does her high school have a day care for toddlers?

— Is there an immunization clinic open on Saturdays or evenings at the public health center?

— Did her primary care center notify her of the inadequate level of immunizations?

Concerning other supervisors or caretakers, the following can be addressed:

— What responsibility, if any, does Sally, the maternal grandmother, have in this issue?

— What about Aunt Shelly. Does she bear any responsibility?

— Have Shelly's toddlers been burned by a curling iron?

— Is the household overcrowded?

Concerning Sara's temperament, or more importantly, Susan's perception of Sara:

— Is she described as a difficult child?

— Is Susan feeling more stress associated with parenting as Sara gets older?

Answers to these questions can help you decide how to proceed in working with Sara and her mother Susan. Most providers would call this neglectful behavior but not neglect.

TREATMENT
GENERIC MEASURES

The goal of any treatment for neglect is to have the child's basic needs met in a manner that fosters the child's ongoing health and well-being. The focus of the evaluation and treatment is to ensure that the child's needs are met in a positive manner. It is ideal to engage the caregiver in how to understand and then meet the child's needs. Unless the child is in immediate danger, efforts should be made to work with the parents/caregivers to optimize their potential for success in meeting the child's basic needs. If the child is believed to be in imminent danger of sustaining harm, immediate actions must be taken to ensure safety, including reporting to CPS.

At times, the child may need to be hospitalized to receive appropriate medical services and allow the CPS investigation to proceed. In such extreme circumstances, actual custody of the child may need to be taken from the parents with the assistance of the courts. In this situation, CPS determines to whom the child is discharged from the hospital. This determination is made as the investigation unfolds. In less critical situations, office-based interventions using the outpatient setting are indicated, which involve a wide range of resources, including home nursing visits along with other community-based services.

The treatment of child neglect begins with a clear assessment of the problem and determination of the family's strengths and challenges they will face in addressing the problems. A positive first step in constructing a treatment plan is communicating concern for the child, showing an interest in helping the parents and family meet the child's needs, and understanding that the family cares about what is best for the child (Schmitt, 1977). It is essential to explain the seriousness of the situation and to communicate clearly that ultimate action will be taken to ensure that the child obtains everything he/she needs. The healthcare provider will hopefully have other disciplines available to assist in treatment planning and ideally will have a working knowledge of what programs and resources are available in the community to help support the child and family.

Once a reasonable plan is designed, ongoing follow-up is necessary. Steps in successfully meeting the plan are identified, and the parents are reinforced for fulfilling each step. The plan should clearly identify what it means to fail in meeting appropriate milestones because caregivers may make multiple attempts to meet the child's needs and fail consistently. After a caregiver makes an appropriate number of failed attempts to meet the child's needs, CPS may need to consider more disruptive solutions, including out-of-home placement.

SPECIFIC MEASURES

Specific interventions for neglect depend on several factors, including the type of neglect, the amount of risk to the child, the developmental level of the child, the abilities of the caregivers, and the types of services available in the community.

For physical neglect, parental education concerning child safety and avoidable environmental hazards is essential, along with follow-up office visits to reinforce the anticipatory guidance. This involves assessment of the child's well-being and provision of additional age-appropriate information as the child grows. Home services such as social work and nursing visits are essential to ensure that the topics discussed in the office setting are carried through once the parent and child return home.

For medical neglect, treatment hinges on the identity of the particular medical condition. Parental education once again is central, with a focus on what symptoms and signs the caregiver needs to know and address. The caregiver must learn the following to understand appropriate care of the child:

1. How and when to contact the healthcare provider

2. What constitutes an emergency

3. The importance of adhering to the treatment plan as outlined

4. Connection to community resources that can help

5. Components of routine care that cannot be ignored

Additional supports such as nursing visits to assist in the child's care may be appropriate, depending on the clinical situation. Follow-up visits should be scheduled, and failure to keep these should be depicted as a serious indicator of the family not being able to care for the child. Finally, some level of case management is essential if the child's medical condition is complex and requires the input of several different healthcare providers.

For FTT cases, the treatment plan depends on identifying the underlying causes. Medical conditions usually require appropriate clinical interventions. Clinicians determine the child's appropriate and necessary nutritional intake, and dietary counseling is provided. Clinicians usually review at frequent intervals the records of what the child is offered and what is consumed. Parental education concerning food preparation, presentation, and assistance is important (Layzer & Goodson, 2001). If nutritional supplements are used, making sure that resources are available to obtain these is important. If technological interventions, such as nasogastric feedings, are suggested, parent training and ongoing home support is essential because sophisticated medical intervention can be challenging to even the most motivated of parents and caregivers. Home nursing visits during which the child's growth parameters are measured and discussed with the family are a critical adjunct to the scheduled office visits (Raynor, Rudolf, Cooper, Marchant, & Cottrell, 1999). The visits provide a set of "eyes" for the healthcare provider into what is actually happening regarding mealtime and nutritional intake (Black, Dubowitz, Hutcheson, Berenson-Howard, & Starr, 1995).

NURSING INTERVENTIONS FOR CHILD NEGLECT

Valuable resources when working with neglectful parents include home visitors (whether nurse or lay people) to determine the state of the home and community-sponsored support groups for parents. In addition, communicating with parents using the term "neglectful" can cement an observation and give the parent an opportunity to respond. One might expect a range of responses from total outrage to total passivity from a parent. But the provider must share the fact that he/she is worried about the child's condition and then determine the parents' position with regard to behavioral change and preventing a repeat event. Based on Henderson's (1966) definition of nursing and Prochaska, Johnson, and Lee's (1998) stages of behavioral change, the nurse could define parents' need for services and education based on a single categorization of willing to change, willing but unable, or unwilling.

Parents willing to change who describe a chaotic home life but do not live in unsafe conditions (such as little food, garbage and excrement in living space, exposed wiring, drugs and poisons within reach of children) are most often open to a change in their behavior to prevent an injury, such as a curling iron burn. Such a parent often states a need of more money or needs to be given ideas on ways to purchase safety gates or a playpen for the toddler. Such parents often benefit from a resourceful nurse who knows the lending closets, second-hand stores, and inexpensive large chain stores that carry such safety devices. This correlates with the Preparation or Action stage of Prochaska et al. (1998).

Willing but unable neglectful parents describe how they do not have the money for safety items or do not have a lending closet in their community. These parents may abuse alcohol or marijuana, have a flat affect, have little education, and have little experience with real-life success. They want the best for their children. They do not see a way to accomplish any change in the next month, but they may see the possibility in the next 6 months. This corresponds to the Contemplation stage (Prochaska et al., 1998).

Unwilling neglectful parents are outraged at the implication that a minor burn on their infant could be considered neglectful on their part. They do not anticipate any change in their parenting in the next 6 months. This correlates with the Pre-contemplation stage (Prochaska et al., 1998). These parents have many emotional needs that were not met by their parents. Their overall tendency is to react with passivity, but they become outraged if called neglectful. They have little motivation or skill to effect change in their lives. In fact, they are usually impulsive and seek immediate gratification without regard for long-term consequences. Therefore, saving for a future purchase of safety equipment is beyond their comprehension.

THE AMERICAN NURSES ASSOCIATION

Included among the position statements that guide nurses' practice is a statement on "Home Care for Mother, Infant, and Family Following Birth" (American Nurses Association [ANA], 1995). Many studies have documented the benefit of home visiting to new families with no known risk factors (Arnold & Bakewell-Sachs, 1991; Brooten, Roncoli, Finkler, Arnold, Cohen, & Mennuti, 1994; Carty & Bradley, 1990; Evans, 1995; Jansson, 1985; Norr & Nacion, 1987; Williams & Cooper, 1993; Yanover, Jones, & Miller, 1976). In addition, numerous studies have demonstrated the importance of home visits by registered nurses, to infants and families identified as at risk, to reduce risk factors that result in preterm births, neglect and abuse, or maternal health problems (Gomby, Larson, Lewit, & Behrman, 1993; Hardy & Streett, 1989; Olds, 1992; Olds, Henderson, Phelps, Kitzman, & Hanks, 1993).

In addition to the ANA, 3 additional policy-influencing boards have recommended home visiting as a cost-saving way to promote and protect the health of pregnant women and children and to prevent child neglect and abuse. These include the US Advisory Board on Child Abuse and Neglect (1993), the National Commission to Prevent Infant Mortality (1989), and the Public Health Service Expert Panel on the Content of Prenatal Care (1989).

CONCLUSION

Wodarski's (1981) early literature review identified that treatment approaches to neglect must address the multifaceted nature of the problem. Nurses are ideally suited to a holistic approach to this comprehensive undertaking. The most ideal approach consists of programs that combine child management, relationship enrichment, caregiver vocational skills enrichment, and interpersonal skill enhancement. Such comprehensive treatments require a significant investment of time and energy on everyone's part, especially the child's caregiver.

Looking beyond the specific case at hand, the nurse may also need to work on system-wide efforts to deal with neglect. The role of such system building, capacity enhancing advocacy is particularly important for the nurse working with neglect. Policies from professional organizations can give additional guidance to the practice of healthcare professionals in this area.

The number of children and families in the child welfare systems has grown out of proportion to the services available for this population; thus, child advocates have witnessed a crisis in the child protection system. In 1999, the National Association of Child Advocates (NACA) released an issue brief titled *A Child Advocate's Guide to State*

Child Protection Services Reform (Epstein, 1999). The new CPS approach focuses on a family's needs and strengths and has a caseworker assess a family for risks, strengths, and service needs. Cases are not classified or placed on a central registry, and the caseworker and family develop a cooperative relationship. Services are voluntary and not ordered by the court but are provided to families with a history of neglect and to support at-risk families.

The National Association of Pediatric Nurse Associates and Practitioners, Inc. (NAPNAP) has a distinct position statement on child abuse and neglect (1992). It affirms the following:

Child abuse and neglect is recognized as a national emergency. Many factors affecting family life contribute to child abuse and/or neglect. These factors are: (1) Increased violence in society; (2) Poverty; (3) Inadequate parenting skills; (4) Unrealistic parental expectations of childhood behavior; (5) Single parent families; (6) Substance and/or alcohol abuse; (7) Stress/isolation; (8) Cultural factors; (9) Delay in identification and intervention; and (10) Inadequate family support groups or extended families. (p. 1.)

For the nurse to affect these factors, multidisciplinary efforts are needed because no one discipline has the full complement of expertise to comprehensively address every factor for every family. Ells (1998) challenges us all to form such multidisciplinary teams and to marshal all community resources to favorably affect children and families in the area of child maltreatment.

APPENDIX: REPORT OF SUSPECTED NEGLECT FORM

(Contributed by Charles F. Johnson, MD; Columbus, Ohio.)

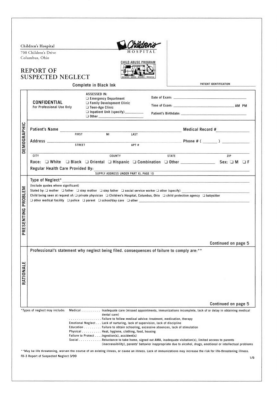

CONFIDENTIAL

For Professional Use Only

Child's Name _____

Medical Record Number _____

Complete in Black Ink.

PATIENT IDENTIFICATION

MEDICAL HISTORY

Immunizations up to date: N Y _____

Allergy: N Y _____

Chronic Illness: N Y _____

Acute Illness: N Y _____

Development: Normal Other _____

Current Medicaitons: N Y _____

Previous Injuries: N Y _____

Previous Hospitalizations: N Y _____

PHYSICAL EXAMINATION & DOCUMENTATION OF INJURIES

T _____ P _____ R _____ BP _____ / _____

Admission Weight _____ pounds/kgm _____ % Length _____ inches/cm _____ % H.C. _____ cm _____ %

General: _____

Norm.	Abn.	Not Exam.	COMMENTS
☐	☐	☐	Head/Face/Hair _____
☐	☐	☐	Eyes _____
☐	☐	☐	Ears _____
☐	☐	☐	Nose _____
☐	☐	☐	Mouth/Throat _____
☐	☐	☐	Teeth _____
☐	☐	☐	Neck/Nodes _____
☐	☐	☐	Chest/Lungs _____
☐	☐	☐	Heart _____
☐	☐	☐	Abdomen _____
☐	☐	☐	Skin _____
☐	☐	☐	Neurological _____
☐	☐	☐	Extremities _____
☐	☐	☐	Genitalia _____
☐	☐	☐	Speech _____
☐	☐	☐	Development _____

LABORATORY TESTS

Tests(s) Performed: Results:

FD-3 Report of Suspected Neglect 3/99

3/9

MEDICAL TREATMENT AND PLAN

Diagnosis:

Treatment:

Plan:

Consults to: _____ Orthopedics _____ Neurosurgery _____ Neurology _____ Surgery

_____ Pedondontics _____ Ophthalmology _____ Other _____

Admitted to the Hospital? ☐ Yes ☐ No If yes, which unit _____

Medical Follow-up: ☐ Yes ☐ No Where _____ When _____

Where _____ When _____

Where _____ When _____

Comments:

This form can be signed by a PL2 or 3. **A co-signature of an attending physician is required.**

Physician's Signature _____ ☐ PL2, ☐ PL3, ☐ Other _____

Print Name _____ Phone _____

Attending Signature _____ Print Name _____

Neglect is an act of omission which results in harm to a child's well being. It may be due to 1) ignorance (doesn't know), 2) economics; (knows but can't), 3) intent (knows can, but won't) or various combinations. Generally, the law requires reporting of #3. Ignorance should respond to education if guardian is mentally capable; a lack of physical resources may require service. Filing of intentional neglect may require documentation that #1 and #2 are not factors in non-compliance.

Neglect is difficult to diagnose because its definition – or its severity – tends to be subjective. Guidelines have been proposed to aid you in determining when to file. The purpose of filing is to bring services to a child whose parents, despite education and resources, do not act to preserve or promote a child's well being.

Prenatal neglect, including substance abuse, which threatens the well being of the fetus, may require reporting.

FD-3 Report of Suspected Neglect 3/99

4/9

CONFIDENTIAL

For Professional Use Only

Child's Name _____

Medical Record Number _____

Complete in Black Ink.

PATIENT IDENTIFICATION

CONTINUED FROM PAGE 1:

Type of Neglect:

Professional's statement why neglect being filed. Consequences of failure to comply are:

FD-3 Report of Suspected Neglect 3/99

5/9

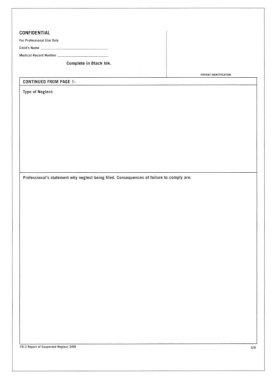

CONFIDENTIAL

For Professional Use Only

Child's Name _____

Medical Record Number _____

Complete in Black Ink.

PATIENT IDENTIFICATION

PSYCHOSOCIAL ASSESSMENT

I. Family Dynamics

NAME FIRST	LAST	DOB/AGE	RELATIONSHIP TO CHILD	EDUCATION	EMPLOYMENT OCCUPATION
1.					
2.					
3.					
4.					
5.					
6.					
7.					

Child lives with: ☐ mother ☐ father ☐ step mother ☐ step father ☐ foster parent ☐ other _____

IIa. Significant Others

NAME FIRST	LAST	DOB/AGE	RELATIONSHIP TO CHILD	EDUCATION	EMPLOYMENT OCCUPATION
1.					
2.					
3.					
4.					

*Place asterisk beside the name(s) of those accompanying child to the hospital for assessment.

IIb. Suspected Perpetrator: Name _____ DOB/Age _____

Info from: ☐ Child ☐ Mother ☐ Father ☐ Other _____

Relationship to child: _____

Sex: ☐ M ☐ F Race: ☐ B ☐ W ☐ Or ☐ Hisp ☐ Combo (specify) _____ ☐ Other _____

Employed: ☐ Yes ☐ No ☐ ? Occupation: _____

IIc. Married Status of Biological Parents

Father: ☐ single ☐ married ☐ separated ☐ divorced ☐ remarried ☐ widowed ☐ unknown

Mother: ☐ single ☐ married ☐ separated ☐ divorced ☐ remarried ☐ widowed ☐ unknown

IId. Name of Child's Legal Guardian: _____

IIe. Child's School System: ☐ Columbus Public ☐ Other _____

Name of School _____ Grade _____

Teacher _____

Performance _____

IIc.

FD-3 Report of Suspected Neglect 3/99

6/9

VII. Pertinent Information: (family and patient background, additional history of abuse, i.e. disclosure process)

VIII. Identified Stress Factors. Family and patient background, relationships, and dynamics. Include known stress factors, such as adverse economic conditions, illness, mental health status of family members, and <u>stress management style</u>.

☐ Family history of sexual or physical abuse?
☐ Domestic Violence?
☐ Criminal behavior?
☐ Substance Abuse?

FD-3 Report of Suspected Neglect 3/99   7/9

CONFIDENTIAL
For Professional Use Only
Child's Name _____
Medical Record Number _____
Complete in Black Ink.

PATIENT IDENTIFICATION

IX. Behavioral Observations: (parent-child interaction, parent affect, child's behavior while in the hospital)

X. Family Support Systems. Include parents, friends, relatives and church affiliations.

FD-3 Report of Suspected Neglect 3/99   8/9

XI. Community Referrals

*1. Child Protection Agency (county where legal guardian resides) _____
   Code # _____ (only active/open FCCS cases)
   Address _____   Contact Person _____

   Currently serviced: ☐ Yes ☐ No _____   Previous contact: ☐ Yes ☐ No

*2. Law Enforcement Agency _____
   Address _____   Contact Person _____
   Address where suspected neglect occurred _____   OR ☐ unknown.

3. Private Physician _____
   Address _____

4. Other Agency Contacted _____
   Address _____   Contact Person _____

XII. Recommended discharge planning:

Recommendations:
☐ Counseling for child
☐ Counseling for parent
☐ Emergency Court Order
☐ Homemaker
☐ Infant Stimulation Program
☐ Protective Day Care
☐ Psychological or developmental evaluation of child
☐ Psychological evaluation of parent
☐ Public Health Nurse
☐ Separate alleged perpetrator from child
☐ Other (specify) _____
Comments _____
_____
_____
_____
_____
_____

Pictures taken? ☐ Yes ☐ No   If yes, ☐ 35mm ☐ Polaroid? How many? _____   By whom? _____
Please contact Stephanie Barry at 614-722-3279 for duplicates.

XIII. Child discharged to: _____
   Social worker's signature _____   Date _____
   Print name _____   Phone _____

*Under Ohio Law (O.R.C Section 2(5).42) suspected child abuse/neglect (which includes non-organic FTT) cases must be reported to the protective agency and police (in county where abuse/neglect occurred).

FD-3 Report of Suspected Neglect 3/99   9/9

REFERENCES

American Nurses Association. *Home Care for Mother, Infant, and Family Following Birth.* Washington, DC: American Nurses Association; 1995.

Arnold LS, Bakewell-Sachs S. Models of perinatal home follow-up. *J Perinat Neonatal Nurs.* 1991;5:18-26.

Belsky J. Etiology of child maltreatment: a developmental-ecological analysis. *Psychol Bull.* 1993;114:413-34.

Berwick DM, Levy JC, Kleinerman R. Failure to thrive: diagnostic yield of hospitalisation. *Arch Dis Child.* 1982;57:347-351.

Black MM, Dubowitz H, Hutcheson J, Berenson-Howard J, Starr RH. A randomized clinical trial of home intervention for children with failure to thrive. *Pediatrics.* 1995;95:807-814.

Bonfenbrenner U. Toward an experimental ecology of human development. *Am Psychol.* 1977;32:512-531.

Bonner BL, Crow SM, Logue MB. Fatal child neglect. In: Dubowitz H, ed. *Neglected Children: Research, Practice, and Policy.* Thousand Oaks, Calif: Sage Publications; 1999:156-173.

Bridges CL. The nurse's evaluation. In: Schmitt BD, ed. *The Child Protection Team Handbook.* New York, NY: Garland Publishing; 1978:65-81.

Brooten D, Roncoli M, Finkler S, Arnold L, Cohen A, Mennuti M. A randomized trial of early hospital discharge and home follow-up of women having cesarean birth. *Obstet Gynecol.* 1994;84:832-838.

Brown J, Cohen P, Johnson JG, Salzinger S. A longitudinal analysis of risk factors for child maltreatment: findings of a 17-year prospective study of officially recorded and self-reported child abuse and neglect. *Child Abuse Negl.* 1998;22:1065-1078.

Burke J, Chandy J, Dannerbeck A, Watt JW. The parental environment cluster model of child neglect: an integrative conceptual model. *Child Welfare.* 1998;77:389-405.

Cantwell HB. The neglect of child neglect. In: Helfer ME, Kempe RS, Krugman RD, eds. *The Battered Child.* 5th ed. Chicago, Ill: University of Chicago Press; 1997:347-373.

Carty E, Bradley C. A randomized, controlled evaluation of early postpartum hospital discharge. *Birth.* 1990;17:199-204.

Chatoor I, Schaefer S, Dickson L, Egan J. Non-organic failure to thrive: a developmental perspective. *Pediatr Ann.* 1984;13:829-843.

Crittenden PM. Child neglect: causes and contributors. In: Dubowitz H. *Neglected Children: Research, Practice, and Policy.* Thousand Oaks, Calif: Sage Publications; 1999:47-68.

Crouch JL, Milner JS. Effects of child neglect on children. *Crim Justice Behav.* 1993;20:49-65.

Daro D. *Confronting Child Abuse: Research for Effective Program Design.* New York, NY: The Free Press; 1988.

Dubowitz H, ed. *Neglected Children: Research, Practice, and Policy.* Thousand Oaks, Calif: Sage Publications; 1999.

Dubowitz H, Black M, Starr RH, Zuravin S. A conceptual definition of child neglect. *Crim Justice Behav.* 1993;20:8-26.

Dubowitz H, Giardino A, Gustavson E. Child neglect: guidance for pediatricians. *Pediatr Rev.* 2000;21:4, 111-116.

Dubowitz H, Klockner A, Starr RH, Black MM. Community and professional definitions of child neglect. *Child Maltreat.* 1998;3:235-243.

Dumas R. Validating a theory of nursing practice. *Am J Nurs.* 1963;63:52.

Ells M. Forming a multidisciplinary team to investigate child abuse. *Portable Guides to Investigating Child Abuse.* Washington, DC: US Dept of Justice; 1998:1-23.

English D. Evaluation and risk assessment of child neglect in public child protection services. In: Dubowitz H, ed. *Neglected Children: Research, Practice, and Policy.* Thousand Oaks, Calif: Sage Publications; 1999:191-210.

Epstein H. *A Child Advocate's Guide to State Child Protective Services Reform.* Washington, DC: National Association of Child Advocates; 1999.

Evans C. Postpartum home care in the United States. *J Obstet Gynecol Neonatal Nurs.* 1995;24:180-186.

Garbarino J. The human ecology of child maltreatment: a conceptual model for research. *J Marriage Fam.* 1977a;39:721-736.

Garbarino J. The price of privacy in the social dynamics of child abuse. *Child Welfare.* 1977b;56:565-575.

Garbarino J, Barry F. The community context of child abuse and neglect. In: Garbarino J, Eckenrode J, eds. *Understanding Abusive Families: An Ecological Approach to Theory and Practice.* San Francisco, Calif: Jossey-Bass Publishers; 1997:56-85.

Garbarino J, Collins CC. Child neglect: the family with a hole in the middle. In: Dubowitz H, ed. *Neglected Children: Research, Practice, and Policy.* Thousand Oaks, Calif: Sage Publications; 1999:1-23.

Garbarino J, Crouter A. Defining the community context for parent-child relations: the correlates of child maltreatment. *Child Dev.* 1978;69:604-615.

Garbarino J, Sherman D. High-risk neighborhoods and high-risk families: the human ecology of child maltreatment. *Child Dev.* 1980;51:188-198.

Gaudin JM Jr. *Child Neglect: A Guide for Intervention.* Washington, DC: US Dept of Health & Human Services, Administration for Children and Families, Westover Consultants (Contract No. HHS-105-89-1730); 1993.

Gaudin JM Jr. Child neglect: short-term and long-term outcomes. In: Dubowitz H, ed. *Neglected Children: Research, Practice, and Policy.* Thousand Oaks, Calif: Sage Publications; 1999:89-108.

Gomby DS, Larson JD, Lewit JD, Behrman RE. Home visiting: analysis and recommendations. *Future Child.* 1993;3:6-22.

Haecker T, Cockerill M, Giardino AP, Christian CW, Giardino ER. Neglect and failure to thrive. In: Giardino AP, Christian CW, Giardino ER, eds. *A Practical Guide to the Evaluation of Child Physical Abuse and Neglect.* Thousand Oaks, Calif: Sage Publications; 1997:169-210.

Hardy JB, Streett R. Family support and parenting education in the home: an effective extension of clinic-based preventive health care services for poor children. *J Pediatr.* 1989;115:927-931.

Hawley A. *Human Ecology: A Theory of Community Structure.* New York, NY: Ronald; 1950.

Henderson V. *The Nature of Nursing—A Definition and Its Implications for Practice, Research and Education.* New York, NY: The Macmillan Company; 1966:15.

Hobbs CJ, Hanks HGI, Wynne JM. Failure to thrive. In: Hobbs CJ, Hanks HGI, Wynne JM, eds. *Child Abuse and Neglect: A Clinician's Handbook.* New York, NY: Churchill Livingstone; 1993a:25-28.

Hobbs CJ, Hanks HGI, Wynne JM. Neglect. In: Hobbs CJ, Hanks HGI, Wynne JM, eds. *Child Abuse and Neglect: A Clinician's Handbook.* New York, NY: Churchill Livingstone; 1993b:89-105.

Homer C, Ludwig S. Categorization of etiology of failure to thrive. *Am J Dis Child.* 1981;135:848-851.

Jansson P. Early postpartum discharge. *Am J Nurs.* 1985;85:547-550.

Johnson CF, Coury DL. Child neglect: general concepts and medical neglect. In: Ludwig S, Kornberg AE, eds. *Child Abuse: A Medical Reference.* New York, NY: Churchill Livingstone; 1992:321-331.

Kaplan SJ. Child and adolescent abuse and neglect research: a review of the past 10 years. Part I: Physical and emotional abuse and neglect. *J Am Acad Child Adolesc Psychiatry.* 1999;38:1214-1222.

LaGreca AM. Issues in adherence with pediatric regimens. *J Pediatr Psychol.* 1990;5:423-436.

Layzer JI, Goodson BD. *Parenting Education and Support: A Review of Research and Recommendations for Practice.* Philadelphia, Pa: Department of Human Services, Division of Community-Based Prevention Services; 2001:1-28.

Ludwig S. Defining child abuse: clinical mandate—evolving concepts. In: Ludwig S, Kornberg AE, eds. *Child Abuse: A Medical Reference.* New York, NY: Churchill Livingstone; 1992a:1-12.

Ludwig S. Failure-to-thrive/starvation. In: Ludwig S, Kornberg AE, eds. *Child Abuse: A Medical Reference.* New York, NY: Churchill Livingstone; 1992b:303-319.

Ludwig S, Rostain A. Family function and dysfunction. In: Levine MD, Carey WB, Crocker AC, eds. *Developmental-Behavioral Pediatrics.* 2nd ed. Philadelphia, Pa: WB Saunders; 1992:147-159.

Lutzker JR, Bigelow KM, Doctor RM, Gershater RM, Greene BF. An ecobehavioral model for the prevention and treatment of child abuse and neglect: history and applications. In: Lutzker JR, ed. *Handbook of Child Abuse Research and Treatment.* New York, NY: Plenum Press; 1998:239-266.

Magura S, Moses S. *Outcome Measures for Child Welfare Services: Theory and Application.* Washington, DC: Child Welfare League of America; 1986.

Matsui DM. Drug compliance in pediatrics. Clinical and research issues. *Pediatr Clin North Am.* 1997;44:1-14.

McCleery JT, Pinyerd BJ. Nursing evaluation and treatment planning. In: Bross DC, Krugman RD, Lenherr MR, Rosenberg DA, Schmitt BD, eds. *The New Child Protection Team Handbook.* New York, NY: Garland Publishing; 1988:127-135.

NAPNAP position statements. *J Pediatr Health Care.* 1992;6:226.

National Clearinghouse on Child Abuse and Neglect Information. *Prevention Pays: The Costs of Not Preventing Child Abuse and Neglect.* Washington, DC: National Clearinghouse on Child Abuse and Neglect Information; 1998:1-5. Available at: http://www.calib.com/nccanch. Accessed February 26, 2003.

National Clearinghouse on Child Abuse and Neglect Information. *Child Maltreatment 2000.* Washington, DC: US Dept of Health & Human Services; 2000. Available at: http://www.acf.hhs.gov/programs/cb/publications/cm00/index.htm. Accessed April 22, 2003.

National Commission to Prevent Infant Mortality. *Home Visiting: Opening Doors for America's Pregnant Women and Children.* Washington, DC: National Commission to Prevent Infant Mortality; 1989.

Norr KF, Nacion K. Outcomes of postpartum early discharge, 1960-1986. A comparative review. *Birth.* 1987;14:135-141.

Oates RK. Neglect and nonorganic failure to thrive. In: Oates RK, ed. *The Spectrum of Child Abuse: Assessment, Treatment and Prevention.* New York, NY: Brunner/Mazel Publishers; 1996:15-19.

Oates RK, Kempe RS. Growth failure in infants. In: Helfer ME, Kempe RS, Krugman RD. *The Battered Child.* Chicago, Ill: The University of Chicago Press; 1997:374-391.

Olds DL. Home visitation for pregnant women and parents of young children. *Am J Dis Child.* 1992;146:704-708.

Olds DL, Henderson CR, Phelps C, Kitzman H, Hanks C. Effect of prenatal and infancy nurse home visitation on government spending. *Med Care.* 1993;31:155-174.

Olds D, Kitzman H. Review of research on home visiting for pregnant women and parents of young children. *Future Child.* 1993;3:53-92.

Olds D, Eckenrode J, Henderson CR, et al. Long-term effects of home visitation on maternal life course and child abuse and neglect. *JAMA.* 1997;278:637-643.

Olds D, Hill PL, Mihalic SF, O'Brien RA. *Blueprints for Violence Prevention.* Boulder, Colo: Center for the Study and Prevention of Violence; 1998:3-96.

Owen M, Coant P. Other forms of neglect. In: Ludwig S, Kornberg AE, eds. *Child Abuse: A Medical Reference.* New York, NY: Churchill Livingstone; 1992:349-355.

Pence D, Wilson C. *Team Investigation of Child Sexual Abuse: The Uneasy Alliance.* Thousand Oaks, Calif: Sage Publications; 1994.

Polansky NA. *Damage Parents: An Anatomy of Child Neglect.* Chicago, Ill: The University of Chicago Press; 1981:1-2.

Polansky NA, Gaudin JM, Ammons PW, Davis KB. The psychological ecology of the neglectful mother. *Child Abuse Negl.* 1985;9:265-275.

Prochaska JO, Johnson S, Lee P. The transtheoretical model of behavior change. In: Shumaker SA, Schron EB, eds. *The Handbook of Health Behavior Change.* 2nd ed. New York, NY: Springs Publishing Company; 1998:59-84.

Public Health Service Expert Panel on the Content of Prenatal Care. *Caring for Our Future: The Content of Prenatal Care.* Washington, DC: US Dept of Health & Human Services; 1989.

Raynor P, Rudolf MC, Cooper K, Marchant P, Cottrell D. A randomised controlled trial of specialist health visitor intervention for failure to thrive. *Arch Dis Child.* 1999;80:500-506.

Reece RM, Ludwig S, eds. *Child Abuse: Medical Diagnosis and Management.* 2nd ed. Philadelphia, Pa: Lippincott Williams & Wilkins; 2000.

Rose SJ. Reaching consensus on child neglect: African American mothers and child welfare workers. *Child Youth Serv Rev.* 1999;21:463-479.

Rose SJ, Meezan W. Variations in perceptions of child neglect. *Child Welfare.* 1996;75:139-160.

Runyan DK, Hunter WM, Everson MD, et al. *Longitudinal Studies of Child Abuse and Neglect. LONGSCAN: The First Five Years at the Coordinating Center, North Carolina and Seattle Site, 1991-1996.* Washington, DC: National Center on Child Abuse and Neglect; 1997.

Schmitt B. *The Child Protection Team Handbook.* New York, NY: Garland, STPM Books; 1977.

Schmitt B. Child neglect. In: Ellerstein NS, ed. *Child Abuse and Neglect: A Medical Reference.* New York, NY: John Wiley and Sons; 1981:297-306.

Sedlak AJ, Broadhurst DD. *Third National Incidence Study of Child Abuse and Neglect.* Washington, DC: US Dept of Health & Human Services; 1996.

US Advisory Board on Child Abuse and Neglect. *Neighbors Helping Neighbors: A New National Strategy for the Protection of Children (Vol. Fourth Report).* Washington, DC: US Dept of Health & Human Services, Administration for Children and Families; 1993.

US Department of Health & Human Services. *Child Abuse and Neglect State Statutes Elements: Reporting Laws: Number 1: Definitions of Child Abuse and Neglect.* National Clearinghouse on Child Abuse and Neglect Information; 1999. Available at: http://www.calib.com/nccanch/pubs/stats02/define/index.cfm. Accessed February 27, 2003.

US Department of Health & Human Services. Administration on Children, Youth and Families. *Child Maltreatment 1999.* Washington, DC: US Government Printing Office; 2001.

Wilcox WD, Nieburg P, Miller DS. Failure to thrive: a continuing problem of definition. *Clin Pediatr.* 1989;28:391-394.

Williams LR, Cooper MK. Nurse-managed postpartum home care. *J Obstet Gynecol Neonatal Nurs.* 1993;22:25-31.

Wodarski JS. Treatment of parents who abuse their children: a literature review and implications for professionals. *Child Abuse Negl.* 1981;5:351-360.

Wolfe DA. Child abuse prevention blending research and practice. *Child Abuse Review.* 1993;2:153-165.

Wolock I, Horowitz B. Child maltreatment as a social problem: the neglect of neglect. *Am J Orthopsychiatry.* 1984;54:530-543.

Yanover M, Jones D, Miller M. Perinatal care of low risk mothers and infants: early discharge with home care. *N Engl J Med.* 1976;294:702-705.

Zenel JA. Failure to thrive: a general pediatrician's perspective. *Pediatr Rev.* 1997;18:371-379.

Zuravin SJ. Child neglect: a review of definitions and measurement research. In: Dubowitz H, ed. *Neglected Children: Research, Practice, and Policy.* Thousand Oaks, Calif: Sage Publications; 1999:24-46.

Chapter 9

DOCUMENTATION OF THE EVALUATION IN CASES OF SUSPECTED CHILD MALTREATMENT

Jennifer Pierce-Weeks, RN, CEN
Eileen R. Giardino, PhD, RN, CRNP

The medical evaluation of a child in cases of suspected maltreatment is an essential area of the overall evaluation, which is part of a multidisciplinary approach to the child and family. The findings for the medical evaluation are important to the investigation of suspected child maltreatment and may be an essential component in judicial or legal proceedings. Additionally, the medical evaluation is a central step in the healthcare process that has as its goal the emotional and physical healing and well-being of the child. Therefore, accurate documentation of the history, physical findings, and laboratory assessment in children suspected of maltreatment is vital to preserve the data developed for the evaluation. The thoroughness and accuracy of the history, physical examination, laboratory findings, and formulation of diagnostic impression are important because the medical record stands as a legal document. It is used by law enforcement, district attorneys, and child protective services (CPS) to make decisions concerning the child's welfare (Dubowitz & Bross, 1992; Limbos & Berkowitz, 1998). One can expect that the medical chart will be scrutinized in legal procedures for decisions regarding the child's welfare or a perpetrator's fate (Jenny, 1996).

The medical evaluation of a child in cases of suspected abuse or neglect first requires examination skills in performing a sensitive and developmentally appropriate history and physical examination. Data such as a developmental history in younger children, witnesses to injury, sketches and photographs of physical injuries, genital examination findings, and documentation of specific history questions and answers are the components of a complete record in child abuse. Thorough documentation of appropriate data in cases of child abuse and neglect is a learned skill; the nurse needs to understand the legal implications surrounding abuse situations and the components of a complete medical evaluation.

GENERAL CONSIDERATIONS FOR THE HISTORY AND PHYSICAL EXAMINATION

Meticulous documentation of the findings of the medical evaluation is essential in suspected child abuse cases. The examiner should never rely on memory to reconstruct the details of the history and physical findings (Giardino, Christian, & Giardino, 1997). The purpose of the medical history is multifaceted to accomplish the following 3 specific goals: gather information that leads to a diagnosis, evaluate the physical safety of the child, and determine if medical treatment is necessary (Barnes, 2001).

Accurate documentation of the child's history and the questions asked and answers given are critical because the record is a legal document and the data may be admitted as evidence in court trials. When court testimony is necessary, a well-documented chart serves to refresh the clinician's memory and possibly decrease the time taken for court proceedings (Bar-on & Zanga, 1996; Dubowitz & Bross, 1992). It is less likely that the examiner may need to testify in civil court proceedings when the documents reflect detailed reports of the evaluation and explicit opinions of the findings (American Academy of Pediatrics [AAP], 1999). Furthermore, CPS uses the record during investigation of the case to make decisions regarding the child's placement in protective care with parents, caregivers, or foster care (Dubowitz & Bross, 1992).

DOCUMENTATION GUIDELINES

The history process begins with obtaining subjective data from the child and the child's caregivers to provide background information concerning the situations surrounding the abuse and the health status of the child. In sexual abuse evaluations, the history provides extremely important data related to the case because there are often few to no physical findings. As much as possible, the examiner documents the patient's subjective statements using quotations rather than paraphrasing the statements. This allows the reader, jury, attorney, or child protection worker to get a sense of the child's own words. Quotations prove helpful in legal proceedings to reflect in the chart the questions the examiner asked (Lahoti, McClain, Girardet, McNeese, & Cheung, 2001). The interpretation of a statement can change dramatically depending on the context and question asked. Additionally, some states have enacted "hearsay" exceptions that may allow healthcare providers to present the child's descriptions in court. This is enhanced if documentation in the record is done carefully (Jenny, 1996).

The standards set for the questioning process require that questions be nonleading and asked without coercion of the child (Dubowitz & Bross, 1992). The court is always concerned that there may have been improper or suggestive questioning methods and may request a pretrial "taint" hearing to determine if information was obtained in appropriate ways. The court may challenge the admissibility of the child's history if it is determined that questioning was not done appropriately (Finkel & Ricci, 1997). The professional does not record personal opinions regarding the caregiver or the situation because such information undermines the credibility of the professional and of the medical record (Marx, 1997).

Because the medical record is a legal document that can be subpoenaed for any court proceedings, it is important that the handwriting be legible, the data be comprehensive, and the events be documented chronologically when necessary (Dubowitz & Bross, 1992; Jenny, 1996). Any corrections made in the notes should be inserted as addenda and marked as such. The signature of the writer of the notes should be clear and followed by the printed name. Dubowitz and Bross (1992) suggest that it is reasonable in some descriptions to use "plain English" rather than medical terms that may be misunderstood by nonmedical people who need to read and use the findings of the medical evaluation. One can also put nonmedical explanations in parentheses to clarify certain findings. For example, for the finding of ". . . subdural hematoma, one could put in parentheses (a collection of blood inside the skull, around the brain. . .)" (Dubowitz & Bross, 1992).

The medical record should reflect the examiner's knowledge of specific aspects of physical abuse and neglect as they are manifest in children, as well as an understanding of growth and development (Barnes, 2001). In child sexual abuse, the history is a critical component of the evaluation (Heger, Emans, & Muram, 2000) because the physical examination findings are usually normal or nonspecific.

Some general information should be entered into the record. It is recommended that the healthcare provider document that the child was informed that the purpose of questioning was for medical diagnosis and treatment and that the child was told of the importance of providing accurate information (Myers, 1996). Other information about the examiner, background to the assessment, and those who are present during an evaluation should also be entered into the medical record as follows (Dubowitz & Bross 1992; Marx, 1997):

— Qualifications of the person completing the medical evaluation

— Name of the person making the statement or demonstrating the documented behavior and that person's relationship to the child

— Name(s) of accompanying adult(s) and relationship to the child

— Date and time of the assessment

— Referral source

— Reason for referral or chief complaint

— Names of people present at the time the statement was made or the behavior was observed

— Name of the person making the entry into the record or chart; include the phone number of that person when possible

DOCUMENTATION OF CONSENT
The consent issue for authorization to complete an examination of suspected child abuse and neglect is complicated and may vary from state to state. The nurse must be aware of what the consent laws are in both the institution and the state. For example, an emergency healthcare situation in which the child comes to the emergency department for care often implies consent for urgent care. In less urgent situations, parental consent is essential. However, when child maltreatment is suspected, the healthcare provider is obligated to act upon suspicions and may need to pursue other avenues for obtaining consent, should the parents deny permission for an examination, to protect the interests of the child and keep him or her safe.

The authorizing party usually signs his or her name in the medical record, followed by a statement that he or she consented to the evaluation. The status of the consenting party may be complicated and depends on the details of the child's case. In child maltreatment settings, the child may come for medical evaluation on the request of a parent/caregiver, CPS/law enforcement personnel, or the agency that assigned physical custody of the child from the court. (See Chapter 14, Legal Issues, for further discussion.)

FORMAT OF ASSESSMENT DOCUMENTATION
Studies looking at the quality of documentation of child physical and sexual abuse have found that clinicians do not always document the overall interaction and findings in the clearest or most complete manner (Limbos & Berkowitz, 1998; Parra, Huston, & Foulds, 1997). Child abuse clinicians can benefit from training in all aspects of documentation because of the complexity of the specific abuse-related data that should be written in the record. In reviewing child abuse records, the quality was shown to be improved by using structured records to aid in the documentation process (Socolar, Champion, & Green, 1996). Checklists can remind the examiner of what details should be documented in the medical record. Structured forms help to increase collected information in the medical records, particularly in the area of dates and times and the illustration of physical injuries on provided diagrams (Limbos & Berkowitz, 1998).

DOCUMENTATION OF TAPED INTERVIEWS

The guidelines of the American Professional Society on the Abuse of Children (APSAC) suggest that the use of videotapes or audiotapes is determined by clinical considerations, logistics, and professional preference (Faller, 1996). Documentation of a taped interview requires careful notation of what occurred. An audiotape of the interview should include information that makes it clear who was doing what and who was present during the taping. Details made explicit via voice recordings on tape are the following (Ledray, 1999):

— Name of the child in question

— Name of the interviewer

— Date, time, and location of the interview

— Other person(s) present during the taping and history taking

Videotapes can decrease the number of interviews a child must undergo when his or her case is being investigated, because other investigators may view the child's statements and responses. Taping allows the practitioner to give the client full attention without concern for writing anything during the session. The tape can be used to show the child's affect during the interview and may enable other professionals to evaluate the strengths of the case (Faller, 1996). It also allows for later review of the tape and critique of the methods with colleagues (Finkel & Ricci, 1997; Pence & Wilson, 1994).

Guidelines for audiotaping and videotaping of history taking in child abuse evaluations continue to be controversial and lack apparent consensus among professionals. Prosecutors have concerns for videotaping or audiotaping interviews because of the ability of those who perform the interviews and the potential for flaws in the techniques. The tape makes interviewer errors evident and documents misphrased or leading questions. Also, defense experts are able to critique the tape and characterize the actions and interactions of the interviewer in a negative perspective to favor the alleged perpetrator (Pence, Wilson, & Broadhurst, 1992). The use of videotape testimony is not permitted in certain states and jurisdictions, so it is imperative to know the details of what certain states allow. It is recommended that examiners using audio and video technology follow accepted practice guidelines for taping, storage, and release of information (Monteleone & Brodeur, 1998; Pence et al., 1992).

DOCUMENTATION OF THE HISTORY

Documentation of the interview should be detailed and complete. Included in the chart are specific questions asked along with the child's verbatim answers (Ledray, 1999), nonverbal behaviors, and emotional responses. Any drawings of the child are labeled with the appropriate heading as to what the diagram is. Then, they are dated and signed by the interviewer and child and made a part of the permanent record (Ledray, 1999). It is especially important to include a statement to indicate that the interviewer asked the child to state the words he or she uses to name body parts: ". . . words describing body parts are the words used by the child . . ." (Poyer, 1997). When an interpreter is used, it is important to document the name of the person and the language interpreted (American College of Emergency Physicians [ACEP], 1999).

In cases of physical abuse, specific information should be documented in the medical history. Much of this information is asked of the caregiver because it relates to how the injury occurred and whether the reasons provided for the injury seem plausible or reasonable given the type of injury sustained and the degree of injury evaluated.

Because the child's story of what occurred as obtained by the examiner can be admitted in court trials, it is critical to document questions and answers thoroughly during the evaluation (Lahoti et al., 2001). During the history and interview process of a child who has sustained injuries, certain indicators from both caregiver and child raise the suspicion of abuse. The following are such areas of suspicion that should be documented in the record (Cheung, 1999; Giardino et al., 1997; Myers, 2001):

— Caregiver's explanation for injury

— History of injury that changes with time or is vague

— No reasonable explanation of injury

— History seems inappropriate for observed injury

— History is developmentally incompatible with child

— Trauma history incongruous or not plausible with physical examination

— Inappropriate caregiver concerns for severe injury

— Nonspecific behavioral indicators from child or caretaker

— Injury cannot be explained by caregiver

— Claim that injury was inflicted by a sibling

— Delay in seeking medical care for life-threatening or serious injury

History From the Caregiver

A common practice for the healthcare provider is to first take a medical history from the child's caregiver before talking with the child. The caregiver's information forms the initial basis for the examination of the child. This history should be obtained from the caregiver without the child present whenever possible (Sorenson, Bottoms, & Perona, 1997). The primary history is usually obtained from the caregiver when the client is an infant, a young child, or developmentally delayed.

The documentation of the history should reflect that the interviewer did not use blaming or accusatory statements or that assumptions or speculations were made. Documentation of the history should include the following information:

— When and how injury occurred

— Whether injury was witnessed; if so, by whom

— Person responsible for the child at time of injury

— If the injury was not witnessed by the caregiver, how the caregiver came to know of the incident

— General health of the child

— Child's previous surgeries and hospitalizations

— Child's significant medical history

— Whether the child previously has been evaluated for this complaint; if so, where

DOCUMENTING NEGLECT

Documentation of neglect involves charting the clues evident from the history and observation of the child. This includes noting aspects of the child's basic needs such as shelter, food, clothing, and medical care. Neglect that stems from a caregiver's lack of knowledge or developmental or psychological deficits still must be documented and reported. It is appropriate to note observations of the child's appearance, physical or developmental concerns, and home environment concerns (Chiocca, 1998). Generally, neglect becomes apparent over time. Therefore, the medical record should contain the history, physical examination, and laboratory and diagnostic information that confirm a pattern of the caregiver failing to meet the child's basic needs.

DOCUMENTING CAREGIVER-CHILD INTERACTIONS

It can be especially important to document the child's demeanor during the history and examination, as well as his or her interactions with the accompanying caregiver. Such data not only indicate to the record reader how the child and caregiver were interacting during the evaluation, but they can also trigger the examiner's memory during testimony. The interactions and relationships between and among the people who are part of the history and physical examination may have bearing on the overall investigation of suspected child abuse and maltreatment (Dubowitz & Bross, 1992). The following are guidelines for information to include in the record when describing particular interactions noted during the assessment either between the caregiver and history taker or the caregiver and child (Dubowitz & Bross, 1992; Marx, 1997):

— Describe actions or questions of the healthcare provider that immediately preceded the behavior/statement.

— Detail demeanor of person making the statement or exhibiting the behavior.

— Include exact words of the person, using quotation marks.

— Describe behavior the child or adult exhibited.

— Note caregiver's concern over, knowledge of, and support for child.

— Note caregiver's indifference or hostility toward child, if applicable.

PHYSICAL FINDINGS

Documentation of the physical examination includes descriptions of the physical findings and specifics of each injury observed and evaluated. The medical chart reflects documentation of any signs of trauma using detailed diagrams, as well as photographic documentation whenever possible. Of course, because of the possibility of civil or criminal court action, all records, drawings, and/or photographs are kept as part of the chart record (AAP, 1999).

In cases of physical abuse, the examiner carefully and legibly records descriptions of each injury. A chart **(Table 9-1)** is helpful for documenting the type, size, shape, color, and age of each injury (Johnson, 1990). Included in the documentation of injuries is an explanation for how the injury occurred as stated by both the child and the caregiver(s). Any incompatibilities between the history of how the injury occurred and its physical manifestations are recorded on the chart. Caregiver inconsistencies regarding how an injury occurred are a major reason for filing a report of abuse to CPS agencies. Detailed information concerning injuries is essential when the examiner must appear in court. (See Appendix: Child Abuse Evaluation Form.)

PHOTOGRAPHIC DOCUMENTATION OF FINDINGS

All traumatic injuries, new and old, should be photographed as an adjunct to written, descriptive documentation. Visual findings are valuable in influencing court proceedings and for peer review and teaching efforts (Ricci, 2001). When second opinions are required, photographs may save the child from the need for reevaluation. Pictures communicate quickly and effectively to all who see them and add credibility to what the patient has stated. Medical providers are usually responsible for determining whether all appropriate areas on the child's body are photodocumented appropriately, even when other professionals such as law enforcement or child

Table 9-1. Chart for Documenting Injuries

Injury Number	Type of Injury	Size	Shape	Object	Color	Observed Age of Injury	Stated Age of Injury	Explanation By: mother, father, child, or other	Is Injury Compatible With History?		
									Yes	No	Uncertain

Reprinted with permission from Johnson CF. Inflicted injury versus accidental injury. Pediatr Clin North Am. 1990;37:809.

protective workers may have taken the photographs (Ricci, 2001). Photographic documentation becomes a permanent part of the medical record and can last indefinitely when stored properly.

There is much discussion about the types of camera equipment that can and should be used to photograph injuries **(Table 9-2)**. Systems vary from more traditional 35-mm fixed-focus or compact cameras to more sophisticated single-lens reflex cameras that offer varied lenses and zoom capability (Ricci, 2001). Less expensive 35-mm integrated lens-flash cameras, as well as self-processing Polaroids, are still used (Finkel & Ricci, 1997). An instant processing Polaroid camera with film that has enhanced color reproduction and resolution exists for medical documentation (Finkel & Ricci, 1997). Polaroid photographs are a good choice because they are tamper proof and do not need to be processed in a laboratory (McCracken, 2000). The best cameras for clear photographic documentation include those that allow control of aperture, shutter speed, and focus. It is wise to consult with people who are familiar with excellent photodocumentation before buying expensive equipment for use in abuse evaluations. Most recently, digital cameras have become available, and their role in photodocumentation in child maltreatment continues to evolve. Initial criticism revolved around the ability to manipulate the images. Therefore, 35-mm photos and slides at present remain the gold standard.

The composition of the photograph should reflect proper arrangement of significant injuries and body part elements to document the patient's condition **(Table 9-3)**. The picture should realistically show injuries without overly exaggerating the trauma (Ricci, 2001). "Before" and "after" pictures are helpful to show the change in condition of the skin and injuries over a stated time frame. Photographs taken before the cleaning of wounds show the original condition of the child, while after shots reveal the child at a different stage. Photographing a bruise from different angles may help to show the amount of bruising or swelling present compared to the natural structures of the body. Such angles provide perspective within the photograph to show the relationship of the bruises to the anatomical structures. Proper perspective helps to accurately depict the full impact of the injuries or bruises (Ricci, 2001).

Photographs remain supplemental to the written record, despite the value of photography. Written descriptions of all injuries or abnormalities must accompany the pictures and must include the location, type, size, and color of the injury. It is appropriate to include descriptive text and hand-drawn diagrams with each photograph because the quality of the photograph cannot be guaranteed (Marx, 1997). The written record should never be in conflict with the photographs taken. Proper documentation of all photographic evidence includes a form with the child's name, case number, and date and time the photographs were taken (Marx, 1997; Ricci & Smistek, 1996). It is helpful to include any outline drawings of the child's body to show the specific photographed areas. A measuring device should be positioned above or below the injury to clearly depict the size of the injury (Ricci, 2001).

It is a challenge to visualize injuries photographically that have not yet bruised or those in which the bruise is clearing (Finkel & Ricci, 1997). Ultraviolet and infrared photography are the best approaches to obtaining visual documentation of such findings. However, the equipment is technologically advanced and expensive, and it requires a level of photographic skill that most people do not have (Finkel & Ricci, 1997).

For photographic documentation of injury to be used as court evidence, the photographs must show proper verification and be relevant to the issue (Myers, 2001). The photographs must accurately portray a complete and fair representation of the

Table 9-2. Advantages and Disadvantages of Types of Cameras Used in Photodocumentation

TYPE OF CAMERA	ADVANTAGES	DISADVANTAGES
Instant processing cameras	Simple operation and low cost	Poor resolution/poor color with 35-mm film
Fixed-focus lens "point-and-shoot" or "compact" 35-mm cameras	Inexpensive and easy to use	Limited close-up capability and expendability Viewfinder does not view the same image as the lens; creates blurred images when the photographer attempts to magnify the image by moving in closer (6-7 feet) than the focusing limit of the lens
Colposcopic cameras	Accurate, standardized equipment for examination or photography of sexual abuse injuries; able to document findings not otherwise seen with the naked eye	Expensive, not portable, and cumbersome to operate; require training usually reserved for health-care providers (i.e., physicians); not equipped for photography of large areas of the body
35-mm format cameras	Provide choice of cameras, lenses, and accessories that offer excellent resolution and close-up capabilities Offer integrated (dedicated) flash that automatically adjusts during photo sessions; compare favorably with and are significantly less expensive than colposcopic cameras for photographing sexually abused children Require little training and offer comfortable operating distance from the subject Provide accurate color balance, automatic exposure, film advance and rewind, built-in flash, and quick flash recharge	Generally no disadvantages

(continued)

Table 9-2. *(continued)*

TYPE OF CAMERA	ADVANTAGES	DISADVANTAGES
"Bridge" cameras	Combine the simplicity and easy use of a point-and-shoot camera with the versatility, expendability, and close-up capability of a 35-mm prepackaged camera system, "bridging the gap" between these 2 kinds of equipment Relatively inexpensive, fully automatic, with telephoto (35-70 mm or 35-105 mm) capability, built-in flash, autofocus, motor drive, and optional databack	Cannot attach specialized lenses or flash units for optional documentation of some injuries (intraoral, intravaginal, ophthalmic)

Reprinted from US Department of Justice. Photodocumentation in the Investigation of Child Abuse. Portable Guides to Investigating Child Abuse. *1996. Available at: http://www.ncjrs.org/html/ojjdp/portable_guides/photodoc/images/tbl_01.gif. Accessed March 12, 2003.*

Table 9-3. Photographing the Injuries

— Photograph all injuries with and without a color/measure standard.

— Label each photograph with the patient's name, medical record number, date and time taken, and name of photographer.

— If close-up photographs are taken, also indicate the location of injury on the patient's body.

— Do not write directly on the back of Polaroid photographs, because this can distort or destroy the image.

— Take follow-up photographs if injuries have not fully developed, usually several hours to days later.

— Do not throw away any photographs in a series, regardless of how well or poorly they develop.

— Make certain the entire injury is viewed in the photograph.

— Respect the patient's modesty by draping any uninvolved breast or genital areas.

— Check photographs before discharging patient.

scene. Verification means that a photographer or medical evaluator can verify that the pictures are an accurate portrayal of the original findings (Myers, 2001). The image must reflect the original abuse findings. It is important that the health professional who examined the child (if other than the photographer) is able to verify during court proceedings that the photographs accurately represent the actual findings of the child's injuries (Finkel & Ricci, 1997; Ricci & Smistek, 1996). Proper verification of photographs is essential so that they can be shown to be relevant to the case; it is also important when reconstructing the case for court purposes. Verification involves keeping meticulous records of photographic data, including date, time, location, case number, camera, lens, aperture, shutter speed, film, light source, subject distance, and macro lens magnification (Ricci, 2001). Also, the record should include documentation that proper chain of custody procedures were followed according to state and local law enforcement procedures (ACEP, 1999). Finally, photographs and negatives should be carefully stored and preserved because proper prosecution may depend on the medical photographs (Marx, 1997).

With regard to obtaining consent for photodocumentation in cases of child abuse, most state laws regarding child abuse evaluations do not require permission from the guardian to photograph the child. It is wise to know the laws of the state in which one practices and in some situations to request consent even if it is not required (Myers, 2001).

USE OF COLPOSCOPE

In cases of child sexual abuse, the colposcope or a fiberoptic scope using light enhancement enables the examiner to visualize anal and genital anatomy to a much greater degree than with the naked eye. The advantage of the colposcope is its ability to photograph the anatomy and findings (Finkel & DeJong, 2001). The colposcope enables the field of vision to be illuminated and magnified, and the examiner may conduct the examination and documentation at the same time (Ricci, 2001). Video cameras attached to colposcopes have advantages over still photography because the examiner can view the scene on a television or computer monitor and achieve greater visibility (Finkel & Ricci, 1997). Use of a video camera also enables the child to view the examination. For some children, being able to view the examination decreases their anxiety because it takes away some of the fear of the unknown (Finkel & Ricci, 1997). When a camera is used to photograph the findings, a 35-mm camera is preferable to a Polaroid (ACEP, 1999).

FORENSIC EVIDENCE COLLECTION

Although most examiners of child maltreatment focus on the medical examination and treatment, the forensic evidence collection component cannot be separated, eliminated, or forgotten. Forensic evidence collection is a component of the complete examination whenever child maltreatment is suspected. Proper documentation of the evidence collected is important to maintain the integrity of the process in the event of legal proceedings. The following are data to be recorded in the medical record (ACEP, 1999):

— Name(s) of the person(s) completing the examination

— Signature and license, credential, and telephone numbers of the examiner(s)

— Description of all evidence sent to the forensic laboratory (see Chapter 5, Laboratory Findings, Diagnostic Testing, and Forensic Specimens in Cases of Child Sexual Abuse)

— Distribution of the evidence, including name of persons accepting the evidence, date, and time

— Name and signature of person who receives the evidence

— Distribution of the medicolegal report; to whom the report has been given

— Name and telephone number of the person to whom the child was discharged

DOCUMENTING CONCLUSIONS, OPINIONS, OR DIAGNOSES FROM THE MEDICAL EVALUATION

Healthcare professionals normally form conclusions from the data gathered during the history, physical examination, and laboratory assessment of a patient. In suspected abuse, it is appropriate to form a conclusion and document whether the physical findings are consistent or inconsistent with a given history (Marx, 1997). The examiner should be as definitive as possible in stating a diagnosis or formulation of opinion (Dubowitz & Bross, 1992). When findings are conclusive for physical abuse, it is acceptable to diagnose child abuse and state that injuries are consistent with a specific situation, such as battered child syndrome. When the findings are not clear, it is acceptable to use terms such as "possible" or "probable" (Dubowitz & Bross, 1992).

In many types of abuse, especially child sexual abuse, few to no physical examination findings support the allegation. In cases of neglect in which physical findings are absent, the best legal approach to documenting conclusions is to give a detailed description of findings for each system so that they can be compared to former or future examinations of the child (Marx, 1997). Most victims of child sexual abuse have nonspecific or normal genital and anogenital findings; thus, it is appropriate to state the conclusions of the history and objective findings in a way that does not negate the possibility that sexual abuse did occur. The following are examples of how to formulate diagnostic assessments in the presence or absence of physical findings (Finkel & DeJong, 2001):

"The history/behavior is descriptive of inappropriate sexual contact; however no diagnostic residual is evident." (p. 256.)

"The history/observations are limited, and although the behaviors observed by the parents have raised concern, there are insufficient historical or behavioral details to support a concern of inappropriate sexual contact." (p. 256.)

It is best to avoid the documentation of assessment findings using statements such as "no evidence of abuse" or "evidence confirms abuse" because they may be used to support an opposite conclusion in legal proceedings (Marx, 1997). Both examples stress the importance of the history in evaluating the child and the findings. One example of documenting normal examination findings but concern for sexual abuse is "the results of the examination were normal but this does not rule out the possibility of sexual abuse" (Dubowitz & Bross, 1992).

When the history and physical examination findings do not support each other, it is appropriate to document that "the examination is inconsistent with the history and an alternative explanation should be sought" (Finkel & DeJong, 2001).

DOCUMENTATION OF THE TREATMENT AND PLAN
The complete plan of treatment and recommendations for follow-up are an important part of the medical record. Careful documentation of the specific healthcare needs of the child, as well as the prognosis, is a useful part of the record. Included are reports to public agencies, such as CPS or police, and recommended consultations (Dubowitz & Bross, 1992).

REPORTING REQUIREMENTS
All states require nurses to report cases of suspected child abuse or neglect. Many also grant immunity from liability when such a report is made in good faith. The healthcare professional can also be held accountable in many states for failure to report. Although it is important to follow institutional policies and procedures, it is equally important to know the reporting requirements of the state in which the nurse works. Of course, state and federal law override institutional policy, and those policies should be in accordance with governmental laws (Sullivan & Mattera, 1997). Therefore, when the examiner makes a report to law enforcement or CPS, the record should reflect why the report was made and to whom the report was given.

Table 9-4. Key Points in Documentation

— Accurate documentation of the history and physical findings in child maltreatment is essential to preserve the evidence.

— Accurate documentation of the child's history and the questions and answers given are critical because the record is a legal document and the data may be admitted as evidence in court trials.

— The examiner documents subjective statements made by the patient, in quotes.

— It can be especially important to describe the demeanor of the child during the history and examination, as well as his or her interactions with the accompanying caregiver.

— In child sexual abuse, the history is a critical component of the evaluation because the physical examination findings are usually within normal limits or nonspecific.

— The information obtained by the presenting adult forms the initial basis for the examination of the child.

— This history should be obtained from the caregiver without the child present whenever possible.

— If the child is developmentally able, the examiner should obtain a history of the incident from the child without the accompanying caregiver.

— Whenever the child asks the examiner to stop, the examiner will stop.

— Allowing for the narrative and slowly approaching more specific questions when the child is having difficulty is appropriate in an effort to ascertain the information needed for a medical evaluation with appropriate evidence collection.

— The chart reflects documentation of any signs of trauma using detailed diagrams illustrating the findings, as well as photographic documentation whenever possible.

— Individual preparation for court usually involves review of the following: the medical record, treatment of the patient, policies and procedures in effect at the time the patient was seen, and the scope and standard of nursing practice.

— No healthcare professional should be willing to testify in a case without meeting with the requesting attorney.

— Remaining professional at all times is the most important component of testifying effectively.

— Forensic evidence collection is a component of the complete examination whenever child maltreatment is suspected.

— Whenever there is doubt as to the acute or chronic nature of the event, evidence collection should occur.

— At all times, the safety of the child should be the utmost concern of the caregiver.

— State and federal law override institutional policy, and those policies should be in accordance with governmental laws.

— It is important to be familiar with the state Nurse Practice Act, know the established standard of practice in one's nursing specialty, and ensure that appropriate policies and procedures are in place at the institution where the nurse practices and evaluates child abuse and neglect.

Adapted from American Nurses Association and the International Association of Forensic Nurses. Scope and Standards of Forensic Nursing Practice. *Washington, DC: American Nurses Association; 1997; American Nurses Association and the Society of Pediatric Nurses.* Statement on the Scope and Standards of Pediatric Clinical Nursing Practice. *Washington, DC: American Nurses Association; 1996.*

COURT TESTIMONY AND DOCUMENTATION

The prospect of testifying in court about a case often elicits stress and concern among healthcare professionals. Testifying can certainly be a stressful experience; however, the witness should always keep in mind that he or she is not expected to be an attorney, judge, or juror, but rather a professional who is asked to tell the truth. There are approaches the nurse can take to lessen the stress of court testimony.

Few attorneys are willing to call a witness for their case without at least one prior conversation with that witness to review what will occur during testimony. By the same token, no healthcare professional should be willing to testify in a case without meeting with the requesting attorney. Preparation is the key to comfort in the courtroom, and meeting with the attorney before testimony is paramount. At a minimum, advanced preparation with the attorney should allow the witness to know whether or not the professional will be testifying as an expert and what the general line of questioning will be.

It is a common and frustrating experience to be called to testify, only to wait for hours because some other situation related to the court process has held up that testimony. To testify in court the healthcare professional often has to clear and rearrange his or her daily schedule to be available for the court time. Furthermore, the compensation given is usually not comparable to the work time missed. Therefore, the nurse called to testify should be aware that the given schedule might change. Concerning documentation, the nurse must review all written documentation of the case and be familiar with the details and conclusions of the examination. Relying on one's memory of a case can be detrimental to the process; it is the witness' responsibility to be clear about the details of the case. Whether expert or fact witness, nervous or calm, remaining professional at all times is the most important component of testifying effectively.

DEPOSITIONS

A deposition is testimony under oath that is recorded for use in court at a later date. The purpose of a deposition is to obtain information that cannot be learned as readily through written records or general investigation. The lawyer for one side orally questions a witness on the opposing side. This testimony allows attorneys involved to find out as much as possible about the case, its strengths and weaknesses, and a witness' credibility.

Depositions take place outside the courtroom; oral testimony is taken under oath, and the proceedings are transcribed. All deposition information is recorded and can be used as official testimony at a later trial. The deposition transcript may be introduced as evidence in court if and when a case proceeds to trial. It is important that the nurse be as prepared for the deposition as she or he is for a factual court case. Preparation first involves talking with the attorney to discuss what the expectations of reviewing the case should be. Then the nurse who is to testify prepares by reviewing the medical record, treatment of the patient, policies and procedures in effect at the time the patient was seen, and scope and standard of nursing practice. Of course, the medical record should not be altered in any way from its original format. (See Chapter 14, Legal Issues, for further discussion.)

CONCLUSION

The implications of an abuse allegation for the child, the child's family, the alleged perpetrator, and the community are profound. The forensic nurse evaluating suspected cases of child maltreatment must make documentation a priority. Its goal is to preserve the valuable information uncovered during the healthcare evaluation for use during the investigation and possible judicial process (**Table 9-4**).

APPENDIX: CHILD ABUSE EVALUATION FORM
CHILDREN'S MEDICAL CENTER OF DALLAS CHILD ABUSE EVALUATION FORM
(Contributed by Benjamin Retta, LMSW; Children's Medical Center of Dallas; Dallas, Tex.)

CAEV
CHILDREN'S MEDICAL CENTER OF DALLAS
1935 Motor Street • Dallas, Texas 75235 • (214) 456-7000
CHILD ABUSE EVALUATION

MED REC NO. _____ ACCT NO. _____
PATIENT _____
DATE _____ LOCATION _____
DOB _____

PART A - MEDICAL REPORT

Sex: ☐ Male ☐ Female Brought by: _____ Relationship: _____
Reason for Evaluation: _____

PLACE OF EXAM	MOST RECENT ALLEGED INCIDENT	EXAMINATION
☐ Reach Clinic	Date: _____	Date: _____
☐ Emergency Center	Time: _____	Time: _____
☐ Inpatient	☐ Check if <72 hours between alleged incident and exam	
☐ Other:		

REFERRING AGENCY	AGENCY PERSONNEL
☐ Dallas Child Protective Services	
☐ Police: City: _____ Case #: _____	Name: _____
☐ Other:	
☐ None	Identification / Badge Number

PART B - AUTHORIZATION

I hereby authorize CMC and Dr. _____ to perform a medical examination for evidence of physical and/or sexual abuse and request medical treatment if indicated. I understand this may include the following:

1. Medical examination of the genital area, which may include pelvic (internal) examination on post pubertal females.
2. Collection of blood, urine, tissues and related specimens as needed.
3. Photographs which may include the genital area for the purpose of documentation.
4. Establishment of a file of information.

I further understand the hospital and physicians are required by law to notify child protection authorities of known or suspected child abuse. All medical reports, including laboratory reports, photographs and forensic results, may be released to Child Protection Services and/or the police department and the District Attorney having jurisdiction, or as otherwise allowed by law.

X_____   X_____
☐ Patient ☐ Parent ☐ Guardian   Date   Agency Representative   Date
X_____
Witness   Date

CMC 64016-003 (589 03/01)   Registration / Consent Page 1 of 6

CAEV
CHILDREN'S MEDICAL CENTER OF DALLAS
1935 Motor Street • Dallas, Texas 75235 • (214) 456-7000
CHILD ABUSE EVALUATION

MED REC NO. _____ ACCT NO. _____
PATIENT _____
DATE _____ LOCATION _____
DOB _____

PART C - SOCIAL INFORMATION

PATIENT (VICTIM)	AGE (years)	SEX (M / F)	RACE
☐ Mother			
☐ Stepmother			
☐ Guardian			
☐ Father			
☐ Stepfather			
☐ Guardian			
Siblings			

Previous involvement of family with child protection authorities? ☐ Yes ☐ No ☐ Unknwon

DATE	TIME	SOCIAL NOTES

Signature: X_____

CMC 64016-003 (589 09/98)   Social Page 2 of 6

CAEV
CHILDREN'S MEDICAL CENTER OF DALLAS
1935 Motor Street • Dallas, Texas 75235 • (214) 456-7000
CHILD ABUSE EVALUATION

MED REC NO. _____ ACCT NO. _____
PATIENT _____
DATE _____ LOCATION _____
DOB _____

PART D - MEDICAL HISTORY
PAST HISTORY

Usual Health Provider: _____
Hospitalization / Surgery / Trauma: _____
Birth / Development: _____
Past Health Problems: _____
Medicines: _____

SEXUAL HISTORY (☐ Check if Not Applicable to Patient)

Hx of voluntary sexual intercourse? . . . ☐ Yes ☐ No
Use of contraception? . . . . ☐ Yes ☐ No
Hx of prior STD? . . . . ☐ Yes ☐ No

FEMALE:
Menarche? . . . . ☐ Yes ☐ No
  Age menses: _____ Date LMP: _____
Use of tampons? . . . . ☐ Yes ☐ No
Hx vaginitis? . . . . ☐ Yes ☐ No
Hx pregnancy(s)? . . . . ☐ Yes ☐ No

BEHAVIOR / EMOTIONAL SYMPTOMS	PHYSICAL SYMPTOMS / HISTORY
Sleep Disturbances . . . . ☐ Yes ☐ No ☐ Unknown	Abdominal / Pelvic Pain . . . . ☐ Yes ☐ No ☐ Unknown
Eating Problems . . . . ☐ Yes ☐ No ☐ Unknown	Vomiting . . . . ☐ Yes ☐ No ☐ Unknown
School Problems . . . . ☐ Yes ☐ No ☐ Unknown	Genital Discomfort or Pain . . . . ☐ Yes ☐ No ☐ Unknown
Sexual Acting Out . . . . ☐ Yes ☐ No ☐ Unknown	Dysuria . . . . ☐ Yes ☐ No ☐ Unknown
Fear . . . . ☐ Yes ☐ No ☐ Unknown	Urinary Tract Infection . . . . ☐ Yes ☐ No ☐ Unknown
Anger . . . . ☐ Yes ☐ No ☐ Unknown	Enuresis . . . . ☐ Yes ☐ No ☐ Unknown
Signs of Depression . . . . ☐ Yes ☐ No ☐ Unknown	Vaginal Itching or Penile Irritation . . . ☐ Yes ☐ No ☐ Unknown
Other Symptoms (Describe): . . ☐ Yes ☐ No ☐ Unknown	Vaginal Discharge or Penile Discharge ☐ Yes ☐ No ☐ Unknown
	Vaginal Bleeding or Penile Bleeding ☐ Yes ☐ No ☐ Unknown
	Rectal Pain . . . . ☐ Yes ☐ No ☐ Unknown
	Rectal Bleeding . . . . ☐ Yes ☐ No ☐ Unknown
	Constipation . . . . ☐ Yes ☐ No ☐ Unknown
	Stool Incontinence . . . . ☐ Yes ☐ No ☐ Unknown

FURTHER HISTORY

CMC 64016-003 (589 09/98)   Medical History Page 3 of 6

CAEV
CHILDREN'S MEDICAL CENTER OF DALLAS
1935 Motor Street • Dallas, Texas 75235 • (214) 456-7000
CHILD ABUSE EVALUATION

MED REC NO. _____ ACCT NO. _____
PATIENT _____
DATE _____ LOCATION _____
DOB _____

PART E - GENERAL PHYSICAL EXAMINATION

Immunizations: _____
Allergies: _____
Pulse _____ /min Respirations _____ /min Temperature: _____ Blood Pressure _____ / _____
Include percentiles of children under age six
Height: _____ %tile Weight: _____ %tile FOC (< age 3): _____ %tile

EXAM	NORMAL	ABNORMAL	COMMENTS
General			
HEENT			
Lungs			
CV			
Abdomen			
GU			
Neurologic			

SKIN

Record any injuries and findings on diagrams: Erythema, Abrasions, Bruises, Contusions, Induration, Lacerations, Fractures, Bites, Burns. Record Size, Appearance and Color of injuries / findings.

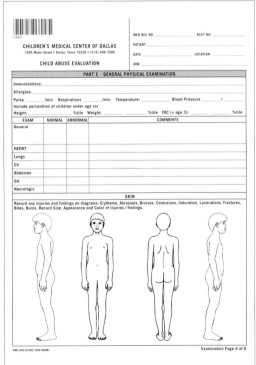

CMC 64016-003 (589 09/98)   Examination Page 4 of 6

Page 5 (top left)

CAEV
CHILDREN'S MEDICAL CENTER OF DALLAS
1935 Motor Street • Dallas, Texas 75235 • (214) 456-7000
CHILD ABUSE EVALUATION

MED REC NO. _____ ACCT NO. _____
PATIENT _____
DATE _____ LOCATION _____
DOB _____

PART F - GENITAL EXAM (Describe all abnormal findings in spaces. Use illustrations when appropriate.)

GENITAL EXAM DONE BY	PATIENT DEMEANOR	TANNER STAGING
❏ Direct visualization only ❏ Colposcopy ❏ Hand held magnifier	❏ Full cooperation ❏ Partial cooperation ❏ Uncooperative ❏ Other	Breast 1 2 3 4 5 N/A Genitals 1 2 3 4 5

GENITAL (Female / Male)

SKIN FINDINGS:
Thighs . . . . ❏ Normal ❏ Abnormal
Perineum . . . . . ❏ Normal ❏ Abnormal
Buttocks . . . . . . ❏ Normal ❏ Abnormal

OTHER:
Genital Warts . . . . . ❏ Yes ❏ No
Other abnormalities . . ❏ Yes ❏ No
If yes, explain: _____

ANAL EXAM (Female / Male)

Exam position used: ❏ Supine ❏ Prone ❏ Lateral ❏ Knee-chest

EXTERNAL FINDINGS:
Perianal Skin . . . . ❏ Normal ❏ Abnormal
Anal verge / folds / rugae . . . . . . ❏ Normal ❏ Abnormal

ANAL TONE:
Anal spasm . . . . ❏ Yes ❏ No
Anal laxity . . . . ❏ Yes ❏ No
Anal dilation > 20 mm . . . . ❏ Yes ❏ No
If yes, stool present? . . . . ❏ Yes ❏ No
Anal wink . . . . ❏ Yes ❏ No
Assessment of tone as normal . . . ❏ Yes ❏ No
Exam method for anal tone: ❏ Observation ❏ Digital exam

GENITAL - FEMALE

(Draw shape of hymen; note any lesions)

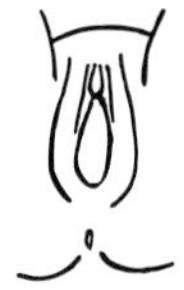

Exam position used: ❏ Supine ❏ Knee-chest ❏ Both
Labia majora . . . . ❏ Normal ❏ Abnormal
Clitoris . . . . ❏ Normal ❏ Abnormal
Labia minora . . . . ❏ Normal ❏ Abnormal
Periurethral tissue / urethral meatus . ❏ Normal ❏ Abnormal
Hymen . . . . ❏ Normal ❏ Abnormal
Describe:

Orifice measurement: Vertical _____ mm
Horizontal _____ mm
How measured: ❏ Visual ❏ Other: _____
Vagina . . . . ❏ Normal ❏ Abnormal
Fossa Navicularis . . . . ❏ Normal ❏ Abnormal
Posterior Fourchette
Other abnormalities:
Discharge? ❏ Yes ❏ No If yes, describe: _____
Pelvic exam done ❏ Yes ❏ No

GENITAL - MALE

(Draw any lesions)

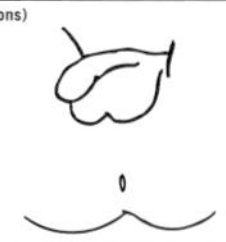

Penis . . . . ❏ Normal ❏ Abnormal
Circumcised . . . . ❏ Yes ❏ No
Urethral meatus . . . . ❏ Normal ❏ Abnormal
Urethral discharge . . . . ❏ Yes ❏ No
If yes, describe:
Scrotum . . . . ❏ Normal ❏ Abnormal
Testes . . . . ❏ Normal ❏ Abnormal
Other . . . . ❏ Normal ❏ Abnormal

CMC 64016-003 (S89 09/98)

Examination Page 5 of 6

Page 6 (top right)

CAEV
CHILDREN'S MEDICAL CENTER OF DALLAS
1935 Motor Street • Dallas, Texas 75235 • (214) 456-7000
CHILD ABUSE EVALUATION

MED REC NO. _____ ACCT NO. _____
PATIENT _____
DATE _____ LOCATION _____
DOB _____

PART G - EVALUATION

❏ **PHYSICIAN NOTES** (Check if history of acute event(s) recorded by physician and filed in REACH office)
❏ **FORENSIC COLLECTION** (Check if samples collected for forensic evaluation; complete Forensic form)
❏ **LABORATORY COLLECTION** (Check if samples collected. Document results when available)

GC CULTURES:	CHLAMYDIA CULTURE:		
❏ Cervical / Vaginal	❏ Cervical / Vaginal	❏ Urinalysis	❏ VDRL
❏ Urethral	❏ Urethral	❏ Urine Culture	❏ Hep B
❏ Rectal	❏ Rectal	❏ KOH prep	❏ HIV (Consent)
❏ Oral		❏ Wet mount	❏ CBC
			❏ PT / PTT

❏ Pregnancy: ❏ Urine ❏ Blood
❏ Other: _____

❏ X-RAYS: ❏ Skeletal Survey ❏ Other: _____
Preliminary Results: _____

PART H - IMPRESSIONS FROM EXAM (All positive findings should be further described in non-medical terms)

❏ No physical findings suggestive of abuse at this time. A normal genital exam does not rule out sexual abuse.
❏ Nonspecific findings: Could be consistent with physical abuse or sexual abuse, but also seen in non-abused children.
❏ Specific physical findings consistent with physical abuse or sexual abuse.

X _____
Physician Signature   Printed last name of physician

_____

Other Medical Diagnoses: _____
Agencies Notified: ❏ Child Protective Service ❏ Law Enforcement ❏ Other: _____

PART I - TREATMENT AND FOLLOW UP

PRESCRIBED TREATMENTS	MEDICAL FOLLOW UP	NOTARIZATION
	❏ Hospitalization ❏ F/U Appointment (REACH Office 640-6134) ❏ Return to primary care system ❏ Other:	*(Optional, only if requested)* I have personal knowledge of the above and I swear it is true and just. Affiant Date Notary Public in and for the State of Texas

CMC 64016-003 (S89 9/98)

Summary Page 6 of 6

Addendum - Forensic Evaluation (bottom left)

CAEV
CHILDREN'S MEDICAL CENTER OF DALLAS
1935 Motor Street • Dallas, Texas 75235 • (214) 456-7000
CHILD ABUSE EVALUATION

MED REC NO. _____ ACCT NO. _____
PATIENT _____
DATE _____ LOCATION _____
DOB _____

Forensic Evaluation For use by Southwestern Institute of Forensic Sciences if alleged assault <72 hours and if forensic specimen obtained. Not part of medical record of patient.

Estimate number of hours since incident: _____

History of Ejaculate? (circle one): YES   Probable/Possible   NO   UNK

Condom used? (circle one): YES   NO

Since the assault has the patient:
Wiped / washed off   YES   NO   UNK
Bathed / showered   YES   NO   UNK
Urinated   YES   NO   UNK
Defecated   YES   NO   UNK
Rinsed mouth / brushed teeth   YES   NO   UNK
Eaten / drank   YES   NO   UNK
Changed clothes   YES   NO   UNK

Evidentiary Collection

Specimen Collected?	Step	Evidence to Crime Lab	Taken by (signature or name)
YES NO	4	Outer clothing	
YES NO	5	Underwear	
YES NO	6	Debris (mark source on drawing) ❏ Fingernail scraping ❏ Blood on body ❏ Dried secretions on body ❏ Dirt ❏ Other (fibers, hair, etc.)	
YES NO	8	Pubic hair combings	
YES NO	9	Cut pubic hair	
YES NO	10	Known blood sample on patient (optional)	
YES NO	11	Pelvic swabs and smears	
YES NO	12	Vaginal swabs and smears	
YES NO	13	Sperm motility (optional on children)	
		OPTIONAL	
YES NO	15a	Oral rinse	
YES NO	15b	Rectal smears	

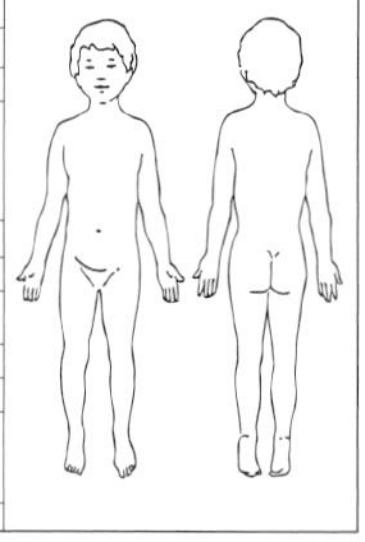

I certify that this is a true and correct record concerning examination of the patient _____ (name)
The completed sexual assault kit was placed in the evidence lock box on _____ at _____ am-pm.

Nurse present during examination _____ Date _____
Examiner's signature _____ Date _____
Examiner's name (printed) _____

CMC 64016-003 (5/99)

Addendum - Forensic Evaluation

Addendum - Physical Notes (bottom right)

CAEV
CHILDREN'S MEDICAL CENTER OF DALLAS
1935 Motor Street • Dallas, Texas 75235 • (214) 456-7000
CHILD ABUSE EVALUATION

MED REC NO. _____ ACCT NO. _____
PATIENT _____
DATE _____ LOCATION _____
DOB _____

Physician Notes For use by Physician to document history of alleged acute abuse event for legal purpose. NOT PART OF MEDICAL RECORD of patient.

Name of person providing history _____ Relationship _____

History or description of event(s) by historian (if person is different than patient)	History or description of event(s) in child's own words

Summary of History

Alleged perpetrator (a.p.) _____ Relationship _____
Location of events _____ Is a.p. in frequent contact w/victim at this time? _____
Number or events: ❏ Once ❏ Est. number _____ ❏ Multiple, but unknown ❏ UNK

If history includes events of alleged sexual abuse, continue (circle all applicable)

Primary alleged activity?	Penetration of orifice	Oral copulation	Touch/rub	Kiss/lick	Unk	Other
Primary area on child involved?	Genitalia/perineum	Anus	Mouth	Breast	Unk	Other
Primary object used by perpetrator(s)?	Finger(s)	Penis	Mouth	Object	Unk	Other

Clothes removed?   YES   NO   UNK   if yes, ❏ from patient ❏ from perpetrator(s)
History of ejaculate?   YES   NO   UNK   if yes, ❏ inside body orifice ❏ outside body orifice? Location _____
Use of surface agent?   YES   NO   UNK   if yes, ❏ lubricant ❏ foam ❏ condom ❏ other _____
Force used on patient?   YES   NO   UNK
Drugs / alcohol use at time of alleged event(s)? YES NO UNK   if yes, ❏ by patient ❏ by perpetrator
Photographs taken of patient during acts? YES NO UNK

Physician signature _____ Date _____

CMC 64016-003 (5/99)

Addendum - Physical Notes

REFERENCES

American Academy of Pediatrics, Committee on Child Abuse and Neglect and Committee on Community Health Services. Investigation and review of unexpected infant and child deaths. *Pediatrics.* 1999;104:1158-1160.

American College of Emergency Physicians. *Evaluation and Management of the Sexually Assaulted or Sexually Abused Patient.* Dallas, Tex: US Dept of Health & Human Services; 1999.

American Nurses Association and the International Association of Forensic Nurses. *Scope and Standards of Forensic Nursing Practice.* Washington, DC: American Nurses Association; 1997.

American Nurses Association and the Society of Pediatric Nurses. *Statement on the Scope and Standards of Pediatric Clinical Nursing Practice.* Washington, DC: American Nurses Association; 1996.

Barnes M. Child abuse histories: what you need to know. *Patient Care for the Nurse Practitioner.* 2001;4:17-18, 21, 25-27.

Bar-on ME, Zanga JR. Child abuse: a model for the use of structured clinical forms. *Pediatrics.* 1996;98(3 Pt 1):429-433.

Cheung K. Identifying and documenting findings of physical child abuse and neglect. *J Pediatr Health Care.* 1999;13:142-143.

Chiocca EM. Documenting suspected child abuse, Part II. *Nursing.* 1998;28:25.

Dubowitz H, Bross DC. The pediatrician's documentation of child maltreatment. *Am J Dis Child.* 1992;146:596-599.

Faller KC. *Evaluating Children Suspected of Having Been Sexually Abused: The APSAC Study Guides 2.* Thousand Oaks, Calif: Sage Publications; 1996.

Finkel M, DeJong A. Medical findings in child sexual abuse. In: Reece R, Ludwig S, eds. *Child Abuse: Medical Diagnosis and Management.* 2nd ed. Philadelphia, Pa: Lippincott Williams & Wilkins; 2001:207-286.

Finkel M, Ricci L. Documentation and preservation of visual evidence in child abuse. *Child Maltreat.* 1997;2:322-330.

Giardino A, Christian C, Giardino E. *A Practical Guide to the Evaluation of Child Physical Abuse and Neglect.* Thousand Oaks, Calif: Sage Publications; 1997.

Heger A, Emans SJ, Muram D. *Evaluation of the Sexually Abused Child: A Medical Textbook and Photographic Atlas.* Oxford, NY: Oxford University Press; 2000.

Jenny C. *Medical Evaluation of Physically and Sexually Abused Children: The APSAC Study Guides 3.* Thousand Oaks, Calif: Sage Publications; 1996.

Johnson CF. Inflicted injury versus accidental injury. *Pediatr Clin North Am.* 1990;37:809.

Lahoti SL, McClain N, Girardet R, McNeese M, Cheung K. Evaluating the child for sexual abuse. *Am Fam Physician.* 2001;63:883-892.

Ledray LE. SANE development guide. *J Emerg Nurs.* 1999;24:197-198.

Limbos MA, Berkowitz CD. Documentation of child physical abuse: how far have we come? *Pediatrics.* 1998;102(1 Pt 1):53-58.

Marx S. Legal issues and documentation. In: Giardino A, Christian C, Giardino E, eds. *A Practical Guide to the Evaluation of Child Abuse and Neglect.* Thousand Oaks, Calif: Sage Publications; 1997:247-273.

McCracken L. Photodocumentation of victim injury. *On the Edge.* 2000;6:5.

Monteleone J, Brodeur A. *Child Maltreatment: A Clinical Guide and Reference.* 2nd ed. St. Louis, Mo: GW Medical Publishing; 1998.

Myers J. Expert testimony. In: Briere J, Berliner L, Bulkley J, Jenny C, Reid T, eds. *The APSAC Handbook on Child Maltreatment.* Thousand Oaks, Calif: Sage Publications; 1996:319-340.

Myers J. Medicolegal aspects of child abuse. In: Reece R, Ludwig S, eds. *Child Abuse: Medical Diagnosis and Management.* Philadelphia, Pa: Lippincott Williams & Wilkins; 2001:545-562.

Parra JM, Huston RL, Foulds DM. Resident documentation of diagnostic impression in sexual abuse evaluations. *Clin Pediatr (Phila).* 1997;36:691-694.

Pence D, Wilson C. *Team Investigation of Child Sexual Abuse: The Uneasy Alliance.* Thousand Oaks, Calif: Sage Publications; 1994.

Pence D, Wilson C, Broadhurst D. *The Role of Law Enforcement in the Response to Child Abuse and Neglect.* Washington, DC: US Dept of Health & Human Services, National Center on Child Abuse and Neglect; 1992.

Poyer K. *Child Victims and Witnesses Interviewing and Investigating.* Washington, DC: US Attorney's Office; 1997.

Ricci L. Photodocumentation of the abused child. In: Reece R, Ludwig S, eds. *Child Abuse: Medical Diagnosis and Management.* 2nd ed. Philadelphia, Pa: Lippincott Williams & Wilkins; 2001:385-404.

Ricci LR, Smistek BS. Photodocumentation in the investigation of child abuse. *Portable Guides to Investigating Child Abuse.* Washington, DC: Office of Juvenile Justice and Delinquency Prevention; 1996.

Socolar RR, Champion M, Green C. Physicians' documentation of sexual abuse of children. *Arch Pediatr Adolesc Med.* 1996;150:191-196.

Sorenson E, Bottoms B, Perona A. *Handbook on Intake and Forensic Interviewing in the Children's Advocacy Center Setting.* Washington, DC: US Dept of Justice; 1997.

Sullivan GH, Mattera M. *RN's Legally Speaking: How to Protect Your Patients and Your License.* Montvale, NJ: Medical Economics; 1997.

US Department of Justice. *Photodocumentation in the Investigation of Child Abuse. Portable Guides to Investigating Child Abuse.* 1996. Available at: http://www.ncjrs.org/html/ojjdp/portable_guides/photodoc/images/tbl_01.gif. Accessed March 12, 2003.

Chapter 10

MENTAL HEALTH ASPECTS OF CHILD SURVIVORS OF ABUSE AND NEGLECT

Paul T. Clements, PhD, APRN-BC, DF-IAFN
Kathleen M. Benasutti, MCAT, ATR-BC, LPC

On any given day, people are able to pick up a newspaper or turn on a television set and hear yet another report of a battered or otherwise abused or neglected child. One of the greatest challenges for child survivors of abuse, their families, and their healthcare providers is grappling with the perception of the abused child as "damaged goods" (Oldham & Riba, 1994; US Department of Health & Human Services [USDHHS], 2003). Because survivors of child abuse must learn to cope with the issues of growth and development within an altered context, they can have role confusion and problems determining what are typical developmental tasks encountered by most children and what are additional threats to their integrity. Indeed, they may embrace the concept of being damaged goods and believe that they can never be "like other kids" (Diaz, Simantov, & Rickert, 2002).

Although significant advances have occurred in identifying and treating child abuse, professional providers are still attempting to grasp the extent of the psychological impact of child maltreatment. One of the largest issues confronting healthcare providers in addressing the psychological impact of child abuse and maltreatment is consistent identification, terminology, and definition (Benasutti, 1993; Flaherty, Sege, Mattson, & Binns, 2002; Hinds & Baskin, 2002; Ludwig, 1992; USDHHS, 2003). Historically, a fine line has been drawn between appropriate physical punishment and abuse. Typically, spanking a child with a hand has not been defined to be abusive, and whipping a child with a belt or rope may also be viewed as parental discipline. However, the same action that leaves marks on bare skin might be legally prosecuted as child abuse in some jurisdictions. This variation in definitions spanning the decades makes the definition, treatment, and intervention of child abuse a complicated issue.

Ludwig (1992) attempted to define the complexity of the concept of child abuse, categorizing it into legal, institutional, and personal definitions. He offered the definitions listed in **Table 10-1**.

Child abuse, regardless of the actual mechanism, is typically a result of either inappropriate use of power and control over a child, typically driven by anger from various issues and dynamics, or insufficient and ineffective parenting stemming from poor parenting skills or lack of commitment to parenting and ensuring the well-being of the child (Dosomething.org, 2003; Finkelhor, 1979; Gordon, Gordon, & Cohen, 1992; Hartley, 2002; Malchiodi, 1990). Inherently, it is against all social expectations to injure a child purposefully, which suggests that the dynamics that lead to abusive

Table 10-1. Definitions of Child Abuse		
DEFINITION OF ABUSE	OVERVIEW	INDICATORS
Legal	Serious bodily injury creates a substantial risk of death or causes serious permanent disfigurement or protracted loss or impairment of the function of a body organ.	Causes the child severe pain, significantly impairs the child's physical functioning (whether temporarily or permanently), and is accompanied by physical evidence of a continuous pattern of separate, unexplained injuries to the child.
Sexual	Defined as any of the following when committed on a child by a perpetrator.	1. *Statutory rape:* sexual intercourse with a child who is less than age 14 years by a person age 18 years or older. 2. *Involuntary or voluntary deviate sexual intercourse:* intercourse by mouth, by rectum, or with an animal. 3. *Sexual assault:* sexual involvement, including the touching or exposing of sexual or other intimate parts of a person for the purpose of arousing or gratifying sexual desire in either the perpetrator or the subject child. 4. *Incest:* sexual intercourse with an ancestor or descendent by blood or adoption. 5. *Promoting prostitution:* inducing or encouraging a child to engage in prostitution. 6. *Rape:* sexual intercourse by force or by compulsion. 7. *Pornography:* Includes the obscene photographing, filming, or depiction of children for commercial purposes or for arousal of self, subject child, or viewing audience.
Neglect	Serious physical neglect.	A physical condition caused by the acts or omissions of a perpetrator that endanger the child's life or development or impair physical functioning. Serious physical neglect is the result of prolonged or repeated lack of supervision or failure to provide essentials of life, including adequate medical care.

(continued)

Table 10-1. *(continued)*

Definition of Abuse	Overview	Indicators
Emotional/ psychological	Serious mental injury is a psychological condition diagnosed by a physician or licensed psychologist.	Caused by the acts or omissions—including the refusal of appropriate treatment—of the perpetrator that: 1. Render the child chronologically and severely anxious, agitated, depressed, socially withdrawn, psychotic, or in reasonable fear that his or her life or safety are threatened. OR 2. Seriously interfere with the child's ability to accomplish age-appropriate developmental and social tasks.
Institutional	Beyond legal definitions, clinicians are also subject to institutional or operational definitions. Although all institutions are bound to state laws, the practical interpretation of that legality may vary among institutions.	These definitions are determined by institutional policy or procedure. This may include community policies regarding the procedure for reporting suspected and actual child abuse. What one institution may determine to be abuse may not be defined as such by another institution.
Personal	The definitions for abuse, especially determining when to file a report, may have varying levels of individual and acceptable parental behaviors.	Definitions may vary based on family background, child-rearing history, socioeconomic status, religious background, racial background, cultural beliefs, the surrounding environment, and other subjective factors.

Adapted from Ludwig S. Defining child abuse: clinical mandate—evolving concepts. In: Ludwig S, Kornberg AE, eds. Child Abuse: A Medical Reference. 2nd ed. New York, NY: Churchill Livingstone; 1992:1-12.

situations are powerful enough to make the perpetrator override and disregard social and moral safeguards that are set forth to avoid such situations, whether via the commission of violence or omission of sufficient care. This chapter explores the dynamics that may potentially result in child abuse. It provides a theoretical framework for understanding the cycle of violence and describes select indicators that will guide nurses during client interviews to screen for potentially abusive situations and the need for additional mental health assessment and referral.

HISTORICAL PERCEPTIONS

Just the word "child" can evoke strong emotional responses. These might include an instantaneous smile at the innocence and joy associated with childhood, or there may be fond memories of one's own childhood days. There may even be laughter at the funny things that children sometimes say and do as they work their way toward understanding and exerting social appropriateness. Parents, probably more than anyone, can easily connect with these strong associations.

It is a seemingly worldwide normative expectation that parents are in the best position to provide for the welfare and well-being of their children as they navigate through the growth and development process. It is a commonly held belief that parents have an obligation to raise their children until they reach adulthood. Included in this responsibility is the use of discipline as a method of instilling morals, understanding right and wrong, making appropriate choices, and developing a sense of self, family, and community.

Although discipline is an expected facet of raising children and although this discipline may include a parental belief that physical punishment is required to reinforce certain tenets of emotional and behavioral discipline, most parents do not purposefully intend to inflict permanent injury on their children. Commonly, when parents overexert the basic tenets of effective child discipline, abusive situations arise. According to the American Academy of Pediatrics Policy Statement (Stein & Perrin, 1998):

An effective discipline system must contain three vital elements: 1) a learning environment characterized by positive, supportive parent-child relationships; 2) a strategy of systematic teaching and strengthening of desired behaviors (proactive); and 3) a strategy for decreasing or eliminating undesired or ineffective behaviors (reactive). Each of these components needs to be functioning adequately to result in improved child behavior. (p. 723.)

Although incidents of child abuse and neglect can frequently be found in today's literature and media, child abuse is not a new phenomenon. For population control, as well as the elimination of children with birth defects, many societies, past and present, have practiced infanticide (Lagaipa, 1990; Radbill, 1987). Abandonment, smothering, and drowning were common forms of terminating children's lives. Moreover, spiritual and political factors motivated the abuse and elimination of certain children. Some societies continue to engage in certain forms of abuse, such as tattooing, genital mutilation, exaggeration of certain body parts, or piercing of body parts with sharp objects. These forms of abuse continue to be debated worldwide in terms of perpetuating and upholding religious and cultural heritage versus purposeful infliction of pain and suffering on children (Annas, 1996; Lagaipa, 1990; Milner, 1998; Toubia, 1994).

American society struggles with the parental rights and control of children versus the rights of the child, especially in regard to seemingly abusive practices. As a healthcare society, there have been significant efforts to make unilateral definitions of abuse: physical, sexual, emotional, and neglect. At times, however, in light of the strong respect for family rights and a stance of cautious noninterference, it is conceivable that many children suffer the consequences of abuse on a regular basis and receive little or no treatment because they "do not tell" or their clues are overlooked or ruled away during assessment (Asher, 2003).

STEREOTYPICAL BELIEFS

Even with all of the advances in nursing education and treatment surrounding child abuse, it is imperative for nurses to confront their own perceptions and beliefs about abuse because these may ultimately have an impact upon the level of care provided to abused and neglected children. There are many myths and stereotypes regarding child abuse that must be challenged, explored, and understood by nurses who are in a position to uncover abuse and provide effective care to abused children. **Table 10-2** lists some common myths.

PERCEPTIONS OF CHILD ABUSE

SOCIAL PERCEPTIONS

Multifaceted and complex issues arise in survivors of child abuse; each of these issues is seemingly monumental and ominous. Issues typical of child survivors are an impaired ability to trust, blurred role boundary and role confusion, and pseudomaturity coupled with failure to accomplish developmental tasks, self-mastery, and control. These issues may vary depending on whether the child represses the abuse, there is immediate intervention and therapy after abuse or an assault, or the therapy continues as mediated by existing support systems and understanding (Burgess, Hartman & Clements, 1995b; Gil, 1991). It is critical to understand that all victims of child abuse and neglect will benefit from having a clinician focus on these issues during assessment and treatment. Additionally, clinicians must protect against the "throwaway child syndrome," which leads to the belief that some children are so "damaged" they cannot be helped. Competent clinicians must be in touch with their own issues and perceptions in order to provide compassion and understanding regarding the nature of abuse. They can also provide a neutral, yet supportive environment that will start the process of undoing self-blame by the child and avoiding perception of the child as damaged goods. All survivors require and deserve treatment and the opportunity to heal emotionally and physically.

It is important to diminish the child's anxiety and engender trust as a first step in the treatment process (Burgess et al., 1995b; Burgess, Holmstrom, & McCausland, 1978; Clements, Benasutti, & Henry, 2001). The abused child should sense the clinician's belief that there is a sense for future orientation and hope for a "normal" life. In addition, the clinician can encourage and guide the child to communicate feelings because the child may be hesitant to express those feelings of fear and loss by virtue of age and position within the family (Clements, 2001a). Without these basic tenets, the therapeutic relationship is immediately in jeopardy, and all attempts at assessment and intervention are at risk for failure.

Mental Health Principles to Keep in Mind During the Abuse Evaluation

Points to Remember During History Taking

Mental health aspects of the healthcare evaluation of child maltreatment begin with the actual healthcare encounter and may be viewed parallel to the medical and physical healthcare aspects. The following discussion highlights several areas the nurse should consider during the healthcare evaluation.

The abused or neglected child is often in a position of significant inequity of control. Someone (typically a "grown-up") has exerted his or her power and control to the disadvantage of the child. Additionally, the child has probably been told that he or she can never tell anyone about what is happening or else something more terrible will occur. It is important to use the knowledge of this inequity of control as a guide for clinical assessment. The supportive environment of the history and physical examination or other clinical assessment can provide a conduit for children to reveal abuse and to seek an anchor for safety (Burgess et al., 1995b; Clements et al., 2001). It is also critical to remember that information gleaned from the assessment may be used to prosecute an alleged abuser. This means that the techniques used to gain the most accurate and reliable information, as well as detailed documentation, may be among the most important things the professional nurse can do for the child. The suggestions in **Table 10-3** can enhance the assessment interview and maximize the potential for gaining pertinent data from a suspected victim of child abuse.

Table 10-2. Myths and Realities About Child Abuse

MYTH	REALITY
Child abuse is a recent phenomenon that, as evident in the media, has occurred much more often in the past 10 years.	Child abuse has occurred at all points in the historical continuum. The difference in this past decade has been an increase in reporting, education, and understanding, not necessarily an increase in abuse. Historically, victims do not report for fear of being disbelieved, fear of threats (to hurt or kill someone they love if they "tell"), or fear of physical reprisal by the perpetrator.
Child abuse typically occurs with strangers.	Various people can abuse children. Whoever has repeated access to a child can be a potential perpetrator. Adult perpetrators may include parents, neighbors, babysitters, schoolteachers, bus drivers, or strangers at a playground. Typically, physical abuse, sexual abuse, emotional abuse, and neglect occur by persons in a "caregiving" role. If the perpetrator is a stranger, it is a criminal assault. Children and adolescents can also be perpetrators, including older children or even same-age peers. Much to the surprise of many professionals, the abuser may even be a businessman, clergy person, school teacher, or healthcare professional, which adds to the difficulty of assessment and treatment of child victims who face disbelief and fear of "false accusation" by care providers that any abuse could have occurred from such an "upstanding member of society" (Allen, 2000; Bagley & King, 1990; Melton, 1994).
Child abuse happens in unusual places.	Children are abused in obvious places. Although there are attempts to maintain secrecy of the abuse, the abuse itself typically occurs in a place where the child commonly is (Barnard, 1989; Henry, 1999; Jenkins, 1998). Although this seems counterintuitive, most parents or other caregiving adults would have their suspicions aroused or become fearful if the child is not where he or she is supposed to be, which, in turn, would potentiate the likelihood of discovering the perpetrator in the act of abuse. Because this is exactly what the perpetrator does not want to happen, he or she will make attempts to merge the abuse into the child's typical environment or schedule, thereby promoting an illusion of normalcy and decreasing the chance of discovery. This situation is typically compounded by secrecy imposed on the child by the perpetrator, with threats of reprisal or harm if the child reveals the abuse.
Some children behave in such a way that they provoke child abuse.	Any type of abuse is the sole responsibility of the perpetrator. Children do not ask for abuse, and they do not "deserve" abuse (Bagley & King, 1990; Helfer, 1984, 1987; Meier, 1985; Rasmussen, 1999).

(continued)

Table 10-2. *(continued)*

MYTH	REALITY
Perpetrators of child abuse are mentally ill or have fantasies about hurting children.	There is no "typical" child abuser. Most are "ordinary" people who come from all economic, ethnic, and social groups. The presence of a mental health disorder is not a prerequisite for abuse. Actually, child abuse is a very complex and organized system of behaviors and secrecy that may make it difficult for mentally ill people to proceed without detection (Burgess, Hartman, & Baker, 1995a; Burgess et al., 1995b; Butler-Smith, 1985; Elliot & Briere, 1994; Sherkow, 1990). There is, however, a small segment of sexual predators who are classifiable as mentally ill; however, their behaviors typically result in more significant damage or death to the child, including any combination of sexual, physical, or emotional abuse of a severe nature (Salter, 1988, 1995, 1998).
Most victims of child abuse are female.	Although the majority of reported cases of abuse are female, this may be a result of the social barometer that projects an ongoing stigma for males who fear shame and questions regarding their masculinity if the secret is revealed (Bagley & King, 1990; Groth & Loredo, 1981; Singer, 2003; Watkins & Bentovim, 1992).
Children with emotional or physical challenges or deformities are not typically targets of abuse.	Statistical data may still reflect a significant level of under-reporting of children with developmental, physical, or emotional disability. These children may be unaware that the abuse is wrong, unable to communicate the abuse, or fearful for their own safety because they are already in an ongoing position of dependence for their safety and security needs (Ammerman, 1992, 1997; Ammerman & Baladerian, 1993; Mitchell & Buchele-Ash, 2000; Tomison, 1996).
It cannot be considered abuse if a child consents to sexual intercourse, or if the child says he or she deserves to be beaten because of being bad.	First and foremost, a child cannot consent to any sexual acts, because this contradicts the "age of consent" laws in the United States (Protection of Children From Sexual Predators Act, 1998). This is compounded by the fact that children, although experiencing sexual urges and drives, do not possess the emotional and cognitive tools to encompass the dynamics involved in sexual relationships with others. Physical abuse, such as beating, is never acceptable or justified. Children may truly believe and may say that the beating was "deserved." However, such a statement is a significant warning sign that the child has now embraced the position of inequity and, as a result, may even purposefully provoke additional abusive episodes (Johnson, 1987).

Points to Remember During Physical Evaluation
A certain level of discomfort may arise during the assessment of a child who has been abused. There may be hesitation to provide a thorough physical assessment for fear of creating additional stress and trauma. This becomes more readily evident during assessment of the child who has been sexually abused. However, a thorough assessment, performed in a matter-of-fact, nonreactive manner can assess the level of physical trauma related to the abuse, check for additional physiological and psychological issues that require intervention, and promote the therapeutic

Table 10-3. Dos and Don'ts for the Assessment Interview

Dos	Don'ts
Get out from behind the desk.	Stay behind the desk in the adult "power position."
Get down to the child's physical level.	Act as if this situation has ruined the child's chances for a normal life.
Be casual and matter of fact. Talk about other things first that are developmentally appropriate (e.g., school, friends, hobbies).	Use clinical terminology that might cause confusion and create a sense of anxiety in the child. Remember, children often want to "please" the therapist or provider and may provide answers that are seemingly "positive" or "okay."
Play, laugh, and create an age-appropriate environment.	Act as if the child is "damaged," "sick," or "different."
Treat the child as you would any child in any healthcare setting.	Jump to the conclusion that the child hates the perpetrator.
Treat the subject with a matter-of-fact approach. Maintain a calm and steady stream of tone and conversation. Take a break if needed.	React negatively to the words or subject matter. Do be aware of your body language since children are just as savvy at interpreting what is not said.
Take the lead in asking questions (but avoid "leading" questions). Obtain as much detail as the child is willing to provide.	Neglect or disregard the interviews of the entire family. Collateral interviews can provide unique perspectives for the assessment.
Assure the child that this is not his or her fault.	Give up if there is some initial resistance and become angry if the child "tests" your limits or tries to "push your buttons."
Believe what the child tells you even when seemingly inconsistent. Remember, children perceive the world differently than adults based on their repertoire of life experience.	Ever doubt a small child who tells you he or she has been abused.

Adapted from Butler-Smith S. Children's Story: Sexually Molested Children in Criminal Court. Walnut Creek, Calif: Launch Press; 1985.

relationship while building the child's self-esteem. Abused children always benefit from a healthcare provider who communicates concern and respect for the child's rights as an individual.

Children watch adults for behavioral and verbal cues to self-assess the seriousness of the situation. The assessment must be completed without a charged affective environment and the attitude must be one of future orientation and attainment of eventual healing. This is best accomplished by nurses maintaining a neutral but supportive stance during their conversation, reinforcing that the child can indeed live a "normal" life, and discussing age-appropriate behaviors and activities as part of their interaction.

DEVELOPMENTAL LEVEL

Children change rapidly during their 18 years of development, so the healthcare provider should assess and intervene at a level that matches the child's cognitive and emotional abilities. Communication with and education of the child should be geared toward instilling skills and tools for self-preservation, self-esteem, and communication. Approaches to this interaction vary greatly across the childhood developmental continuum including, for example, play for younger children and groups or journaling for adolescents. Children should identify activities that they enjoy and that the healthcare provider believes are conduits toward building self-esteem, safety, and communication. Healthcare providers should also educate children regarding the need to avoid maladaptive methods of coping, such as fighting, sibling violence, cigarettes, drugs, or alcohol, and instruct them to seek out adult guidance and support when impulses toward these behaviors arise.

FAMILY STRUCTURE

Exploring dynamics that may increase the likelihood for abusive situations is imperative because all children are inherently members of a larger family system. When assessing the family system, the perception of a child as being intrinsically problematic, "special," or "different" from other children or siblings is often seen in abuse and neglect situations. This may be because of a caregiver's negative attitude toward the child or inadequate knowledge of child development, which encourages unrealistic expectations of behavioral, emotional, and psychological needs (Hunka, O'Toole, & O'Toole, 1985). Additionally, parents may experience intense difficulty with unconditional acceptance of a child who may have been of low birth weight, premature, handicapped, or illegitimate.

Most parents do not intend to abuse their child, yet abuse is a typical cycle that reflects a counterintuitive situation wherein positive behaviors are not useful in meeting the child's emotional needs, resulting in provocative behavior and the risk of painful contact being chosen by the abused child as opposed to feeling ignored (Scharer, 1978).

Parents who abuse or neglect may exhibit certain behaviors, which should indicate to the nurse the necessity of additional assessment. These include the following:

— Chaotic household

— Marital discord

— Minimal interaction and attachment between parent and child

— Inappropriately leaving the child at home alone

— Apparent or expressed disregard for the child's needs or safety

— Exaggerated anger response to child behavior (extreme and unrealistic approaches at discipline)

— Unilateral negativity when speaking about or referring to the child

— Anger regarding the "inconvenience" that the child's legitimate needs create in the parent's life (e.g., getting sick, going to therapy, driving the child to school)

— Poor understanding of childhood developmental tasks and behaviors

— Overtly protective of the child

— Exhibiting or expressing jealousy over "all the attention" the child is getting

Lack of Resources

There are common factors in abuse and neglect of children that are related to financial stressors and lack of emotional and social support. A tremendous amount of pressure can be put on a family system with limited financial resources or a poor distribution of social and family responsibility. A caregiver in this family system may experience a sense of failure that may lead to low self-esteem and poor emotional control. This can result in poor frustration tolerance and anger management during overwhelming crises, which can easily result in abusive episodes. Unless the financial and social stressors are alleviated, or there is education and intervention regarding anger management and impulse control, a destructive "circuit" is created and used for relief during conflicts. This circuit includes a charged emotional atmosphere in the adult, which seeks an outlet for the negative energy; the conduit for energy release is an act of abuse, and the outlet is the child (Kerr & Bowen, 1988).

Social isolation can also promote abusive situations. Many families live in a paucity of knowledge regarding resources available to them within the community. Families who are accused of child abuse may be unaware of the myriad social services that could have alleviated the potential for abuse, or they may admit that they were too ashamed to ask for help for fear that they would be perceived as parental failures.

Trauma Response Patterns

Van der Kolk (1987) cites 5 major characteristics of human responses to trauma:

1. A persistence of startle response and irritability

2. Proclivity toward explosive outbursts of aggression

3. Fixation on the trauma

4. Generally constricted level of personality function

5. An atypical dream life

These symptoms represent a few of the multitude of traumatic presentations and behaviors exhibited by victims of abuse and violence across the childhood continuum.

Emotional and Behavioral Aspects: Attempts at Mastery and the Compulsion to Repeat the Trauma

Posttraumatic Stress Disorder

The *Diagnostic and Statistical Manual of Mental Disorders, Fourth Edition* [DSM-IV] classifies posttraumatic stress disorder (PTSD) as an anxiety disorder, characterized by a cluster of symptoms that result from the impact of a significantly traumatic experience (American Psychiatric Association [APA], 1994). These symptoms are disruptive and disturbing to the survivor of the trauma and can derail the usual developmental trajectory and the ability to complete the activities required in daily life (Burgess et al., 1995b; Clements, 2001b; Clements & Burgess, 2002; Freud, 1969; van der Kolk, 1988, 1989).

Children who have been exposed to abuse or violence are at significant risk to develop PTSD-related symptoms (Clements, 2001b; Clements & Burgess, 2002; Clements & Weisser, in press; Vigil & Clements, 2003). "Within the first hours after the event a child may crystallize an altered and restricted view of his or her personal future" (Eth & Pynoos, 1994). Such a response requires treatment to reduce the symptom intensity and potentially to integrate the event into the child's life history.

According to the DSM-IV, a child is at risk for PTSD (Diagnostic Category 309.81) (APA, 1994) after there has been exposure to a traumatic event in which both of the following are present: (1) the child experienced, witnessed, or was confronted with an event or events that involved actual or threatened death or serious injury, or a threat to the physical integrity of others, and (2) the child's response involved intense fear, helplessness, or horror. In children, this may also be expressed by disorganized or agitated behaviors.

In addition to the existence of the recognizable stressor, the traumatic event is persistently reexperienced, as described in one or more of the following groups of symptoms **(Table 10-4)**.

The first group of symptoms listed in **Table 10-4** involves reexperiencing the event through recurrent and intrusive distressing memories of the event as images, thoughts, or perceptions. In children, this may manifest itself in repetitive play during which themes of the trauma are expressed. There may be recurrent dreams described as frightening dreams without recognizable content. Additionally, a child may act or feel

---

Table 10-4. Posttraumatic Stress Disorder Diagnostic Criteria

1. One or more of the following reexperiencing symptoms:
   — Involuntary intrusive thoughts related to the event
   — Recurrent upsetting dreams
   — Flashbacks of the event
   — Distressing psychological reactions to trauma cues
   — Physiological reactions to trauma cues

2. At least 3 of the following avoidant symptoms:
   — Avoids thoughts, feelings, or talk related to the traumatic event
   — Avoids activities, persons, or places associated with the event
   — Fails to remember significant portions of the event
   — Has decreased interest in activities
   — Feels estranged from others
   — Has difficulty feeling emotions
   — Has difficulty trusting others
   — Has feelings of impending doom/lack of future orientation

3. At least 2 of the following symptoms of increased arousal:
   — Sleep disturbance
   — Irritability/mood swings
   — Difficulty with concentration
   — Hypervigilance to surroundings
   — Pronounced startle response

Adapted from American Psychiatric Association. Diagnostic and Statistical Manual of Mental Disorders. 4th ed. Washington, DC: American Psychiatric Association; 1994.

as if the traumatic event were recurring again. This can include a sense of reliving the experience, illusions, hallucinations, and dissociative flashback episodes. There may be intense psychological or physiological distress at exposure to internal or external cues that symbolize or resemble an aspect of the traumatic event.

The second group of symptoms is characterized by persistent avoidance of associated stimuli and a numbing of responsiveness in thought and activity. This may be presented via difficulty with memory retrieval, affective and cognitive blunting, interpersonal detachment, and a pessimistic outlook on the future. There are efforts to avoid all thoughts and feelings or conversations associated with the traumatic event. Additionally, attempts are made to avoid activities, places, or people that arouse recollection of the trauma. There may be an inability to recall an important aspect of the traumatic event or a markedly diminished interest and participation in significant activities. The child may express and display feelings of detachment and estrangement from others. Additionally, the child may display a restricted range of affect and may express a sense of a foreshortened future (e.g., does not expect to have a career, marriage, children, or a normal life span).

The third group of symptoms is manifested by an increased level of arousal not present before the traumatic event. These symptoms may include sleep pattern disturbances (difficulty falling asleep or staying asleep), irritability or outbursts of anger, hypervigilance, difficulty concentrating, and exaggerated startle response (APA, 1994; Garrick, Eth, Morrow, Marciano, & Shalev, 1998). The startle response is a critical indicator of PTSD. This primitive response to noise is evident as early as 24 to 36 hours after birth and typically disappears by age 4 months (Boback & Jensen, 1987; Whaley & Wong, 1997). Children with PTSD have demonstrated an autonomic arousal related to a traumatic event, with the salient feature being absence of an extinction of a symptomatic response to traumatic cues (Clements & Burgess, 2002). There is a reflex exaggerated startle response to auditory, visual, tactile, or olfactory cues that are reminders of the traumatic event (CC Publishing, 1998; Clements & Burgess, 2002; Clements et al., 2001; Garrick et al., 1998).

Characteristics of PTSD have been identified as common in children who have experienced sexual or physical abuse. Typical responses include increased misperception of the duration and sequencing of time and events, premonition formation, reenactment or the unknowing performance of acts similar to the traumatic occurrence, marked and enduring personality alterations, and changes in the recognition and tolerance of the affective response of fear, contributing to inhibition or counterphobic behaviors (Burgess et al., 1995a; Burgess et al., 1995b; Clements & Burgess, 2002; Eth & Pynoos, 1985; Eth, Silverstein, & Pynoos, 1985; Sherkow, 1990; van der Kolk, 1989; Vigil & Clements, 2003).

A diagnosis of PTSD must be considered in abused children. This disorder is a physiological and psychological response pattern to overwhelming trauma. Child abuse is clearly classifiable as such an overwhelming trauma. In fact, child abuse inevitably raises the issue of human accountability, which supports the statement that the risk for "PTSD is apparently more severe and longer lasting when the stressor is of human design" (APA, 1987, p. 248).

If a child is unable to integrate the traumatic event into his or her life history, then an acute PTSD response may ensue. This is identified by a display of intrusive or avoidant behaviors. Exposure to stimuli may induce a state of hyperarousal and numbing, which may cause the child to experience highly emotional states with lower levels of thinking. In many cases, the ego cannot adapt to the trauma and becomes disorganized, flooded, and overwhelmed (Kris, 1956; Osofsky, Cohen, & Drell, 1995; Winnicott, 1958). Rainey,

Aleem, Ortiz, Yaragani, Pohl, and Berchow (1987) describe the visual and motoric reliving of traumatic events with nightmares and flashbacks generally preceded by physiological arousal. The disruptions also may impact sensory, perceptual/cognitive, and interpersonal performance levels. Symptoms of sensory disruption may include hyperactivity, headaches, stomachaches, back pain, genitourinary distress, and nightmares.

Perceptual and cognitive disruptions may include internal and external cues that produce intrusions of images and auditory and kinesthetic information associated with the trauma. These may be related to future concerns about repeated danger. Symptoms of interpersonal disruption include avoidant behaviors, such as an excessive fear of others and an inability to assert or protect oneself. Other disruptions may be masked as aggressive behaviors, including aggression toward peers, family members, and pets.

The patterns of *acute* PTSD symptoms are typically noted by the child's caregiver or other adults who interact with the child on a regular basis (e.g., schoolteacher, daycare worker, grandparent).

The *avoidant* pattern is characterized by denial of the event. This child appears distant and alienated with a lack of energy for learning and living. Often his or her behavior has a preoccupied daydreaming quality. These children may turn to substance abuse, display phobic behavior, encounter adjustment problems at home and school, display affect and behaviors of depression, and exhibit conduct disorders.

The *aggressive* pattern is characterized by externalized and typically angry behavioral displays. This acting out may be bold or secret. The child may test and break rules. Impulsivity increases, and the child may fight with peers and siblings or show overt defiance toward adults.

Eventually, when the body and mind become overwhelmed with the traumatic event and can no longer successfully manage the impact that it has on the child's daily life, trauma learning may occur. Trauma learning emphasizes the repetition of behavior, which Freud (1939) discussed in *Moses and Monotheism*, exploring the positive and negative effects of trauma. This repetition can be observed in traumatized children in several presentations, each of which will be reviewed in the following section. These include integration of the traumatic event, reenactment of the trauma, repetition of the trauma as either victim or victimizer, or displacement of the aggression (Burgess & Hartman, 1988; Burgess et al., 1995b; DeRanieri, Clements, & Henry, 2002; van der Kolk, 1989; Vigil & Clements, 2003).

Emotional and Behavioral Presentations

Burgess and Hartman's (1988) conceptual framework describes information processing of traumatic events and a suggested path of symptom responses. This anatomy of trauma is predicated on neuropsychosocial concepts of information processing and the role of the neuromodulatory systems on cognition and memory (van der Kolk, 1989). Burgess et al. (1995b) developed a framework based on the work of Burgess and Hartman (1988) to look at information processing of traumatic events in children. This framework suggests the progression of patient symptom responses as sequelae to a traumatic event. This framework is congruent with the tenets currently set forth in the DSM-IV for a diagnosis of PTSD and provides a continuum for the emotional and behavioral responses after a traumatic event. It can provide a model for assessing the psychological and behavioral aftermath for children who have been victims of abuse.

The model represents a continuum of responses that a child may have after a traumatic event. This spectrum ranges from *integration* (no subsequent sequelae) to *displacement* (psychotic reactions).

Integration

The optimal response pattern after a traumatic event is no resultant PTSD and the subsequent integration of the traumatic event into the victim's life experience. In the integrated pattern, the child is able to acknowledge the traumatic event but is not compelled to dwell on it or avoid it through psychological defenses. Rutter (1985) has speculated that a child's ability to incorporate a traumatic event into his or her belief system depends on several factors, including appraisal of the situation and his or her capacity to process the life event.

It is unclear how many children can readily integrate trauma without experiencing PTSD. Clinically, these children are typically not encountered for therapeutic intervention because it is usually the disruptive behaviors and emotional responses, and not necessarily the traumatic event itself, that lead caregivers to bring children to healthcare professionals for evaluation and treatment.

Reenactment

The literature suggests that an abused child may be driven to compulsively reenact the traumatic event. Johnson (1987) writes: "Victims of trauma often find themselves repeatedly reenacting abusive relationships throughout their lives. It was in the study of such disorders that Freud (1959) first described 'repetition compulsion'" (Johnson, 1987, p. 8). Reenactment is experienced by children as a recollection of the traumatic event. This may occur as flashbacks, which may contain fragmented detail and an intense sensory experience. In young children, there may be repetitive themes and aspects of the traumatic event expressed via play (Burgess et al., 1995b; Clements et al., 2001; Clements & Weisser, in press). There may be frightening dreams that have unrecognizable content. The verbal or play behaviors demonstrate that the child is acting as if the trauma is happening again. During this stage, the child continues to identify with the role of the victim. The child may fear that the perpetrator will come and "get" him or her just as the person did before.

Repetition

During the repetition stage of the trauma learning process, behavior patterns generally are noted in the child's play with others. The behavioral repetition of the trauma may be played out in either the role of the trauma victim or the role of the victimizer. Repetition of the trauma in the role of the victimizer is a major cause of aggression and violence. The traumatized child may attempt to act out the dynamics of the event on other children, who are usually smaller and weaker, in an attempt to gain a sense of control or mastery over the trauma that originally happened to him or her.

Displacement

During the displacement stage, behaviors and thoughts of the trauma are elaborated symbolically. The elaboration may manifest as a dream or fantasy, and this may include symbolic representations of the violent act. Ultimately, this symbolic elaboration may lead to psychotic reactions that have patterns of the original trauma embedded in them.

When a child is unable to link ongoing, self-defeating, disrupting behaviors to the original trauma, there is no resolution or integration, and the underlying fear persists. This leads to an inability to use new experiences to develop and grow. Instead, the flexibility of the child to discriminate new information may be lost, and the child is either numb to the new information or hyperalert, or he or she may perceive it as dangerous.

THE ISSUE OF BELIEF

The role of the healthcare provider is to assess and evaluate the need for intervention. It is not the healthcare provider's role to determine the veracity of the child's allegation. It is far more dangerous to not believe a child and send him or her home to the abuser than to investigate the child's allegations and have the result of an exoneration of the alleged abuser. It is critical to understand that for an abused child, telling may represent the most difficult and daring act of his or her entire existence. In this light, if the child tells and is indeed telling the truth, but no additional assessment occurs, the healthcare provider has potentially reinforced the child's belief that the situation is without hope of rescue.

INTERVENTIONS

There are myriad interventions for working with children who have experienced abuse. Traditional talk therapy is appropriate, although not necessarily the modality of choice or preference, especially for children. Options for intervention should include consideration of the child's developmental level and trauma-related behaviors. Such interventions can include experiential approaches, such as art therapy, play therapy, storytelling, and doll play (Clements et al., 2001; Clements & Weisser, in press; Gil, 1991).

It has been said that the work of children is play. In this light, approaching children on their level can provide a valuable conduit toward gleaning pertinent information or tailoring effective interventions. Additionally, it can promote an exchange of significant information and allow an opportunity for children to ask questions of the healthcare provider. This alone can be substantial in establishing a sense of trust while strengthening the therapeutic alliance.

Abused, neglected, or emotionally abused children are frequently overstimulated or understimulated; therefore, they may lack the ability to explore, experiment, and even play. The caregiver must facilitate these natural and now constricted or disorganized tendencies (Burgess et al., 1995b; Gil, 1991). Expressive therapies can be used to discover and resolve problems and are best used for nonpsychotic children. The expressive approach combines both directed and nondirected expression to facilitate communication concerning traumatic issues (Clements et al., 2001; Clements & Weisser, in press; Clunn, 1991; Gil, 1991).

SHORT-TERM GOALS

The short-term goals of age-appropriate and expressive therapies include establishment and promotion of therapeutic rapport between the nurse and the child and creation of an anchor for safety (Burgess et al., 1995b; Clements & Burgess, 2002). By communicating to the child, either verbally or through collaborative expressive methods (e.g., drawing pictures, play therapy, story telling), that the nurse is interested in what the child has to say about anything traumatic that has happened, the child is more likely to reveal relevant information for assessment and intervention (Clements et al., 2001; Clements & Weisser, in press) **(Figure 10-1)**. Violation of trust is one of the basic tenets to all abuse, and thus, dealing with it is the first and most critical step in providing effective treatment. Children can learn from the provider that adults can be trusted and that their words and actions are performed within an environment of honesty and with a display of healthy interpersonal boundaries. Strategies for attaining this trust include the following:

— Telling the child what you are going to do before you do it

— Clarifying that the child understands what you are going to do

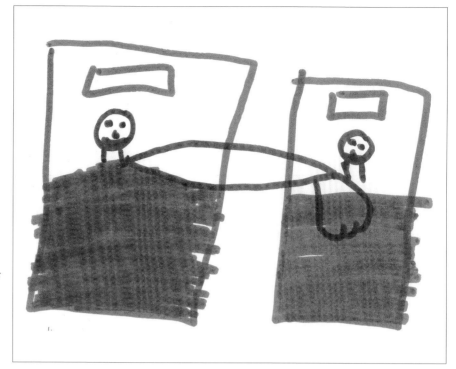

Figure 10-1.
Drawing by an 11-year-old boy during a therapeutic session with a nurse revealing an episode of sexual abuse by a male relative who was spending the night at his house.

— "Checking in" with the child during the process to assess the level of anxiety and understanding

— Providing the opportunity for the child to control the therapeutic environment whenever feasible

Regardless of the expressive modality, it is important to remember that the child has encountered a real or perceived lack or loss of control, and that allowing the child to regain a sense of some control can only enhance trust and communication.

With assistance and guidance, goals for those who treat abused and neglected children are to help the child integrate the traumatic event into his or her life history and to facilitate the ability to reinvest in mastering age-appropriate developmental tasks and goals. Although there may be some early evidence of this in the short term, in behaviors such as improved affect, increased play and verbalizations, and improved levels of trust, probably no other kind of therapy requires ongoing assessment to monitor for these sometimes subtle changes. Additionally, children may unfold during therapeutic interactions and share their emotions more freely as they begin to trust (Clements et al., 2001; Clements & Weisser, in press; Gil, 1991). This requires the care provider to continue to assess the perceptions of the child regarding his or her level of autonomy, empowerment, and safety.

LONG-TERM GOALS
Unlike the adult client, the child is experiencing more developmental changes and expected tasks as therapeutic interventions progress. Depending on the child's age, inherent developmental tasks and expectations may provide additional dynamics that can make integration of the trauma more problematic. This can include things such as peer pressure, establishment of identity and role perceptions, ongoing expansion of ego structure, and moral development. Depending on the length of treatment, the child may face dealing with the past trauma while simultaneously facing the challenges inherent in the next development level.

The length of treatment varies among children relative to the nature, severity, and duration of the abuse and to the child's preabuse methods of coping (Burgess et al., 1995b; Clements & Weisser, in press). The goal of integration can be easily conveyed by the clinician to the child if expressed in everyday language such as the following:

— It was a terrible thing that happened to you.

— You didn't ask for it to happen to you.

— It wasn't your fault that it happened to you.

— Sometimes adults make bad decisions and do things that are wrong.

— Now it is time to focus on yourself and to figure out how to get back to your everyday life.

— Forgetting what happened isn't really the answer. Remembering what happened may be scary at first, but thinking about it in a new way can help you learn to live with it and continue to do the things that other children do.

SUMMARY

Maltreatment and abuse are words that clinicians may hear daily. One of the greatest challenges for clinicians is to provide comprehensive assessment, intervention, and referral to the child survivors of abuse and their families. Survivors of child abuse must learn to cope adaptively with their own growth and development within the context of the loss of power and control with which they had to contend previously. This can lend itself to role confusion and lack of clarity regarding what are typical developmental tasks encountered by most children and what are misperceptions of additional threats to their integrity.

Children benefit from assessment strategies and interventions, which can help promote adaptive coping and healing. As mental health professionals expand and then apply their understanding of the identification and treatment of child abuse, they potentially prevent the derailment of a child's emotional growth and development and minimize the extent of the psychological impact of the maltreatment.

This chapter has provided an overview of the basic tenets necessary for the psychological assessment and guidance required in planning interventions for children who survive abusive situations. Ultimately, the therapeutic relationship between the child, the child's family, and the clinician can be the strongest intervention of all. Trust facilitates assessment, successful intervention, and ultimately healing.

REFERENCES

Allen D. Abusers: a personal construct psychology. *Nursing & Residential Care*. 2000;2:134-137.

American Psychiatric Association. *Diagnostic and Statistical Manual of Mental Disorders*. 3rd ed. (Revised). Washington, DC: American Psychiatric Association; 1987:248.

American Psychiatric Association. *Diagnostic and Statistical Manual of Mental Disorders*. 4th ed. Washington, DC: American Psychiatric Association; 1994.

Ammerman RT. Sexually abused children with multiple disabilities: each is unique, as are their needs. *NRCCSA News*. 1992;1:13-14.

Ammerman RT. Physical abuse and childhood disability: risk and treatment factors. In: Geffner R, Sorenson SB, Lundberg-Love PK, eds. *Violence and Sexual Abuse at Home: Current Issues in Spousal Battering and Child Maltreatment*. New York, NY: The Hawthorne Press; 1997:207-224.

Ammerman RT, Baladerian NJ. *Maltreatment of Children With Disabilities.* Chicago, Ill: National Committee to Prevent Child Abuse; 1993.

Annas C. Irreversible error: the power and prejudice of female genital mutilation. *J Contemp Health Law Policy.* 1996;12:325-353.

Asher JB. Moving beyond a don't-ask–don't-tell approach. In: Giardino AP, Datner E, Asher J, eds. *Sexual Assault Victimiztion Across the Life Span: A Clinical Guide.* St. Louis, Mo: GW Medical Publishing; 2003:447-457.

Bagley C, King K. *Child Sexual Abuse.* New York, NY: Tavistock/Routledge; 1990.

Barnard G. *The Child Molester: An Integrated Approach to Evaluation and Treatment.* New York, NY: Brunner/Mazel; 1989.

Benasutti KM. *Childhood Psychological Maltreatment and the Use of Art Expressions* [unpublished masters thesis]. Philadelphia, Pa: Hahnemann University; 1993.

Boback I, Jensen M. *Essentials of Maternity Nursing: The Nurse and the Childbearing Family.* 2nd ed. St. Louis, Mo: Mosby; 1987.

Burgess A, Hartman C. Information processing of trauma. *J Interpers Violence.* 1988;3:443-457.

Burgess A, Hartman C, Baker T. Memory presentations of childhood sexual abuse. *J Psychosoc Nurs.* 1995a;33:9-16.

Burgess A, Hartman C, Clements P. Biology of memory and childhood trauma. *J Psychosoc Nurs.* 1995b;33:16-26.

Burgess A, Holmstrom L, McCausland M. Counseling young victims and their families. In: Burgess WA, Groth AN, Holmstrom LL, Sgroi SM, eds. *Sexual Assault of Children and Adolescents.* Lexington, Mass: Lexington Books; 1978:181-204.

Butler-Smith S. *Children's Story: Sexually Molested Children in Criminal Court.* Walnut Creek, Calif: Launch Press; 1985.

CC Publishing. Acute stress disorder. Available at: http://www.ccpublishing.com/journals2/acute_stress_disorder.html. Accessed August 29, 1998.

Clements PT. Homicide bereavement: scary tales for children. In: Cox G, Bendiksen R, Stevenson R, eds. *Understanding and Treating Complicated Grief.* Amityville, NY: Baywood; 2001a:41-52.

Clements PT. Kids in chaos: how to help children deal with family homicide and bereavement. *Nurs Spectrum.* 2001b;2:20w-21w.

Clements PT, Benasutti KM, Henry GC. Drawing from experience: utilizing drawings to facilitate communication and understanding with children exposed to sudden traumatic deaths. *J Psychosoc Nurs.* 2001;39:12-20.

Clements PT, Burgess AW. Children's responses to family homicide. *Fam Community Health.* 2002;25:1-11.

Clements PT, Weisser SM. Cries from the morgue: guidance for assessment, evaluation, and intervention with children exposed to homicide of a family member. *J Child Adolesc Psychiatr Nurs.* In press.

Clunn P. *Child Psychiatric Nursing.* St. Louis, Mo: Mosby; 1991.

DeRanieri JT, Clements PT, Henry GC. When catastrophe happens: assessment and intervention after sudden traumatic deaths. *J Psychosoc Nurs Ment Health Serv.* 2002; 40:30-37.

Diaz A, Simantov E, Rickert VI. Effect of abuse on health: results of a national survey. *Arch Pediatr Adolesc Med*. 2002;156:811-817.

Dosomething.org. Why does child abuse happen? Available at: http://www.do something.org/newspub/section.cfm?SID=36&cid=5. Accessed February 10, 2003.

Elliot D, Briere J. Childhood and adolescent development. In: Stoudemire A, Klunman B, eds. *An Introduction to Medical Students*. 2nd ed. Philadelphia, Pa: JB Lippincott; 1994:261-317.

Eth S, Pynoos R. Developmental perspective on psychic trauma in childhood. In: Figley CR, ed. *Trauma and Its Wake*. New York, NY: Brunner/Mazel; 1985:36-52.

Eth S, Pynoos R. Children who witness the homicide of a parent. *Psychiatry*. 1994;57:287-306.

Eth S, Silverstein S, Pynoos R. Mental health consultation to a preschool following the homicide of a mother and child. *Hosp Community Psychiatry*. 1985;36:73-76.

Finkelhor D. *Sexually Victimized Children*. New York, NY: Free Press; 1979.

Flaherty GE, Sege R, Mattson CL, Binns HJ. Assessment of suspicion of abuse in the primary care setting. *Ambul Pediatr*. 2002;2:120-126.

Freud A. *The Writings of Anna Freud*. Vol. V. New York, NY: International University Press; 1969.

Freud S. Moses and monotheism. In: Strachey J, ed. *The Standard Edition of the Complete Psychological Works of Sigmund Freud*. London: Hogarth Press; 1939 (Original work published in 1905):3-137.

Garrick T, Eth S, Morrow N, Marciano D, Shalev A. A startle habituation model of post-traumatic stress disorder in rats. FTP: Traumatology: The international electronic journal of innovations in the study of the traumatization process and methods for reducing or eliminating related human suffering. Available at: http://rdz.acor.org/ lists/trauma//art2vli2.html. Accessed August 29, 1998.

Gil E. *The Healing Power of Play: Working With Abused Children*. New York, NY: The Guilford Press; 1991.

Gordon S, Gordon J, Cohen V. *Better Safe Than Sorry Book: A Family Guide for Sexual Assault Prevention*. Amherst, NY: Prometheus Books; 1992.

Groth A, Loredo C. Juvenile sexual offenders: guidelines for assessment. *Int J Offender Ther Comp Criminol*. 1981;25:31-39.

Hartley CC. The co-occurrence of child maltreatment and domestic violence: examining both neglect and child physical abuse. *Child Maltreat*. 2002;7:349-358.

Helfer R. The epidemiology of child abuse and neglect. *Pediatr Ann*. 1984;13:747-751.

Helfer R. The developmental basis of child abuse and neglect: an epidemiological approach. In: Helfer R, Kempe R, eds. *The Battered Child*. Chicago, Ill: University of Chicago Press; 1987:60-80.

Henry J. Videotaping child disclosure interviews: exploratory study of children's experiences and perceptions. *J Child Sex Abus*. 1999;8:35-49.

Hinds A, Baskin LS. Child sexual abuse: when to suspect it and how to assess for it. *Contemp Urol*. 2002;14:31-32, 35-36, 39.

Hunka CD, O'Toole AW, O'Toole R. Self-help therapy in Parents Anonymous. *J Psychosoc Nurs Ment Health Serv*. 1985;23:24-32.

Jenkins P. *Moral Panic: Changing Concepts of the Child Molested in Modern America.* New Haven, Conn: Yale University Press; 1998.

Johnson DR. The role of creative arts therapies in the diagnosis and treatment of psychological trauma. *Arts Psychother.* 1987;14:7-13.

Kerr M, Bowen M. *Family Evaluation: An Approach Based on Bowen Theory.* New York, NY: WW Norton; 1988.

Kris E. The recovery of childhood memories in psychoanalysis. *Psychoanal Study Child.* 1956;11:54-88.

Lagaipa SJ. Suffer the little children: the ancient practice of infanticide as a modern moral dilemma. *Issues Compr Pediatr Nurs.* 1990;13:241-251.

Ludwig S. Defining child abuse: clinical mandate—evolving concepts. In: Ludwig S, Kornberg AE, eds. *Child Abuse: A Medical Reference.* 2nd ed. New York, NY: Churchill Livingstone; 1992:1-12.

Malchiodi C. *Breaking the Silence.* New York, NY: Brunner/Mazel; 1990.

Meier H, ed. *Assault Against Children: Why It Happens, How to Stop It.* San Diego, Calif: College-Hill Press; 1985.

Melton G. Doing justice and doing good: conflicts for mental health professionals, *Future Child.* 1994;2:102-118.

Milner LS. *Hardness of Heart: Hardness of Life—The Stain of Human Infanticide.* Kearney, Neb: Morris Publishing; 1998.

Mitchell LM, Buchele-Ash A. Abuse and neglect of individuals with disabilities: building protective supports through public policy. *Journal of Disability Policy Studies.* 2000;10:225-243.

Oldham JM, Riba MB, eds. *American Psychiatric Press Review of Psychiatry.* Arlington, Va: American Psychiatric Press; 1994.

Osofsky JD, Cohen G, Drell, M. The effects of trauma on young children: a case study of 2-year-old twins. *Int J Psychoanal.* 1995;76:595-607.

Protection of Children From Sexual Predators Act. October, 1998. Available at: http://www.ageofconsent.com/childsexlaws.htm. Accessed February 3, 2003.

Radbill S. Children in a world of violence: a history of child abuse. In: Helfer R, Kempe R, eds. *The Battered Child.* Chicago, Ill: University of Chicago Press; 1987:3-22.

Rainey J, Aleem A, Ortiz A, Yaragani V, Pohl R, Berchow, R. Laboratory procedures for inducement of flashbacks. *Am J Psychiatry.* 1987;144:1317-1319.

Rasmussen LA. The trauma outcome process: an integrated model for guiding clinical practice with children with sexually abusive behavior problems. *J Child Sex Abus.* 1999;8:3-33.

Rutter M. Resilience in the face of adversity: protective factors and resistance to psychiatric disorder. *Br J Psychiatry.* 1985;147:598-611.

Salter A. *Treating Child Sex Offenders and Victims: A Practical Guide.* Thousand Oaks, Calif: Sage Publications; 1988.

Salter A. *Transforming Trauma: A Guide to Treating Adult Survivors of Sexual Abuse.* Thousand Oaks, Calif: Sage Publications; 1995.

Salter A. *Sadistic Versus Grooming Sex Offenders*. Available on video [0761914676]. Thousand Oaks, Calif: Sage Publications; 1998.

Scharer K. Rescue fantasies: professional impediments in working with abused families. *Am J Nurs*. 1978;78:1483-1484.

Sherkow S. Evaluation and diagnosis of sexual abuse of little girls. *J Am Psychoanal Assoc*. 1990;38:347-369.

Singer K. Characteristics observed in male sexual abuse victims. Available at: http://www.malesurvivor.org/articles/char.htm. Accessed February 10, 2003.

Stein MT, Perrin EL. Guidance for effective discipline. American Academy of Pediatrics. Committee on Psychosocial Aspects of Child and Family Health. *Pediatrics*. 1998;101:723-728.

Tomison AM. Child maltreatment and disability. *Issues in Child Abuse Prevention*. 1996;7:1-11.

Toubia N. Female circumcision as a public health issue. *N Engl J Med*. 1994;331:712.

US Department of Health & Human Services. *Definitions, Scope, and Effects of Child Sexual Abuse*. National Clearinghouse on Child Abuse and Neglect Information. Available at: http://www.calib.com/nccanch/pubs/usermanuals/sexabuse/effects.cfm. Accessed February 10, 2003.

van der Kolk B. *Psychological Trauma*. Washington, DC: American Psychiatric Press; 1987.

van der Kolk B. The trauma spectrum: the interaction of biological and social events in the genesis of trauma response. *J Trauma Stress*. 1988;1:274.

van der Kolk B. The compulsion to repeat the trauma: re-enactment, repetition, and masochism. *Psychiatr Clin North Am*. 1989;12:389-405.

Vigil GJ, Clements PT. Child and adolescent homicide survivors: complicated grief and altered worldviews. *J Psychosoc Nurs Ment Health Serv*. 2003;41:30-39.

Watkins B, Bentovim A. The sexual abuse of male children and adolescents: a review of current research. *J Child Psychol Psychiatry*. 1992;33:197-248.

Whaley L, Wong D. *Essentials of Pediatric Nursing*. 5th ed. St. Louis, Mo: Mosby; 1997.

Winnicott DW. Psychogenesis of a beating fantasy. In: Winnicott C et al., eds. *Psychoanalytic Explorations*. Cambridge, Mass: Harvard University Press; 1958:45-48.

Chapter 11

Sexual Abuse of Adolescents

Barbara Speller-Brown, RN, MSN, CPNP
Suzanne P. Starling, MD, FAAP

Sexual abuse is a common problem affecting adolescents in our society. Awareness of sexual abuse has increased over the past decade, and medical providers frequently are asked to evaluate adolescents with abuse allegations. The sexual abuse of adolescents presents a challenge for the examiner. The unique psychological and physical aspects of the adolescent require special consideration on the part of healthcare providers working with them. This chapter explores the unique aspects of the sexual abuse of adolescents.

Epidemiology

According to the National Child Abuse and Neglect Data System in 1997, 13% of the nearly 1 million cases of child abuse substantiated by child protective services (CPS) were sexual abuse. Of the sexual abuse cases, 77% of the victims were girls and 23% boys, with a large proportion of the children over age 8 years (US Department of Health & Human Services [USDHHS], 1999). Adolescents have a higher rate of sexual assault than any other age group. In 1998, the US Department of Justice reported rates of sexual assault at 1.7 per 1000 for persons age 24 to 29 years. The rates per 1000 for adolescents were 3.5 for 12 to 15 years, 5.0 for those age 16 to 19 years, and 4.6 for those age 20 to 24 years. More than half of all reported sexual assaults were in victims younger than age 25 years (Rennison, 1999).

The adolescent age group has one of the highest rates of sexual assault in the United States. Retrospective studies find that 27% to 32% of adult women and 13% to 26% of adult men report experiencing some form of sexual abuse before age 18 years (Elliot & Briere, 1994; Finkelhor & Baron, 1986). Other studies conservatively suggest that 1 in 4 girls and 1 in 7 boys will be sexually abused by the time they reach age 18 years (Peipert & Domagalski, 1994).

Regardless of socioeconomic status, the risk of adolescent sexual abuse increases in less cohesive, more disorganized, or dysfunctional families. Living without one of the biological parents, absence of the mother for girls, and absence of the father for boys also increase the risk for sexual abuse. Disabled adolescents have 1.75 times the rate of abuse seen in nondisabled teens (Briere, 1992; Elliot & Briere, 1994; Hymel & Jenny, 1996). Adolescents with developmental delay in the mildly retarded range are at particular risk for date and acquaintance rape (Quint, 1999).

Sexual Maturity

Adolescence is the transitional stage between childhood and adulthood. Adolescent boys and girls undergo a series of pubertal changes during this stage. Providers need to evaluate stages of sexual maturation when examining adolescents for sexual abuse. Sexual maturation ratings (SMRs), also referred to as Tanner stages, are useful for understanding and evaluating sexual maturation in this age group. The stages of pubertal changes for each secondary sexual characteristic are outlined in **Figures 11-1** to **11-6**. Breast and pubic hair development is evaluated in girls, and genital and pubic hair development is evaluated in boys. It is important to stage breast and pubic hair development separately to determine any discrepancy between the stages. Breast development is primarily controlled by ovarian estrogen secretion, and pubic hair development is stimulated by adrenal androgen secretion (Wheeler, 1991).

Sexual development in girls involves the enlargement of the ovaries, uterus, vagina, labia, and breasts and the growth of pubic hair. With the onset of puberty, estrogen causes changes in breast tissue and the hymen in most girls. Breast development is usually the first manifestation of puberty in girls and begins in stage 2 with breast budding, which takes place before pubic hair appears. Menarche usually occurs in breast stage 3 or 4 and generally occurs within 2 years of the onset of breast development (Seidel, Ball, Dains, & Benedict, 1995; Wheeler, 1991). The same estrogenization that causes breast changes also causes the hymen to become elastic, thickened, and redundant, thus allowing the hymen to stretch during penetration without injury in many cases. Therefore, many adolescents will have a normal hymenal examination even after a history of vaginal penetration.

Secondary development in boys involves genital development and pubic hair growth. A change in genital development usually precedes the appearance of pubic hair, which generally appears 18 to 24 months after the onset of testicular growth. Enlargement of the scrotum and testes occurs in stage 2, with little or no enlargement of the penis. Ejaculation generally first occurs in SMR stage 3, with semen appearing between SMR 3 and 4 (Seidel et al., 1995; Wheeler, 1991).

Figures 11-1 to 11-5. Male and female stages of pubertal changes. Reprinted with permission from van Wieringen JC. Growth Diagrams 1965 Netherlands. Second National Survey on 0–24-year-olds. The Netherlands: ©Wolters-Noordhoff Groningen; 1971.

Adolescent Risk-Taking Behaviors

Adolescence is a period of rapid physical, emotional, and cognitive growth (Slap, 1986). It is a time when teenagers are trying to establish their own identity and decide their futures. They are preoccupied with the physical changes taking place with their bodies and how they are similar to or different from their friends. Self-identity, self-esteem, and body image are important issues for this age group. Adolescents may believe they are

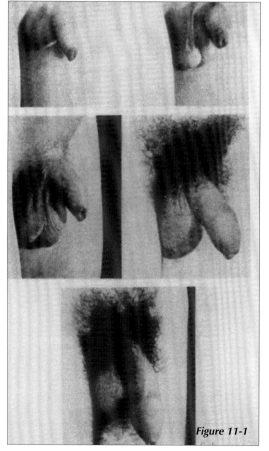

Figure 11-1

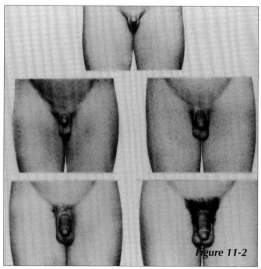

Figure 11-2

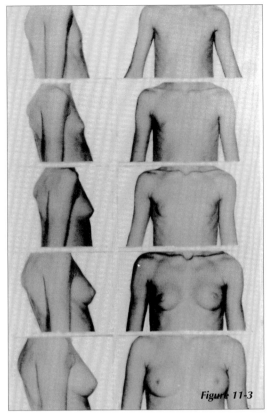

Figure 11-3

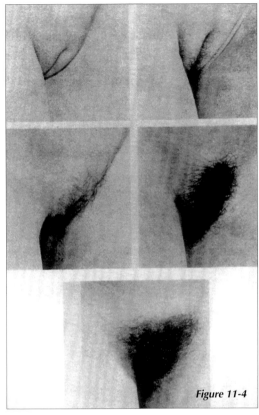

Figure 11-4

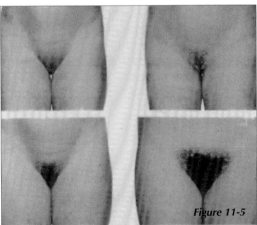

Figure 11-5

indestructible, and their risk-taking behaviors present a challenge to healthcare providers (Reif & Elster, 1998; Slap, 1986).

Prior sexual abuse has been shown to affect later sexual activity. Female adolescents who report prior sexual abuse are at increased risk for pregnancy. They are more likely to have a boyfriend pressuring them to conceive and to have fears about infertility (Rainey, Stevens-Simon, & Kaplan, 1995). A sexually active teen may believe she will not get pregnant and may experiment with sex because her friends are doing it. The opinion of peers is extremely important in determining behavior and the choices adolescents make.

Immaturity and the influence of peer pressure play roles in the inability of adolescents to comprehend the implications of their actions. The possibility of pregnancy or acquisition of sexually transmitted diseases (STDs) may seem remote to a teen. Reif and Elster (1998) reviewed a national survey of adolescent sexual behaviors and found that of the 53% of adolescents who reported sexual intercourse, 32% had intercourse by grade 9 and 66% by grade 12. Nearly 17% had 4 or more sexual partners, and 7% of the teens reported a pregnancy.

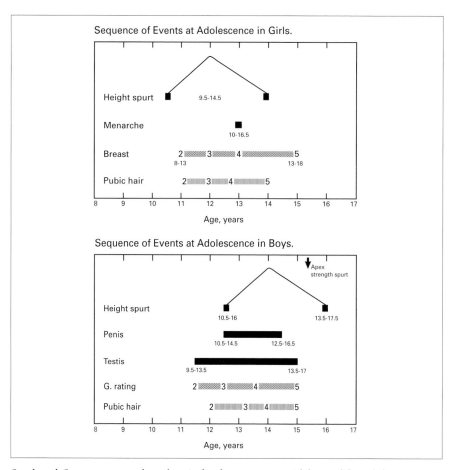

Figure 11-6.
Sequence of events at adolescence in girls and boys. The average girl and boy are represented. The range of ages within which each event charted may begin and end is given by the figures placed directly below its start and finish. Reprinted with permission from Marshall WA, Tanner JM. Variations in the pattern of pubertal changes in boys. Arch Dis Child. 1970;45:22.

Segal and Stewart report that chemical substances are widely used by adolescents as a means of excitement, consolation, and rebellion and as a symbol of social and sexual maturity and independence. Peer pressure, permissiveness, and the decline of self-esteem are the essential causes of adolescent substance use and abuse (Segal & Stewart, 1996).

DATING VIOLENCE

Date rape and acquaintance rape are increasing problems among adolescents. The term ***date rape*** has been defined as a nonconsensual sexual act between 2 persons in a romantic relationship (Mills & Granoff, 1992). ***Acquaintance rape*** is defined as nonconsensual sex between individuals who knew one another before the sexual act (Parrot, 1989). The majority of offenses involve female victims but acquaintance rapes of male victims do occur, involving both male and female perpetrators (Holmes & Slap, 1998). (See also Chapter 15, The Relationship Between Domestic Violence and Child Maltreatment.)

The perception of when rape has occurred varies among adolescents. The American College of Obstetricians and Gynecologists' Committee on Adolescent Health Care showed that some adolescent females believe forced sex is acceptable if the couple dated a long time, others believe it acceptable if the woman agreed to have sex but later changed her mind, and still others believe it acceptable if the woman "led him on." Of the adolescent men in the study, 54% believed that forced sex was acceptable if the young woman said yes and later changed her mind, and 40% believed that forced sex was acceptable if the man spent a lot of money on the date (ACOG Committee on Adolescent Health Care, 1993).

Date rape is more likely to involve verbal coercion for males and females, as well as physical pressure, such as fondling and unwanted kissing, and alcohol or drugs. Girls age 16 to 19 years are 4 times more likely to be victims of sexual assault than women of other age groups (Rickert & Wiemann, 1998). In the majority of cases, the perpetrator is an acquaintance. The highest incidence of acquaintance rape is among women in the twelfth grade of high school and the first year of college. Most know their assailant, and many of the attacks occur during a date (Bechtel & Podrazik, 1999). Studies indicate that teenagers in rural communities are as much at risk as university freshmen.

Many adolescents have not yet developed the skills needed to recognize and avoid potentially dangerous dating situations. Demographic characteristics that increase vulnerability to date rape include younger age at first date, early sexual activity, earlier age of menarche, a past history of sexual abuse, or prior sexual victimization. Acceptance of violence toward women also increases the risk (Rickert & Wiemann, 1998). Alcohol and drugs have been identified as contributing factors in the date and acquaintance rape of adolescents. Nearly half of adolescent assaults involve alcohol or drug use (Kaplan et al., 2001). Chemical substance use lowers inhibitions, decreases mental capacity, and may decrease the person's ability to defend against any unwanted advances. The "date rape drugs," such as flunitrazepam (Rohypnol) and similar drugs, have received a great deal of media attention. These drugs are sedative hypnotics, generally mixed in beverages, and can cause somnolence, decreased anxiety, or profound sedation. They can be associated with amnesia during the period of drug action (Schwartz & Weaver, 1998). Although the use of these drugs is concerning, their use is less common compared to that of alcohol.

SEXUAL ABUSE OF MALES

Sexual abuse of boys is common but is underreported and underdiagnosed. In 1990, Finkelhor found that 16% of men over age 18 years reported sexual abuse at some point in their lives (Finkelhor, Hotaling, Lewis, & Smith, 1990). Most assaults in adolescent boys are extrafamilial (Faller, 1989). Male perpetrators are identified in up to 90% of young adolescent male assaults (Holmes & Slap, 1998), with perpetrators most commonly identified as heterosexual (Holmes & Slap, 1998; Jenny, Roesler, & Poyer, 1994). Studies of older adolescents and young adults reveal a decrease in the percentage of male assailants as the rates of female perpetration against males rises with victim age (Holmes & Slap, 1998). Male victims typically describe 3 or more acts, which may include forced anal penetration of the victim or perpetrator, vaginal penetration of the perpetrator, orogenital contact of or by the perpetrator, and manual genital contact of or by the perpetrator. Anal penetration is described in up to 70% of male victims (Holmes & Slap, 1998).

MEDICAL EVALUATION OF ACUTE SEXUAL ASSAULT

Acute sexual assault in the adolescent is typically defined as an assault occurring within 72 hours of the evaluation. Some teens immediately report the assault and seek medical attention; however, many do not disclose the event for days or weeks, making an acute assault examination unnecessary in some cases. Adult protocols have typically indicated that a forensic evidence kit is not necessary after 72 hours, basing this time frame on the length of time seminal products could be collected from the victim's body after the assault (Willott & Allard, 1982). However, with recent advances in the DNA amplification technology used for the identification of seminal products, the forensic evidence kit may be useful even after the typical acute assault period. Teenagers should be evaluated on a case-by-case basis for evaluation as an acute or nonacute sexual abuse victim. Those examined within only a few days from the assault may benefit from evidence collection. **Table 11-1** contains an overview of acute assault protocols.

Table 11-1. Acute Assault Examination Protocol

IDENTIFYING INFORMATION

— Patient's name, date of birth, address, parents' names

— Alleged perpetrator's name, age, address (if known)

HISTORY OF PRESENT EVENT (OBTAIN SEPARATE HISTORIES FROM PATIENT AND PARENT/CARETAKER)

— Description of the event: sexual acts, exact place and time

— Physical complaints: discharge, bleeding, pain

— Other injuries sustained in event: cuts, bruises, fractures, bite marks

— Behavioral concerns: nightmares, anorexia, school failure, runaway behavior

PAST MEDICAL HISTORY

— Previous illnesses, including previous sexually transmitted diseases (STDs)

— Previous surgeries

— Medications, including birth control

— Onset of menarche and last menstruation

— Allergies and immunizations, including tetanus and hepatitis B

— History of previous sexual abuse or assault

— History of consensual sexual activity

SOCIAL HISTORY

— Names/relationships of people in the patient's home

— Educational level, including any developmental delay or special classes

— Support of friends and family members (obtain separate histories)

GENERAL PHYSICAL EXAMINATION

— Thorough general examination, including vital signs, height, and weight

— Special attention to skin, mucous membranes, hair

— Photographs of nongenital injuries

GENITAL EXAMINATION

— SMR (Tanner) stage of breasts and genitals

— Indicate examination position and use of any instrumentation

(continued)

Table 11-1. *(continued)*

— Description of labia majora and minora, urethra, clitoris, periurethral and perihymenal tissue

— Description of hymen: configuration, margins, evidence of trauma

— Description of posterior fourchette and fossa navicularis

— Internal speculum examination if needed to describe injury to vaginal walls and cervix

— For males, description of penis and scrotum

— Collection of specimens for STDs

— Forensic evidence kit (see text for details)

— Photographs—colposcopy or 35 mm, videography, or other image capture

ANAL EXAMINATION

— Description of examination position and any instrumentation

— Description of buttocks and surrounding skin

— Documentation of anal tone, tags, tears, fissures, lesions, or other evidence of trauma

— Photographs—colposcopy or 35 mm, videography, or other image capture

STD TESTING AND PROPHYLAXIS

— See text and **Table 11-3**

PREGNANCY PROPHYLAXIS

— 2 tablets of Ovral (50 μg ethinyl estradiol, 0.5 mg DL-norgestrel) within 72 hours of assault*

— 2 tablets 12 hours after first dose

— Consider antiemetic before both doses

FOLLOW-UP

— Consider follow-up for acute assault with injury to assess healing

— Repeat rapid plasma reagin (RPR), HIV, hepatitis B antibody tests at recommended intervals

— Mental health counseling for patient and family members

— Provide detailed, written follow-up instructions

Other drugs are being approved in the United States and may supplant use of Ovral.

Drug dosage recommendations listed herein are those of the authors and are not endorsed by the US Public Health Service or the US Department of Health & Human Services.

HISTORY AND INTERVIEW

As with all evaluations for sexual abuse, the history of the event is paramount. The client interview with adolescents is important, because the teen may be the only available witness to the event and may give details that had been previously undisclosed to his or her parents or the investigators. The examiner should clarify that the information will need to be shared with the appropriate authorities.

Laws pertaining to adolescent confidentiality and reproductive health vary from state to state. In many medical situations, adolescents have a right to confidentiality when seeking healthcare, particularly related to reproductive health and contraception issues. However, when sexual abuse is being investigated, the adolescent must be informed that the same confidentiality does not apply. Voluntarily disclosed information, such as consensual intercourse that the teen wishes to conceal from her parents, must be shared with investigating authorities. The practitioner should inform the teen before the interview that many issues are not confidential and the teen may wish not to discuss those issues.

As with all forensic interviews, adolescents should be interviewed alone and the questions should be open-ended and nonleading. Initial history from the teen should include the timing and chronology of the assault. An examiner must determine whether the assault has been reported to the authorities. Additional information such as timing of menstrual cycle, painful urination, and genital bleeding or discharge **(Table 11-2)** is best elicited from the patient. Other history includes any type of sexual contact, including consensual acts, contraceptive use, use of tampons, and pertinent history of anogenital injuries, surgeries, or diagnostic procedures. Previous or concurrent consensual intercourse and the time frame in which it occurred is helpful in making assessments

---

Table 11-2. Complete Evaluation of Vaginal Discharge in Teenagers

Saline Mount	*Trichomonas*	— Motile cells
	Candida	— Hyphae and yeast
	Gardnerella	— Clue cells
Gram's Stain	Gonorrhea	— Intracellular diplococci
	Gardnerella	— Clue cells
Potassium Hydroxide (KOH)	*Candida*	— Hyphae and yeast
	Gardnerella	— Whiff test
Giemsa Stain	Herpes	
Culture	*Candida*	
	Gonorrhea	
	Gardnerella	
	Chlamydia	
	Herpes	

Reprinted with permission from Wald ER. Gynecologic infections in the pediatric age group. Pediatr Infect Dis. *1984;3(3 Suppl):s12. ©Lippincott Williams & Wilkins.*

---

regarding the etiology of any injury found on examination. Examination findings alone cannot distinguish between injury resulting from consensual intercourse and injury resulting from assault. In many cases, the examiner can only conclude that injuries are present, not which activity may have resulted in the injuries. The court is the venue where the issues of consent in sexual assault are decided.

The interview of the adolescent may give the examiner a clue to the state of mind of the teen and his or her ability to tolerate the examination procedures. Assault victims may be suffering from acute traumatic stress and may display a variety of emotional behaviors. Some may have hysterical crying or giggling, whereas others may appear calm and in control. Every effort should be made to be sensitive to the victim's mental state. Male victims may be embarrassed by their inability to prevent the assault or may harbor fears of homosexuality.

The parent interview will include the patient's past medical history and family history. In addition, parents often are able to offer insight and observations not elicited from the adolescent. Although the parent may wish to be present during the examination, adolescents should be allowed to choose who accompanies them during their examinations. Some teens may be embarrassed, while some comforted by the presence of parents in such examinations.

PHYSICAL EXAMINATION

The examination procedures are explained to the teen, and he or she should be made familiar with instruments, such as the colposcope, that may be used during the examination. Teenage girls who have not experienced a gynecological examination may need preparation consisting of explanation of the examination technique and use of the vaginal speculum. The examiner also should explain the use of any culture swabs and forensic kit evidence collection that may occur in the examination. The adolescent should be encouraged to ask questions, so that any misconceptions may be clarified before the examination.

Once preparation is complete, the examination should consist of a careful head-to-toe examination of the body. During the acute evaluation, it is important to examine the skin carefully for areas of abrasion, bruising, or bite marks that may have occurred during the assault. Bite marks can prove to be valuable forensic evidence. The neck should be examined for linear bruising or ligature marks that may indicate strangulation injuries. Other areas of consideration are the oropharynx for petechiae or lacerations, the breasts for bruising or suck marks, and the hands, forearms, and knees for abrasions. (See Chapter 4, The Physical Examination in the Evaluation of Suspected Child Maltreatment: Physical Abuse and Sexual Abuse Examinations, for further details regarding examinations.)

Genital examination should include inspection of the thighs and external genitalia for injury. Common injuries in sexual assault of females include abrasions or lacerations of the fossa navicularis and posterior fourchette, bruising or petechiae of the hymen, and injury to the perineal body or labia (Girardin, Seneski, Faugno, Slaughter, & Whelan, 1997). Acute transections of the hymen can be seen. The distensibility of the hymen allows a great deal of manipulation without injury, and in many cases the examination will not reveal acute injuries. Although the use of instrumentation in prepubertal children is not recommended, the estrogenization of adolescent hymens makes the hymen more difficult to examine, and specialized techniques are applied. Cotton swabs may be used to examine the rim of the adolescent hymen by carefully running the swab over the entire rim to look for transections or acute injury. Some examiners have found the use of a Foley catheter inserted into the hymen and then distended with water or air allows better visualization of the hymenal leaflets (Persaud,

Squires, & Rubin-Remer, 1997; Starling & Jenny, 1997). Speculum examination, which may be performed to rule out injury to the vaginal vault or cervix, is also used to obtain necessary forensic evidentiary swabs from the cervix.

A thorough anal examination is required for female and male victims. The anus is examined for indications of injury or infection, such as bruises and abrasions, tears, edema, and discharge. Normal distensibility of the anus can allow penetration without injury, and most anal examinations are normal. As with genital examinations, the closer to the time of the assault that the adolescent is examined, the more likely that acute injury will be noted. Males should have a careful inspection of the penis and scrotum for signs of acute injury or infection, such as bite marks, bruising, or discharge.

The acute examination often includes collection of a forensic evidence kit for analysis by the crime laboratory. Cultures of the vagina, anus, and oral cavity should be considered in all acute assaults. A wet prep for identification of infection and sperm is recommended. Because sexually transmitted infection in the adolescent population could have been acquired before the assault, some centers do not culture adolescent assault victims for forensic purposes.

DOCUMENTATION

Careful documentation of the history and examination is imperative. Statements made by the patient should be differentiated from those made by the parent. It may be helpful to have different documentation sections to differentiate between the patient and parent histories. The history should be documented in direct quotes as much as possible. Physical examination should include the nongenital and genital portions of the examination. Documentation of the genital examination should include descriptions of all the genital structures and detailed descriptions of any injuries. Use of such terminology as "intact hymen" is insufficient, and use of specific descriptions is more appropriate. Photographic documentation of injury is standard of care in sexual assault centers but not mandatory for legal purposes. (See Chapter 9, Documentation of the Evaluation in Cases of Suspected Child Maltreatment.) Use of colposcopy improves the assessment of injury by allowing magnification and illumination of potential injuries, as well as providing the ability for photodocumentation of the examination (Slaughter & Brown, 1992). Use of 35-mm photography, digital photography, and videocolposcopy is practiced in many centers as well.

The medical provider's assessment should reflect whether the examination results are consistent with the history. A normal-appearing examination does not exclude the possibility of sexual assault because findings on physical examination depend on factors related to the circumstances during the assault. It is important for medical providers to know that *rape* is a legal term describing forced intercourse and not a medical diagnosis.

LABORATORY EVALUATION

Adolescents being evaluated for possible acute assault should be tested for STDs. Among sexually active adolescents, sexually transmitted infection could have been acquired before the assault, and STD testing is more for medical and psychological well-being than for forensic documentation. A detailed history of the assault, including the areas of the body involved, is essential to appropriate testing.

If mucous membrane contact is involved, swabs should be obtained for *Neisseria gonorrhoeae* and *Chlamydia trachomatis*. The gold standard for laboratory evaluation in sexual abuse is collection of cultures, using swabs of the genital, oral, and anal cavities as directed by history. A DNA probe for STD testing in children and adolescents, although felt to be accurate by most researchers, has not been adequately tested in children and adolescents and is currently recommended only as a secondary test to increase diagnostic sensitivity. Antigen testing is not an acceptable alternative because it has a high rate of false positive and negative results. Positive cultures for *N. gonorrhoeae* should be followed by additional confirmatory tests by the laboratory, such as carbohydrate degradation, enzyme substrate, or immunological methods. A wet prep should be collected for identification of bacterial vaginosis and *trichomonas*. At the initial examination, the concentration of infectious agents acquired in the assault may not be enough to produce a positive test. If prophylactic antibiotics are not offered for STDs during the acute examination, adolescents should be retested with a wet prep and cultures for *N. gonorrhoeae* and chlamydia 2 weeks after the assault. In centers that do not culture for STDs in acute adolescent assault, the teens are treated prophylactically with antibiotics.

Additional potentially sexually transmissible diseases to consider are syphilis, hepatitis B, and human immunodeficiency virus (HIV) infection. These blood-borne pathogens may be transmitted more frequently in adolescent victims than in children because genital penetration is more common in adolescent assault victims. Serological testing requires repeated testing over weeks to months to rule out later conversion. The Centers for Disease Control and Prevention (CDC) provides guidelines for the testing, follow-up, and treatment of STDs in sexual assault (CDC, 2002). See the CDC website for further information (http://www.cdc.gov/STD/treatment).

FORENSIC EVIDENCE COLLECTION KIT

A forensic evaluation with evidence collection generally takes place if a victim seeks medical care within 72 hours of an assault. The forensic evidence evaluation includes the collection of body fluids from the victim for identification of foreign DNA. A typical kit contains swabs and slides for vaginal, anal, and oral fluid collection. A wet prep is examined for evidence of motile or nonmotile sperm. Detailed instructions for specimen collection generally are included in the kits. Areas of contact with semen or other bodily fluids are swabbed. Bite marks should be swabbed with a saline-moistened swab for saliva. Paper bags are provided for stained clothing that may contain genetic material or may have trace debris useful for analysis. A new, clean paper bag should be used for storage of genetic material; plastic bags may cause degradation and should be avoided. A comb is provided to collect potential foreign hairs from the victim's pubic hair. Some kits require plucking or cutting head hair for comparison. Blood is collected for the victim's blood type to compare with potential foreign blood types. The kits should be labeled with the victim's name, examiner's name, and date and time of collection, and then sealed. It is important to maintain careful chain of custody to avoid contamination of evidence.

As noted previously, the advancement of DNA technology may change the time frames in which forensic evidence is collected. In cases in which seminal material could be found in the cervix, forensic kits may be collected even after several days or weeks. These procedures vary by locality and crime laboratory procedure and may change as the science advances. (See Chapter 5, Laboratory Findings, Diagnostic Testing, and Forensic Specimens in Cases of Child Sexual Abuse.)

SEXUALLY TRANSMITTED DISEASE PROPHYLAXIS

Adolescents seen in acute examinations require prophylaxis for STDs. **Table 11-3** contains recommendations on testing and treatment. After acute assault, prophylaxis is offered for gonorrhea, chlamydia, and *trichomonas* infections. In cases in which the assault places a nonimmune teen at risk for acquiring hepatitis B, immunization must be considered. Although the CDC does not recommend routine HIV prophylaxis, a consult with an infectious disease specialist may be warranted if the patient is at special risk. In more chronic sexual abuse evaluations, cultures generally are performed and the child is treated only if positive by culture (CDC, 2002).

Table 11-3. Sexually Transmitted Disease Testing and Prophylaxis		
INFECTIOUS AGENT	TEST SITE	RECOMMENDED PROPHYLAXIS
Neisseria gonorrhoeae	Culture of genitals, mouth, and/or anus	Ceftriaxone 125 mg IM in a single dose
Chlamydia trachomatis	Culture of genitals, mouth, and/or anus	Azithromycin 1 g PO in a single dose OR Doxycycline 100 mg PO twice a day for 7 days
Trichomonas vaginalis	wet prep of vaginal fluid	Metronidazole 2 g PO in a single dose
Bacterial vaginosis	wet prep of vaginal fluid	
Syphilis	serum	None recommended
Hepatitis B	serum	Consider immunization
HIV	serum	None recommended (see text)

Adapted from Centers for Disease Control and Prevention. Sexually transmitted disease treatment guidelines 2002. MMWR Morb Mortal Wkly Rep. 2002;51(RR-6):1-80. Available at: http://www.cdc.gov/ STD/treatment. Accessed February 19, 2003.

Drug dosage recommendations listed herein are those of the authors and are not endorsed by the US Public Health Service or the US Department of Health & Human Services.

PREGNANCY PROPHYLAXIS

Adolescents are at risk for unwanted pregnancy resulting from assault. Adolescent menstrual cycles are often erratic and may go unnoticed by a teen for several months. Teens who are SMR or Tanner stage 3 or above but not yet reporting the onset of menarche may be experiencing unrecognized menstrual cycles and should be tested for pregnancy. If the teen has a negative pregnancy test, prophylaxis can be offered. A contraceptive such as Ovral (50 μg ethinyl estradiol and 0.5 mg DL-norgestrel) may be given at the time of acute presentation as 2 pills acutely and 2 pills 12 hours after the first dose. The actual mechanism of pregnancy prevention for contraceptives is unknown. The majority of evidence suggests that the mechanism of action is inhibition or delay of ovulation. When started within 72 hours of the assault, it is reported to be safe and at least 75% effective (Glasier, 1997). Newer drug regimens are being approved in the United States and may supplant traditional contraceptives for use in pregnancy prophylaxis.

The decision to administer this prophylaxis must be discussed with the family because the parent or teen's ethical and moral beliefs may factor into the decision. Occasionally, a situation will arise in which the teen and parent disagree on the administration of pregnancy prophylaxis. Although laws pertaining to adolescent confidentiality, reproductive health, and rights to contraception vary from state to state, mature minors in the United States have the right to obtain birth control without specific parental consent (Levesque, 2000). Therefore, in cases in which the adolescent's wishes do not correspond to the parents' wishes, the rights of the adolescent generally prevail.

MEDICAL EVALUATION OF NONACUTE SEXUAL ABUSE

Adolescents may delay disclosure of sexual abuse or assault for a variety of reasons. They may feel ashamed or helpless or their safety may be compromised if they disclose. An adolescent may make a spontaneous disclosure to a friend, relative, or counselor months to years after abuse has occurred. Sexual abuse may manifest itself as depression or school failure, chronic vague medical complaints, or onset of substance abuse. Still others may have feelings of helplessness, anger, and grief. **Table 11-4** lists common nonspecific presenting complaints of sexually abused adolescents (Hunter, Kilstrom, & Loda, 1985).

Providers should recognize this as a time of crisis for most adolescents, and a multidisciplinary approach to care is optimal. Referral to a center that specializes in sexual abuse evaluation is preferable. If this is not an option, a social worker or child psychologist with experience in abuse dynamics should perform a mental health evaluation. Medical providers should be aware of referral resources for psychological intervention.

At presentation for medical care, the teen and parents should be interviewed separately to determine the nature and extent of the abuse and to determine if CPS or law enforcement has been involved. Careful history may elicit a medical concern for STDs. The adolescent or his or her parents may harbor concerns such as unwanted pregnancy, fear of genital disfigurement, or fear of future infertility, which should be addressed in a sensitive, age-appropriate manner.

Medical examination in the nonacute evaluation is similar to that in the acute evaluation. A complete examination is performed. Examination findings usually do not include acute injury such as bruising and abrasions, but may include healing or healed transections of the hymen or other genital structures. Often the examinations are normal. Normal examinations may be the result of complete healing of injury; however, sexual abuse of the adolescent anogenital structures may not produce injury at all because of the elasticity of the hymen and anus. Cultures often are obtained in cases involving genital-genital, genital-anal, or genital-oral contact **(Table 11-5)**. In nonacute cases in which a great deal of time has passed, the biochemical markers on the skin and in the anogenital area may have degraded (Duenhoelter, Stone, Santos-Ramos, & Scott, 1978). A forensic evidence collection kit is usually unnecessary. However, the availability of DNA amplification technology has expanded the time frame for collection of forensic evidence, and individual consideration should be made for each case (Ledray & Netzel, 1997). If the clothing worn during the assault has not been laundered, this may have forensic value and should be collected as evidence for law enforcement.

SEQUELAE OF SEXUAL ABUSE

Adolescent sexual abuse and assault often result in severe psychological trauma that may continue into adulthood. Many adolescent victims experience feelings of embarrassment, guilt, grief, and fear. These feelings cause reluctance to report the assault. A violation of trust may be experienced if the adolescent is a victim of date rape or had a social relationship with the assailant. Adolescent sexual abuse victims may blame themselves, especially if alcohol or drugs were involved or if they felt that they encouraged the act in any way with voluntary sexual play or provocative dress. Adolescents who were abused as children are more likely to abuse tobacco and alcohol, attempt suicide, and exhibit violent or criminal behavior (US Preventive Services Taskforce, 1996).

Table 11-4. Common Presenting Complaints of Sexually Abused Adolescents

PHYSICAL SIGNS AND SYMPTOMS

Genital discharge and bleeding	Genital skin lesions
Genital itching	Genital or urethral trauma
Pregnancy	STDs
Recurrent urinary tract infections	Other genital infections
Abdominal pain	Fatigue or exhaustion
Seizures	Sleep disturbances
Appetite disturbance	Drug overdose

PSYCHOSOMATIC DISORDERS

Diffuse somatic complaints	Abdominal pain
Anorexia	Headaches
Hysterical or conversion reactions	

SEXUAL PROBLEMS

Promiscuity or prostitution	Sexual dysfunction
Sexual perpetration of others	Fear of intimacy
Sexual revictimization	

SOCIAL OR BEHAVIORAL PROBLEMS

School adjustment problems	Family conflicts
Mood swings	Neurotic or conduct disorders
Phobias, avoidance behaviors	Social withdrawal
Aggressive behavior	Impulsive behavior
Truancy or runaway behavior	Substance abuse
Self-mutilating behavior	Suicidal ideation, gestures, or attempts

OTHER PSYCHOLOGICAL PROBLEMS

Excessive guilt	Anxiety
Irritability	Depression
Feelings of helplessness	Self-hate, self-blame
Low self-esteem	Mistrust
Amnesia	Hyperalertness
Fear of criticism or praise	Terrified of rejection
Rage	Flashbacks
Obsessive ideas	Dissociation

OTHER

Asymptomatic sibling of a victim or association with a known perpetrator

Adapted from Hunter RS, Kilstrom N, Loda F. Sexually abused children: identifying masked presentations in a medical setting. Child Abuse Negl. *1985;9:17-25.*

Consequences of adolescent sexual abuse or assault include promiscuity, pregnancy, prostitution, running away from home, and attempted suicide. The US Department of Health & Human Services estimates that annually 730 000 to 1.3 million youths age 12 to 21 years run away from home. Although many return within 30 days, approximately 25% will become permanently homeless. More than half of those who run away list sexual abuse as one of the precipitating causes. Recent estimates suggest that 50% of runaways engage in prostitution or survival sex, 50% have significant alcohol problems, and 80% use illicit drugs (MacKenzie, 1992). To survive, most will participate in other illegal activities, such as using and dealing drugs, selling sex for drugs, engaging in pornography, and theft. Many are homeless. The risk of unprotected sex is apparent in increased rates of STDs and pregnancy in the homeless adolescent population.

The reaction of medical providers, parents, and other adults can be more psychologically damaging than the physical aspects of sexual abuse. If adolescents disclose abuse and are blamed, disbelieved, or unprotected, they may recant their disclosures. This leaves them vulnerable to repeated abuse and prevents them from getting necessary psychological intervention.

Posttraumatic stress disorder (PTSD), cognitive distortions, altered emotionality, dissociation, impaired self-reference, and avoidance are major types of psychological disturbances frequently found in adolescents who have been abused. Posttraumatic stress refers to certain enduring psychological symptoms that occur in reaction to the abuse, with sudden and uncontrollable flashbacks being the most disturbing and intrusive symptom. The repetitive intrusive thoughts that include themes of danger, humiliation, sex, and guilt make it difficult to concentrate for extended periods or have a normal mental life (Briere & Elliott, 1993). PTSD is thought to affect at least 80% of all adolescent rape victims (Pynoos & Nader, 1992).

After sexual abuse, adolescents may develop distorted self-perceptions and assumptions about themselves, others, and their environment. These cognitive distortions cause adolescents to underestimate their self-worth, resulting in feelings of guilt, self-blame, and low self-esteem (Briere & Elliott, 1993). Adolescents with sexual abuse histories are also more likely to have major depression (Lanktree, Briere, & Zaidi, 1991). Other psychological and behavioral complaints include aggression, anxiety, eating disorders, and school failures. See **Table 11-4** for other nonspecific symptoms.

Table 11-5. Culture Criteria for Adolescent Sexual Assault/Abuse

— All acute assaults

— Adolescents with allegation of genital-genital, genital-oral, or genital-anal contact

— Adolescents abused by unknown perpetrators or perpetrators with risk factors for STDs

— Adolescents with a genital or anal discharge

Note: some centers do not culture acute assaults; see text.

Prevention and Anticipatory Guidance

Adolescents may delay seeking healthcare because of embarrassment, shame, guilt, denial, and issues surrounding their right to confidentiality. Medical evaluation should include not only adolescent well-care, but also an understanding of the dynamics of adolescent risk-taking behaviors. The practitioner should perform a complete health assessment to include analysis of physical and psychological growth; immunization history; sexual practices, including risk for HIV, STDs, and pregnancy; and assessment of the need for psychological intervention.

Medical providers treating adolescents are in a unique situation to provide preventive services (Kaplan et al., 2001). Teens should be informed about normal growth and development; screened for behavioral and medical risks, including dating violence; and given guidance on how to avoid unhealthy behaviors and relationships. Providers need to be aware of local community resources for the psychological treatment of sexually abused adolescents.

Discussion of sexual abuse with adolescents should include prevention strategies for sexual assault. The teen should be aware of the prevalence and nature of date and acquaintance rape. Jenny (1989) studied 100 adolescent female rape victims and found that most sexual assaults occurred at night when the adolescent voluntarily agreed to go out with a young man she had known less than 24 hours, was impaired by drugs or alcohol, or was hitchhiking. This information should be shared with teens. Adolescents need to know that they have the right to say "no" in any situation. Providers need to emphasize the importance of adolescents keeping themselves safe and reducing the risk of personal harm. They should avoid the use of alcohol or drugs, which can interfere with judgment. They should avoid abusive or disrespectful partners. Adolescents should know that they are vulnerable to assault and try to avoid risky situations, such as walking alone at night, being alone in poorly lit areas, and use of alcohol and other substances (American Academy of Pediatrics Committee on Adolescence, 1994).

Summary

Adolescents present a unique population for the medical provider. An understanding of sexual maturity level and risk-taking behaviors of adolescents is necessary to provide the proper framework for the evaluation of sexual abuse and assault. The evaluation of the adolescent should include a sensitive history and thorough medical examination, followed by appropriate mental health evaluation. Medical providers possess the unique ability to provide education and intervention for adolescents to help treat and prevent sexual abuse.

References

ACOG Committee on Adolescent Health Care. Adolescent acquaintance rape. ACOG committee opinion: Committee on Adolescent Health Care Number 122—May 1993. *Int J Gynaecol Obstet.* 1993;42:209-211.

American Academy of Pediatrics Committee on Adolescence. Sexual assault and the adolescent. *Pediatrics.* 1994;94:761-765.

Bechtel K, Podrazik M. Evaluation of the adolescent rape victim. *Pediatr Clin North Am.* 1999;46:809-823, xii.

Briere J. Types and forms of child maltreatment. In: Briere J, ed. *Child Abuse Trauma: Theory and Treatment of the Lasting Effects.* Thousand Oaks, Calif: Sage Publications; 1992:3-18.

Briere J, Elliott DM. Sexual abuse, family environment, and psychological symptoms: on the validity of statistical control. *J Consult Clin Psychol.* 1993;61:284-288;

discussion 289-290.

Centers for Disease Control and Prevention. Sexually transmitted disease treatment guidelines 2002. *MMWR Morb Mortal Wkly Rep.* 2002;51(RR-6):1-80. Available at: http://www.cdc.gov/STD/treatment. Accessed February 19, 2003.

Duenhoelter JH, Stone IC, Santos-Ramos R, Scott DE. Detection of seminal fluid constituents after alleged sexual assault. *J Forensic Sci.* 1978;23:824-829.

Elliot DM, Briere J. Forensic sexual abuse evaluations: disclosures and symptomatology. *Behav Sci Law.* 1994;12:261-277.

Faller KC. Characteristics of a clinical sample of sexually abused children: how boy and girl victims differ. *Child Abuse Negl.* 1989;13:281-291.

Finkelhor D, Baron L. Risk factors for child sexual abuse. *J Interpers Violence.* 1986;1:43-71.

Finkelhor D, Hotaling G, Lewis IA, Smith C. Sexual abuse in a national survey of adult men and women: prevalence, characteristics, and risk factors. *Child Abuse Negl.* 1990;14:19-28.

Girardin BW, Seneski PC, Faugno DK, Slaughter L, Whelan M. *Color Atlas of Sexual Assault.* St. Louis, Mo: Mosby; 1997.

Glasier A. Emergency postcoital contraception. *N Engl J Med.* 1997;337:1058-1064.

Holmes WC, Slap GB. Sexual abuse of boys: definition, prevalence, correlates, sequelae, and management. *JAMA.* 1998;280:1855-1862.

Hunter RS, Kilstrom N, Loda F. Sexually abused children: identifying masked presentations in a medical setting. *Child Abuse Negl.* 1985;9:17-25.

Hymel KP, Jenny C. Child sexual abuse. *Pediatr Rev.* 1996;17:236-249; quiz 249-250.

Jenny C. Adolescent risk-taking behavior and the occurrence of sexual assault. *Am J Dis Child.* 1989;142:770-772.

Jenny C, Roesler TA, Poyer KL. Are children at risk for sexual abuse by homosexuals? *Pediatrics.* 1994;94:41-44.

Kaplan DW, Feinstein RA, Fisher MM, et al. Care of the adolescent sexual assault victim. *Pediatrics.* 2001;107:1476-1479.

Lanktree CB, Briere J, Zaidi LY. Incidence and impacts of sexual abuse in a child outpatient sample: the role of direct inquiry. *Child Abuse Negl.* 1991;15:447-453.

Ledray LE, Netzel L. DNA evidence collection. *J Emerg Nurs.* 1997;23:156-158.

Levesque RJR. *Adolescents, Sex, and the Law: Preparing Adolescents for Responsible Citizenship.* Washington, DC: American Psychological Association; 2000.

MacKenzie R. At-risk youth. In: McAnarney ER, Kreipe RE, Orr DP, Comerci GD, eds. *Textbook of Adolescent Medicine.* Philadelphia, Pa: WB Saunders; 1992:237-240.

Marshall WA, Tanner JM. Variations in the pattern of pubertal changes in boys. *Arch Dis Child.* 1970;45:22.

Mills CS, Granoff BJ. Date and acquaintance rape among a sample of college students. *Soc Work.* 1992;37:504-509.

Parrot A. Acquaintance rape among adolescents: identifying risk groups and intervention strategies. *J Soc Work Hum Sexuality.* 1989;8:47-61.

Peipert JF, Domagalski LR. Epidemiology of adolescent sexual assault. *Obstet Gynecol.* 1994;84:867-871.

Persaud DI, Squires JE, Rubin-Remer D. Use of Foley catheter to examine estrogenized hymens for evidence of sexual abuse. *J Pediatr Adolesc Gynecol.* 1997;10:83-85.

Pynoos RS, Nader K. Post-traumatic stress disorder. In: McAnarney ER, Kreipe RE, Orr DP, Comerci GD, eds. *Textbook of Adolescent Medicine.* Philadelphia, Pa: WB Saunders; 1992:1003-1009.

Quint EH. Gynecological health care for adolescents with developmental disabilities. *Adolesc Med.* 1999;10:221-229, vi.

Rainey DY, Stevens-Simon C, Kaplan DW. Are adolescents who report prior sexual abuse at higher risk for pregnancy? *Child Abuse Negl.* 1995;19:1283-1288.

Reif CJ, Elster AB. Adolescent preventive services. *Prim Care.* 1998;25:1-21.

Rennison CM. *Criminal Victimization 1998: Changes 1997-1998 With Trends 1993-1998.* Washington, DC: Bureau of Justice Statistics; 1999.

Rickert VI, Wiemann CM. Date rape among adolescents and young adults. *J Pediatr Adolesc Gynecol.* 1998;11:167-175.

Schwartz RH, Weaver AB. Rohypnol, the date rape drug. *Clin Pediatr (Phila).* 1998;37:321.

Segal BM, Stewart JC. Substance use and abuse in adolescence: an overview. *Child Psychiatry Hum Dev.* 1996;26:193.

Seidel H, Ball J, Dains J, Benedict G. *Mosby's Guide to Physical Examination.* 3rd ed. St. Louis, Mo: Mosby; 1995:84-130.

Slap GB. Normal physiological and psychosocial growth in the adolescent. *J Adolesc Health Care.* 1986;7(suppl 6):13S-23S.

Slaughter L, Brown CR. Colposcopy to establish physical findings in rape victims. *Am J Obstet Gynecol.* 1992;166(pt 1):83-86.

Starling SP, Jenny C. Forensic examination of adolescent female genitalia: the Foley catheter technique. *Arch Pediatr Adolesc Med.* 1997;151:102-103.

US Department of Health & Human Services. National Center on Child Abuse and Neglect. *Child Maltreatment 1997: Reports From the States to the National Child Abuse and Neglect Data System.* Washington, DC: US Government Printing Office; 1999.

US Preventive Services Taskforce. Guidelines. Section I. Screening. Part I. Mental health disorders and substance abuse. *Guide to Clinical Preventive Services.* 2nd ed. Baltimore, Md: Williams & Wilkins; 1996.

van Wieringen JC. *Growth Diagrams 1965 Netherlands. Second National Survey on 0–24-year-olds.* The Netherlands: Wolters-Noordhoff Groningen; 1971.

Wald ER. Gynecologic infections in the pediatric age group. *Pediatr Infect Dis.* 1984;3 (3 Suppl):s12.

Wheeler MD. Physical changes of puberty. *Endocrinol Metab Clin North Am.* 1991;20:1-14.

Willott GM, Allard JE. Spermatozoa—their persistence after sexual intercourse. *Forensic Sci Int.* 1982;19:133-154.

Chapter 12

MUNCHAUSEN SYNDROME BY PROXY

Julie Pape, CPNP
Eileen R. Giardino, PhD, RN, CRNP
Angelo P. Giardino, MD, PhD, FAAP

Munchausen syndrome by proxy (MSBP) is a form of child abuse that occurs when a caregiver either fabricates or induces illness in another person. The offending caregiver is usually the mother, while the victim is usually a child. MSBP typically affects children by their third birthday and takes an average of 15 months to diagnose. MSBP has a 75% fatality rate when the children are young and the caregiver induces the symptoms, especially suffocation. The term Munchausen syndrome by proxy refers to the child's victimization, the caregiver's disorder, and the interactions that occur between caregiver and child (Ayoub & Alexander, 1998).

HISTORY

A 1951 article titled "Munchausen's Syndrome" described Munchausen as a common syndrome in which the patient showing the syndrome is admitted to a hospital with an apparent acute illness (Asher, 1951). The patient provides a history mostly made up of falsehoods and, on closer look, has been successful in deceiving an astonishing number of hospitals and professionals. The patient usually discharges himself or herself from the hospital against medical advice and is usually only discovered when someone recognizes the patient or the patient's story as one witnessed at a different hospital. Asher identified one of the possible motives for this syndrome as a desire of the patient to be the center of interest and attention.

Twenty-six years later, Meadow (1977) described Munchausen syndrome by proxy as another expression of the dynamics seen in Munchausen's syndrome by highlighting 2 case reports. In both cases, the child's mother provided false stories and altered specimens even with close supervision, causing unpleasant and serious consequences for the children. Both children developed illness, and the second child died.

Meadow's description of MSBP recognizes that a syndrome is a cluster of signs and/or symptoms that may have many different etiologies. The following 4 aspects constitute the syndrome cluster:

1. Illness in a child that is simulated (faked) and/or produced by a parent or someone who is *in loco parentis*

2. Presentation of the child for medical assessment and care, usually persistently, often resulting in multiple medical procedures

3. Denial of knowledge by the perpetrator as to the etiology of the child's illness

4. Acute symptoms and signs of the child abate when the child is separated from the perpetrator

Meadow's early descriptions of MSBP continue to provide useful and necessary information regarding common characteristics in these cases.

Belief that MSBP occurs may be one of the most challenging dilemmas for healthcare providers to overcome. Bursch, Weinberg, and Shilkoff (1996) found that although 95% of the pediatric nurses responded it was "very important" to know about MSBP, only about half of the respondents had heard of MSBP. Most pediatric nurses had learned about MSBP from direct experience (23.5%). The challenge, therein, lies with the first case nurses may encounter. If recognition is most often based on past experience, this uphill battle is a dynamic that must be factored in during the diagnostic process. Knowledgeable professionals must take time early on to discuss the dynamics of MSBP with other members of the multidisciplinary team so everyone is able to determine that their approach is based on the most current information possible.

VICTIM AND PERPETRATOR CLASSIFICATION

MSBP is also known more formally as factitious disorder by proxy (FDP) as classified by the American Psychiatric Association (APA, 2000) in the *Diagnostic and Statistical Manual of Mental Disorders* (DSM-IV-TR). The perpetrator who inflicts false signs and symptoms on a child may be diagnosed with FDP. The DSM-IV-TR criteria for FDP are as follows (APA, 2000, p. 783):

— Intentional production or feigning of physical or psychological signs or symptoms in another person who is under the individual's care.

— The motivation for the perpetrator's behavior is to assume the sick role by proxy.

— External incentives for the behavior (such as economic gain) are absent.

— The behavior is not better accounted for by another mental disorder.

The DSM-IV-TR discusses internal and external incentives that motivate a person to engage in harmful, manipulative, and deceptive behaviors that place a child at risk for illness and death (Ayoub & Alexander, 1998). The child is a victim of this form of maltreatment secondary to the illness, impairment, or symptom complex that is imposed on him or her. Ayoub and Alexander (1998) propose that this form of maltreatment be designated as abuse by pediatric condition falsification (PCF) and describe the following forms of deception related to the child's condition:

— Directly causing the healthcare condition

— Over-reporting or under-reporting of signs and symptoms

— Creating a false appearance of signs and symptoms

— Coaching the victim (or others) to misrepresent the victim as ill

Cases involving this form of illness fabrication typically have the parent as perpetrator and the child as victim. However, MSBP may be seen in older individuals and in other people in a dependent situation, such as adults with special needs. In any event, by whatever terminology is used, this phenomenon represents a serious healthcare emergency that requires careful evaluation and intervention (APA, 2000; Ayoub & Alexander, 1998; Pasqualone & Fitzgerald, 1999).

MEDICAL HISTORY

A most difficult challenge in the diagnosis of MSBP is the absence of an accurate history as given by the caregiver. The presenting history in cases of suspected MSBP is often not accurate, just as the history may not be true or accurate in cases of child physical abuse. The caretaker either misrepresents or creates symptoms the child is not really experiencing naturally. The history is of paramount importance in MSBP because it provides the foundation for appropriate testing and eventual diagnosis. Healthcare providers must at least consider the possibility that when faced with a diagnostic dilemma, the given history may not be accurate.

Obtaining an accurate history in cases of MSBP proves challenging to providers. Many perpetrators of MSBP are described as likeable, caring, knowledgeable, and attentive parents. It can be difficult for nurses and other healthcare providers to believe that the caregiver may be misrepresenting the child's history or inducing symptoms. It can be confusing to talk with the parent who may be the perpetrator of MSBP because he or she reports information that is complicated to follow chronologically, difficult to corroborate, and simply atypical. Many of the children who suffer from MSBP are described as seriously ill, chronically ill, or having special healthcare needs. It can take a great deal of determination to obtain an accurate current and past medical history.

The caregiver may give a history of a child who has physical conditions such as allergies, seizures, apnea, and various gastrointestinal problems (Ayoub & Alexander, 1998). The child may present with problems that are not backed up by the findings on physical examination or illnesses that do not have a typical presentation. Other conditions such as delayed healing, failure to thrive (FTT), nonaccidental injuries, or high infection rates are common presentations (Ayoub & Alexander, 1998).

Primary providers should personally review old medical records of the child and other family members as pertinent and not rely on the caregiver to reflect the contents of those records. A caregiver who reports records were "lost" should not be believed at face value; rather, members of the healthcare team should pursue the lost records so they can be properly reviewed.

THE MULTIDISCIPLINARY TEAM APPROACH

The approach to the caregiver in cases of suspected MSBP is key. If the healthcare provider confronts the caregiver too early about suspicion concerning the story, the caregiver typically removes the child from that practice or even the broader medical community in the geographical area. MSBP often takes months to years to diagnose accurately because caregivers frequently leave when suspicion mounts (Rosenberg, 1987). Such actions place children in harm's way because the caregiver's needs outweigh those of the child. Healthcare providers should refrain from confronting the caregiver until the community-based multidisciplinary team (MDT) has met and is able to determine a fully informed course of action.

Much care should be taken, with speed, when children are young and reported symptoms are significant. For example, the greatest fatality rate occurs in children who are victims of either suffocation or poisoning (Rosenberg, 1987). The stakes are high when symptoms are not only reported but also induced. Schreier and Libow (1993a, 1993b) estimate that nearly 10% of mothers who deliberately induce illness in their children ultimately kill them.

Greatest success in cases of MSBP is met when all MDT members have reviewed the information relevant to the case. Failure of the MDT members to effectively communicate leaves the offending parent the opportunity to assume control of the situation. Even if a formal report has not been made to child protective services (CPS) or law enforcement, representatives from each of these agencies, as well as prosecution, mental health care, and other members of the medical diagnostic team should collaborate to determine the best course of action for that particular case. Traditional notification may need to be amended in situations requiring such a high degree of confidentiality. The team must respond rapidly and plan quickly as to how the case should proceed. The immediate and long-term safety needs of a child must be discussed with all team members because MSBP cases are too complicated to have any one agency or professional act in isolation.

It may jeopardize the child's safety if an agency acts independently or another professional informs the family of the concern. Of 117 cases reviewed in the literature, 10 children (9%) died at the hands of their mothers (Rosenberg, 1987). "In 20% of the child death cases, the parents had been confronted with the diagnosis of MSBP and the children had been sent home to them, subsequently to die" (Rosenberg, 1987). Timing and collaboration of all team members may be the main tools healthcare professionals can use to save the child's life.

DOCUMENTATION

Documentation of a child's history and presenting physical symptoms is necessary in providing effective healthcare. In MSBP, patterns regarding the manifestation of possible symptoms, as well as the consistency of the child's physical presentation in relation to the history, provide the necessary information to determine the reliability of the history.

Documentation must be as objective and specific as possible. For example:

> "Mother reports the child stopped breathing at home. Mother reports she provided rescue breathing until the paramedics arrived. Mother reports prior to incident, child was happy and playing on living room floor."

Less specific documentation is as follows:

> "Child apparently stopped breathing at home. Paramedics responded."

In cases of suspected suffocation, additional historical information should include the condition of the child when he or she began breathing (e.g., choking, gasping, spontaneous breathing).

As with all cases of suspected child abuse, the provider must ask and then document whether anyone else responded to or observed the event. Interviewing witnesses separately is important to corroborate information whenever possible.

As with any other diagnostic process, the list of differential diagnoses must be as complete as possible. For example, a differential diagnosis for apnea must include MSBP. MSBP must also be considered in cases of sudden onset of apnea, apnea that has only been documented by one caregiver, and apnea that occurs in an older child (6 months or older) with no documented underlying condition.

There are 5 main consequences for a child falsely labeled as ill, as follows:

1. The child will receive needless and harmful investigations and treatments.

2. A genuine disease may be induced by the mother's actions, for example, renal failure as a result of regular injections of allergic agents given to cause fever.

3. The child may die suddenly as a result of the mother misjudging the degree of insult. For example, mothers who partially suffocate their children to cause unconsciousness may smother the child for too long, thereby causing brain damage or death.

4. The child may develop chronic invalidism because he or she accepts the illness story and believes himself or herself to be disabled and unable to attend school, work, or even walk.

5. The child may develop Munchausen syndrome as an adult; the child has learned and then taken on the lying behavior of the mother (Meadow, 1989).

Table 12-1. Characteristics of Munchausen Syndrome by Proxy

DIAGNOSTIC CHARACTERISTICS

— Illness in a child factitiously reported, simulated, or produced by parent/primary caretaker

— There may be history of unusual illness in other siblings or parent

— Medical complaints may be common or bizarre in nature

— Child's illness defies diagnosis or control of symptoms (e.g., the worst case of its kind, or failure to establish diagnosis at multiple healthcare sites or providers)

— Acute symptoms or signs abate when child is separated from the parent

CHARACTERISTICS OF PARENT PERPETRATOR

— Most often mother

— Father distant, uninvolved, marriage may be troubled

— Mother friendly, calm, cooperative and well liked: a "model parent"

— May have medical background

— May have frequent symptoms, possibly Munchausen syndrome

— Spends long hours at bedside or in the hospital

Reprinted with permission from Ludwig S. The role of the physician. In: Levin AV, Sheridan M, eds. Munchausen Syndrome by Proxy: Issues in Diagnosis and Treatment. *New York, NY: Lexington Books; 1995:289. ©1995 John Wiley & Sons, Inc. Reprinted by permission of John Wiley & Sons, Inc.*

The role of the primary provider is not to figure out how the caregiver could have created the symptoms but rather to recognize when the history and symptoms do not fit. It is essential for a healthcare provider to entertain the possibility that MSBP does happen and that it should be considered in the diagnostic process. **Table 12-1** (Ludwig, 1995) lists the diagnostic characteristics of MSBP. Once the provider is well educated on MSBP characteristics, methods of fabrication and corresponding diagnostic strategies are useful resources (Rosenberg, 1987) **(Table 12-2)**.

HOSPITALIZATION

A telling sign of possible MSBP often occurs when the child is separated from the primary caregiver. Frequently, symptoms disappear when the child is removed from his or her natural environment. Although separation may be a useful approach, it often leaves the team with the knowledge that the caregiver may be harming the child but without any concrete information to prove the suspicion (Foreman & Farsides, 1993). Hospitalization can provide a more diagnostic atmosphere, resulting in a better outcome for the child than separation through foster care. Although separation through foster care may be useful with certain age groups and in certain situations, it will not provide the same level of certainty as covert video surveillance.

COVERT VIDEO SURVEILLANCE

Covert video surveillance has become a useful and enlightening tool during the diagnostic process. However, its use should not be undertaken without careful

PRESENTATION	METHOD OF SIMULATION AND/OR PRODUCTION	METHOD OF DIAGNOSIS
Table 12-2. Munchausen Syndrome by Proxy: Methods of Fabrication and Corresponding Diagnostic Strategies		
Bleeding	— Warfarin poisoning	— Toxicology screen
	— Phenolphthalein poisoning	— Diapers positive
	— Exogenous blood applied	— Blood group typing (major and minor) — Cr labeling of erythrocytes
	— Exsanguination of child	— Single blind study — Mother caught in the act
	— Addition of other substances (paint, cocoa, dyes)	— Testing; washing
Seizures	— Lying	— Other MSBP features/retrospective
	— Poisoning — phenothiazines — hydrocarbons — salt — imipramine	— Analysis of blood, urine, IV fluid, milk
	— Suffocation/carotid sinus pressure	— Witnessed — Forensic photos of pressure points
CNS Depression	— Drugs — Lomotil — insulin — chloral hydrate — barbiturates — aspirin — diphenhydramine — tricyclic antidepressants — acetaminophen — hydrocarbons	— Assays blood, gastric contents, urine, IV fluid; analysis of insulin type
	— Suffocation	— See "Apnea," "Seizures"
Apnea	— Manual suffocation	— Patient with pinch marks on nose — Video camera (hidden) — Mother caught — Diagnosis of exclusion
	— Poisoning — imipramine — hydrocarbon	— Toxicology (gastric/blood) — Chromatography of IV fluid
	— Lying	— Diagnostic process of elimination

(continued)

Table 12-2. *(continued)*

PRESENTATION	METHOD OF SIMULATION AND/OR PRODUCTION	METHOD OF DIAGNOSIS
Diarrhea	— Phenolphthalein/other laxative poisoning — Salt poisoning	— Stool/diaper positive — Assay of formula/gastric content
Vomiting	— Emetic poisoning — Lying	— Assay for drug — Admit to hospital
Fever	— Falsifying temperature — Falsifying chart	— Careful charting, rechecking — Careful charting, rechecking — Duplicating temperature chart in nursing station
Rash	— Drug poisoning — Scratching — Caustic applied/painting skin	— Assay — Diagnosis of exclusion — Assay/wash off

Reprinted with permission from Rosenberg D. Web of deceit: a literature review of Munchausen syndrome by proxy. Child Abuse Negl. *1987;11:554.*

thought and planning. Video surveillance of a caregiver's interactions with a child is associated with the Fourth Amendment to the *Constitution of the United States*, which states that probable cause is needed for the court to issue the use of surveillance (Morrison, 1999). Generally, the rules for wiretapping cover the use of video surveillance. Institutional protocols must be in place to ensure video monitoring is used only when most useful and appropriate. Much like a magnetic resonance imaging (MRI) scan, covert surveillance should not be used for every child who comes to a clinic or hospital, but rather is used according to specific clinical criteria to provide additional information for the provider to make a diagnosis.

Southall, Plunkett, Banks, Falkov, and Samuels (1997) studied 39 children in whom covert video surveillance was used during the diagnostic process. Thirty-six of the children were referred for apparent life-threatening events (ALTEs), one with suspected epilepsy, one with FTT, and one with suspected strangulation. Covert video surveillance documented abuse in 85% of the cases, with intentional suffocation observed in 30 of the children.

Covert video surveillance certainly has importance in possible MSBP. However, the decision to use this approach to aid in the diagnosis of MSBP must be made carefully and after appropriate consultation and discussion. Covert video surveillance should not replace careful history taking, thorough examination, or consultation and collaboration with the members of the entire MDT. Forensic pediatricians must be consulted to be certain that nurses, physicians, and staff follow the most up-to-date approaches. In addition, protocols must be in place to review video documentation, determine the level of monitoring necessary for the child's safety, determine who provides the monitoring, and decide how intervention will occur on a child's behalf if the situation becomes dangerous.

Recommendations for the use and handling of covert electronic surveillance to ensure that the process is legal and ethical are as follows (Catlin, 1997):

— Obtain court order for installation and nonconsensual entry

— State the particulars for which staff are looking

— Describe the need for video surveillance

— Set/restrict time frame for surveillance

— Observe only pertinent activity and prevent observation of noncriminal innocent activity

— Camera is used only when the suspected individual is in the area of observation

— Provide security for handling and sealing of videos

— Contact the hospital's risk management personnel and attorney to ensure proper use of technology

Southall et al. (1997) found that although measures were in place to respond to the concern of apnea or cyanotic episodes, other unpredictable events required modification of the initial protocol for covert video surveillance. In one case of suspected intentional suffocation, the child's mother was observed breaking the infant's arm. This was an unexpected form of abuse, and the institution amended protocols to address responses required in different and unpredictable situations.

Because of the nature of MSBP, as well as the role of the nurse toward patient and family, dilemmas arise when dealing with possible detection of the situation. Brown (1997) describes 4 dilemmas facing nurses:

1. Confidentiality issues regarding invasion of privacy of parents and patients

2. Deceptive measures in dealing with the parent(s)

3. Child endangerment while watching and waiting for enough time to elapse on tape while a caregiver is harming a child

4. Staff division resulting from anger, disbelief, and shock of believing that caregiver is possibly harming the child

Hospitalization has some benefits for the child and family as the diagnostic process occurs. Medical diagnostic testing to rule out organic disorders that may be causing the symptoms often requires at least a short hospital stay. Additionally, trained healthcare observers can provide a great deal of objective information to aid in the diagnostic process. The volume of information a hospital stay can provide far outweighs multiple office visits where concerns are documented but events are unlikely. Care should be taken to use hospitalization as a part of the plan of care in situations in which this level of observation is required.

Uneventful hospital stays should not be the sole determining factor in assessing a child's long-term safety. For example, if a 6-month-old child is reported to have a sudden onset of unexplained apnea episodes and the medical workup reveals a healthy child with no explanation for the episodes, the healthcare provider may consider hospitalizing the child to provide a higher level of skilled observation. If the child has no apnea episodes during the hospital stay, the question arises as to how assured medical care providers should be as to the safety or danger of the child when discharged to the same home environment. Southall et al. (1997) identified that "thirty-nine patients undergoing covert video surveillance had forty-one siblings, twelve of whom had previously died unexpectedly. Eleven of the sibling deaths had been classified as sudden infant death syndrome but after covert video surveillance, four parents admitted to suffocating eight of these siblings" (p.735). Predicting when the situation may become life threatening to the child is difficult. A simple conversation doubting the reality of the events reported may be enough to tip the scale for the abuser to induce an event.

It is relatively common for the symptoms to continue during the hospital stay. Twenty-five percent of cases reported involved simulation of symptoms only (Rosenberg, 1987). In 72% of these cases, the simulation continued during the hospitalization. More dramatic were the cases of produced illness (50%) in which the production of symptoms occurred in 95% of the cases while the child was hospitalized. In 25% of the cases, simulation and production of illness were involved and continued at a rate of 84% while the child was hospitalized.

The perpetrator of MSBP in about 98% of cases is the biological mother (Rosenberg, 1987). She is often described as likeable, caring, attentive, friendly, and a "model parent." The dynamic of multiple hospitalizations, primary nursing, and an attentive parent make the barrier of belief in the possibility difficult. Providers must be prepared to identify and discuss these dynamics with nursing staff who have much more exposure to the child and family. Nursing staff may become divided in its belief and support of a particular approach during the diagnostic process. Discussion of any suspicions regarding the caregivers or the concerns of the case in public places in a hospital is tenuous and unethical. Furthermore, if the perpetrator suspects or hears of staff suspicions, this could further jeopardize the child's immediate and long-term safety. An offender who is aware of suspicions may react by relocating the child and other family members. Nursing staff must be aware of the status of the monitoring when covert video surveillance is used to maintain clearly defined roles and appropriate response and interaction with the child and the family.

PARENTAL PROFILES

Initially, biological mothers were most often found to be the perpetrators of MSBP. Meadow (1998) reports that in the first 10 years of dealing with these families, he did not encounter a single case in which the father was the perpetrator. However, he further states that over the past 10 years, he has been involved in 15 cases involving a male perpetrator. Parnell and Day (1998) provide some insight to this dynamic in that many of the earlier cases of MSBP are more accurately identified as repetitive physical abuse that was unrecognized by the medical community.

One common characteristic of the MSBP perpetrator is that many suffer from personality disorders. Some personality disorders recognized in MSBP have been noted in the literature: hysterical personality disorder was noted several times, and borderline personality, narcissistic personality disorder, and unspecified personality disorder were noted occasionally. In several accounts, the perpetrator and her husband were described as emotionally distant (Rosenberg, 1987). Additionally, psychiatric illness, past histories of abuse, parent-child symbiosis, social disadvantage, and perpetrators who have studied or worked in the healthcare field are common elements. However, every individual with these attributes will not become a perpetrator of

MSBP (Fisher & Mitchell, 1995; Fisher, Mitchell, Meadow, & Morley, 1995). People with these described characteristics may function normally for many years but then be unable to function normally in the presence of triggers. For others, these factors may have been visible their whole lives. Southall et al. (1997) found that many of the histories were thought to be plausible. In one case, the mother who claimed she had suffocated her son because of stress related to his crying was found on video to have premeditatively suffocated her child while he was deeply sleeping.

The role of psychology in cases of MSBP is of great importance. In-depth psychological assessment can provide useful information but should not be considered in isolation. As Southall et al. (1997) demonstrated, the ability of the perpetrator to deceive, misrepresent, fabricate, and maybe even induce events in a child are not characteristics reserved only for his or her interaction with the child. Many case reports include a well-intentioned mental health provider who adamantly believes a perpetrator, allowing an unsafe and often dangerous situation for a young child. Detection of this form of abuse involves collaboration between community child health professionals, hospital, psychiatrists, social workers, and police officers (Southall et al., 1997).

OUTCOMES

Many questions need to be addressed by the multidisciplinary team in cases of suspected and confirmed MSBP. How and when should confrontation take place? How assured are we that young children will be safe and older children will be able to cope and relearn how to be stable, productive members of society? What then should the role of reunification play? For example, it would be very dangerous for the primary provider to confront the mother by telling her the healthcare team suspects she is attempting to smother her child and then to discharge the child to her care. A safer approach is to formulate the plan during a team meeting so that everyone on the team is aware of his or her role. It may be decided that the primary provider is the best person to confront the mother; however, having CPS and law enforcement standing by is an essential element in a successful intervention. A perpetrator who becomes out of control may need to be removed from the premises. The child may be placed in the custody of the courts until a safe environment can be determined. Once confrontation occurs and the child is no longer at risk, the covert video surveillance should cease and the child should be moved to a room with close direct visual observation. Hospital discharge should occur as soon as the child is medically ready and a safe environment can be secured.

If a child is placed in protective custody, how long will he or she remain there? Levin and Sheridan (1995) describe an approach that is based on the level of the team's concern for the child's safety if the child is exposed to the perpetrator. One suggested measure of comfort is whether the perpetrator confessed and if other adults involved are able to identify the risk to the child now that the true cause of the child's symptoms is known. In addition, measures must be in place for trained professionals to monitor the home environment.

Connecting a family to services previously untapped may be a bridge for successful long-term placement for the child. Johnson (1995) identified the following 4 elements for successful family preservation:

1. Families have the potential and desire to change.

2. The safety of the child is ensured.

3. All recommended services are available.

4. The plan is supported by professionals.

No research has confirmed that treatment for perpetrators of MSBP has been successful. The short-term and long-term safety needs of the child are of utmost consideration in making this determination despite the potential benefits of family reunification. Therefore, every case is assessed independently and followed closely.

SUMMARY

Cases of MSBP may be the most difficult a practitioner will ever face. Mistrust, disbelief, and uncertainty are common elements identified by professionals after working on these cases. After dealing with MSBP, the nurse may find it difficult to blindly trust caregivers at their word when taking the patient history, but such skepticism helps to keep skills sharp. Although MSBP is a rare occurrence in light of the staggering statistics of other forms of child maltreatment, it is an astute and knowledgeable practitioner who considers the diagnosis and seeks to find the missing links to an often complicated history.

REFERENCES

American Psychiatric Association. *Diagnostic and Statistical Manual of Mental Disorders, Text Revision*. 4th ed. Washington, DC: American Psychiatric Association; 2000.

Asher R. Munchausen's syndrome. *Lancet*. 1951;1:339-341.

Ayoub C, Alexander R. Definitional issues in Munchausen by proxy. *APSAC Adv*. 1998;11:7-10.

Brown M. Dilemmas facing nurses who care for Munchausen syndrome by proxy patients. *Pediatr Nurs*. 1997;23:416-418.

Bursch B, Weinberg HD, Shilkoff S. Nurses' knowledge of and experience with Munchausen syndrome by proxy. *Issues Compr Pediatr Nurs*. 1996;19:93-102.

Catlin A. Commentary on dilemmas facing nurses who care for Munchausen syndrome by proxy patients. *Pediatr Nurs*. 1997;23:419-421.

Fisher GC, Mitchell I. Is Munchausen syndrome by proxy really a syndrome? *Arch Dis Child*. 1995;72:530-534.

Fisher G, Mitchell I, Meadow R, Morley CJ. Controversy. *Arch Dis Child*. 1995;72:528-529.

Foreman DM, Farsides C. Ethical use of covert videoing techniques in detecting Munchausen syndrome by proxy. *BMJ*. 1993;307:611-613.

Johnson D. Patriarchal terrorism and common couple violence: two forms of violence against women. *J Marriage Fam*. 1995;57:283-294.

Levin AV, Sheridan M, eds. *Munchausen Syndrome by Proxy: Issues in Diagnosis and Treatment*. New York, NY: Lexington Books; 1995.

Ludwig S. The role of the physician. In: Levin AV, Sheridan M, eds. *Munchausen Syndrome by Proxy: Issues in Diagnosis and Treatment*. New York, NY: Lexington Books; 1995:289.

Meadow R. Munchausen syndrome by proxy: the hinterland of child abuse. *Lancet*. 1977;2:342-345.

Meadow R. ABC of child abuse. Munchausen syndrome by proxy. *BMJ*. 1989;299:248-250.

Meadow R. Munchausen syndrome by proxy abuse perpetrated by men. *Arch Dis Child*. 1998;78:210-216.

Morrison C. Cameras in hospital rooms: the Fourth Amendment to the Constitution and Munchausen syndrome by proxy. *Crit Care Nurs Q.* 1999;22:65-68.

Parnell TF, Day DO, eds. *Munchausen by Proxy Syndrome: Misunderstood Child Abuse.* Thousand Oaks, Calif: Sage Publications; 1998.

Pasqualone G, Fitzgerald S. Munchausen by proxy syndrome: the forensic challenge of recognition, diagnosis, and reporting. *Crit Care Nurs Q.* 1999;22:52-64.

Rosenberg D. Web of deceit: a literature review of Munchausen syndrome by proxy. *Child Abuse Negl.* 1987;11:547-563.

Schreier HA, Libow JA. *Hurting for Love: Munchausen by Proxy Syndrome.* New York, NY: The Guilford Press; 1993a.

Schreier HA, Libow JA. Munchausen syndrome by proxy: diagnosis and prevalence. *Am J Orthopsychiatry.* 1993b;63:318-321.

Southall DP, Plunkett MC, Banks MW, Falkov AF, Samuels MP. Covert video recordings of life-threatening child abuse: lessons for child protection. *Pediatrics.* 1997;100:735-760.

Chapter 13

CHILD PROTECTIVE SERVICES AND CHILD ABUSE

Eileen R. Giardino, PhD, RN, CRNP
Anne Lynn, ACSW, MLSP
Angelo P. Giardino, MD, PhD, FAAP

Child abuse and neglect remains a serious problem in the United States despite years of effort by professionals and communities to prevent, investigate, and treat this problem. The majority of reported cases involve child neglect, followed by physical abuse, sexual abuse, and then emotional maltreatment. A smaller number involve other forms of abuse and exploitation (Sedlak & Broadhurst, 1996; Wang & Daro, 1998). Child abuse professionals generally recognize that the reported incidence of abuse and neglect is an underestimate of the actual occurrence of the problem. Community-based incidence studies estimate that reported child abuse constitutes only about 40% of actual reportable cases (US Department of Health & Human Services [USDHHS], 1988, 2000). In fact, over 10 years ago, the US Advisory Board on Child Abuse and Neglect (1990) declared child maltreatment a national emergency. Despite recent statistical decreases in the number of cases of child abuse and neglect, the overall incidence is still too high and much work remains to be done to prevent child maltreatment (USDHHS, 1999b).

Child protective services (CPS) is the agency in a community that serves to protect children and rehabilitate families in need of intervention when there are concerns of child abuse and neglect (DePanfilis & Salus, 1992). The purpose of CPS is multifaceted because it is usually the agency to receive reports of suspected child abuse and neglect and then identify those children who have been abused or neglected or who are at risk of abuse and neglect. CPS also identifies services needed for children and arranges for families to receive interventions that might help the child and reduce the further incidence of abuse or neglect in a specific home. The overall goal of CPS is to protect children and rehabilitate families to provide a safe environment that can address the safety and developmental needs of the child (DePanfilis & Salus, 1992). This chapter addresses the ways in which CPS interacts with families and other agencies to provide a safe environment for the child.

THE HISTORY OF CHILD ABUSE AND NEGLECT POLICY

Although child maltreatment is an old problem, efforts to address the problem in a consistent and meaningful way are a relatively recent phenomenon given the scope of the problem of child abuse and neglect. Although the child welfare movement originated in 1875 with the founding of organizations such as the New York Society for the Prevention of Cruelty to Children and the American Humane Association, child abuse was of less concern than more pressing issues such as infant mortality and maternal health (Levine & Levine, 1992).

Initial public funding for child welfare was established by the Social Security Act of 1935, which provided funding for the protection and care of homeless, dependent, and neglected children (USDHHS, 1998). The impetus for the development of reporting laws was the recognition of a formal medical profile for physically abused children. Physicians published a series of clinical reports, and the American Academy of Pediatrics (AAP) held a symposium in the 1940s to discuss combinations of injuries in infants that would later be seen as related to abuse, such as multiple fractures in the long bones with chronic subdural hematoma where diagnosis remains elusive (Caffey, 1946).

The catalyst for the widespread recognition and identification of child abuse victims came about with the publication of the single most influential report on child maltreatment that described and named the ***battered child syndrome*** (Kempe, Silverman, Steele, Droegemuller, & Silver, 1962). This new medical diagnosis was characterized by "injury to soft tissue and skeleton" accompanied by "evidence of neglect, including poor skin hygiene, multiple soft tissue injuries, and malnutrition" (Kempe et al., 1962, p. 17). In addition to the detailed descriptions of trauma that were often in conflict with the available information from the case histories, Kempe et al. (1962) further speculated that physicians were unwilling to consider parents as the source of harm and were reluctant to report cases to the proper authorities. Kempe et al. (1962) stated "training and personality usually make it quite difficult for [a physician] to assume the role of policeman or district attorney, and start questioning patients as if he were investigating a crime" (p. 107).

Kempe's 1977 address to the AAP identified the increasingly recognized problem of sexual abuse and raised the consciousness of pediatricians about the problem (Kempe, 1978). The severe emotional problems a child faces that result from incestuous relationships were identified as major medical and social problems that healthcare providers needed to recognize and understand. Kempe (1978) described the situation of child sexual abuse as a "hidden pediatric problem and a neglected area" in professional practice (p. 382). This was one of the first calls to this major problem of child abuse.

The recognition of the battered child syndrome and the reluctance of physicians to report was the primary impetus to develop mandatory reporting legislation. The Children's Bureau drafted the first model reporting statute in 1963. Two other model statutes followed in 1965, drafted by the American Medical Association and the Program of State Governments. By 1966, legislation mandating physicians to report suspected child abuse appeared in every state but Hawaii. The first statutes specified the following concerning the physician's responsibility to report suspected abuse (McCoid, 1965):

Any physician . . . having reasonable cause to suspect that a child under the age of [the maximum age of juvenile court] brought to him or coming before him for examination, care or treatment has had serious physical injury or injuries inflicted upon him other than by accidental means by a parent or other person responsible for his care, shall report or cause a report to be made in accordance with the provisions of the Act. (p. 20.)

Every state constructed a system of CPS agencies to intervene in situations of alleged abuse. Individual state legislation broadened most aspects of the early statutes to expand the range of professionals required to report and the types of maltreatment to be reported. Definitions of abuse were expanded to include emotional abuse, sexual abuse, and exploitation, in addition to physical abuse. The Child Abuse Prevention and Treatment Act of 1974 (CAPTA) passed by the United States Congress defined child abuse and neglect and set the standard for state mandatory reporting laws (USDHHS, 1996). This legislation provided funding to the states to establish the capacity in public child welfare agencies to receive and investigate reports of suspected abuse and neglect. The legislation promoted the establishment of statewide central report receiving capabilities and central registry functions to ensure that situations would be investigated and that children could be protected from repeated instances of abuse and neglect. States were required to adopt similar definitions of abuse to qualify for federal child protection funding. The act defined abuse and neglect as follows (CAPTA, 1974):

The physical or mental injury, sexual abuse, negligent treatment, or maltreatment of a child under the age of eighteen by a person who is responsible for the child's welfare under circumstances which indicate the child's health or welfare is harmed or threatened thereby as determined in accordance with regulations prescribed. (Section 3.)

In 1997, Congress passed the first major reform of federal child welfare policy since 1980, known as the Adoption and Safe Families Act of 1997 (ASFA). The Guidelines for Public Policy and State Legislation Governing Permanence for Children were then developed as one of several steps undertaken by the federal government in response to Adoption 2002, President Clinton's Initiative on Adoption and Foster Care. The child protection and foster care system in the United States is primarily governed by state law and a state's implementation of its laws; the guidelines were meant to help states evaluate and modernize their laws that affect children and families who are having difficulties and require intervention by the child welfare system (USDHHS, 1998).

Adoption 2002 is the initiative on adoption and foster care that addresses the problems associated with the long periods that America's foster children spend waiting for permanent and stable homes necessary for their healthy development. Among the proposed action steps recommended in Adoption 2002 is the development of model guidelines for state legislation to advance the goal of giving every child in the nation's public child welfare system a safe and permanent home and a timely decision-making process as to whom the permanent caregivers will be. Therefore, planning for the permanent home begins when a child enters the foster care system because foster care is presumed to be a temporary setting. The goal is to secure a permanent family for the child. Permanency refers to a safe, stable custodial environment for the child with a lifelong relationship with a nurturing caregiver and helps establish the foundation for a child's healthy development (USDHHS, 1998). Permanency planning efforts in the CPS system ideally begin as soon as a child enters care. The law heightens the importance of providing quality services as quickly as possible to enable families in crisis to more quickly address their problems (USDHHS, 1998).

CHILD PROTECTIVE SERVICES

The focus of CPS agencies is concern for the care of children, as expressed through laws that are established in every state. Mandated legal authority that evolved from child abuse laws provides a framework for CPS to take action when needed to protect children and work with in-need families (DePanfilis & Salus, 1992). The focus of child protection is to reduce the risks of a child from further maltreatment while maintaining family integrity as much as possible (Pence & Wilson, 1994b; Wilson & Pence, 2000).

The role of CPS as defined by most state legislation was reactive to the need to receive and investigate reports of suspected child abuse and neglect at the hands of parents or caretakers. Social and protective services were provided to the alleged offending parent(s) on a nonvoluntary basis as an alternative to the removal of their children for placement in protective care (e.g., foster care). Intervention with families in a preventive way or intervention in situations of potential risk to children were generally not the norm because of concerns about family integrity, confidentiality, and intrusiveness on the part of the state. CPS agencies have a difficult task before them in that they have 2 major goals that are not always mutually obtainable, namely, protecting the child from further maltreatment and preserving the family in which the abuse or neglect occurred (Gelles, 2001a, 2001b). Although this may be possible in a large number of cases, it is not possible in all cases. CPS agencies and their caseworkers must constantly assess the future risk to children if they remain with the caregiver who maltreated them, and this determination must be made with imperfect information. Tragic results may occur with misjudgments in either direction (Gelles, 2001a; Smolowe, 1995).

ROLE OF CPS IN THE INVESTIGATION OF CHILD ABUSE

State or county administered CPS services were developed to react to allegations received from mandated reporters, neighbors, parents, relatives, and victims. Allegations are received and assessed for conformity with legal definitions of abuse; the relationship between the victim and perpetrator; the geographical location of the abused, abuser, and incident; and the level of severity. Many states developed child abuse and neglect hotlines to receive reports and route them to local CPS offices for investigation. Generally, CPS receives reports and assigns them to a social worker or investigator, who must begin an investigation immediately or within 24 hours, depending on the nature and severity of the allegations **(Figure 13-1)**.

It is the responsibility of CPS to contact the child victim, parents, caregivers, and alleged perpetrator(s) and then visit them in person during the course of the investigation to determine whether abuse occurred. The investigation time frame varies by state and can be as short as 10 days and as long as 60 days. At the conclusion of the investigation period, the case is deemed substantiated, unsubstantiated, founded, or unfounded. If the findings are substantiated, the investigating agency may provide services to the child and family, whereas unsubstantiated claims warrant closure of the case (DePanfilis & Salus, 1992) **(Figure 13-1)**.

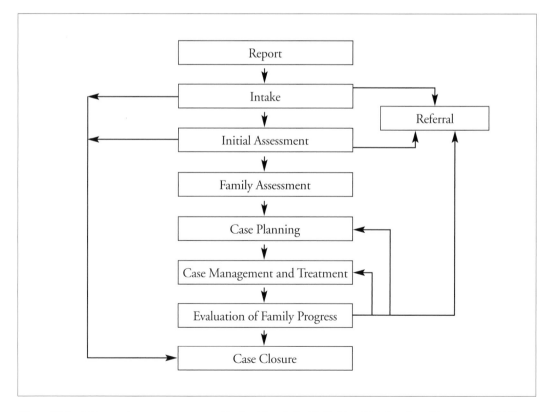

Figure 13-1. *Child protective system case process. Reprinted from DePanfilis D, Salus MK. A Coordinated Response to Child Abuse and Neglect: A Basic Manual. National Clearinghouse on Child Abuse and Neglect Information. Updated April 6, 2001. Available at: http://www.calib.com/nccanch/pubs/usermanuals/basic/figure2.cfm. Accessed February 17, 2003.*

Many state legislatures took great pains to protect the confidentiality of the family and the freedom of the family from unnecessary state intrusion in their homes and lifestyles. For example, in the 1970s, the confidentiality provisions of the CPS law in Pennsylvania prohibited the sharing of information about alleged child abuse cases between the CPS agency and local law enforcement personnel without the written consent of all of the parties involved. This was true even though many cases of child abuse rose to the level of criminal behavior, including homicide, aggravated assault, rape, and incest. These acts of violence were viewed differently because of the nature of the familial relationship between the alleged perpetrator and the victim. Consequently, law enforcement and child protection professionals frequently found themselves at odds in their separate investigations rather than able to work together on behalf of children and their families.

COLLABORATION IN THE INVESTIGATIVE PROCESS

In more recent years, professionals who deal with child abuse and neglect and most state legislatures have come to recognize that the problem of child abuse and neglect is not the domain of a single agency or profession (Wilson & Pence, 2000). No single agency or profession has the resources or mandate to intervene, treat, and prevent child abuse and neglect. Collaborative systems of intervention and treatment have developed, allowing for the sharing of information among professionals of various disciplines that can more effectively provide services and protect children. Multidisciplinary intervention teams, regional diagnostic centers, child assessment centers, and child advocacy centers (CACs) are some innovative examples of coordinated systems of intervention and care that attempt to balance the rights of the family with the rights of children to be free from abuse and neglect.

Models of Collaboration in Child Abuse Investigation

The investigation of child abuse is ideally a multidimensional process involving CPS, law enforcement, police and prosecution, healthcare and mental health professionals, and other community agencies. In maltreatment cases, CPS often takes a lead role in organizing and overseeing the collaborative relationships with potential referral sources and the agencies involved in the investigation. It requires coordinated efforts to include the broad range of services of individuals and organizations involved in the process.

When child abuse investigations take place in a fragmented manner, with CPS, police, healthcare providers, and the district attorney's office gathering information concerning the details of the case, the child may be subjected to many interviews. Realizing this situation is not ideal, models have been developed in which these agencies and disciplines work together to coordinate their respective mandated and professional responsibilities in a way that puts the interests of the child at the center of the child protection effort. In an effort to promote joint investigations, several governmental agencies convened a symposium to consider recommendations focused on fostering interdisciplinary work in child maltreatment investigations and treatment (Dinsmore, 1993). A coordinated response to child maltreatment was recommended based on the understanding that such an approach would lead to the following (Dinsmore, 1993):

— Reducing the number of interviews the child must endure

— Minimizing the number of people involved in the case

— Enhancing the quality of the evidence discovered for criminal prosecution and civil litigation

— Providing information essential to CPS and other family service organizations

— Decreasing the likelihood of conflicts between and among various involved agencies

Multidisciplinary and interdisciplinary work regarding professional activity dealing with the evaluation and management of child maltreatment led to the development of the concept of the multidisciplinary team (MDT) (Pence & Wilson, 1994b; Wilson, 1992). An MDT exists when a group of professionals agree to work together in a collaborative, coordinated manner to address the problems that arise as a result of child abuse and neglect (Pence & Wilson, 1994a, 1994b). The MDT's goal is to ensure that the multidimensional needs of the child and family are addressed during the child maltreatment investigation and treatment interventions (Pence & Wilson, 1994a; Rowe, Leonard, Seashore, Lewiston, & Anderson, 1970; Wilson & Hilbert, 1973). A variety of MDT models exist; they vary depending on need, locality, and setting.

CHILD ADVOCACY CENTER JOINT INVESTIGATIONS

One model of collaborative agency involvement in the investigation of child sexual abuse that has evolved over the past 2 decades is that of CACs. These centers offer an approach to services for victims and families by bringing together a multidisciplinary team to evaluate the child and coordinate services between CPS, law enforcement, and the family (National Children's Alliance [NCA], 2003). The child-centered approach tries to coordinate the interviews needed so that a child does not have to tell his or her story multiple times to the different agencies involved in the investigation and prosecution of a case (NCA, 2003).

The CAC model brings together CPS, law enforcement, and other agencies to interview children in a comfortable and friendly environment (NCA, 2003). The goal of a CAC is to decrease the number of interviews and the associated trauma of the interview process by facilitating joint interviews between the agencies that need to hear the child's story. The number of CACs in the United States is increasing as cities recognize the value of helping the child through the difficult process when child abuse is suspected. Many CACs have specialists in forensic interviewing to assist the process and help the agencies involved. It is ideal for the CAC to house both CPS and police, to facilitate the investigative process (NCA, 2003). Because of constraints in the structures of some city governments, the co-location of the agencies is not always possible.

According to NCA, CACs "stress coordination of investigation and intervention services by bringing together professionals and agencies as a multidisciplinary team to create a child-focused approach to child abuse cases. The goal is to ensure that children are not revictimized by the very system designed to protect them" **(Table 13-1)**. In addition to the joint interviews of the suspected child sexual abuse victim, most CACs provide the following formal processes to promote effective team functioning:

— Pre/post interview conferences that include the collaborating agencies

— Scheduled case reviews with the entire MDT

— Joint interdisciplinary training programs

— System of case tracking and follow-up that keeps each team member aware of case activities and outcome

Some communities are unable to create a formal organization such as a CAC but are still able to get agencies and disciplines to conduct joint interviews. This initial collaboration may form the groundwork for a future CAC should local factors be such that a more formal collaboration would be possible.

The benefits of effective joint investigations, including the ideal performed within a CAC are described as follows (Ells, 1998):

— Less "system-inflicted" trauma to children and families

— Increased agency performance, including enhanced accuracy of investigations and more appropriate interventions

— Efficient use of limited community resources

— More capable professionals as they develop collaborative skills

— Recognition of the difficulty inherent in the maltreatment-related work and the opportunity to develop a professional network that decreases the sense of isolation and risk of professional burnout

CHILD ABUSE REPORTS

The role of CPS in receiving reports of child abuse and neglect varies among states, from being the sole receiver to sharing responsibility with law enforcement. Some states require notification of CPS and police in certain forms of maltreatment such as physical or sexual abuse (DePanfilis & Salus, 1992). Healthcare professionals must refer to local and state guidelines for specific reporting procedures.

CPS agencies receive referrals daily alleging that a child has been neglected or abused. After a referral is "screened in," the agency conducts an investigation to determine whether the child has been maltreated or is at risk of maltreatment (National Clearinghouse on Child Abuse and Neglect Information [NCCANI], 2001). CPS screened in and screened out an estimated 2.97 million reports in 1999. CPS agencies in 1999 screened in an estimated 1.79 million family-based referrals from 50 states and screened out an estimated 1.17 million referrals. CPS agencies investigated approximately 60.4% of the nearly 3 million referrals they received and screened out approximately 39.6% of the referrals (NCCANI, 2001).

Reports to CPS of child abuse and neglect are often initiated by telephone contact from a number of sources. Nonhealthcare-related sources might experience even more fear in reporting to officials than those who are mandated to report signs of possible abuse or maltreatment. In all cases, it is ideal for CPS staff to offer support and encouragement to all persons who decide to report because there are usually concerns and fears regarding what the family might do to retaliate or concerns with having to testify in court (DePanfilis & Salus, 1992) **(Table 13-2)**.

The content of the report from state to state includes some common information **(Table 13-3)**. Detailed information regarding the condition and location of the child, the parents, and the alleged abuser; details of the nature and character of the maltreatment; and information regarding the reporter are vital aspects of the formal report (DePanfilis & Salus, 1992). When potential maltreatment occurs in settings other than the home (e.g., foster home, daycare center), specific information about that setting or facility is also included in the report.

In the process of investigating maltreatment reports, CPS must determine the credibility of the reported information, whether from professionals or lay people in the community. CPS must determine whether the complaint is valid and should be accepted for an initial assessment/investigation. CPS caseworkers ask questions to evaluate the credibility of the report (DePanfilis & Salus, 1992) **(Table 13-4)**.

Table 13-1. Description of National Children's Alliance and Member Child Advocacy Centers

National Children's Alliance (formerly the National Network of Children's Advocacy Centers) is a not-for-profit organization whose mission is to provide training, technical assistance, and networking opportunities to communities seeking to plan, establish, and improve child advocacy centers (CACs).

In 1987, National Children's Alliance was founded by Congressman Bud Cramer, then District Attorney of Madison County Alabama, in response to the needs of a growing number of facility-based child abuse intervention programs and the demand for guidance from grassroots organizations working with child victims. Today, the Alliance is a membership organization providing services to CACs, multidisciplinary teams, and professionals across the country.

The purpose of CACs is to provide a comprehensive, culturally competent, multidisciplinary team response to allegations of child abuse in a dedicated, child-friendly setting. A child-appropriate, child-friendly setting and a multidisciplinary team are essential for accomplishment of the mission of CACs and for full membership in National Children's Alliance.

A team response to allegations of child abuse includes forensic interviews, medical evaluations, therapeutic interventions, victim support/advocacy, case review, and case tracking. These components may be provided by CAC staff or other members of the multidisciplinary team. To the maximum extent possible, components of the team response are provided at the CAC to promote a sense of safety and consistency to the child and family.

The following program components are necessary for full membership in National Children's Alliance:

— Child-appropriate and child-friendly facility: a CAC provides a comfortable, private, child-friendly setting that is physically and psychologically safe for clients.

— Multidisciplinary team (MDT): a multidisciplinary team for response to child abuse allegations includes representation from law enforcement, child protective services (CPS), prosecution, mental health, medical, victim advocacy, and CAC.

— Organizational capacity: a designated legal entity responsible for program and fiscal operations has been established and implements basic sound administrative practices.

— Cultural competency and diversity: the CAC promotes culturally competent policies, practices, and procedures. Cultural competency is defined as the capacity to function in more than one culture, requiring the ability to appreciate, understand, and interact with members of diverse populations within the local community.

— Forensic interviews: forensic interviews are conducted in a neutral, fact-finding manner and coordinated to avoid duplicative interviewing.

— Medical evaluation: specialized medical evaluation and treatment are to be made available to CAC clients as part of the team response, either at the CAC or through coordination and referral with other specialized medical providers.

— Therapeutic intervention: specialized mental health services are to be made available as part of the team response, either at the CAC or through coordination and referral with other appropriate treatment providers.

— Victim support and advocacy: victim support and advocacy are to be made available as part of the team response, either at the CAC or through coordination with other providers, throughout the investigation and subsequent legal proceedings.

(continued)

Table 13-1. *(continued)*

— Case review: team discussion and information sharing regarding the investigation, case status, and services needed by the child and family are to occur routinely.

— Case tracking: CACs must develop and implement a system for monitoring case progress and tracking case outcomes for team components.

Adapted from National Children's Alliance. National Children's Alliance Member Standards. Available at: http//www.nca-online.org. Accessed March 3, 2003.

Table 13-2. Typical Concerns of Caregivers Regarding Reporting Suspected Child Abuse and Neglect

Concern	Response
"The parents seem like very angry people. What if the parents come after me?"	Although there may be a few exceptions, most abusive parents lack the social skills to face adults, especially those whom they perceive to be in authority positions. This inability to confront adults is one of the reasons why their children are vulnerable to being harmed. An occasional parent may yell or threaten, but that usually is as far as it goes.
"I have no right to intervene in a family's affairs."	The laws in your state give you the right to protect the child by reporting your suspicions of child abuse and neglect. It is the only way the child and family can begin receiving the help they need.
"Their cultural practices are different from mine. I have no right to impose my child-rearing beliefs on them."	The definitions of child abuse and neglect included in state laws apply to all families residing in a state or community. These laws do not provide for exceptions when, by legal standards, culturally accepted child-rearing practices are abusive or neglectful.
"I've worked for this director for 5 years. I just can't believe that she would sexually abuse the children. There must be some other explanation."	Adults who abuse or neglect children come from all kinds of backgrounds and are not always easy to identify. You must trust your observation skills and your knowledge of the physical and behavioral signs of child maltreatment. Also, remember that in your report you are not accusing any one person; you are reporting the condition of a child or children that you suspect was caused by child abuse or neglect.

(continued)

Table 13-2. *(continued)*

CONCERN	RESPONSE
"I just started at the center and don't want to be considered a troublemaker ... but Mrs. Littleton is extremely rough with the children, and yesterday she left fingermarks on both of Carmen's arms."	Sometimes, your intervention with a colleague might prevent a child from getting seriously hurt. Most centers have administrative policies for how to report concerns about staff treatment of children.
"The last time I reported, nothing happened. The child is still with his family, and the father is still abusing him. The CPS caseworker never even got in touch with me. I left lots of messages, but he never called me back. This time, I'm not going to bother reporting."	The facts and circumstances of each case are different, and you cannot assume that all cases will be handled in the same way or have the same results. Confidentiality laws and policies often make it difficult for CPS to keep you informed. When you do not get the response you expect from a caseworker, ask to speak with his or her supervisor.
"I really don't think anything will get done, so what's the use of reporting."	It is true that filing the report does not guarantee that the child and family will get help. However, if you do not report, the children may continue to be at risk. At the very least, a record of the report will be made, your legal obligation fulfilled, and the investigative process begun. Abused and neglected children cannot be protected unless they are first identified, and the key is reporting.
"I might be sued by the parents for making a false report."	In every state, mandated reporters are immune from civil liability for making a report in good faith (where knowledge or reasonable suspicion exists), even if it is not substantiated by the investigator. Even if someone does sue you, the court will dismiss the case when they find out that you are a mandated reporter. Some states have provisions to pay your legal fees if you must defend a lawsuit.

Reprinted from Koralek D. Caregivers of Young Children: Preventing and Responding to Child Maltreatment. *Washington, DC: US Dept of Health & Human Services; 1992. Contract No. HHS-105-88-1702.*

SOURCES OF REPORTS

Professionals submitted the majority of the reports of child abuse and neglect in 1999 **(Figure 13-2)**. A professional is someone who had contact with the alleged child victim as part of his or her job (NCCANI, 2001). Education personnel (15.0%), legal or law enforcement personnel (13.6%), and social services personnel (13.2%) were the most common sources of reports.

The remaining 45.3% of screened-in reports were from nonprofessional sources. The largest portion of reports in the nonprofessional category (12.2%) was from anonymous or unknown reporters (NCCANI, 2001). Nonprofessional sources also included parents, relatives, neighbors, friends, alleged victims, alleged perpetrators, and other sources (NCCANI, 2001).

PROCESS OF A CHILD PROTECTIVE SYSTEM CASE

Once a situation is reported to CPS, the caseworker follows a process of steps to intervene and treat the child and family **(Figure 13-1)**. The steps are defined as follows:

— Intake

— Initial assessment

— Family assessment

— Case planning

— Case management and treatment

— Evaluation of family process

— Case closure

The essential decisions at intake concern 2 questions:

1. Does the reported information meet the agency guidelines for child maltreatment?

2. How urgent is the referral?

CPS considers many issues during the initial assessment part of the investigative process because answers to questions may also involve input and collaboration with law enforcement **(Table 13-5)**. Important decisions emerge from analyzing assessment data and talking with people who have information concerning the child, family, and agencies that are also involved in the process. Along with CPS, other systems involved in the assessment process include law enforcement, prosecutors, healthcare professionals, and mental health professionals (Pence & Wilson, 1994b). The intricacies of the process are evident by the number of questions asked of potentially many people in the child's family system.

Family Assessment

CPS caseworkers and other professionals conduct a family assessment after the child's safety is determined and ensured. The goal of the family assessment is to determine the details of possible maltreatment, factors that contributed to the risk of

---

Table 13-3. Content of Report to Child Protective Services

The report to CPS should include the following information:

— Name, age, sex, and address of the child(ren)

— Nature and extent of the child's injuries/condition

— Name and address of the parent or other person responsible for the child

---

Reprinted from DePanfilis D, Salus MK. Child Protective Services: A Guide for Caseworkers. Washington, DC: US Dept of Health & Human Services; 1992.

Table 13-4. Evaluating the Credibility of the Report

The following items should be considered in evaluating the credibility of the report:

— Is the reporter willing to give his or her name, address, and telephone number?

— What is the reporter's relationship to the victim and family?

— How well does the reporter know the family?

— If the reporter knew of previous abuse or neglect, why is he or she reporting now?

— How does the reporter know about the case?

— Does the reporter stand to gain anything for reporting or from the report being validated?

— Has the reporter made previous unfounded reports on this family?

— Is the reporter willing to meet with a caseworker in person if needed?

— Does the reporter appear to be intoxicated, extremely bitter, angry, or exhibiting behavior that would make the caseworker question his or her competency?

— Can or will the reporter refer CPS to others who know about the situation?

— What does the reporter hope will happen as a result of the report?

Reprinted from DePanfilis D, Salus MK. Child Protective Services: A Guide for Caseworkers. *Washington, DC: US Dept of Health & Human Services; 1992.*

---

maltreatment, and the effects of maltreatment on the child and family system. The family assessment uncovers personal and environmental factors that may contribute to child maltreatment, as well as surrounding issues related to the abuse. The assessment addresses the following (DePanfilis & Salus, 1992):

— Nature, extent, and causes of the factors contributing to the risk of maltreatment

— Effects of child's maltreatment and the treatment needs of all family members

— Individual and family strengths that can be tapped in the intervention process

— Conditions and behaviors that must change for the risk of maltreatment to be reduced

— Prognosis for family's ability to change

Case Planning

The case planning process is ideally a collaborative effort developed between the CPS caseworker and family/community professionals who are involved and may continue to be involved with the family. Case planning involves engaging family members in decisions regarding changes they need to make to reduce or eliminate the risk of maltreatment, as well as agreement on what must be done to provide safe living conditions for the child. In some situations, the court orders the family to participate in services or complete certain actions it deems necessary to provide a safe environment (DePanfilis & Salus, 1992).

After completing a family assessment, CPS and other community service providers collaborate to determine strategies to change aspects of the family system that resulted in child abuse and neglect. Considerations in the case planning stage of the process include the following (DePanfilis & Salus, 1992):

— Goals that must be achieved to reduce the risk of maltreatment and meet the treatment needs identified

— Priorities among the goals

— Interventions or services that can be used to achieve the goals

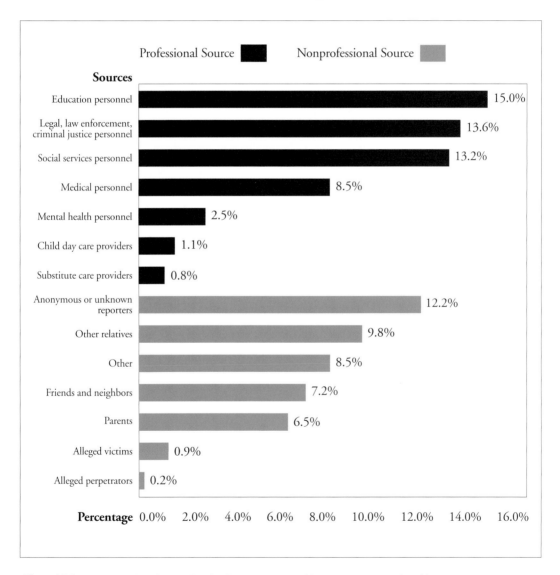

Figure 13-2. *Reporters of child abuse and neglect by source. Reprinted from US Department of Health & Human Services.* Child Maltreatment 1999: Reports From the States to the National Child Abuse and Neglect Data Systems. *1999a. Available at: http://www.acf.dhhs.gov/ programs/cb/publications/cm99/cpt1.htm. Accessed February 17, 2003.*

— Steps or tasks that must be completed for goals to be achieved

— Designated responsibilities of the CPS caseworker

— Determination of the family members' responsibilities

— Responsibilities of other service providers

— Time frames for goal achievement

— How and when the case plan will be evaluated to determine goal accomplishment

The planning process seeks to engage family members in determining changes that should be made to reduce or eliminate maltreatment risks and what client, caseworker, and other service providers can do to ensure that necessary changes occur (DePanfilis & Salus, 1992).

Case Management and Treatment

The case management and treatment stage of the process involves the implementation of the steps and services needed to accomplish the case plan. CPS often coordinates, arranges, and provides the delivery of services to the family. General procedures to follow when child abuse or neglect is suspected include the following (DePanfilis & Salus, 1992):

— Make an oral report to the child abuse hotline/local CPS agency. If there is immediate danger to the child or siblings, this should be emphasized with other report information.

— In the case of serious bodily injury, sexual abuse, or death, a report should also be made to the local police department.

— Perform a physical examination to determine condition, needed treatment, and possible evidence collection. In sexual abuse cases, evidence of physical abuse and neglect should be noted, and efforts should be made to minimize the psychological effects of a genital examination.

— Record all findings.

Evaluation of Family Progress and Case Closure

CPS performs an ongoing assessment process that continues throughout the life of the case. CPS caseworkers evaluate family progress based on the following criteria (DePanfilis & Salus, 1992):

— The safety of the child

— Achievement of goals and tasks in the case plan

— Reduction of the risk of maltreatment

— Success in meeting the child's and other family members' needs resulting from the maltreatment

CPS determines a case can close when risks to the child and within the family have been sufficiently reduced or eliminated so that the child is protected and his or her developmental needs are met sufficiently without societal intervention (DePanfilis & Salus, 1992).

CPS caseworkers involve clients and family in decisions regarding the welfare of the child and closure of the case. Caseworkers should apply specific principles to the case closure process to ensure the best possible outcome for the family and child. The following are steps involved in the closure of a case (DePanfilis & Salus, 1992):

Table 13-5. Child Protective Services Process of Initial Assessment/Investigation

PRIMARY DECISIONS OR ISSUES TO CONSIDER AT INITIAL ASSESSMENT

CPS

— Did the child suffer maltreatment or is he or she threatened by harm as defined by the state reporting law?

— Is the parent(s)/caretaker(s) responsible for the maltreatment?

— Is maltreatment likely to occur in the future? If so, what is the level of risk of maltreatment?

— Is the child safe? If not, what measures are necessary to ensure the child's safety?

— Are there emergency needs in the family that must be met?

— Are continuing agency services necessary to protect the child and reduce the risk of maltreatment occurring in the future?

Law enforcement

— Did a crime occur?

— Who is the alleged offender?

— Is there evidence to arrest the alleged offender? (law enforcement)

CPS and law enforcement

— Do sources of corroboration or witnesses exist?

— Has all physical evidence been obtained/preserved?

— Are there any other victims?

—Should the child be taken into protective custody?

CONSIDERATIONS FOR CASES INVOLVING OUT-OF-HOME CARE ABUSE

Licensing personnel

— Are personnel actions indicated and, if so, are they being initiated appropriately by the child care facility?

— Should the facility's or foster care or other child care provider's license be revoked?

CPS and licensing personnel

— What responsibility do others in the facility have for any incident of maltreatment, and is a corrective action plan needed to prevent the likelihood of future incidents?

(continued)

Table 13-5. *(continued)*

OTHER DISCIPLINES THAT HAVE A ROLE IN THE INITIAL ASSESSMENT PROCESS

— Foster care, residential, or child care licensing personnel may participate in the initial assessment if abuse is allegedly committed by an out-of-home caretaker.

— Medical personnel may be involved in assessing and responding to medical needs of a child or parent and perhaps in documenting the nature and extent of maltreatment.

— Mental health personnel may be involved in assessing the effects of any alleged maltreatment and in helping to determine the validity of specific allegations.

— Teachers may be involved in providing direct information about the effects of maltreatment and in describing information pertinent to risk assessment.

— Military family advocacy personnel may be directly involved by providing information when one of the family members is in the military.

— Other community service providers may have had past experience with the child and/or family and may be a resource in helping to address any emergency needs that the child or family may have.

Adapted from DePanfilis D, Salus MK. Child Protective Services: A Guide for Caseworkers. Washington, DC: US Dept of Health & Human Services; 1992.

---

1. Meet personally with the family to discuss the case closure.

2. Establish time frames (together) for when the case should be closed.

3. Acknowledge the family's (and the caseworker's) feelings about the case closure.

4. Prepare for a family-created crisis that may occur as a reaction to anticipated independence resulting from the planned closure.

5. Review the progress made as a result of CPS involvement, emphasizing efforts that were essential for the resulting changes.

6. Refer the family to any additional resources as needed.

7. Leave the door open for services if needed in the future (including providing information to the family about how to contact the agency and who should be contacted in the future).

CPS AND MANDATORY REPORTING

Mandatory reporting laws share several core components. Reporting laws define abusive situations, reportable circumstances, degree of certainty that reporters must attain before making a report (e.g., reason to suspect, reason to believe), and the age limits of reportable children. The laws define who must report, outline the sanctions for failure to report, and define immunity from civil and criminal liability for reports filed "in good faith." However, state laws differ in important ways such as the definition and specificity of what constitutes abuse and under what conditions a report must be made. State CPS laws impose a penalty for failure to report suspected child abuse.

States have widely expanded the scope of the mandatory reporting requirement to include a broad range of human service providers, social workers, and teachers

(**Table 13-6**). In some states, the requirement extends to commercial film processors who may see examples of sexually explicit photographs of children, indicating possible abuse or exploitation. Animal humane officers may be included because of the association between cruelty to animals and child abuse. When all states are considered, approximately 40 different professions are named in mandatory reporting laws (Wurtele & Miller-Perrin, 1992). Research has shown that various professions respond quite differently to reporting requirements. For example, psychiatric nurses were more likely to report abuse compared with nonmedically trained mental health workers (Kalichman, Craig, & Follingstad, 1988). Nurses and ministers were found to be more likely to report abuse than family practice physicians and psychologists (Williams, Osborne, & Rappaport, 1987). These results suggest differences in compliance with reporting laws among professions and service delivery settings.

For persons who report potential abuse in good faith, reporting laws have provisions to protect reporters from criminal prosecution and civil lawsuits resulting from filing a report. The law provides immunity to protect those who demonstrate concern for the child and family (DePanfilis & Salus, 1992). State laws either presume that reports are filed in good faith or specify that reports must be made without malice. Mandated reporters are rarely determined to have filed reports that are harassing or without just cause (Drake, 1996). The immunity provision is designed to remove the hesitation to report based on uncertainty about whether abuse has occurred. Mandated reporters must only have reasonable cause to suspect that abuse has occurred. It is up to the investigators to make the determination that abuse occurred based on the evidence uncovered in a thorough investigation. A reporter can be sued, but the immunity component for the statute permits him or her to claim the immunity before the judge hearing the case. (See Chapter 14, Legal Issues.)

A uniform application of reporting laws cannot account for particular circumstances, professional discretion, and judgment and can place mandated reporters in circumstances that conflict with basic professional values and ethical principles (Butz,

---

Table 13-6. Mandated Healthcare Reporters According to State Child Abuse Laws

— Physicians and surgeons

— Hospital residents and interns

— Physician's assistants

— Registered nurses and licensed practical nurses

— Dentists

— Optometrists

— Chiropractors

— Podiatrists

— Psychologists

— Mental health practitioners

— Social workers

— Medical examiners/coroners

Redman, Fry, & Kolodner, 1998; Greipp, 1997). This can result in situations in which professionals do not follow the law. And, in some instances, this can result in serious harm to children in need of protection.

The dilemma faced by many professionals about reporting requirements and when they are obligated to report can best be addressed by examining the explicit language of the child abuse law covering the jurisdiction involved. Reasonable grounds may exist to report suspected abuse if a child tells the professional that he or she has been physically or sexually abused, someone else (e.g., relative, sibling, friend) tells the professional that the child has been abused, and the professional's observations of the child's behavior or observation of signs or indicators of abuse leads to the belief that the child has been abused.

Some state laws require a report to be made only if mandated professionals have reason to suspect based on a child's statement, the professional's observation of behavior, or signs or symptoms in a child they have directly examined. In general, healthcare professionals should make a report to the appropriate CPS agency for investigation when they have *reasonable cause to suspect* that a child has been abused or neglected or is at imminent risk of harm. Typically, an oral report should be made immediately to the statewide child abuse hotline, followed by a written report (often on a standardized form provided for this purpose) to the local CPS agency responsible for investigating such reports within a time period established by state law.

Most states have established a mechanism for receiving such reports, with a toll-free hotline number being the most common. State reporting laws are available on the Internet through various legal resource websites, including the National Clearinghouse on Child Abuse and Neglect Information at http://www.calib.com/nccanch (Kalichman, 1999).

What to Report

Many states have written report forms to help professionals determine what information is needed when contacting the hotline or local CPS agency. Examples of information useful to the CPS agency include the following (DePanfilis & Salus, 1992):

— Child's name, address, telephone number, and birth date

— Child's age and gender

— Parents/caregivers' names, addresses, and phone numbers

— Name of the person(s) suspected to have caused the child's injuries

— Nature and extent of the injury(ies), maltreatment, or neglect

— Approximate date and time alleged abuse occurred

— Information about previous injuries, maltreatment, neglect of the child or siblings

— How the information came to light

— Any action taken to treat or help the child

— Any statements made by the child

— Any statements/explanation offered by the parent/caregiver

— Other information that would be useful (e.g., who else lives at home or has caregiving responsibilities for the child and could be potentially helpful in the investigation)

The investigation of cases of sexual abuse requires considerable resources to identify and assess the reported cases because the evidence is less definitive than in physical abuse and neglect and objective witnesses or physical findings are rare (Pence & Wilson, 1994b). Investigation of child sexual abuse cases is time consuming because it involves skillful interviewing of people involved in the situation (Pence & Wilson, 1994b). Likewise, emotional abuse substantiation rates are low, and these situations may be the most difficult to resolve.

Legal definitions of abuse as outlined in state law may have a direct effect on whether cases are reported. A study conducted by Rycraft (1990) found that states with broad and nonspecific definitions have the highest reporting and substantiation rates, and states with narrow and specific definitions of abuse have among the lowest. He concluded that definitions of child abuse are a determining factor in decisions to report and the dispositions of reported cases.

Benefits of Reporting

The reporting of suspected child abuse or neglect can be essential to the protection of children from further abuse or neglect. It can lead to actions that assist the family in obtaining necessary services to improve their parenting skills or their living conditions. It can also help break the intergenerational cycle of child abuse and neglect by treating the child, reducing trauma, and preventing future abuse by that parent or that child victim. Even in the absence of services after a report, the act of investigation and intervention can have positive consequences for the child and family. The child may experience the intervention by child protection professionals or law enforcement as evidence that someone will intervene on the child's behalf. Parents may experience the intervention as evidence that their behavior is not acceptable and may cause further intervention in the future. And, of course, the report may result in the removal of the child from an abusive situation, effectively stopping the abuse.

Critics of mandatory reporting argue that the requirement to report has not had the desired outcome of protecting children in many cases. In fact, mandated reporting may be immobilizing the systems set up to deal with child abuse. By casting a broad net so as not to overlook an abused child, child protection agencies are swamped with reports that are in large part unsubstantiated, wasting limited resources. Also, mandated reporters can become frustrated with making reports that seem to generate little interest and intervention from CPS agencies.

Some professionals believe mandated reporting requires them to violate the confidentiality of their clients and children, thereby undermining the therapeutic relationship they may have with the client. They believe this can endanger children by interfering with opportunities for effective treatment. Some believe reporting is harmful to children and families because the resulting investigation can be destructive and intrusive and should only be pursued when compelling evidence shows abuse is occurring. This is particularly problematic in state laws, in which language and definitions of abuse are vague or overly broad.

By focusing on the child and the child's safety first, mandated reporters can develop a framework for evaluating situations that come before them, knowing when and what to report and how to assist the family in gaining maximum benefit and minimum trauma from the experience whenever possible.

Little, if any, training exists for mandated reporters in dealing with suspected child abuse cases either during professional education and training or as continuing education courses. Most CPS agencies are charged with the responsibility of providing public education about child abuse and methods of reporting for mandated reporters and the larger community. However, most professionals learn from experience about making reports of suspected child abuse, and these experiences are not always positive.

Child abuse reporting sets in motion a chain of events that begins with the acceptance of the report by the hotline. The referral is screened according to the local laws and regulations governing the public child welfare system response. CPS conducts a risk assessment and, if warranted, starts an investigation.

The identity of the mandated reporter is generally kept confidential from the family. In many situations, the person or family can ascertain the identity of the reporting source based on the circumstances and nature of the reported allegations. In the case of a mandated reporter who is a medical provider, informing the family a report is being made in accordance with the CPS law can be beneficial. A mandated reporter should be prepared to address the consequences of making a report. The following are some considerations concerning mandated reporting:

— How will the parents and child(ren) be informed that a report is being made?

— How will the mandated reporter interact with the family and with the child protection agency personnel after making the report?

— What additional information must be collected?

— What information should be shared with CPS and what information should remain confidential between the medical professional and the family and/or child?

Many states have developed materials and publications for mandated reporters that outline local laws and regulations and provide information on responding to child abuse. Mandated reporters must educate themselves about the local community systems, learn about services available to children and families, and attend training on recognizing and responding to child abuse.

The mandated reporter is obligated to inform parents, caregivers, and the child that a report is being made. A report is made out of care and concern for the child and family, as well as the professional's ethical responsibility and legal mandate. Informing the family can help them know what to expect in response to the report, and it involves the family actively in addressing the problem that led to the abuse. Informing about the report can retain the family's trust in helping professionals who interact with them openly and honestly. Of course, there are instances when it would be counterproductive to inform the family before making a report to CPS or law enforcement. This would include situations in which doing so would put the child at risk for further abuse (DePanfilis & Salus, 1992).

OUTCOMES OF CPS INTERVENTIONS

The purpose of CPS is to protect children and strengthen the relationships between the child and caregivers. The greatest concern of CPS is to ensure child safety and make decisions regarding the dangers a child faces and the appropriate services needed for the child and the family to ensure a child is not abused again. The effectiveness of CPS interventions can be measured by the overall outcomes the agencies achieve based on the goals they set. Child welfare agencies are generally held accountable to measure, report, and track results for the children they serve (USDHHS, 1998). An annual summary of child welfare data provides the findings from the 30 states that kept the best outcome measures of the services provided.

The following 8 points are some of the performance data as determined by the 1998 annual report of child welfare outcomes, along with some practice implications of the data (USDHHS, 1998):

1. Eleven percent of child maltreatment victims were then the victims of at least one additional incident of maltreatment within 12 months. In all cases, the CPS agency should evaluate the situation in a timely manner and evaluate the results of all interventions before deciding to close the case.

2. Most children who exit foster care achieve permanency, but the goal of state child welfare agencies is to achieve permanency for all children under their placement and care and ensure that children grow up in safe and stable families. Eighty-two percent of children left foster care to permanent family placements:

   — 66% reunified with their families or other relatives

   — 14% were adopted

   — 2% had legal guardians appointed

3. About four fifths of all children leaving foster care exited to permanent settings, regardless of race or ethnicity.

   — States can work to develop and/or reinforce community supports for families, address cultural differences, and increase parental child-rearing competencies to help parents overcome abusive behavior toward their children. It is important for state child welfare agencies to keep children safe and find them permanent placements as quickly as possible if they are removed from their homes.

4. Approximately 6% of children exited foster care to emancipation. More than one third of children were younger than age 12 years when they entered the foster care system and had spent 6 or more years in care without finding a permanent home.

   — The large number of children growing up in foster care supports the mandate of the Foster Care Independence Act of 1999 requiring states to provide independent living and supportive services to children who remain in foster care and to help them transition to self-sufficiency.

5. Sixty-five percent of children reunited with their parents or other relatives had been in foster care for fewer than 12 months.

   — Although most children were reunited with their families within 12 months of entering foster care, many other children took longer. The state child welfare agency should work for the child's return, when it can be done safely. The agency must identify needed family services of abused or neglected children and take steps to expedite the safe return of children to their families.

6. Seventeen percent of the children who entered foster care in fiscal year 1998 had been in foster care previously.

   — It is important that state child welfare agencies avoid reuniting children with their families without providing necessary support services to the families.

7. Forty-nine percent of adoptions occurred after the children had been in foster care 4 years or more; 16% of adoptions occurred within 2 years of the child's entry into foster care.

   — The waiting time for children to find permanent homes is too long. The Adoption and Safe Families Act strongly promotes timely adoption of children who cannot return to their own homes. Many state child welfare agencies work concurrently to reunite a family while planning for the possibility that reunification will not succeed. CPS needs to work on strategies that expedite adoption, such as listing the child with appropriate adoption exchanges or taking timely steps to complete home studies.

8. Eighty-one percent of children in foster care less than 12 months had 2 or fewer placements; 39% of children in care 48 months or more had 2 or fewer placements.

— The longer a child remained in foster care, the less likely it was for that child to experience a stable placement. It is important that state child welfare agencies provide adequate supports to foster children and their foster parents to prevent the disruption of placements. Appropriate supports help reduce the number of placement settings experienced by children in foster care.

SUMMARY

The role of CPS in the protection of children is essential. Children suspected of having been abused and neglected become part of the CPS system, and CPS is responsible for ensuring the safety and security of those children. The responsibility of CPS is to protect the child and help with the investigation of the alleged charges. CPS remains a part of the case until the best interests of the child are determined.

— Most, if not all, state CPS laws impose a penalty for failure to report suspected child abuse.

— Mandated reporters are protected from civil and criminal liability associated with reporting.

— Most, if not all, state CPS laws impose a penalty for failure to report suspected child abuse.

— CPS agencies and, in some cases, law enforcement authorities conduct an investigation into the facts of the situation and make a determination of whether abuse occurred.

— Child abuse reporting sets in motion a chain of events that begins with the acceptance of the report by the hotline.

REFERENCES

Butz AM, Redman BK, Fry ST, Kolodner K. Ethical conflicts experienced by certified pediatric nurse practitioners in ambulatory settings. *J Pediatr Health Care.* 1998;12:183-190.

Caffey J. Multiple fractures in the long bones of infants suffering from chronic subdural hematoma. *Am J Roentgenol.* 1946;56:163-173.

Child Abuse Prevention and Treatment Act (CAPTA). US Code title 42, chapter 67: 93-247; 1974.

DePanfilis D, Salus MK. *Child Protective Services: A Guide for Caseworkers.* Washington, DC: US Dept of Health & Human Services; 1992.

DePanfilis D, Salus MK. *A Coordinated Response to Child Abuse and Neglect: A Basic Manual.* National Clearinghouse on Child Abuse and Neglect Information. Updated April 6, 2001. Available at: http://www.calib.com/nccanch/pubs/usermanuals/basic/figure2.cfm. Accessed February 17, 2003.

Dinsmore J. *Joint Investigations of Child Abuse: Report of a Symposium.* Washington, DC: US Dept of Health & Human Services, National Center on Child Abuse and Neglect; 1993.

Drake B. Unraveling unsubstantiated. *Child Maltreat.* 1996;1:261-271.

Ells M. Need for a team approach. In: *Forming a Multidisciplinary Team to Investigate Child Abuse: Portable Guides to Investigating Child Abuse.* National Criminal Justice Reference Service; 1998. Available at: http://www.ncjrs.org/html/ojjdp/portable_guides/forming/need.html. Accessed February 20, 2003.

Gelles R. Family preservation and reunification: how effective a social policy? In: White S, ed. *Handbook of Youth and Justice.* New York, NY: Kluwer Academic/Plenum Publishers; 2001a.

Gelles RJ. *CAPTA: Successes and Failures at Preventing Child Abuse and Neglect.* Testimony prepared for US House of Representatives Committee on Education and the Workforce Subcommittee on Select Education. August 2, 2001b. Available at: http://edworkforce.house.gov/hearings/107th/sed/capta8201/gelles.htm. Accessed March 3, 2003.

Greipp ME. Ethical decision making and mandatory reporting in cases of suspected child abuse. *J Pediatr Health Care.* 1997;11:258-265.

Kalichman SC. *Mandatory Reporting of Suspected Child Abuse: Ethics, Law, & Policy.* 2nd ed. Washington, DC: American Psychological Association; 1999.

Kalichman SC, Craig ME, Follingstad DR. Mental health professionals and suspected cases of child abuse: an investigation of factors influencing reporting. *Community Ment Health J.* 1988;24:43-51.

Kempe C. Sexual abuse, another hidden pediatric problem: the 1977 C. Anderson Aldrich Lecture. *Pediatrics.* 1978;62:382-389.

Kempe C, Silverman F, Steele B, Droegemuller W, Silver H. The battered-child syndrome. *JAMA.* 1962;181:17-24.

Koralek D. *Caregivers of Young Children: Preventing and Responding to Child Maltreatment.* Washington, DC: US Dept of Health & Human Services; 1992. Contract No. HHS-105-88-1702.

Levine M, Levine A. *Helping Children: A Social History.* New York, NY: Oxford University Press; 1992.

McCoid AH. The battered child and other assaults upon the family: Part I. *Mil Law Rev.* 1965;50:20.

National Children's Alliance. National Children's Alliance Member Standards. Available at: http://www.nca-online.org. Accessed March 3, 2003.

National Clearinghouse on Child Abuse and Neglect Information. *What Is Child Maltreatment?* National Clearinghouse on Child Abuse and Neglect Information. Available at: http://www.calib.com/nccanch. Accessed May 8, 2001.

Pence DM, Wilson CA. Reporting and investigating child sexual abuse. *Future Child.* 1994a;4:70-83.

Pence DM, Wilson CA. *Team Investigation of Child Sexual Abuse: The Uneasy Alliance.* Thousand Oaks, Calif: Sage Publications; 1994b.

Rowe DS, Leonard MF, Seashore MR, Lewiston NJ, Anderson FP. A hospital program for the detection and registration of abused and neglected children. *N Engl J Med.* 1970;282:950-952.

Rycraft JR. Redefining child abuse and neglect: narrowing the focus may affect children at risk. *Public Welfare.* 1990;48:14-21.

Sedlak AJ, Broadhurst DD. *Third National Incidence Study of Child Abuse and Neglect (NIS-3).* Washington, DC: US Dept of Health & Human Services. Available at: http://www.calib.com/nccanch/pubs/statinfo/nis3.cfm. Accessed September 1, 1996.

Smolowe J. Making the tough calls. *Time.* December 11, 1995.

US Advisory Board on Child Abuse and Neglect. *Child Abuse and Neglect: Critical First Steps in Response to a National Emergency.* Washington, DC: US Government Printing Office; 1990.

US Department of Health & Human Services. *National Study on the Incidence and Prevalence of Child Abuse and Neglect.* Washington, DC: US Government Printing Office; 1988.

US Department of Health & Human Services. *Child Abuse Prevention and Treatment Act,* as amended (October 3, 1996). 42 U.S.C. 5106g et seq. 10-3-1996. P.L. 104-235.

US Department of Health & Human Services. *Child Welfare Outcomes 1998: Annual Report.* Washington, DC: National Clearinghouse on Child Abuse and Neglect Information; 1998.

US Department of Health & Human Services. *Child Maltreatment 1999: Reports From the States to the National Child Abuse and Neglect Data Systems.* Available at: http://www.acf.dhhs.gov/programs/cb/publications/cm99/cpt1.htm. 1999a. Accessed February 17, 2003.

US Department of Health & Human Services. *Child Maltreatment 1999: Reports From the States to the National Child Abuse and Neglect Data Systems.* Washington, DC: US Government Printing Office; 1999b.

US Department of Health & Human Services. Administration on Children, Youth and Families. *Child Maltreatment 1998: Reports From the States to the National Child Abuse and Neglect Data System.* Washington, DC: US Government Printing Office; 2000.

Wang CT, Daro D. *Current Trends in Child Abuse Reporting and Fatalities: The Results of the 1997 Annual Fifty State Survey.* Chicago, Ill: Prevent Child Abuse America; 1998.

Williams HS, Osborne YH, Rappaport NB. Child abuse reporting law: professionals' knowledge and compliance. *Southern Psychologist.* 1987;3:20-24.

Wilson C, Pence D. How should child protective services and law enforcement coordinate the initial assessment and investigation? In: Dubowitz H, DePanfilis, eds. *Handbook for Child Protection Practice.* Thousand Oaks, Calif: Sage Publications; 2000:101-104.

Wilson EP. Multidisciplinary approach to child protection. In: Ludwig S, Kornberg AE, eds. *Child Abuse: A Medical Reference.* 2nd ed. New York, NY: Churchill Livingstone; 1992:79-84.

Wilson EP, Hilbert D. A hospital team approach to child abuse. *Pa Med.* 1973;Sept:419-425.

Wurtele SK, Miller-Perrin CL. *Preventing Child Sexual Abuse: Sharing the Responsibility.* Lincoln: University of Nebraska Press; 1992.

Chapter 14

LEGAL ISSUES

Angelo P. Giardino, MD, PhD, FAAP
Frank P. Cervone, Esq.
Eileen R. Giardino, PhD, RN, CRNP

The healthcare professional evaluating a child for suspected maltreatment will inevitably come in contact with the people and practices of the legal system. Law enforcement personnel may become involved in the investigation and rely on information generated by the healthcare encounter. An arrest may ensue, and the case may be moved to a court setting in which attorneys seek additional information from various professionals involved with the case. The legal system operates differently from the healthcare setting, and the courtroom is often a new and strange environment for the health professional because of law's rich history, governing principles, and unique vocabulary. This chapter seeks to provide the nurse with an overview of the legal issues surrounding child maltreatment that may require the nurse's input and understanding. The chapter will describe the role of the legal system and the courts.

Legal issues arise with the initial suspicion of child maltreatment. The identification and investigation of potential child abuse and neglect will have a set of legal ramifications for medical treatment, social service intervention, and criminal prosecution (Devlin & Reynolds, 1994; Goldner, Dolgin, & Manske, 1996). Each state defines child abuse and child neglect in its laws and regulations. Although wording sometimes differs from state to state, the laws are generally intended to guide the reporting of child maltreatment to appropriate authorities, establish standards for intervention and protective intervention, and outline activities and behaviors that require examination and possible punishment by the criminal justice system (Goldner et al., 1996).

Child abuse laws have specific importance to healthcare providers because they often clarify the responsibilities of professionals and healthcare facilities involved with child maltreatment cases. Issues of family privacy and legal proof compete with the desire to protect children and to serve families (Katner & Plum, 2002; Myers, 2002).

The pediatric health practitioner's goal is to work for the health and well-being of the child. This goal can be advanced through effective interaction and participation in the legal process and careful navigation through the judicial/court system. Nurses need not become experts in the law or in courtroom strategy (Myers JL, 1996). Rather, they will have the greatest opportunity to serve the child's interests if they are familiar with the principles that underlie the intersection of healthcare and legal practice in child maltreatment cases.

MANDATED REPORTING

The nurse's responsibility begins with the identification of potential cases of child maltreatment (Fiesta, 1992). Legislation exists in every state that requires specific professionals—those who are likely to come into contact with children in the course of their work—to report suspected cases of maltreatment to the designated child protective services (CPS) agency (National Clearinghouse on Child Abuse and Neglect

Information [NCCANI], 2000). Lists of professionals who are required to report vary by state, but healthcare providers such as nurses and physicians are required to report in every state (NCCANI, 2000). (See Appendix: Mandatory Reporters, Statutes at-a-Glance.)

Mandated reporters must report cases that reach the level of suspicion that triggers obligatory reporting; such reporters are mandated to report these potential cases (Carlisle, 1991; Murphy, 1995). They are not afforded professional judgment or flexibility in such cases and do not have discretion in this matter (Myers, 1998). The "triggering level" for reporting may be a difficult issue for healthcare professionals, depending on the case. The legal terms that trigger mandated reporting typically include the following (Myers, 1998):

— Cause to believe

— *Reasonable* cause to believe

— *Known or suspected* abuse

— Reason to *suspect*

— Observation or examination that discloses evidence of abuse

One must consider the close distinctions in meaning, for example, evidence that would cause a person to *suspect* something happened versus evidence sufficient to *believe* the event occurred. Each of these phrases is slightly different, but the overarching intent is to ensure that a healthcare professional, such as a nurse, is mandated to report possible maltreatment when the available case material would lead a competent professional to consider child abuse or neglect as a reasonably likely diagnosis to explain the case (Myers, 1998). Across the United States, various phrases are used in the statutes, so each child-serving professional must be familiar with the law in the local jurisdiction (NCCANI, 2002a).

To encourage the often difficult task of reporting suspected child maltreatment, state laws generally include provisions designed to remove barriers that might dissuade a person from the duty to report and penalties to encourage compliance, including the following (Goldner et al., 1996; Zellman & Faller, 1996):

— Immunity for good faith reporting (i.e., the reporter may still be sued in civil court but will be protected from liability [Rhodes, 1996])

— Standards to guide "reasonableness" of opinion (i.e., concern of possible maltreatment need not be absolutely diagnosed before reporting)

— Rules protecting the anonymity of the reporter

— Relaxation of "privileged communication rights" such as the doctor/patient privilege

— Procedures for reporting and how the information is processed

— Power of physicians and police officers to assume protective custody for the child if deemed necessary for the child's safety

— Penalties for failure to report

The intent of the reporting laws is to encourage the protection of children from additional risk of injury via the early identification and investigation of child maltreatment (Pillitteri, 1994). By law, state or county CPS agencies are responsible for the receipt of the report and its investigation (several states also include law enforcement), the assessment of child and family social service needs, the development of an intervention strategy that includes treatment for the child and potentially for the family, and ongoing follow-up and monitoring of cases of child maltreatment until the case is closed. (See Chapter 13, Child Protective Services and Child Abuse, for a description of typical CPS processes.) CPS traditionally works closely with law enforcement in their respective investigations and with the courts on the custody and parental rights issues that arise in the case (Dubowitz & DePanfilis, 2000).

The impact of the reporting laws has been to dramatically increase the number of potential child abuse reports made to CPS annually, for example, from 669 000 reports in 1976 to approximately 3 million in 1998 (US Department of Health & Human Services [USDHHS], 2000). Because some children or some incidents have multiple reports, it is estimated that approximately 2 million children are involved in these reported cases. After investigation and processing, approximately 1 million cases each year are substantiated; that is, CPS concludes that maltreatment *probably* or *is likely* to have occurred. For example, in 1998, of the approximately 3 million reports received by CPS agencies in the United States, approximately 903 000 were substantiated (USDHHS, 2000).

Any person may make a report of suspected abuse to local authorities, using a local, state, or national hotline to provide information and concerns about a child's well-being. Professionals, however, account for the largest number of reports. Among professionals, school personnel make the most reports (30% of professional reports), followed by law enforcement personnel (22%), healthcare personnel (20%), and child-care providers (4%) (Zellman & Fair, 2002).

Reasons that motivate professionals to make reports of suspected maltreatment have been identified as including the following (Zellman & Faller, 1996):

— Stopping maltreatment

— Getting help for a family

— Complying with the mandated reporter law/workplace policies and procedures

— Helping the family see the seriousness of the problem

— Bringing CPS expertise into case

Other issues that influence professionals' decision to report include the seriousness of the injury (professionals are more likely to report if physical injuries are present or if sexual intercourse occurred), the age of the child involved (professionals are more likely to report if child was young versus adolescent), and a history of previous abuse (professionals are more likely to report if previous abuse occurred) (Zellman & Faller, 1996).

Data from the national incidence studies show an apparent discrepancy between the number of cases known to various professionals and the number reported to CPS agencies. Even after possible data collection discrepancies are considered, some recognized cases may not result in reports or CPS investigation. Thus, it would appear that compliance with mandated reporting laws is not one hundred percent. In a recent study examining primary care providers' child abuse reporting patterns that included nurse practitioners, compliance with the reporting mandate was outstanding, with 92% of providers reporting all cases in which abuse was suspected (Flaherty, Sege, Binns, Mattson, & Christoffel, 2000). However, in this same study, 8% of providers did not report on 5% of suspected cases, and it appeared that providers who had some formal child maltreatment education after their initial training were more likely to report than those who had none (Flaherty et al., 2000). Professionals may at times fail to report cases that meet the reporting standards. Zellman and Faller (1996) characterized possible reasons for professionals not reporting cases of suspected child maltreatment to CPS as falling into the following 3 general categories:

1. Perceived cost of reporting to the reporter

   — Takes too much time

   — Lawsuit fears

   — Uncomfortable with family

2. Belief that the professional could do a better job than the system for the child

   — CPS overreaction

   — Poor quality of services

   — Professional felt able to help the child

   — Treatment already accepted by caregiver

   — Treatment already in place will be disrupted if reported

3. Concern does not reach reporting level

   — Insufficient evidence that abuse occurred

   — Maltreatment not serious enough to report

   — Situation resolved on its own

   — Report already made

Although concerns about the value of making reports to overworked agencies may be pertinent in specific locales, mandatory reporting laws do not allow such discretion for the healthcare provider who is mandated to report (Myers, 1998). Healthcare professionals are required to report suspicions of maltreatment regardless of whether they perceive that the CPS agency will make a difference in the child's life. Experiences of inadequate investigation, meager system response, and a relative paucity of services offered to families need to propel advocacy efforts on behalf of children and families in the community and not be used as excuses for failures to make mandated reports in the future (Butz, Redman, Fry, & Kolodner, 1998).

Nursing scholars have addressed the ethical considerations that face the nurse in reaching a decision to make a report (Butz et al., 1998; Greipp, 1997; Hamblet, 1994; Lewin, 1994). In considering the philosophical dimensions that underpin the rich ethical issues implicated in the child maltreatment reporting decision, 2 major theoretical frameworks exist and may be helpful to consider. The first framework is ***teleological***, in which the worth of an action is determined by the value of the ends and consequences of taking such an action (Hamblet, 1994). Child abuse reporting in such a framework would be viewed as valuable or not valuable based on the results such reporting produced. The second framework is referred to as ***deontological***, meaning the worth of an action is determined not by the consequences produced but by characteristics of that action that inherently make it right or wrong (Hamblet, 1994). The characteristics that determine whether an action is right or wrong may be singular, for example, in following a principle such as the Golden Rule, or more multifaceted, such as following the fundamental principles to which nursing professionals are socialized to consider (Hamblet, 1994). During a nurse's professional training, values and professional standards are learned; the commonly understood principles that guide a nurse's clinical practice are summarized as follows (Hamblet, 1994):

— *Autonomy:* the right of self-determination

— *Beneficence:* the duty to do good

— *Nonmaleficence:* the duty to avoid harm

— *Fidelity:* the priority of keeping promises

— *Justice:* the need for fairness

— *Veracity:* the responsibility to tell the truth

Child abuse reporting in a deontological framework would be viewed as valuable or not valuable based on the reporting action's concordance with a principle or set of principles, such as those already discussed, and not necessarily on the actual result of a given report. For example, the reporter might act based on the legal duty to report but also feel compromised or conflicted by the possibility that a child's injuries are not clearly diagnostic of abuse or that family stability might be shaken. Understanding these ethical paradigms may lead to a fuller discussion of the inevitable conflicts that may arise and be experienced by nursing healthcare professionals as they confront the mandated reporting responsibility (Butz et al., 1998; Greipp, 1997; Lewin, 1994).

CRIMINAL INVESTIGATION PROCESS

The focus of the law enforcement investigation is to obtain statements and physical evidence that will corroborate the allegation of child maltreatment (Giardino & Kolilis, 2002). The police interview the suspected victim, the caregivers, and the suspected perpetrator. Police often investigate in tandem with CPS.

The interview of the suspected victim is similar to the history that a healthcare provider would obtain, essentially the who, what, when, where, and how of the occurrence of the abuse. Law enforcement officers, because of their need to uncover evidence and corroborate statements, frequently spend time with the child clarifying times, locations, and the presence of others. Specially trained interviewers, often working in centers known as children's alliances or child advocacy centers (CACs), can perform this role of lead interviewer, while collaborating colleagues from law enforcement and child welfare observe the interview on a video screen or through a mirror.

Rarely does the healthcare provider interview the perpetrator. The police are, by their training, often best positioned to do this, and they pay close attention to the perpetrator's background and history of prior contact with the legal system (Hammond, Lanning, Promisel, Shepherd, & Walsh, 1997). Additionally, law enforcement officers are aware of the constitutional rights of suspected perpetrators, and they collect the interview history in a manner that will allow it to be used in court if necessary (Lanning & Walsh, 1996).

The medical examination is a key piece of the investigation; the diagnostic opinions of the examiner are critical to the case. (See Chapter 5, Laboratory Findings, Diagnostic Testing, and Forensic Specimens in Cases of Child Sexual Abuse, for a full discussion.) Healthcare professionals should take care to preserve physical evidence in accordance with local law enforcement and health institution protocols. For example, for a court to admit physical specimens into the record as evidence, the court and parties must be assured of the chain of custody; that is, the specimen was in the control of person "A" who conveyed it to person "B," and so on, so that one can determine by questioning whether the specimen is in the same condition as when it was collected from the scene or patient at the time of the event. (See Chapter 5, Laboratory Findings, Diagnostic Testing, and Forensic Specimens in Cases of Child Sexual Abuse.)

Once the police interviews and the medical evaluation are complete and this information is presented by the law enforcement investigator to the prosecutor, a decision must be made whether or not to charge the alleged perpetrator. In deciding to arrest, the police will consider whether there is "probable cause" that the crime occurred and that this person is the one responsible for the crime. The constitutionally mandated standard of probable cause is then evaluated by a judicial officer.

The decision to charge is complicated and must be done in a context that has full awareness of the constitutional guarantees that apply in criminal proceedings and the high standard of proof in criminal court and made with the understanding of what may or may not be admissible as evidence (Bulkley, Feller, Stern, & Roe, 1996). Issues a prosecutor may consider in determining a charge include the quality of uncovered evidence and the timing related to the statute of limitations applicable to the crime believed to have been committed.

Once the perpetrator has been charged, the prosecutor and defense attorney may begin plea negotiations to avoid the risks and burdens of a court trial (Bulkley et al., 1996).

THE JUDICIAL SETTING: JUVENILE, DOMESTIC RELATIONS, CRIMINAL, AND CIVIL COURTS

Although many cases of suspected child maltreatment are unsubstantiated, and some are resolved by agreements or other nonadversarial approaches, some child abuse cases find their way into courts of law for prosecution of offenders, continued protection of the child, or resolution of custody disputes. The approach of the American legal system to children and their needs has evolved over the past 3 centuries. The historical approach of Anglo-American common law viewed children as property with parents free to do as they pleased, provided that they avoided extreme punishment or permanent injury. Limited child labor protections and social welfare institutions from the early twentieth century gave rise to the current view of childhood as a unique period of a citizen's development and a willingness to intervene if the parenting of the child is felt to be inadequate (Goldner et al., 1996).

The nation's court systems distinguish cases involving maltreatment of children and youth as matters involving family law, juvenile delinquency and child protection, or prosecution of adult perpetrators (Myers, 1998). Regardless of which court they are involved with, children enter this formal, adult setting that is specifically designed to resolve what may be contentious adult disputes in an adversarial, rule-driven manner (American Academy of Pediatrics [AAP], 1999). Court proceedings may be seen as potentially anxiety-provoking situations for children because of the adversarial nature of the process and the rules that govern fact-finding (AAP, 1999; Bulkley et al., 1996). Children primarily become involved with the court system for the following reasons:

— Concerns over their own possible maltreatment

— Contested parental custody arrangements, often as a corollary to divorce proceedings

— Offenses they are suspected of having committed (often called delinquency offenses)

— Their adoption

— Traffic offenses

Rarely, children may be called as a witness in a nonabuse-related criminal or civil case of which they have some knowledge. Child maltreatment and divorce-related custody disputes account for the majority of child court appearances (AAP, 1999).

JUVENILE AND CHILD PROTECTION COURTS

Juvenile courts, sometimes called children's courts, are governed by state laws and are typically separate from adult courts (Katner & Plum, 2002). The juvenile court exercises its power over minors brought into the system because of all forms of child abuse, neglect, abandonment, unwillingness to submit to parental control (incorrigibility), and delinquency (committing criminal offenses). Whereas social service interventions are often voluntarily accepted by a family or child, the juvenile court's participation is often directive and even coercive.

Two legal doctrines underlie the role of the juvenile court in child maltreatment cases, distinguishing juvenile court from domestic relations and criminal courts (Bulkley et al., 1996). First, under the theory of *parens patriae*, or the "state as parent," the government has the authority to step in and limit a parent's authority over his or her child when the court perceives a danger to the child's physical or mental health. Families are seen to have a right to autonomy over the decisions they make, privacy for their deliberations and actions, and the ability to stay whole or together as they choose (Bulkley et al., 1996). This right is not absolute, however, and the government may intervene if there is a compelling reason to protect the children from harm. Second, the government and its courts must consider what the child needs in order to determine what care or services should be provided for the child's continued healthy development. As part of the doctrine of due process of law, the state or local children and youth agency must create service plans that include assessments, identification of service provider and other resources, and timelines for compliance with the plan. Typically, the parents and the child (or child's representative) participate in the creation of the plan and have the opportunity to challenge the plan in court. The protective and due process doctrines act to balance each other.

The juvenile court has broad discretion in addressing issues and invokes judicial authority to facilitate the social welfare system's goal of rehabilitating and treating the abusive family when possible. The guiding principles that underlie the juvenile court's authority include the following (Goldner et al., 1996):

1. Children (particularly young children) lack the mental competency and maturity possessed by adults.

2. Before intervening, the child's caregivers must be shown to be unfit, unable, unwilling, or unavailable to care adequately for the child.

3. Intervention may be taken to promote the best interests of the child.

The juvenile court, like many of the professionals who work in child welfare and related fields, must pursue 2 goals that are sometimes in conflict: the preservation of families and the protection of children. For some children, the court's involvement will focus on protecting the child from further maltreatment and harm, with termination of parental rights and permanent, alternative family placements as the most severe but necessary remedies. For other children, the court might order the provision of services and treatment to the child and family; it may order mental health evaluation of children and parents as well.

The juvenile court developed alongside the movement toward professional social work and the increased use of social services to support families and protect children. The juvenile court exercises state authority to intervene in a family over the objection of a parent to protect a child and has a tradition of relying on nonlegal professionals for information and assistance in assessing the situation before it. In considering a given case, CPS caseworkers, social workers, physicians, psychiatrists, and psychologists are frequently asked for guidance by the juvenile court. The juvenile court tends to be more involved with the provision of services and treatment and on ensuring long-term monitoring of the interventions with a focus on helping the child and family rather than on punishing the offending parent.

One key difference between juvenile (and domestic relations) cases and the more commonly observed criminal court process lies in the standard of proof required to make a decision. Whereas the finder of fact in a criminal proceeding—the jury or the judge—can convict a criminal defendant only if the evidence is "beyond a reasonable doubt," civil proceedings use lower measures: "preponderance of evidence" (i.e., more likely than not), "clear and convincing evidence" (i.e., compelling but not the only reasonably possible reading of the evidence), or simply "substantial evidence" (i.e., more than a little) (Myers, 1998). In short, proving maltreatment is legally easier in juvenile or family court than in the criminal justice courtroom.

Juvenile court intervention has certain disadvantages. There is often the possibility of multiple out-of-home placements that may be lengthy and disruptive to the child and family. The court sometimes orders the removal of the child, rather than the offender, from the family. Each move to help a child also risks unnecessary intervention. Finally, the paucity of effective services and treatments that the juvenile courts can provide is legendary.

In general, the CPS agency files a petition with the juvenile court asking for the court's involvement on behalf of protecting the child. The initial hearing is to determine whether the child or children should be removed from the family home to keep them safe from further abuse or injury. From here, preparation begins for the trial in which evidence will be presented from both sides to the judge, who will decide if maltreatment has occurred. If the judge decides that abuse or neglect has occurred, then the case moves on to a disposition hearing in which the judge will decide who will have custody of the child and what protection will be put in place. Options include the following (**Figure 14-1**):

— Protective supervision order: wide range of structure

— Removal of child (temporary): foster care, kinship care

— Removal of child (parent): termination of parental rights

DOMESTIC RELATIONS COURT (FAMILY COURT)
Domestic relations court, or family court, addresses the conflicts that may arise between 2 parents or other involved caregivers, such as grandparents or kin. Issues dealt with by such a court include child custody and visitation, child support, divorce, and issues related to marital property. Family violence and domestic abuse may be assigned by law or local practice to family court. In domestic relations proceedings, the standard for decision making in child custody is typically a version of the question, "What is in the best interests of the child?"

Today, across the country, child abuse allegations may arise within families who are involved in divorce or other civil custodial disputes. Approximately 2% of custody disputes include a complaint related to child abuse (Thoennes & Tjaden, 1990). Therefore, domestic relations court may become involved with child maltreatment in regard to such custody-related disputes. If one parent alleges that the other (or someone in the household) is responsible for maltreating the child or children, the parent in such a situation may then, within the divorce/separation process, request specific custody arrangements to limit the likelihood of the child being exposed to further abuse, such as sole custody with no visitation for the other or sole custody

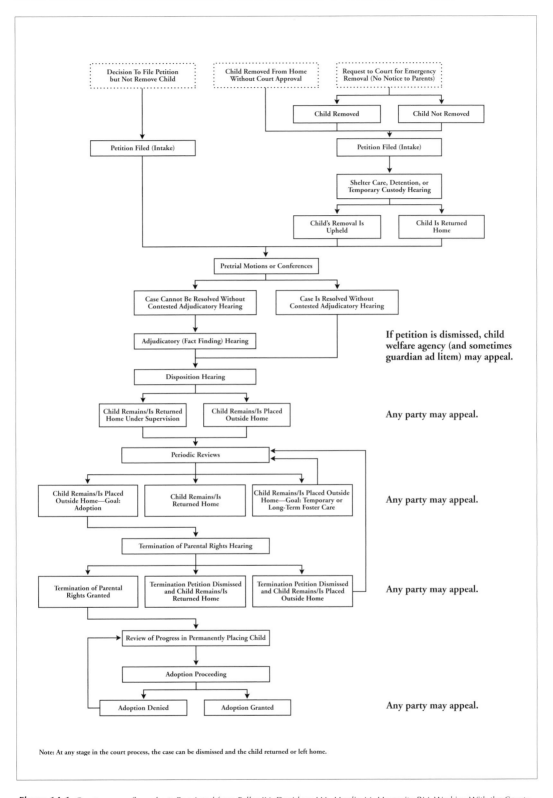

Figure 14-1. *Court process flow chart. Reprinted from Feller JN, Davidson HA, Hardin M, Horowitz RM. Working With the Courts in Child Protection. US Dept of Health & Human Services. 1992. Available at: http://www.calib.com/nccanch/pubs/usermanuals/courts/courts.pdf.*

with supervised visitation (Myers, 1998). If already divorced, the parent may request a modification of the original agreement in view of the alleged maltreatment with an imposition limitation on visitation. In a study that examined a sampling of sexual abuse allegations in the setting of custody/visitation disputes, accusations were brought by mothers 67% of the time, by fathers 28% of the time, and by third parties 11% of the time (Thoennes & Tjaden, 1990). Actual abuse was substantiated in 50% to 67% of the cases, depending on the standard applied, with 33% of the cases having been deemed not to involve abuse. Four factors were significantly associated with the credibility of the allegation, as follows (Thoennes & Tjaden, 1990):

1. Age of the child

2. Frequency of the abuse

3. Existence of prior abuse reports

4. Amount of time between divorce filing and the emergence of the abuse report

Domestic relations courts have been criticized in the past for their handling of child maltreatment issues for reasons such as the following:

— Personnel not having much experience with child maltreatment, having been traditionally more involved with parental rights in divorce proceedings

— Lack of structural coordination with CPS and juvenile courts (i.e., little information sharing, computer systems not interfaced)

— Concern that disputing parents in the context of a divorce situation may deliberately put forward false allegations of child maltreatment

Although there is little evidence of widespread falsification in custody disputes and divorce proceedings, healthcare professionals need to take any concerns about maltreatment seriously and handle this in a careful manner with a focus on the medical and healthcare status of the child in question (Green, 1986; Gunter et al., 2000; Herman & Bernet, 1997). In a study that examined one city's experience with substantiation of sexual abuse allegations cases and concomitant custody or visitation disputes, the allegations tended to be substantiated less frequently in cases with parental conflict but, nevertheless, were substantiated more than half the time (Paradise, Rostain, & Nathanson, 1988).

CRIMINAL COURT: PROSECUTIONS

All states view child abuse as a crime, and through their state penal codes and criminal laws, each state defines specific elements of sexual abuse, physical abuse, emotional abuse, and neglect (NCCANI, 2000). States vary in their definitions, and each healthcare provider should be familiar with the specifics that govern practice in his or her state.

Although many advocates argue for full prosecution of all cases of child maltreatment, this ideal has not been achieved for 3 reasons. First, juvenile courts were traditionally viewed as the ideal place for handling the child abuse and neglect cases because of their focus on the family needs and the provisions of services to the child and family. Second, the ability to prove child maltreatment is challenging in criminal court because of the constitutional protections afforded defendants in a criminal court. For example, rules of evidence, procedures for search and seizure, standards for judging guilt (beyond a reasonable doubt), the right to confront witnesses, and the right to examine and cross examine are stringent. Third, the criminal court is seen as especially threatening and potentially damaging to children because it requires multiple interviews, inevitable delays that extend for years, insensitive questioning, and the need for face-to-face confrontation in court with the defendant (AAP, 1999; Bulkley et al., 1996; Myers, 1998).

The family may also experience emotional trauma during criminal proceedings, especially when the offender is a parent. The prosecution of a parent may lead to loss of employment and income, disruption or dissolution of the family, incarceration of the parent, and the potential feeling of guilt on the part of the child victim or witness. If an acquittal occurs, the child may be held in contempt by other family members and potentially develop a feeling of complete hopelessness. In addition, offender treatment is often inadequate, ineffective, or unavailable.

Some healthcare professionals may ask why family members should be prosecuted at all. Arguments favoring prosecution of intrafamilial abusers include clearly establishing the perpetrator as solely responsible for the maltreatment, recognizing the innocence of the victim and providing him or her with a sense of vindication and fairness, deterring others from maltreating children, and ensuring that offenders are treated or incapacitated, thus preventing or reducing the risk for further episodes of maltreatment (Bulkley et al., 1996; Katner & Plum, 2002).

CIVIL COURT: LAWSUITS

Child maltreatment may be seen as a civil offense open to a civil lawsuit in which a child or adult survivor who has been maltreated seeks monetary damages from the perpetrator or from a professional involved in the case (Myers, 1998). Civil court is the venue where private citizens may seek to address offenses caused by another for intentional negligent or reckless conduct. Several specific legal issues arise when discussing civil suits for child abuse and neglect cases, and they tend to revolve around the quality of care provided the child at the time of the abuse and the failure to protect the child from harm (Katner & Plum, 2002). Classic tort analysis asks 3 questions: Was there a duty? Was the duty breached? Did the breach cause the injury? Additionally, civil actions are also limited by statute of limitation issues; this may be of particular importance regarding child maltreatment cases because of the length of time that may elapse from abuse to disclosure.

CHILDREN AS WITNESSES

Courts increasingly recognize the need to handle children differently from adults, owing mainly to children's dependency on adults, their varying level of understanding about the proceedings, and their ongoing emotional and cognitive development (AAP, 1999; Nurcombe, 1985).

Children have a unique position in the US judicial system, and their functioning as witnesses in their own child maltreatment cases has received professional attention. Opinions span the entire spectrum, with some claiming that having a child facing the accuser in court may have a health-promoting effect while others caution that such face-to-face confrontation in the court setting can damage the child (AAP, 1999). No agreement currently exists in the professional literature about the benefit or harm to a child witness although all children experienced high levels of anxiety before testifying (AAP, 1999; Runyan & Toth, 1991). Proponents of the positive aspects of child testimony claim that when the child sees the perpetrator take responsibility for the abusive actions, the child's sense of self-worth and personal safety may improve. On the other hand, proponents of the potentially negative effects claim that the courtroom experience may cause a high degree of distress in the child and may exacerbate the child's feelings of stigmatization and being a victim. The child may be placed in the no-win situation of having to give damaging testimony against a person (often a family member) with whom there has been a positive attachment but a negative experience (AAP, 1999). Factors associated with the improved mental health of children who testified at their own child maltreatment cases were maternal support and time elapsed from giving the testimony, regardless of whether it was a positive or negative experience.

Researchers looking at children testifying in court have found the following (Saywitz & Goodman, 1996; Saywitz, Goodman, & Lyon, 2002):

— Children as young as 5 years of age understand the need to tell the truth.

— Younger children tell the truth because of fear of punishment, whereas older children understand the need for truthful statements in order to allow the fact-finding of the trial to occur.

— Children age 4 to 7 years rely on their observation of overt behavior to understand court process and the roles of court personnel, and they have difficulty understanding the abstract principles underlying law, evidence rules, and the trial process.

— Children at approximately 10 years of age understand the rudiments of the investigation and court process at trial.

To decrease the amount of stress experienced by the child, some child advocates have employed methods to make the trial process easier for children (Pennsylvania Bar Association, 2002). "Court schools" have been developed to demystify the experience for the child. Before the actual court experience, children are brought into the courtroom and shown where they and others will sit, and the roles of court personnel are explained. The child is permitted to explore the court environment, and any questions the child has are answered. **Table 14-1** lists activities that may be used to minimize the stress of court involvement for children.

PROFESSIONALS IN COURT AS WITNESSES

Healthcare professionals may be called to court in 2 different categories: (1) lay or fact witness or (2) expert witness (Myers & Stern, 2002).

Lay witnesses have personal knowledge of relevant facts for the child maltreatment case. They are called to tell in court what they saw or heard about the case (Myers & Stern, 2002). A nurse could be a fact witness in a case when in the course of providing care he or she is an eyewitness to the disclosure (Myers JL, 1996). The nurse may, therefore, be called as a lay witness to recount the event of the disclosure by the child. An expert witness is someone who has special knowledge and is called to help those in court to understand technical, clinical, or scientific issues related to relevant facts in the case (Myers JEB, 1996).

The expert witness does not necessarily have any personal involvement in the case, as the lay witness does, but the expert has special knowledge that allows testimony in court. The nurse could be an expert in a child maltreatment case if, for example, by virtue of training, he or she was a nurse practitioner and was called to explain the interpretation of the physical examination findings regarding health and possible maltreatment. As the field of forensic nursing continues to develop, nurses may be asked to serve as expert witnesses more and more in the courtroom setting (Ledray, 2003).

In general, criminal courts are stricter in terms of how much the expert is permitted to say during the court proceedings. Judges often allow the experts to speak more broadly in juvenile and domestic relations courts compared to criminal cases.

Myers, JEB (1996) suggests using the acronym HELP to explain the privileges of expert testimony, as follows:

Table 14-1. Matrix of Activities to Reduce Adverse Effects of Court Intervention

	CHILD	COURT	LEGAL PROCESS
Pretrial	— Preparation for process (e.g., "court school")	— Education of lawyers about child development and the way to ask questions	— Pleas and speedy processing — Collection of corroborating evidence — Elimination of competency hearings or fewer preliminary hearings
Trial	— Closed circuit — Simple, clear questions — Frequent breaks	— Child-size furniture — Explanation of oath — Let child sit with parent or support person — Testimony in chambers — Minimize size of audience — Minimize use of objections and legal jargon during testimony	— Use of expert witnesses — Use of hearsay exceptions to corroborate or replace testimony — Minimize continuances and other delays
Post-trial	— Debriefing by counselor — Debriefing by judge — Certificate of award for testimony		

Reprinted with permission from Runyan DK, Toth PA. Child sexual abuse and the courts. In: Krugman RD, Leventhal JM, eds. Child Sexual Abuse: Report of the Twenty-Second Ross Roundtable on Critical Approaches to Common Pediatric Problems. Columbus, Ohio: Ross Laboratories; 1991:57-75.

H—Honesty: derives from the oath the expert says in which he or she swears to tell the truth, the whole truth, and nothing but the truth. At the core of integrity and professionalism is a commitment to be honest and not shade the truth in favor of one side or the other.

E—Evenhandedness: derives from the expert's role of being an objective helper, not a partisan advocate for one side or the other. Whereas the client's attorney is expected to win the case, the expert is expected to say what he or she knows in an honest and professional manner. If any biases exist, these should be disclosed.

L—Limits: knows the limits of expertise in the professional literature and knows one's own limits. The expert should be able to inform those in court about the limits of current knowledge.

P—Preparation: highlights the expert's responsibility to review records and be familiar with the complex issues to be discussed **(Table 14-2).**

CONCLUSION

Healthcare professionals working with children and families involved in cases of actual or suspected child maltreatment have a high likelihood of needing to interact with law enforcement officers and attorneys who become involved in the case. At a minimum, the healthcare provider's status as a mandated reporter will often require some contact with the police and the courts as the case is investigated and potentially prosecuted. Nurses do not need to become legal experts to advocate effectively for the children and families in their care, but familiarity with the legal system and the part that law enforcement and the courts play in dealing with child maltreatment issues will be helpful. Professional practice among the police investigating the case and the courts dealing with custody issues and the potential prosecution of the perpetrator has developed so that special attention is increasingly paid to the emotional burden such proceedings may have on the child. Ultimately, the healthcare professional serves the interests of the child best by performing excellent healthcare evaluations and clarifying the health-related issues that affect the specific child.

Table 14-2. ABCs of Coping With Cross-Examination

Adversary system	Understand the adversary system so you know what makes lawyers tick.
Be calm	Be calm; breathe. Don't let the cross-examiner throw you off. If the attorney intimidates, lower your voice, speak calmly. Resist or restate unfair or ambiguous questions.
Control	Control is the name of the game. The cross-examiner seeks to control you. To avoid undue control: — Admit-deny. Brodsky (1991) describes the admit-deny technique. The cross-examiner focuses on what you could have done differently (e.g., "You could have done additional testing, couldn't you?"). Go ahead and acknowledge whatever is fair to acknowledge. However, stand by your testimony and deny you did anything wrong (e.g., "Although additional testing was possible, further testing was unnecessary in this case because . . .") (Brodsky, 1991). — Leading questions. The cross-examiner controls you with leading questions that require short answers, preferably "yes" or "no." when "yes" or "no" is not the correct answer, try "maybe" or "that depends" or "I can't answer that with a simple yes or no. May I explain myself?" — Communicate with confidence, but don't be a know-it-all. — Don't retreat. Don't change your opinion on cross-examination. — Level the linguistic playing field. The cross-examiner refers to you by name. If you refer to the attorney as "Sir" or "Ma'am," your deference gives a measure of control to the attorney. Why not refer to the attorney by name? Doing so puts you on a linguistic par with the attorney.

(continued)

Table 14-2. *(continued)*	
Do not get defensive	Getting defensive undermines your credibility. Acknowledge your limits, and confidently reaffirm your expertise and testimony. When you are attacked, borrow from the martial arts—redirect the attacker's energy to your advantage. For example, if the cross-examiner asks, "Don't you think your assessment would have been more complete if you had contacted additional people?" Your answer could be, "There are additional people I could have contacted. In this case, however, I contacted everyone necessary for a complete and thorough assessment."
Eye contact	Look the jury in the eye. Maintain frequent—although not continuous—eye contact with them. The cross-examiner may try to divert your gaze away from them.
Fishing expeditions	A cross-examiner who has little to work with may go on a fishing expedition, seeking a chink in your armor. The cross-examiner asks general questions to reveal weaknesses or lack of knowledge. Do not get hooked.
Goofs and gaffes	When you make a mistake, correct it quickly during cross-examination, let it slide, or fix it during redirect examination.
Holes in your testimony	One of the most effective cross-examination techniques is to poke a few holes in your testimony—to raise a few doubts about you—and to leave those holes unfilled and those doubts unexplained until closing arguments.
I don't know	"I don't know" is sometimes the correct answer. Remember, though, that a string of "I don't knows" looks bad.
Junk science	The cross-examiner who cannot think of anything better to do may attack the entire field as junk science. Acknowledge the limits of the field's knowledge but confidently reassert what is known.
Keep it simple	Avoid jargon that will confuse the jury.
Learned treatises	Do not let the lawyer take things out of context; insist on reading it: "I cannot comment on one sentence in a 20-page article. If you will give me an hour to read the entire article, I'll be happy to discuss it."

Reprinted with permission from Myers JEB. Legal Issues in Child Abuse and Neglect Practice. 2nd ed. Thousand Oaks, Calif: Sage Publications; 1998:364-365.

APPENDIX: MANDATORY REPORTERS, STATUTES AT-A-GLANCE

MANDATORY REPORTERS OF CHILD ABUSE AND NEGLECT

(Current through December 31, 2001)

| STATE | PROFESSIONS THAT MUST REPORT | | | | | OTHERS WHO MUST REPORT | | STANDARD FOR REPORTING | PRIVILEGED COMMUNICATIONS |
	Health Care	Mental Health	Social Work	Education/ Child Care	Law Enforcement	All Persons	Other*		
ALABAMA §§ 26-14-3(a) 26-14-10	✓	✓	✓	✓	✓		• Any other person called upon to give aid or assistance to any child	• Known or suspected	• Attorney/client
ALASKA §§ 47.17.020(a) 47.17.023 47.17.060	✓	✓	✓	✓	✓		• Paid employees of domestic violence and sexual assault programs and drug and alcohol treatment facilities • Members of a child fatality review team or multidisciplinary child protection team • Commercial or private film or photograph processors	• Have reasonable cause to suspect	
ARIZONA §§ 13-3620(A) 8-805(B)-(C)	✓	✓	✓	✓	✓		• Parents • Anyone responsible for care or treatment of children • Clergy	• Have reasonable grounds to believe	• Clergy/penitent • Attorney/client
ARKANSAS § 12-12-507(b)-(c)	✓	✓	✓	✓	✓		• Prosecutors • Judges • Div. of Youth Services employees • Domestic violence shelter employees and volunteers	• Have reasonable cause to suspect • Have observed conditions which would reasonably result	
CALIFORNIA Penal Code §§ 11166(a),(c) 11165.7(a)	✓	✓	✓	✓	✓		• Firefighters • Animal control officers • Commercial film and photographic print processors • Clergy • Court appointed special advocates (CASAs)	• Have knowledge of or observe • Know or reasonably suspect	• Clergy/penitent

Readers should not rely on this summary for legal advice.

National Clearinghouse on Child Abuse and Neglect Information, February 2002

MANDATORY REPORTERS OF CHILD ABUSE AND NEGLECT

(Current through December 31, 2001)

STATE	PROFESSIONS THAT MUST REPORT					OTHERS WHO MUST REPORT		STANDARD FOR REPORTING	PRIVILEGED COMMUNICATIONS
	Health Care	Mental Health	Social Work	Education/ Child Care	Law Enforcement	All Persons	Other*		
COLORADO §§ 19-3-304(1), (2), (2.5) 19-3-311	✓	✓	✓	✓	✓		• Christian Science practitioners • Veterinarians • Firefighters • Victim advocates • Commercial film and photographic print processors	• Have reasonable cause to know or suspect • Have observed conditions which would reasonably result	
CONNECTICUT §§ 17a-101(b) 17a-103(a)	✓	✓	✓	✓	✓		• Substance abuse counselors • Sexual assault counselors • Battered women's counselors • Clergy • Child advocates	• Have reasonable cause to suspect or believe	
DELAWARE tit. 16, § 903 tit. 16, § 909	✓	✓	✓	✓		✓		• Know or in good faith suspect	• Attorney/client • Clergy/penitent
DISTRICT OF COLUMBIA §§ 4-1321.02(a), (b), s(d) 4-1321.05	✓	✓	✓	✓	✓			• Know or have reasonable cause to suspect	
FLORIDA §§ 39.201(1) 39.204	✓	✓	✓	✓	✓	✓	• Judges • Religious healers	• Know or have reasonable cause to suspect	• Attorney/client
GEORGIA §§ 19-7-5(c)(1), (g) 16-12-100(c)	✓	✓	✓	✓	✓		• Persons who produce visual or printed matter	• Have reasonable cause to believe	
HAWAII §§ 350-1.1(a) 350-5	✓	✓	✓	✓	✓		• Employees of recreational or sports activities	• Have reason to believe	
IDAHO §§ 16-1619(a), (c) 16-1620	✓		✓	✓	✓	✓		• Have reason to believe • Have observed conditions which would reasonably result	• Clergy/penitent • Attorney/client

Readers should not rely on this summary for legal advice.

National Clearinghouse on Child Abuse and Neglect Information, February 2002

MANDATORY REPORTERS OF CHILD ABUSE AND NEGLECT

(Current through December 31, 2001)

STATE	PROFESSIONS THAT MUST REPORT					OTHERS WHO MUST REPORT		STANDARD FOR REPORTING	PRIVILEGED COMMUNICATIONS
	Health Care	Mental Health	Social Work	Education/ Child Care	Law Enforcement	All Persons	Other*		
ILLINOIS 325 ILCS 5/4 720 ILCS 5/11-20.2	✓	✓	✓	✓	✓		• Homemakers, substance abuse treatment personnel • Christian Science practitioners • Funeral home directors • Commercial film and photographic print processors	• Have reasonable cause to believe	
INDIANA §§ 31-33-5-1 31-33-5-2 31-32-11-1	✓	✓	✓	✓	✓	✓	• Staff member of any public or private institution, school, facility, or agency	• Have reason to believe	
IOWA §§ 232.69(1)(a)-(b) 728.14(1) 232.74	✓	✓	✓	✓	✓		• Commercial film and photographic print processors • Employees of substance abuse programs • Coaches	• Reasonably believe	
KANSAS § 38-1522(a), (b)	✓	✓	✓	✓	✓		• Firefighters • Juvenile intake and assessment workers	• Have reason to suspect	
KENTUCKY §§ 620.030(1), (2) 620.050(2)	✓	✓	✓	✓	✓	✓		• Know or have reasonable cause to believe	• Attorney/client • Clergy/penitent
LOUISIANA Ch. Code art. 603(13) Ch. Code art. 609(A)(1) Ch. Code art. 610(F)	✓	✓	✓	✓	✓		• Commercial film or photographic print processors • Mediators	• Have cause to believe	• Clergy/penitent • Christian Science practitioners
MAINE tit. 22, § 4011(1) tit. 22, § 4015	✓	✓	✓	✓	✓		• Guardians *ad litem* and CASAs • Fire inspectors • Commercial film processors • Homemakers	• Know or have reasonable cause to suspect	• Clergy/penitent

Readers should not rely on this summary for legal advice.

National Clearinghouse on Child Abuse and Neglect Information, February 2002

MANDATORY REPORTERS OF CHILD ABUSE AND NEGLECT

(Current through December 31, 2001)

| STATE | PROFESSIONS THAT MUST REPORT | | | | OTHERS WHO MUST REPORT | | STANDARD FOR REPORTING | PRIVILEGED COMMUNICATIONS |
	Health Care	Mental Health	Social Work	Education/ Child Care	Law Enforcement	All Persons	Other*		
MARYLAND Family Law §§ 5-704(a) 5-705(a)	✓		✓	✓	✓	✓		• Have reason to believe	• Attorney/client • Clergy/penitent
MASSACHUSETTS ch. 119, § 51A ch. 119, § 51B	✓	✓	✓	✓	✓		• Drug and alcoholism counselors • Probation and parole officers • Clerks/magistrates of district courts • Firefighters	• Have reasonable cause to believe	
MICHIGAN § 722.623 (1), (8) 722.631	✓	✓	✓	✓	✓			• Have reasonable cause to suspect	• Attorney/client
MINNESOTA §§ 626.556 Subd. 3(a), 8	✓	✓	✓	✓	✓			• Know or have reason to believe	• Clergy/penitent
MISSISSIPPI § 43-21-353(1)	✓	✓	✓	✓	✓	✓	• Attorneys • Ministers	• Have reasonable cause to suspect	
MISSOURI §§ 210.115(1) 568.110 210.140	✓	✓	✓	✓	✓		• Persons with responsibility for care of children • Christian Science practitioners • Probation/parole officers • Commercial film processors • Internet service providers (ISPs)	• Have reasonable cause to suspect • Have observed conditions which would reasonably result	• Attorney/client • Clergy/penitent
MONTANA § 41-3-201(1)-(2), (4)	✓	✓	✓	✓	✓		• Guardians *ad litem* • Clergy • Religious healers • Christian Science practitioners	• Know or have reasonable cause to suspect	• Clergy/penitent

Readers should not rely on this summary for legal advice.

National Clearinghouse on Child Abuse and Neglect Information, February 2002

MANDATORY REPORTERS OF CHILD ABUSE AND NEGLECT

(Current through December 31, 2001)

STATE	PROFESSIONS THAT MUST REPORT					OTHERS WHO MUST REPORT		STANDARD FOR REPORTING	PRIVILEGED COMMUNICATIONS
	Health Care	Mental Health	Social Work	Education/ Child Care	Law Enforcement	All Persons	Other*		
NEBRASKA §§ 28-711(1) 28-714	✓		✓	✓		✓		• Have reasonable cause to believe • Have observed conditions which would reasonably result	
NEVADA §§ 432B.220(3), (5) 432B.250	✓	✓	✓	✓	✓		• Clergy • Religious healers • Alcohol/drug abuse counselors • Christian Science practitioners • Probation officers • Attorneys • Youth shelter workers	• Know or have reason to believe	• Clergy/penitent • Attorney/client
NEW HAMPSHIRE §§ 169-C:29 169-C:32	✓	✓	✓	✓	✓	✓	• Christian Science practitioners • Clergy	• Have reason to suspect	• Attorney/client • *Clergy/penitent privilege denied*
NEW JERSEY § 9:6-8.10				✓	✓	✓		• Have reasonable cause to believe	
NEW MEXICO §§ 32A-4-3(A) 32A-4-5(A)	✓		✓	✓	✓	✓	• Judges	• Know or have reasonable suspicion	
NEW YORK Soc. Serv. Law § 413(1)	✓	✓	✓	✓	✓		• Alcoholism/substance abuse counselors • District Attorneys • Christian Science practitioners	• Have reasonable cause to suspect	
NORTH CAROLINA §§ 7B-301 7B-310						✓	• Any institution	• Have cause to suspect	• Attorney/client • *Clergy/penitent privilege denied*

Readers should not rely on this summary for legal advice.

National Clearinghouse on Child Abuse and Neglect Information, February 2002

MANDATORY REPORTERS OF CHILD ABUSE AND NEGLECT

(Current through December 31, 2001)

STATE	PROFESSIONS THAT MUST REPORT					OTHERS WHO MUST REPORT		STANDARD FOR REPORTING	PRIVILEGED COMMUNICATIONS
	Health Care	Mental Health	Social Work	Education/ Child Care	Law Enforcement	All Persons	Other*		
NORTH DAKOTA §§ 50-25.1-03 50-25.1-10	✓	✓	✓	✓	✓		• Clergy • Religious healers • Addiction counselors	• Have knowledge of or reasonable cause to suspect	• Clergy/penitent • Attorney/client
OHIO § 2151.421(A)(1), (A)(2), (G)(1)(b)	✓	✓	✓	✓			• Attorneys • Religious healers	• Know or suspect	• Attorney/client • Physician/patient
OKLAHOMA tit. 10, § 7103(A)(1) tit. 10, § 7104 tit. 10, § 7113 tit. 21, § 1021.4	✓			✓		✓	• Commercial film and photo-graphic print processors	• Have reason to believe	
OREGON §§ 419B.005(3) 419B.010(1)	✓	✓	✓	✓	✓		• Attorneys • Clergy • Firefighters • CASAs	• Have reasonable cause to believe	• Mental health/ patient • Clergy/penitent • Attorney/client
PENNSYLVANIA § 23-6311(a),(b)	✓	✓	✓	✓	✓		• Funeral directors • Christian Science practitioners • Clergy	• Have reasonable cause to suspect	• Clergy/penitent
RHODE ISLAND §§ 40-11-3(a) 40-11-6(a) 40-11-11	✓					✓		• Have reasonable cause to know or suspect	• Attorney/client • *Clergy/penitent privilege denied*
SOUTH CAROLINA §§ 20-7-510(A) 20-7-550	✓	✓	✓	✓	✓		• Judges • Funeral home directors and employees • Christian Science practitioners • Film processors • Religious healers • Substance abuse treatment staff • Computer technicians	• Have reason to believe	• Attorney/client • Priest/penitent

Readers should not rely on this summary for legal advice.

National Clearinghouse on Child Abuse and Neglect Information, February 2002

MANDATORY REPORTERS OF CHILD ABUSE AND NEGLECT

(Current through December 31, 2001)

STATE	PROFESSIONS THAT MUST REPORT					OTHERS WHO MUST REPORT		STANDARD FOR REPORTING	PRIVILEGED COMMUNICATIONS
	Health Care	Mental Health	Social Work	Education/ Child Care	Law Enforcement	All Persons	Other*		
SOUTH DAKOTA §§ 26-8A-3 26-8A-15	✓	✓	✓	✓	✓		• Chemical dependency counselors • Religious healers • Parole or court services officers • Employees of domestic abuse shelters	• Have reasonable cause to suspect	
TENNESSEE §§ 37-1-403(a) 37-1-605(a) 37-1-411	✓	✓	✓	✓	✓	✓	• Judges • Neighbors • Relatives • Friends • Religious healers	• Knowledge of/reasonably know • Have reasonable cause to suspect	
TEXAS Family Code §§ 261.101(a)-(c) 261.102	✓			✓		✓	• Juvenile probation or detention officers • Employees or clinics that provide reproductive services	• Have cause to believe	• *Clergy/penitent privilege denied*
UTAH §§ 62A-4a-403(1)-(3) 62A-4a-412(5)	✓					✓		• Have reason to believe • Have observed conditions which would reasonably result	• Clergy/penitent
VERMONT tit. 33, § 4913(a)	✓	✓	✓	✓	✓		• Camp administrators and counselors • Probation officers	• Have reasonable cause to believe	
VIRGINIA § 63.1-248.3(A) 63.1-248.11	✓	✓	✓	✓	✓		• Mediators • Christian Science practitioners • Probation officers • CASAs	• Have reason to suspect	

Readers should not rely on this summary for legal advice.

National Clearinghouse on Child Abuse and Neglect Information, February 2002

MANDATORY REPORTERS OF CHILD ABUSE AND NEGLECT

(Current through December 31, 2001)

STATE	PROFESSIONS THAT MUST REPORT					OTHERS WHO MUST REPORT		STANDARD FOR REPORTING	PRIVILEGED COMMUNICATIONS
	Health Care	Mental Health	Social Work	Education/ Child Care	Law Enforcement	All Persons	Other*		
WASHINGTON §§ 26.44.030 (1), (2) 26.44.060(3)	✓	✓	✓	✓	✓		• Any adult with whom a child resides • Responsible living skills program staff	• Have reasonable cause to believe	
WEST VIRGINIA §§ 49-6A-2 49-6A-7	✓	✓	✓	✓	✓		• Clergy • Religious healers • Judges, family law masters or magistrates • Christian Science practitioners	• Reasonable cause to suspect • When believe • Have observed	• Attorney/client • *Clergy/penitent privilege denied*
WISCONSIN § 48.981(2), (2m)(c), (2m)(d)	✓	✓	✓	✓	✓		• Alcohol or drug abuse counselors • Mediators • Financial and employment planners • CASAs	• Have reasonable cause to suspect • Have reason to believe	
WYOMING §§ 14-3-205(a) 14-3-210						✓		• Know or have reasonable cause to believe or suspect • Have observed conditions which would reasonably result	• Attorney/client • Physician/patient • Clergy/penitent
TOTALS, ALL STATES	48	40	44	46	41	18	N/A	N/A	26

*For a complete listing of individuals mandated to report suspected child maltreatment, see Department of Health and Human Services, Child Abuse and Neglect State Statute Compendium of Laws: Reporting Laws: Mandatory Reporters of Child Abuse and Neglect (2002).

Reprinted from National Clearinghouse on Child Abuse and Neglect Information. Statutes at-a-Glance: Mandatory Reporters of Child Abuse and Neglect. Washington, DC: US Dept of Health & Human Services; February 2002b:1-9.

National Clearinghouse on Child Abuse and Neglect Information, February 2002

Readers should not rely on this summary for legal advice.

REFERENCES

American Academy of Pediatrics. The child in court: a subject review (RE9923). *Pediatrics.* 1999;104:1145-1148.

Brodsky SL. *Testifying in Court: Guidelines and Maxims for the Expert Witness.* Washington, DC: American Psychological Association; 1991.

Bulkley JA, Feller JN, Stern P, Roe R. Child abuse and neglect laws and legal proceedings. In: Briere J, Berliner L, Bulkley JA, Jenny C, Reid TA, eds. *The APSAC Handbook on Child Maltreatment.* Thousand Oaks, Calif: Sage Publications; 1996:271-296.

Butz AM, Redman BK, Fry ST, Kolodner K. Ethical conflicts experienced by certified pediatric nurse practitioners in ambulatory settings. *J Pediatr Health Care.* 1998;12:183-190.

Carlisle D. Accountability: to tell or not to tell. *Nurs Times.* 1991;87:46-47.

Devlin BK, Reynolds E. Child abuse: how to recognize it; how to intervene. *Am J Nurs.* 1994;94:26-32.

Dubowitz H, DePanfilis D, eds. *Handbook for Child Protection Practice.* Thousand Oaks, Calif: Sage Publications; 2000.

Feller JN, Davidson HA, Hardin M, Horowitz RM. *Working With the Courts in Child Protection.* US Dept of Health & Human Services. 1992. Available at: http://www.calib.com/nccanch/pubs/usermanuals/courts/courts.pdf.

Fiesta J. Protecting children: a public duty to report. *Nurs Manage.* 1992;23:14-17.

Flaherty EG, Sege R, Binns HJ, Mattson CL, Christoffel KK. Health care providers' experience reporting child abuse in the primary care setting. *Arch Pediatr Adolesc Med.* 2000;154:489-493.

Giardino AP, Kolilis G. The role of law enforcement in the investigation of child maltreatment. In: Giardino AP, Giardino ER, eds. *Recognition of Child Abuse for the Mandated Reporter.* 3rd ed. St. Louis, Mo: GW Medical Publishing; 2002:279-308.

Goldner JA, Dolgin CK, Manske SH. Legal issues. In: Monteleone JA, ed. *Recognition of Child Abuse for the Mandated Reporter.* 2nd ed. St. Louis, Mo: GW Medical Publishing; 1996:171-210.

Green AH. True and false allegations of sexual abuse in child custody disputes. *Am Acad Child Psychiatry.* 1986;25:449-456.

Greipp ME. Ethical decision making and mandatory reporting in cases of suspected child abuse. *J Pediatr Health Care.* 1997;11:258-265.

Gunter M, duBois R, Eichner E, et al. Allegations of sexual abuse in child custody disputes. *Med Law.* 2000;19:815-825.

Hamblet JL. Ethics and the pediatric perioperative nurse. *Inside OR.* 1994;16:15-21.

Hammond CB, Lanning KV, Promisel W, Shepherd JR, Walsh B. *Law Enforcement Response to Child Abuse: Portable Guide to Investigating Child Abuse.* Washington, DC: US Dept of Justice; 1997.

Herman SP, Bernet W. AACAP Official Action. Summary of the practice parameters for child custody evaluation. *J Am Acad Child Adolesc Psychiatry.* 1997;36:1784-1787.

Katner D, Plum HJ. Legal issues. In: Giardino AP, Giardino ER, eds. *Recognition of Child Abuse for the Mandated Reporter.* 3rd ed. St. Louis, Mo: GW Medical Publishing; 2002:309-350.

Lanning KV, Walsh B. Criminal investigation of suspected child abuse. In: Briere J, Berliner L, Bulkley JA, Jenny C, Reid TA, eds. *The APSAC Handbook on Child Maltreatment.* Thousand Oaks, Calif: Sage Publications; 1996:246-270.

Ledray LE. SANE-SART history and role development. In: Giardino AP, Datner EM, Asher JB, eds. *Sexual Assault Victimization Across the Life Span: A Clinical Guide.* St. Louis, Mo: GW Medical Publishing; 2003:471-486.

Lewin L. Child abuse: ethical and legal concerns for the nurse. *J Psychosoc Nurs.* 1994;32:15-18.

Murphy SS. Legal issues for nurses: reporting child abuse—a nurse's duty. *Texas Nurs.* 1995;69:1-4.

Myers JEB. Expert testimony. In: Briere J, Berliner L, Bulkley JA, Jenny C, Reid TA, eds. *The APSAC Handbook on Child Maltreatment.* Thousand Oaks, Calif: Sage Publications; 1996:319-340.

Myers JEB. *Legal Issues in Child Abuse and Neglect Practice.* 2nd ed. Thousand Oaks, Calif: Sage Publications;1998.

Myers JEB. The legal system and child protection. In: Myers JEB, Berliner L, Briere J, Hendrix CT, Jenny C, Reid TA, eds. *The APSAC Handbook on Child Maltreatment.* 2nd ed. Thousand Oaks, Calif: Sage Publications; 2002:305-327.

Myers JEB, Stern P. Expert testimony. In: Myers JEB, Berliner L, Briere J, Hendrix CT, Jenny C, Reid TA, eds. *The APSAC Handbook on Child Maltreatment.* 2nd ed. Thousand Oaks, Calif: Sage Publications; 2002:379-401.

Myers JL. Workshop effectiveness: nurses as witnesses in court cases involving physical child abuse. *J Nursing Law.* 1996;3:35-44.

National Clearinghouse on Child Abuse and Neglect Information. *Child Abuse and Neglect State Statutes Elements: Reporting Laws. Number 1: Definitions of Child Abuse and Neglect. Definition Document.* Washington, DC: US Dept of Health & Human Services; May 2000. Available at: http://www.calib.com/nccanch. Accessed January 1, 2003.

National Clearinghouse on Child Abuse and Neglect Information. *Child Abuse and Neglect State Statues Elements: Reporting Laws. Number 2: Mandatory Reporters of Child Abuse and Neglect.* Washington, DC: US Dept of Health & Human Services; 2002a. Available at: http://www.calib.com/nccanch/pubs/stats02/mandrep.cfm. Accessed March 11, 2003.

National Clearinghouse on Child Abuse and Neglect Information. *Statutes at-a-Glance: Mandatory Reporters of Child Abuse and Neglect.* Washington, DC: US Dept of Health & Human Services; February 2002b:1-9.

Nurcombe B. The child as witness: competency and credibility. *Am Acad Child Psychiatry.* 1985;24:473-480.

Paradise JE, Rostain AL, Nathanson M. Substantiation of sexual abuse charges when parents dispute custody or visitation. *Pediatrics.* 1988;81:835-839.

Pennsylvania Bar Association. *How to Handle a Child Abuse Case: A Manual for Attorneys Representing Children.* Course Code FL 13. April, 1997. Vol 1. Mechanicsburg, Pa: Pennsylvania Bar Association; 2002.

Pillitteri AR. The role of the nurse as a mandated reporter of child abuse. In: Bullough B, Bullough VL, eds. *Nursing Issues for the Nineties and Beyond.* New York, NY: Springer Publishing; 1994:95-109.

Rhodes AM. Legal issues: immunity for reporting child abuse. *MCN Contents.* 1996;21:169.

Runyan DK, Toth PA. Child sexual abuse and the courts. In: Krugman RD, Leventhal JM, eds. *Child Sexual Abuse: Report of the Twenty-Second Ross Roundtable on Critical Approaches to Common Pediatric Problems.* Columbus, Ohio: Ross Laboratories; 1991:57-75.

Saywitz KJ, Goodman GS. Interviewing children in and out of court: current research and practice implications. In: Briere J, Berliner L, Bulkley JA, Jenny C, Reid TA, eds. *The APSAC Handbook on Child Maltreatment.* Thousand Oaks, Calif: Sage Publications; 1996:297-318.

Saywitz KJ, Goodman GS, Lyon TD. Interviewing children in and out of court. In: Myers JEB, Berliner L, Briere J, Hendrix CT, Jenny C, Reid TA, eds. *The APSAC Handbook on Child Maltreatment.* 2nd ed. Thousand Oaks, Calif: Sage Publications; 2002:349-377.

Thoennes N, Tjaden PG. The extent, nature, and validity of sexual abuse allegations in custody/visitation disputes. *Child Abuse Negl.* 1990;14:151-163.

US Department of Health & Human Services. *Child Maltreatment 1998: Reports From the States to the National Child Abuse and Neglect Data System.* US Dept of Health & Human Services, Administration on Children, Youth and Families.Washington, DC: US Government Printing Office; 2000.

Zellman GL, Fair CC. Preventing and reporting abuse. In: Myers JEB, Berliner L, Briere J, Hendrix CT, Jenny C, Reid TA, eds. *The APSAC Handbook on Child Maltreatment.* 2nd ed. Thousand Oaks, Calif: Sage Publications; 2002:449-475.

Zellman GL, Faller KC. Reporting of child maltreatment. In: Briere J, Berliner L, Bulkley JA, Jenny C, Reid TA, eds. *The APSAC Handbook on Child Maltreatment.* Thousand Oaks, Calif: Sage Publications; 1996:359-382.

Chapter 15

THE RELATIONSHIP BETWEEN DOMESTIC VIOLENCE AND CHILD MALTREATMENT

Holly M. Harner, CRNP, PhD, MPH

It is estimated that almost 4 million women each year are victims of domestic violence (The Commonwealth Fund, as cited by the Family Violence Prevention Fund, 2003). Although men may be victims of domestic violence, women are the primary targets of violence in dating relationships, marriage, and pregnancy (Crowell & Burgess, 1996). Research indicates that as the violent relationship continues, physical, sexual, and emotional abuse often occur with increasing frequency, duration, and intensity. Other factors occurring within the family may also affect domestic violence, including substance use, financial stress and job loss, mental or physical illness in the family, the birth of a child, and separation and divorce.

Women are not the sole victims of violence in the home. In the 1990s, approximately 3 million children were reported to child protective agencies annually for suspected child abuse and maltreatment (Kelley, Thornberry, & Smith, 1997). Children in homes plagued by domestic violence are likely to suffer similar abuse and maltreatment, either directly or indirectly. An estimated 3 to 10 million children whose mothers are abused witness her abuse (Carlson, as cited by the American Bar Association, 1994). These children may not only witness domestic violence but may also suffer directly from abuse and maltreatment by either parent. Of children who are in a domestically violent home, at least two thirds directly experience abuse at the hand of the mother's abuser (McKay, 1994). According to the US Advisory Board on Child Abuse and Neglect (USABCAN, 1995), "some experts argue that domestic violence is the *single major precursor* to child abuse and neglect fatalities in the United States" (p. 124).

Despite the relationship between domestic violence and child abuse, only recently have advocates for battered women and abused children viewed these crimes as interconnected (Beeman, Hagemeister, & Edleson, 1999; Shipman, Rossman, & West, 1999). These newly formed alliances have become stronger as empirical evidence pointing toward the intergenerational transmission of violence in families has grown (Green, 1998; Thormaehlen & Bass-Feld, 1994). Still, a need remains for nurses caring for families to protect and advocate for adults and children vulnerable to abuse. This can best be done by comprehensive, universal screening for domestic violence and child abuse, documentation of forensic findings, and providing appropriate referrals to victim service organizations and child welfare agencies as indicated (Campbell & Lewandowski, 1997).

This chapter will assist nurses caring for families to understand the relationship among domestic violence and child abuse and maltreatment. The crimes of domestic violence, child abuse, and maltreatment are briefly reviewed, and various patterns of children's exposure to violence, including the child as witness to domestic violence and the child as the target of abuse, are explored. Implications of various family stressors on children in the violent home, including divorce and substance abuse, are described. Trauma response patterns, including physical, cognitive, psychosocial, and behavioral responses, of children in violent homes are addressed, as is the role of nurses caring for victims of domestic violence and child abuse.

DOMESTIC VIOLENCE

Inquiry into violence against women, including the rape of women and children, domestic violence and homicide, and stalking, has grown dramatically over the last 3 decades (Crowell & Burgess, 1996). Researchers, nurses, and victim advocates, in their work with survivors of domestic violence, have dramatically altered the way violence in the home is viewed by healthcare providers, public policy makers, and the criminal justice system. Today, domestic violence is regarded as a progressively dangerous, criminal pattern of activity occurring between intimate partners in marital, as well as dating and cohabiting, relationships. Within these relationships, one partner, usually the male, uses various behaviors to exercise power and control over the other. These behaviors may include physical and/or sexual assault or battery, psychological or financial abuse, and isolation from friends, family members, and co-workers (Orloff, 1996).

Domestic violence crosses racial, social, and economic boundaries, negating stereotypes to the contrary (Campbell & Campbell, 1996; Crowell & Burgess, 1996). Although research on domestic violence occurring among gay and lesbian couples is in its infancy, early data suggest that domestic violence occurs at rates similar to that of heterosexual couples (Cruz & Firestone, 1998). Domestic violence occurring during pregnancy has become an area of increased research interest over the last decade, with nurses pioneering this area of inquiry (Campbell, Oliver, & Bullock, 1993; Campbell, Poland, Waller, & Ager, 1992; McFarlane, 1989; McFarlane & Parker, 1994; McFarlane, Parker, & Soeken, 1996a, 1996b). In particular, domestic violence during pregnancy as an indicator of the potential for the abuse of children has received increased attention among those aiming to decrease the intergenerational transmission of violence through early prenatal and postpartum intervention (Campbell & Parker, 1992; McFarlane & Soeken, 1999; Overpeck, Brenner, Trumble, Trifiletti, & Berendes, 1998). Additionally, domestic violence within vulnerable populations, including pregnant and parenting teenagers (Parker, 1993) and minority women (Campbell & Campbell, 1996; McFarlane, Kelly, Rodriguez, & Fehir, 1994; McFarlane, Parker, Soeken, Silva, & Reed, 1999) has also been explored.

CHILD ABUSE AND MALTREATMENT

According to the National Child Abuse and Neglect Data System (US Department of Health & Human Services [USDHHS], 2002), almost 3 million children were reported to statewide child abuse and prevention programs in 2000. Of these reports, almost two thirds were deemed sufficiently credible to warrant an investigation. It was estimated that 1200 children died in 2000 as a result of child abuse and maltreatment (USDHHS, 2002). The true incidence of child abuse fatalities is unknown because deaths may be underreported, evidence poorly handled, and cases inaccurately diagnosed or inadequately investigated (Herman-Giddens et al., 1999). It does appear that those children who are most at risk for fatal child abuse and neglect are younger, usually under age 5 years (USDHHS, 2002). Although no uniform typology of the abusive parent exists, it is thought that most physical abuse resulting in child fatalities is perpetrated by males, including fathers, stepfathers, and boyfriends. In most cases, the causes of nonaccidental death to children include head trauma and internal injuries (USABCAN, 1995).

Death at the hands of a parent or caregiver is not the outcome of all cases of child maltreatment. Hundreds of thousands of children each year are subject to repetitive violence in the home, surviving the brutality that has killed others (USABCAN, 1995). Physical, sexual, and emotional abuse, as well as neglect of basic life-sustaining needs, have both immediate and long-term sequelae for child survivors (Burgess, Hartman, & Clements, 1995; Famularo, Fenton, Kinscherff, Ayoub, & Barnum, 1994; Widner-Kolberg, 1997).

THE LINK BETWEEN DOMESTIC VIOLENCE AND CHILD MALTREATMENT

The exposure of children to violence on television, in cinema, on the Internet, and even in video games has been postulated to increase violent behavior among American youth (Strasburger & Donnerstein, 1999). Over the last decade, children's exposure to violence within the family, particularly domestic violence, has been increasingly addressed by nurses and other healthcare providers (Attala, Bauza, Pratt, & Vieira, 1995; Erikson & Henderson, 1992; McKay, 1994; Ryan & King, 1997; Thormaehlen & Bass-Feld, 1994; Wolfe & Korsch, 1994). Historically, the effect of domestic violence on children went largely unnoticed, if not completely disregarded, by those caring for victims of domestic violence. Often regarded as extensions of the battered woman, children were rarely viewed as potential victims of abuse and neglect (Rhea, Chafey, Dohner, & Terragno, 1996). As nurses and researchers began to approach the family from a broader systems perspective, the physical and psychosocial effects of violence on the marital dyad, on the children, and on future generations became of increasing concern.

Children in domestically violent homes are often referred to as the "unseen," "silent," or "secondary" victims of violence (Rhea et al., 1996). Understandably, battered women may be unaware of the degree to which their children witness their abuse (Campbell & Lewandowski, 1997; Hilton, 1992; Wolfe & Korsch, 1994). Additionally, fear of losing custody for failing to protect children in the violent home may cause mothers to minimize the abuse their children have witnessed (Magan, 1999). However, in most domestically violent homes, children witness violence between their parents either directly or indirectly. Although the presence of these children during episodes of violence may go unnoticed by many parents, the consequences of their exposure to domestic violence can be difficult to ignore.

Children may overhear violently loud arguments between their parents, many regarding their own care or well-being. They may hear threats and accusations of infidelity made from one parent to the other. While hiding under tables and behind chairs, they may dodge objects thrown through the air. They may see slaps, punches, and blows exchanged (Rhea et al., 1996; Wolfe & Korsch, 1994). Additionally, children, especially younger children, may suffer accidental injures while in the arms of the victim parent (Christian, Scribano, Seidl, & Pinto-Martin, 1997). Older children, especially boys, may suffer accidental injuries when trying to intervene in parental violence or while trying to protect the victim parent during an attack.

Frequently, children are witnesses to more than one act of violence between their parents. On average, children in domestically violent homes are aware of at least 9 incidents of violence and are able to remember 4 attacks distinctly (Straus, 1992). As the violent relationship continues, children are exposed to violence that is greater in intensity, frequency, duration, and lethality. Almost half of the children exposed to domestic violence witness potentially life-threatening violence (McCloskey, Figueredo, & Koss, 1995). These children may wake in the aftermath of the violence to find broken furniture, shards of glass, and injured loved ones. Older children may be required to call the police and an ambulance for the victim parent.

Children in domestically violent homes may also suffer from nonaccidental injuries inflicted by either parent. The USABCAN (1995) reported that child abuse is involved in 40% to 60% of domestically violent homes. In these homes, males abuse almost 70% of physically abused children (Sedlak & Broadhurst, 1996). Some evidence shows that the severity of domestic violence is often predictive of the severity of child abuse (McKay, 1994). Ross (1996) noted that the greater the number of violent behaviors used by a husband against his wife, the greater the likelihood that children in the home would be physically abused. Despite these correlations, child abuse typically does not occur at the same time as domestic violence. In many violent homes, each violent episode is seen as a "temporarily separate crisis" (Bowker, Arbitell, & McFerron, 1988, p. 160), each necessitating a separate resolution.

FAMILY STRESSORS IN THE VIOLENT HOME

Family stressors, including birth, death, job loss and financial strain, substance abuse, and mental and physical illnesses may challenge the adaptive nature of any family. However, the violent family, which may have fewer resources for adequate coping, may be even more vulnerable to family stressors (Shipman et al., 1999; Widner-Kolberg, 1997). Few stressors cause such a profound impact on violent families as separation and divorce. Separation violence, including physical and sexual violence, harassment, and stalking, is of particular concern for victims of domestic violence. Current research points to an increased risk of homicide for the female victim and her children after leaving an abusive relationship (Campbell, 1994).

When separation culminates in divorce, custody and visitation issues can continue to pose problems for victims of domestic violence. When violent ex-husbands are permitted visitation with their children, they may use visitation as an opportunity to continue harassing and even abusing their former spouse (Shalansky, Eriksen, & Henderson, 1999). Domestic violence may escalate to include child abuse, with children serving as surrogate victims for their mothers. In some cases, children may even be manipulated or coerced into abusing their mother on behalf of their father.

The creation of blended families resulting from a parental death, separation, or divorce may also place a child at risk for exposure to domestic violence or child maltreatment. With the addition of new family members, children who have never been exposed to violence may find themselves as the direct or indirect targets of abuse and maltreatment by a stepparent. Jealousy over a previous marriage may be exhibited by abuse of children born of a prior relationship (Campbell & Lewandowski, 1997). These children may also be targeted by a new partner envious of the attention and caregiving they are paid by their mother. Jealousy, especially in cases of real or perceived questionable paternity, may also place future pregnancies at risk.

In addition to separation and divorce, other familial factors that stress the already violent home may include use of substances, including illicit drugs and alcohol. Although no substance is the direct cause of domestic violence or child abuse, violence in the home is significantly correlated with substance use. It has been estimated that in 25% to 85% of domestic violence cases, substances have been used before an attack. In most cases, more than one substance is used; the most common combination is a mixture of alcohol and cocaine (Bennett, 1995). Children in homes where substances are used are at an increased risk of neglect and maltreatment because caregivers are less able to supervise children adequately while under the influence.

RESPONSE PATTERNS OF CHILDREN IN VIOLENT HOMES

The response of victims after a traumatic event has been described for various crimes, including cases of rape (Burgess & Holmstrom, 1974) and domestic violence (Walker, 1984). With the recognition of posttraumatic stress disorder (PTSD), trauma response patterns have become one of the leading psychiatric diagnoses of this decade. Application of traumatic response patterns to children who have been exposed to violence has been addressed by numerous investigators (Davies & Flannery, 1998; Famularo, 1997; Perry, 1994; Schwarz & Perry, 1994). Like their adult counterparts, children may also suffer from intrusive thoughts, including nightmares, as a result of experiencing violence or witnessing abuse. They may also display strong avoidance tendencies, especially when an event or location avoided is a reminder of the traumatic event. Emotional numbing or feelings of apathy toward parents, peers, and others may also be a characteristic noted in children after trauma. Finally, hyperactive startle responses or responses that are far more dramatic than what the situation calls for are also a characteristic of children who have witnessed or experienced violence (Famularo, 1997).

To varying degrees, physical, cognitive, psychosocial, and behavioral responses predictably follow victimization. Additionally, various trauma-specific factors affect the degree to which victims respond. When the victim of a traumatic event is a child, several specific considerations must be weighed in evaluating his or her response (Wolak & Finkelhor, 1998). These can include the child's age and developmental level; the frequency, duration, and lethality of the trauma; past trauma history; relationship to the perpetrator; and the individual family characteristics supporting the child.

PHYSICAL RESPONSE

Physical response patterns in the form of physical injuries are frequently the initial presentation of child abuse and maltreatment recognized by nurses as signs of abuse (Cheung, 1999; Davis & Zitelli, 1995). Obvious injuries, including bilateral orbital hematomas (Cheung, 1999; Monteleone & Brodeur, 1998), spiral fractures (Patterson, 1998), and immersion burns (Scalzo, 1998), should raise the index suspicion for child abuse in most pediatric nurses (Monteleone & Brodeur, 1998). Nurses are also likely to be suspicious of injures when an inadequate or developmentally inappropriate explanation for the injury is given by the parent (Cheung, 1999). However, accidental injuries, which may occur in the course of developing various motor skills, such as walking, running, and riding a bike, may prove more difficult to distinguish from those that are intentionally inflicted (Patterson, 1998).

Injuries to areas of bony prominences, especially the forehead, palms of the hands, elbows, shins, and knees, are frequently associated with accidental or nonintentional injuries (Monteleone & Brodeur, 1998; Patterson, 1998). A toddler learning to walk may present with a contusion or abrasion located on his forehead or chin if he were to trip or fall forward. His hands, in an attempt to break his fall, may also suffer visible abrasions or cuts. Likewise, his knees may also show the signs of an unsuccessful attempt at walking or running. Accidental injuries in children, as in adults, tend to be located in the distal areas of the body, including the arms, the hands, or the legs. Rarely do accidental injuries present in central areas of the body, such as the abdomen or the back.

Conversely, intentionally inflicted injuries are typically directed to targeted areas of the child's victim's body, including the abdomen, the back, or the genital area, as well as the face (Brockmeyer & Sheridan, 1998; Monteleone & Brodeur, 1998). ***Patterned injuries***, or injuries with a characteristic size, shape, or texture, are also likely to be present in cases of intentional injuries (Brockmeyer & Sheridan, 1998). Common patterned injuries include bite marks, slap marks, ligature marks from choking or strangulation, ring imprints from punching, strap or belt marks from whipping, and cigarette burns. Intentional scald burns, which may be inflicted as punishment for unsuccessful toilet training, will present with well-demarcated areas of tissue injury and tissue sparing and are indicative of abuse (Patterson, 1998; Scalzo, 1998). Common burns consistent with intentional injuries include stocking and glove patterned burns to the hands and feet, as well as donut-shaped burns to the buttocks (Scalzo, 1998).

The **pattern of injury**, which indicates old as well as recently inflicted injuries, can also help distinguish between accidentally and intentionally inflicted injuries (Brockmeyer & Sheridan, 1998). Common patterns of injury can include bruises in different stages of healing, as well as evidence of broken and healing rib fractures, which are most commonly the result of severe physical abuse among infants under age 2 years (Cadzow & Armstrong, 2000). Old injures for which medical care was not sought should also raise the index of suspicion for nurses (Monteleone & Brodeur, 1998). Additionally, patterns of neglect, including malnutrition, decubitus ulcers, infestations, chronic urine burns, and muscle wasting are also indicators of chronic maltreatment and neglect.

Some preliminary evidence shows that children who witness domestic violence, but are not directly targeted, may present with different injuries than those children who are the primary targets of abuse. Specifically, child witnesses may present with injuries more typically resembling accidental injuries. Child witnesses to domestic violence may be accidentally injured in the course of their mother's abuse, thus resulting in a less typical injury presentation (Christian et al., 1997). Because these injuries may not raise the same degree of suspicion as injuries consistent with targeted violence, all injuries in children must be thoroughly evaluated by nurses.

COGNITIVE RESPONSE

Children who witness domestic violence, as well as those who are directly abused, may also have various trauma-related symptoms affecting their cognitive abilities (Famularo et al., 1994; Schwarz & Perry, 1994). Hypervigilance and increased arousal and startle responses, symptoms diagnostic of posttraumatic stress response in adults, may be seen in children from violent homes (Famularo et al., 1994; Schwarz & Perry, 1994). Avoidance of events and places associated with abuse may also be seen in children. For example, children exposed to violence in the later evening hours may be more avoidant of bedtime rituals because of the association between abuse and nighttime (Famularo, 1997).

Children of violent homes may have mild to severe developmental delays. Largely as a result of living in a chronically unpredictable and dangerous family environment, children may be required to shift their attention from normal developmental tasks to survival (Perry, 1999). Older children may have decreased concentration, coupled with difficulty focusing their attention on various tasks. They may be easily distracted from daily activities and routines. These symptoms may manifest in school-age children and adolescents as poor grades and academic skill levels below their expected abilities (Rhea et al., 1996). When a child's cognitive abilities are compromised, poor grades and unfavorable reports may place him or her at even further risk for harsh discipline.

PSYCHOSOCIAL RESPONSE

Recent research indicates that children who witness domestic violence suffer similar psychosocial sequelae to those who are physically abused. Like other responses to trauma, psychological responses of children exposed to violence and those who have been abused will vary from one child to the next, may change over time, and may manifest after certain events or situations that may trigger abusive memories. Early psychological responses of children in violent homes can include confusion, fear, and sadness. Guilt, particularly in the egocentric child, may also predominate. Guilt, in this case, often results from the child feeling responsible for the violence, as well as his or her inability to stop the abuse (Wolfe & Korsch, 1994). For older children, shame and guilt may be replaced by anger at either parent and depression. Some children may grow to associate with the violent parent as a way to protect himself or herself from future abuse, whereas others may learn to associate with the victim stance (Thormaehlen & Bass-Feld, 1994).

The psychological responses of children in violent homes often influence future social interactions. Early fear may manifest into anxiety, particularly regarding separation from their primary caregiver. Anxiety and distrust of unfamiliar people may also be present in some children. This may be seen with transitions into preschool or daycare. As the child gets older, defensive withdrawal from social situations may also occur. Older children may present as the proverbial "loner child" who does not engage in normal developmental play with other children (Thormaehlen & Bass-Feld, 1994).

BEHAVIORAL RESPONSE

Children's behavioral responses after trauma, especially violence in the home, are often characterized as ***externalizing*** or ***internalizing*** behaviors (Rhea et al., 1996). Perry (1999) has also referred to this as hyperarousal and dissociation, respectively. Externalizing behaviors, or behaviors typically expressed outwardly, can be seen in children of all ages. Externalizing behaviors seen in the toddler and school-age child can begin with periods of increased restlessness and whining and may culminate in crying, yelling, and temper tantrums. Older children who have learned that using violence is an acceptable way to meet their needs may use violence in their everyday lives. They may begin to engage in more delinquent types of behaviors, including lying, stealing, and truancy. Invariably, these types of behaviors result in other deleterious consequences in the home and possibly in the criminal justice system.

Rather than expressing trauma outwardly, some child victims may exhibit internalizing behaviors in response to the trauma (Rhea et al., 1996). Toddlers and school-age children may regress behaviorally, secluding themselves from other children. Older children may internalize trauma and act out through sexual promiscuity and early pregnancy. For some teenagers, pregnancy may be seen as a way to disconnect from the family system. Ironically, though, early pregnancy generally serves only to reinforce dependence on the family of origin. In addition to early pregnancy, substance use, isolation, or self-directed violence are also forms of internalization. In severe cases, children may completely dissociate from traumatic events, separating emotional from physical feelings.

Behavioral regression as a result of trauma deserves further mention. Developmental milestones, including toilet training, cessation of self-soothing behaviors such as thumb sucking, and sleeping alone or with the lights off, can be compromised after trauma in children. Such behavioral regression, seen by some parents as child failures or even intentional, may also increase the risk of abuse and maltreatment by parents.

IMPLICATIONS FOR NURSING PRACTICE

Every nurse, regardless of specialty, will interact with and care for members of a family. Families will present in various stages of development and transitions. Over the years, the definition of family has expanded to include more than the traditional 2-parent household. Various family compositions will require care, including the single-parent family, the gay or lesbian family, families in which the primary caregiver is a grandmother or other relative, or adoptive or foster families. Nurses caring for all family types must capitalize on the family's strengths while attempting to minimize or eradicate their weaknesses. This is especially true when working with the violent family.

PEDIATRIC NURSES

Like other healthcare professionals, pediatric nurses are required to assess for and intervene in cases of suspected child abuse and maltreatment. However, their role in caring for adult victims of violence, typically the mothers of abused or neglected children, has recently been addressed (American Academy of Pediatrics, 1998; Barkan & Gary, 1996). Because of the danger domestic violence poses for children in the home, pediatric nurses must incorporate routine screening and assessment for domestic violence among the parents of their patients. This is especially necessary when the nurse suspects child abuse or maltreatment coinciding with domestic violence.

A study of 154 women screened for domestic violence in a pediatric setting over a 3-month period reported 31% (n = 47) had experienced domestic violence at some time in their lives, and 17% (n = 25) reported domestic violence within the previous 2 years. Also, 5 episodes of child abuse were identified in women who reported recent domestic violence, and 2 of these episodes had not been reported before the domestic violence screen (Siegel, Hill, Henderson, Ernst, & Boat, 1999).

Assessing for domestic violence in a private, nonthreatening, nonblaming manner can allow for greater disclosure by the victim mother (Campbell & Lewandowski, 1997). Easy-to-use, reliable screening methods, such as the Abuse Assessment Screen (McFarlane & Parker, 1994) or the RADAR screening tool (Philadelphia Family Violence Working Group, 1998) can assist the nurse in assessing for domestic violence **(Figures 15-1 to 15-3)**.

Healthcare providers caring for older adolescents and teenagers, especially those entering into dating relationships, must begin screening for teenage dating violence as soon as their adolescent clients begin to date. Dating violence, including acquaintance rape, has been reported to occur in 19% to 55% of adolescent dating relationships (Gray & Foshee, 1997). For many of these teenagers the lessons learned in early dating relationships might serve as relationship "scripts" for the future. The nurse must inquire about the safety of romantic or intimate relationships in which the teenage patient is involved. Nonjudgmental and confidential inquiry into the nature of any sexual activity, including exposure risks for unplanned pregnancy and sexually transmitted infections, as well as any concurrent drug and alcohol use, is important **(Figure 15-4)**.

WOMEN'S HEALTH NURSES

Nurses caring for women in family planning, prenatal, obstetric, and postpartum settings have a duty to screen for domestic violence among all female patients **(Figure 15-5)**. Currently, it is recommended that all female patients be screened for domestic violence at their family planning or yearly gynecologic visits (McFarlane & Parker, 1994). Additionally, women who present frequently for treatment of sexually transmitted infections, emergency contraception, and unplanned pregnancies should be screened at every clinical encounter because these conditions may be associated with pressured or coerced sex as well as violence.

Women receiving prenatal care should be screened a minimum of 3 times during pregnancy for domestic violence because current research indicates that domestic violence increases as the pregnancy progresses. Women who frequently miss prenatal appointments or who are screened late in pregnancy should be routinely assessed at

RADAR: A DOMESTIC VIOLENCE INTERVENTION

R = ROUTINELY SCREEN FEMALE PATIENTS
Victims of violence are very likely to disclose abuse to a Health Care Provider, but only if they are asked about it. Always interview the patient alone.

A = ASK DIRECT QUESTIONS
Ask simple direct questions in a non-judgmental way. "Is there anyone who has physically or sexually hurt you or frightened you?" "Have you ever been hit, kicked, or punched by your partner?" "Does your partner try to control your activities or your money?" "I notice you have a number of bruises; did someone do this to you?" "Because violence is so common in many women's lives, we've begun to ask about it routinely:"

IF PATIENT ANSWERS YES, SEE OTHER SIDE FOR RESPONSES AND CONTINUE WITH THE FOLLOWING STEPS:

D = DOCUMENT YOUR FINDINGS
Record a description of the abuse as she has described it to you. Use statements such as "the patient states she was..." If she gives the specific name of the assailant use it in your record. "She says her boyfriend John Smith struck her..." Record all pertinent physical findings. Use a body map to supplement the written record. Offer to photograph injuries. When serious injury or sexual abuse is detected, preserve all physical evidence. Document an opinion if the injuries were inconsistent with the patient's explanation.

A = ASSESS PATIENT SAFETY
Before she leaves the medical setting, find out if she is afraid to go home. Has there been an increase in frequency or severity of violence? Have there been threats of homicide or suicide? Have there been threats to her children or pets? Is there a gun or other weapon present?

R = RESPOND, REVIEW OPTIONS & REFERRALS
If the patient is in imminent danger, find out if there is someone with whom she can stay. Does she need immediate access to a shelter? Offer her the opportunity of a private phone to make a call. If she does not need immediate assistance, offer information about hotlines and resources in the community (see other side). Remember that it may be dangerous for the woman to have these in her possession. Do not insist that she take them. Make a follow-up appointment to see her.

IF THE PATIENT ANSWERS YES:
Encourage her to talk about it.
"Would you like to talk about what has happened to you? or "Would you like help?"
Listen non-judgmentally.
This serves both to begin the healing process for the woman and to give you an idea of what kind of referrals she may need.
Validate her experience.
"You are not alone." "You do not deserve to be treated this way." "You are not to blame." "What happened to you is a crime." "Help is available to you." "The violence is likely to get worse, and I am worried about you." "If you are not safe, your children are not safe."

IF THE PATIENT ANSWERS NO, OR WILL NOT DISCUSS THE TOPIC:
Be aware of any clinical signs that may indicate abuse:
Injury to the head, neck, torso, breasts, abdomen, or genitals; bilateral or multiple injuries; delay between onset of injury and seeking treatment; explanation by the patient which is inconsistent with the type of injury; any injury during pregnancy; prior history of trauma; chronic pain symptoms for which no etiology is apparent; psychological distress such as depression, suicidal ideation, anxiety, sleeping or eating disorders; a partner who seems overly protective or who will not leave the woman's side; frequent health care visits; substance abuse.
If any of these clinical signs are present, ask more specific questions. Make sure she is alone.
"I am worried about you. It looks as though someone may have hurt you. Can you tell me how it happened?" "Sometimes when people feel the way you do, it may be because they are being hurt at home. Is this happening to you?"
If the patient denies abuse, but you strongly suspect it, document your opinion, and let her know there are resources available to her should she choose to pursue such options in the future. Make a follow-up appointment to see her.

RESOURCES
215/386-7777	Women Against Abuse, 24 hr. Hotline & Shelter
215/686-7082	Women Against Abuse Legal Center
215/751-1111	Women In Transition, 24 hr. Hotline
215/739-9999	English 24 hr. Hotline/Lutheran Settlement
215/235-9992	Espanol 24 hr. Hotline/Lutheran Settlement
215/978-1174	Congreso de Latinos Unidos
215/886-8725	Korean Women's Support
215/627-3922	SEWAA (for women from Pakistan, Nepal, Sri Lanka, India)

© 1998, 1995 RADAR Pocket Card developed by Phila. Family Violence Working Group, c/o Physicians for Social Responsibility 215/765-3630. Adapted from NY Office for Prevention of Domestic Violence. RADAR action steps developed by the Mass Medical Society. © 1992 Mass Medical Society. Used with permission.

Figure 15-1. *RADAR pocket card used for domestic violence screening. (Contributed by the Institute for Safe Families; Philadelphia, Pa.)*

RADAR FOR PEDIATRICIANS: A DOMESTIC VIOLENCE INTERVENTION

R = ROUTINELY SCREEN MOTHERS FOR ABUSE
Intervening on behalf of battered women is an active form of preventing child abuse. Victims of violence are very likely to disclose abuse to a health care provider, but only if they are asked about it. Always interview the parent alone if the child is over two.

A = ASK DIRECT QUESTIONS
Ask questions routinely in the course of taking a social history in the context of safety and discipline. "The safety of moms can affect the health and safety of children, so I want to ask you some personal questions." "Because violence is common in so many women's lives, I've begun to ask about it routinely:" "Is there anyone who has physically or sexually hurt you or frightened you?" "Have you ever been hit, kicked, or punched by your partner?" "I notice you have a number of bruises; did someone do this to you?"

IF THE MOTHER ANSWERS "YES", SEE OTHER SIDE FOR RESPONSES AND CONTINUE WITH THE FOLLOWING STEPS:

D = DOCUMENT YOUR FINDINGS
Document in the pediatric chart that RADAR screening was done. Indicate response as "+", "-", or "suspected". Ask Mom if it's safe to document in chart. If yes, use statements such as "the child's mother states she was..." Include the name of the assailant in your record. "She says her boyfriend, John Smith, struck her..." Note any obvious injuries to the mother. Offer her help in arranging for appropriate medical services.

A = ASSESS SAFETY OF MOTHER AND CHILDREN
Before she leaves the medical setting, find out if it is safe for her and her children to go home. Has there been an increase in frequency or severity of violence? Have there been threats of homicide or suicide? Is there a gun or other weapon present? Have there been threats to children or pets? Are the children currently being abused or in immediate danger?

R = RESPOND, REVIEW OPTIONS & REFER
Know in-house and local resources for referral. If the patient is in imminent danger, find out if there is someone with whom she can stay. Does she need immediate access to a shelter? Offer her the opportunity to use a private phone. If she does not need immediate help, offer information about hotlines and resources in the community (see other side). Offer to write down phone numbers if it is unsafe to take information. Remember that it may be dangerous for her to have these in her possession. Discuss the effects of family violence on children. Do the children need a referral? Make a follow-up appointment to see her and her children and document the options discussed

IF THE MOTHER ANSWERS "YES":
Encourage her to talk about it.
"Would you like to talk about what has happened?" or "What help do you need?" "What would you do if this happens again?" "How do you think this has affected your children?"
Listen non-judgmentally.
This will begin the healing process for the woman and give you an idea about what kind of referrals she needs.
Validate her experience.
"You are not alone." "You do not deserve to be treated this way." "You are not to blame." "What happened to you is a crime." "Help is available to you." "The violence is likely to get worse, and I am worried about you." "If you are not safe, your children are not safe."

BE AWARE OF A CONNECTION BETWEEN CERTAIN CLINICAL SIGNS AND DOMESTIC VIOLENCE:
If clinical signs such as depression, suicidal ideation, anxiety, sleeping/eating disorders, or substance abuse are present, ask more specific questions. Make sure she is alone.
"I am worried about you. It looks as though someone may have hurt you. Can you tell me how it happened?" "Sometimes when people feel the way you do, it's because they are being hurt at home. Is this happening to you?"
If the mother denies abuse, but you strongly suspect it, let her know there are resources available to her when she chooses to pursue such options in the future. Discuss the effects of family violence on children. Being exposed to violence in the home can be as traumatic for a child as being a direct victim of violence. Let her know that she can come to you in the future if she has questions or needs help. Make a follow-up appointment to see her and the children.

RESOURCES
215-386-7777	Women Against Abuse, 24 hr. Hotline & Shelter
215-686-7082	Women Against Abuse Legal Center
215-751-1111	Women In Transition, 24 hr. Hotline
215-739-9999	Lutheran Settlement House - English 24 hr. Hotline
215-235-9992	Lutheran Settlement House - Spanish 24 hr. Hotline
215-978-1174	Congreso de Latinos Unidos
215-886-8725	Korean Women's Support
215-627-3922	SEWAA (for Women from Pakistan, Nepal, Sri Lanka, India)
800-932-0313	Childline: To report child abuse
215-683-6100	Child Protective Services (DHS): To report

© 2002 RADAR Pocket Card for Pediatricians developed by The Institute for Safe Families and the PA Chapter, American Academy of Pediatrics. Philadelphia, PA, 215-765-3630. RADAR acronym developed by the Mass Medical Society. © 1992 Mass Medical Society. Used with permission.

Figure 15-2. *Pediatric RADAR card. (Contributed by the Institute for Safe Families; Philadelphia, Pa.)*

WHERE TO TURN FOR HELP

No one deserves to be beaten or hurt at home. The violence is not your fault. You did not make it happen. You are not alone. You have choices. There are people to help and support you. You have legal choices, too, because domestic violence is a crime. If you or your children are involved in a relationship in which you are being hurt and abused, review the safety tips below and the places you can call for help on the other side of this card. For other forms of family violence, see additional resources on this card.

Printed by the Philadelphia Family Violence Coordinating Council c/o The Institute for Safe Families, a division of Physicians for Social Responsibility 215/765-3630

SAFETY TIPS: IF YOUR PARTNER IS VIOLENT

If planning to leave, choose the safest time to get away. Keep spare keys, a set of clothes, important papers, prescriptions and money in a safe place (or with someone you trust) in case you leave.

When being treated for injuries, ask medical personnel to document your visit. Keep any evidence of physical abuse (ripped clothing, photos of bruises and injuries, etc.)

Know where you can go for help; tell someone what is happening to you. Have phone numbers of friends, relatives, and domestic violence programs with you.

Plan with your children and identify a safe place for them: a room with a lock or a neighbor's house where they can go for help. Reassure them their job is to stay safe, not to protect you.

Call the police (or arrange a signal with a neighbor to call the police) if you are in danger and need help.

Hotlines are always available to you during a crisis; however, it's helpful to try and contact a domestic violence hotline about laws, support groups, shelter, and other resources available to you before you have to use them.

PARTNER ABUSE/DOMESTIC VIOLENCE

Women Against Abuse, 24 hr. Hotline	215/386-7777
Women Against Abuse, Legal Center	215/686-7082
Women In Transition, 24 hr. Hotline	215/751-1111
Lutheran Settlement-Women's Program, 24 hr. Hotline English 215/739-9999 Espanol	215/235-9992
Congreso de Latinos Unidos	215/978-1174
SEWAA (for women from Pakistan, Nepal, Sri Lanka, India)	215-627-3922
Korean Women's Support Committee	215/886-8725
National Domestic Violence Hotline	800/799-7233

EMERGENCY SERVICES

Women Against Abuse, (24-hour hotline)	215/386-7777
Eliza Shirley House (24-hour accessibility)	215/568-5111
Suicide Hotline (24-hour hotline)	215/686-4420
JFK Mobile Crisis Unit (24-hour service)	215/685-6440
Pet Net (for your animals)	215/426-6304 Ext. 244

ADOLESCENT VIOLENCE

Voyage House, Hotline	215/545-2910
Youth Emergency Service, Hotline/Shelter	800/371-7233
The Attic (Gay, Lesbian, HIV Youth Issues)	215/545-4331

CHILD ABUSE/CHILD SEXUAL ABUSE-INCEST

Childline: To report Child Abuse	800/932-0313
Child Protective Services: To Report	215/683-6100
Women Organized Against Rape	215/985-3333

ELDER ABUSE

Older Adult Protective Services	215/765-9033
CARIE (Advocates for the elderly)	215/545-4437
Judicare (Legal assistance)	215/238-8943

SEXUAL ASSAULT/RAPE

Women Organized Against Rape, Hotline	215/985-3333
Allegheny/MCP Rape Victims' Program	215/842-4010

FOR HELP TO STOP BEING VIOLENT

Menergy (for men who are violent)	215/242-2235
Project RAP (for men who are violent)	215/629-3990
Men's Resource Center	610/971-9310
Parents' Anonymous, Support	800/448-4906
Family Support Services Center	215/387-0832
Sunnycrest Family Support Center	215/387-2050

Figure 15-3. *"Where to Turn for Help" card. (Contributed by the Institute for Safe Families; Philadelphia, Pa.)*

every clinical encounter for violence. Positive responses to screening during pregnancy should alert the nurse to the potential for continued abuse of the women and future child abuse and maltreatment. Safety planning measures for leaving an abusive relationship should be discussed following a positive response to violence screening, regardless of the woman's immediate intention to leave the relationship. These plans should be reviewed and revised as needed at every successive clinical encounter.

SUMMARY

In conclusion, the violent family is one that can pose challenges for nurses charged with their care. Although nurses and other healthcare providers working with families are in a unique situation to assess for violence occurring in the home, there may be both real and perceived barriers to providing appropriate care to victims of abuse. In some cases, nurses may be reluctant to screen for violence and abuse within families because of inadequate training and lack of experience with high-conflict families. The frustration on the part of the medical team that may arise when working with a woman who has suffered abuse at the hand of her partner on numerous occasions is real and must be recognized as a potential barrier to continued screening or service referral. Caring for children who have suffered abuse may make it difficult to provide services for a violent parent who herself may also have been victimized in the home. Finally, the nurse's own experience with violence in the home must also be recognized as having the potential to affect the care the nurse gives to victims or perpetrators of violence (Shea, Mahoney, & Lacey, 1997).

INTERPERSONAL VIOLENCE C.Q.I. TOOL
FOR MEDICAL FACILITIES
Created By: Lisa Leiding, RN, SANE
Hospital or Clinic: St. Vincent Hospital

GENERAL INFORMATION

Incident(s) (CHECK ALL THAT APPLY)
- ❏ Domestic violence
- ❏ Intimate partner
- ❏ Teen dating violence
- ❏ Sibling abuse
- ❏ Parent abuse
- ❏ Child abuse
- ❏ Elder abuse

Presentation to Hospital

❏ January ❏ February	❏ Saturday
❏ March ❏ April	❏ Sunday
❏ May ❏ June	❏ Monday
❏ July ❏ August	❏ Tuesday
❏ September ❏ October	❏ Wednesday
❏ November ❏ December	❏ Thursday
	❏ Friday

- ❏ 0701 - 1500
- ❏ 1501 - 2300
- ❏ 2301 - 0700
- ❏ Private Vehicle
- ❏ Ambulance
- ❏ Law Enforcement

REPORTING

MANDATORY REPORTING
- ❏ Child Abuse
- ❏ Elder Abuse

Interpersonal Violence with:
- ❏ Shooting
- ❏ Stabbing
- ❏ Blunt Force Objects
- ❏ Unconscious Patient
- ❏ Death

AGENCY:
- ❏ City Police
- ❏ County Sheriff
- ❏ NM State Police
- ❏ Tribal Police
- ❏ BIA
- ❏ Children, Youth and Families (CYFD)
- ❏ SANE

WEAPONS
- ❏ Gun
- ❏ Knife
- ❏ Bat
- ❏ Car
- ❏ Phone calls
- ❏ _____
- ❏ _____

DISCLOSURE
- ❏ Screened
- ❏ Self-Disclosure
- ❏ Suspected D. V.

PATIENT TYPE:
- ❏ Trauma Patient
- ❏ Abuser
- ❏ Victim

VICTIM INFORMATION

Ethnicity: _____
Immigration Status:
- ❏ Documented
- ❏ Undocumented

Age: _____

Sex: Male   Female
Pregnant: Yes   No
              Not Known

Injury Assessment:
- ❏ Psychological Abuse
- ❏ Economic Abuse
- ❏ Spiritual Abuse
- ❏ Sexual Assault / Abuse

- ❏ Physical Abuse
- ○ Bruises ○ Scratches ○ Abrasions
- ○ Lacerations ○ Broken Bones ○ GSW
- ○ Burns ○ Bites ○ Internal Organ Injury
- ○ Head Trauma ○ Unconscious
- ○ Abortion: Spontaneous or Threatened

Victim Prescription Drug Use:
- ❏ None ❏ _____
- ❏ _____

ABUSER INFORMATION

Ethnicity: _____
Immigration Status:
- ❏ Documented
- ❏ Undocumented

Age: _____
- ❏ Unknown age
Sex: Male   Female
Pregnant: Yes   No
              Not Known

- ❏ Same Sex relationship
- ❏ Relationship to Victim
  _____
- ❏ Recent Separation/Divorce
- ❏ Never Married
- ❏ Children Present
- ❏ 1st Violent Incident
- ❏ 2 + Violent Incidents
- ❏ Violence in other relationships

Substance Use

What was in system at time of incident?

	Victim	Abuser
None	❏	❏
Illegal Drugs	❏	❏
Alcohol	❏	❏

Abuser Prescription Drug Use:
- ❏ None
- ❏ _____
- ❏ _____

DISPOSITION AND REFERRALS

- ❏ Discharged   ❏ Morgue
  - ❏ Home
  - ❏ To friend's house
- ❏ Admitted unit: _____
  - ❏ Critical Care
  - ❏ Med - Surg
  - ❏ Mental Health

- ❏ Transferred to:
  _____
- ❏ Shelter
- ❏ Follow-up Pictures
- ❏ Other:

- ❏ Restraining Order
- ❏ Legal Aide
- ❏ Law Enforcement

Counseling
- ❏ Rape Crisis Center
- ❏ D.V. Counseling

THIS FORM IS NOT PART
OF THE PATIENT'S MEDICAL RECORD.
CONFIDENTIAL; Pursuant to Section 41-9-5, NMSA

Figure 15-4. *Interpersonal violence Continuous Quality Improvement (CQI) tool.*
Reprinted with permission from Leiding L. Domestic violence. On the Edge. 2001;7:5-6.

DOMESTIC VIOLENCE C.Q.I. TOOL page 2

☐ Refused to discuss domestic violence (Given hotline number and shelter information)
☐ Safety plan only
☐ Exam without photographs
☐ Full exam (examination, photographs, safety planning)

| Identified problems in transportation, examination or referral process: _____ _____ _____ _____ _____ | FOR OFFICE USE ONLY | Health Care System Implications: Private Insurance: ☐ Yes ☐ No Carrier: _____ Medicaid: ☐ Medicare: ☐ Self Pay: ☐ Yes ☐ No Indigent Fund: ☐ Yes ☐ No |

RECOMMENDED SOLUTIONS:

| _____ _____ _____ _____ _____ _____ _____ _____ | FOR OFFICE USE ONLY | How many prior visits? (2 years) Medical: _____ Trauma related: _____ |
| | | How many subsequent visits? Medical: _____ Trauma related: _____ |

Domestic Violence Team Comments or Suggestions:
(EMS, MD, Nursing, Advocate, Shelter, Law Enforcement, Charge Nurse etc...)

_____
_____
_____
_____
_____

PATIENT'S PRIMARY MD: _____

STAFF	PATIENT'S STICKER
MD: _____ PRIMARY NURSE: _____ CRISIS COUNSELOR: _____	OR (for employees) Patient Initials: _____ Date of Birth: _____ Date of Exam: _____ Medical Record Number OR Employee Number: _____

This C.Q.I. tool must be removed from the Domestic Violence Flow Sheet after completed. This tool will be routed to the Trauma Program Office ASAP. Statistics will be made available at the completion of every quarter.   **THIS FORM IS NOT PART OF THE PATIENT'S MEDICAL RECORD.**
                                        Confidential; Pursuant to Section 41-9-5, NMSA

Figure 15-5. *Domestic violence CQI tool.*
Reprinted with permission from Leiding L. Domestic violence.
On the Edge. *2001;7:5-6.*

Despite these barriers, nurses in a variety of settings, including family planning clinics, prenatal and obstetric departments, and pediatric settings, work with violent families on a daily basis. Some families resemble the recognizable patterns and presentations associated with violence in the home and others do not. However, only through routine assessment for violence among all families can the degree of safety be established. Routine assessment is an intervention that may encourage families to report victimization and consider safe, nonviolent alternatives. Although not all women will leave an abusive relationship, the knowledge that the healthcare setting is a safe environment may make it easier to return for care and counseling in the future. When children are identified as either being abused or at high risk for experiencing violence, assessment of and mandatory referral to local child advocacy organizations, such as the Department of Health & Human Services, further demonstrates that violence is an unacceptable way to handle conflict.

Finally, screening can also be a productive intervention that can have important implications for the nonviolent family as well. As stated previously, recognition on the part of the nurse that violence in the home occurs and places women and children at risk reinforces the message that violence is unacceptable and can have long-term physical, psychological, behavioral, and legal ramifications for everyone involved. Broaching the subject of violence in the home can open dialogues between the nurse and the client and can also foster dialogue between the client and others outside the clinical setting.

REFERENCES

American Academy of Pediatrics. The role of the pediatrician in recognizing and intervening on behalf of abused women: American Academy of Pediatrics Committee on Child Abuse and Neglect. *Pediatrics*. 1998;101:1091-1092.

American Bar Association. *The Impact of Domestic Violence on Children: A Report to the President of the American Bar Association*. Washington, DC: ABA; 1994.

Attala J, Bauza K, Pratt H, Vieira D. Integrative review of effects on children of witnessing domestic violence. *Issues Compr Pediatr Nurs*. 1995;18:163-172.

Barkan S, Gary L. Woman abuse and pediatrics: expanding the web of detection. *J Am Med Womens Assoc*. 1996;51:96-100.

Beeman S, Hagemeister A, Edleson J. Child protection and battered women's services: from conflict to collaboration. *Child Maltreat*. 1999;4:116-126.

Bennett L. Substance abuse and the domestic assault of women. *Soc Work*. 1995;40:760-769.

Bowker LH, Arbitell M, McFerron JR. On the relationship between wife beating and child abuse. In: Yllo K, Bograd M, eds. *Perspectives on Wife Abuse*. Newbury Park, Calif: Sage Publications; 1988:158-174.

Brockmeyer D, Sheridan D. Domestic violence: a practical guide to the use of forensic evaluations in clinical examination and documentation of injuries. In: Campbell J, ed. *Empowering Survivors of Abuse*. Thousand Oaks, Calif: Sage Publications; 1998:214-228.

Burgess AW, Hartman CR, Clements PT Jr. Biology of memory and childhood trauma. *J Psychosoc Nurs Ment Health Serv*. 1995;33:16-26, 52-53.

Burgess AW, Holmstrom L. Rape trauma syndrome. *Am J Psychiatry*. 1974;131:981-986.

Cadzow S, Armstrong KL. Rib fractures in infants: red alert. The clinical features, investigations and child protection outcomes. *J Paediatr Child Health*. 2000;36:322-326.

Campbell JC. Child abuse and wife abuse: the connections. *Md Med J*. 1994;43:349-350.

Campbell JC, Campbell DW. Cultural competence in the care of abused women. *J Nurse Midwifery*. 1996;41:457-462.

Campbell JC, Lewandowski LA. Mental and physical health effects of intimate partner violence on women and children. *Psychiatr Clin North Am*. 1997;20:353-374.

Campbell JC, Oliver C, Bullock L. Why battering during pregnancy? *AWHONNS Clin Issues Perinat Womens Health Nurs*. 1993;4:343-349.

Campbell JC, Parker B. Battered women and their children. *Annu Rev Nurs Res*. 1992;10:77-94.

Campbell JC, Poland ML, Waller JB, Ager J. Correlates of battering during pregnancy. *Res Nurs Health*. 1992;15:219-226.

Cheung K. Practice guidelines: identifying and documenting findings of physical child abuse and neglect. *J Pediatr Health Care*. 1999;13:142-143.

Christian C, Scribano P, Seidl T, Pinto-Martin J. Pediatric injury resulting from family violence. *Pediatrics*. 1997;99:e8. Available at: http://www.pediatrics.org/cgi/content/fukll/99/2/e8. Accessed February 19, 2003.

Crowell N, Burgess AW. *Understanding Violence Against Women*. Washington, DC: National Academy Press; 1996.

Cruz J, Firestone J. Exploring violence and abuse in gay male relationships. *Violence Vict*. 1998;13:159-173.

Davies WH, Flannery DJ. Post-traumatic stress disorder in children and adolescents exposed to violence. *Pediatr Clin North Am*. 1998;45:341-353.

Davis H, Zitelli B. Childhood injuries: accidental or inflicted? *Contemp Pediatr*. 1995;12:94-102.

Erikson J, Henderson A. Witnessing family violence: the children's experience. *J Adv Nurs*. 1992;17:1200-1209.

Family Violence Prevention Fund. Domestic Violence Is a Serious, Widespread Social Problem in America: THE FACTS. 2003. Available at: http://www.fvpf.org/facts/. Accessed January 21, 2003.

Famularo R. What are the symptoms, causes, and treatments of childhood posttraumatic stress disorder? *Harv Ment Health Lett*. 1997;13:8.

Famularo R, Fenton T, Kinscherff R, Ayoub C, Barnum R. Maternal and child posttraumatic stress disorder in cases of child maltreatment. *Child Abuse Negl*. 1994;18:27-36.

Gray H, Foshee V. Adolescent dating violence: differences between one-sided and mutually violent profiles. *J Interpers Violence*. 1997;12:126-141.

Green A. Factors contributing to the generational transmission of child maltreatment. *J Am Acad Child Adolesc Psychiatry*. 1998;37:1334-1335.

Herman-Giddens M, Brown G, Verbiest S, et al. Underascertainment of child abuse mortality in the United States. *JAMA*. 1999;282:463-467.

Hilton Z. Battered women's concerns about their children witnessing wife assault. *J Interpers Violence*. 1992;7:77-86.

Kelley B, Thornberry T, Smith C. *In the Wake of Childhood Maltreatment*. Juvenile Justice Bulletin. Washington, DC: US Dept of Justice, Office of Juvenile Justice and Delinquency Prevention; 1997. NCJ 165257.

Leiding L. Domestic violence. *On the Edge*. 2001;7:5-6.

Magan R. In the best interest of battered women: reconceptualizing allegations of failure to protect. *Child Maltreat*. 1999;4:127-135.

McCloskey LA, Figueredo AJ, Koss MP. The effects of systemic family violence on children's mental health. *Child Dev*. 1995;66:1239-1261.

McFarlane J. Battering during pregnancy: tip of an iceberg revealed. *Women Health*. 1989;15:69-84.

McFarlane J, Kelly E, Rodriguez R, Fehir J. De Madres a Madres: women building community coalitions for health. *Health Care Women Int*. 1994;15:465-476.

McFarlane J, Parker B. Preventing abuse during pregnancy: an assessment and intervention protocol. *MCN Am J Matern Child Nurs*. 1994;19:321-324.

McFarlane J, Parker B, Soeken K. Abuse during pregnancy: associations with maternal health and infant birth weight. *Nursing Res*. 1996a;45:37-42.

McFarlane J, Parker B, Soeken K. Physical abuse, smoking, and substance use during pregnancy: prevalence, interrelationships, and effects on birth weight. *J Obstet Gynecol Neonat Nurs*. 1996b;25:313-320.

McFarlane J, Parker B, Soeken K, Silva C, Reed S. Research exchange: severity of abuse before and during pregnancy for African American, Hispanic, and Anglo women. *J Nurse Midwifery*. 1999;44:139-144.

McFarlane J, Soeken K. Weight change of infants, age birth to 12 months, born to abused women. *Pediatr Nurs*. 1999;25:19-23, 35-36, 108.

McKay MM. The link between domestic violence and child abuse: assessment and treatment considerations. *Child Welfare*. 1994;73:29-39.

Monteleone J, Brodeur A, eds. *Child Maltreatment: A Clinical Guide and Reference*. 2nd ed. St Louis, Mo: GW Medical Publishing; 1998.

Orloff L. Effective advocacy for domestic violence victims: role of the nurse midwife. *J Nurse Midwifery*. 1996;41:473-490.

Overpeck M, Brenner R, Trumble A, Trifiletti L, Berendes H. Risk factors for infant homicide in the United States. *N Engl J Med*. 1998;339:1211-1216.

Parker B. Abuse of adolescents: what can we learn from pregnant teenagers? *AWHONNS Clin Issues Perinat Womens Health Nurs*. 1993;4:363-370.

Patterson M. Child abuse: assessment and intervention. *Orthoped Nurs*. 1998;17:49-56.

Perry B. Neurobiological sequelae of childhood trauma: post traumatic stress disorders in children. In: Marburg M, ed. *Catecholamine Functions in Post Traumatic Stress Disorder: Emerging Concepts*. Washington, DC: American Psychiatric Press; 1994:253-276.

Perry B. *Effects of Traumatic Events on Children: An Introduction.* 1999. Available at: http://www.bcm.tmc.edu/cta/effects_I.htm. Accessed January 21, 2003.

Philadelphia Family Violence Working Group. *RADAR Pocket Card.* Philadelphia, Pa: American Academy of Pediatrics; 1998.

Rhea M, Chafey K, Dohner V, Terragno R. The silent victims of domestic violence: who will speak? *J Child Adolesc Pediatr Nurs.* 1996;9:7-15.

Ross S. Risk of physical abuse to children of spouse abusing parents. *Child Abuse Negl.* 1996;20:589-598.

Ryan J, King M. Child witnesses of domestic violence: principles of advocacy. *Clin Excell Nurse Pract.* 1997;1:47-56.

Scalzo A. Burns and child maltreatment. In: Monteleone J, Brodeur A, eds. *Child Maltreatment: A Clinical Guide and Reference.* 2nd ed. St Louis, Mo: GW Medical Publishing; 1998:105-128.

Schwarz E, Perry B. The posttraumatic response in children and adolescents. *Psychiatr Clin North Am.* 1994;17:311-326.

Sedlak A, Broadhurst D. *The Third National Incidence Study of Child Abuse and Neglect.* 1996. Available at: http://www.calib.com/nccanch/pubs/statinfo/nis3.cfm. Accessed January 21, 2003.

Shalansky C, Eriksen J, Henderson A. Abused women and child custody: the ongoing exposure to abusive ex-partners. *J Adv Nurs.* 1999;29:416-426.

Shea C, Mahoney M, Lacey J. Breaking through the barriers to domestic violence intervention. *Am J Nurs.* 1997;97:26-33.

Shipman K, Rossman R, West J. Co-occurrence of spousal violence and child abuse: conceptual implications. *Child Maltreat.* 1999;4:93-102.

Siegel R, Hill T, Henderson V, Ernst H, Boat B. Screening for domestic violence in the community pediatric setting. *Pediatrics.* 1999;104(pt 1):874-877.

Strasburger V, Donnerstein E. Children, adolescents and the media: issues and solutions. *Pediatrics.* 1999;103:129-139.

Straus MA. Children as Witnesses to Marital Violence: A Risk Factor for Lifelong Problems Among a Nationally Representative Sample of American Men and Women—A Report of the 23rd Ross Roundtable on Critical Approaches to Common Pediatric Problems. September, 1992. Available at: http://pubpages.unh.edu/~mas2/VB48.pdf. Accessed January 21, 2003.

Thormaehlen DJ, Bass-Feld ER. Children: the secondary victims of domestic violence. *Md Med J.* 1994;43:355-359.

US Advisory Board on Child Abuse and Neglect. *A Nation's Shame: Fatal Child Abuse and Neglect in the United States.* Washington, DC: US Dept of Health & Human Services, US Government Printing Office; 1995.

US Department of Health & Human Services. Administration on Children, Youth, and Families. *Child Maltreatment 2000.* Washington, DC: US Government Printing Office; 2002.

Walker L. *The Battered Woman Syndrome.* New York, NY: Springer; 1984.

Widner-Kolberg M. Child abuse. *Crit Care Nurs Clin North Am.* 1997;9:175-182.

Wolak J, Finkelhor D. Children exposed to partner violence. In: Jasinski JL, Williams LM, eds. *Partner Violence: A Comprehensive Review of 20 Years of Research*. Thousand Oaks, Calif: Sage Publications; 1998:73-111.

Wolfe D, Korsch B. Witnessing domestic violence during childhood and adolescence: implication for pediatric practice. *Pediatrics*. 1994;94:594-599.

Chapter 16

RISKS TO CHILDREN IN THE DIGITAL AGE

Eileen M. Alexy, MSN, RN, CS

Child sexual victimization facilitated by the use of a computer is a relatively recent and poorly understood phenomenon. In response to the discovery of this new conduit for promoting illicit sexual activity with children, in 1998 the Office of Juvenile Justice and Delinquency Prevention began to label online sexual crimes directed toward children as Internet Crimes Against Children (ICAC). ICAC were defined as any computer-facilitated sexual exploitation of children, including online solicitation and child pornography (Office for Victims of Crime, 2001; Office of Juvenile Justice and Delinquency Prevention, 1998).

To date, only 2 studies have investigated the online victimization of children (Finkelhor, Mitchell, & Wolak, 2000; Mitchell, Finkelhor, & Wolak, 2001). Data were gathered for both studies from a telephone survey of a national sample of 1501 youths age 10 to 17 years, who were regular Internet users. The investigators found that 1 in 5 children received a sexual solicitation or approach over the Internet in the last year. Finkelhor et al. (2000) also reported that 1 in 33 children received an **aggressive sexual solicitation**, meaning a solicitor asked to meet them somewhere, called them on the telephone, and/or sent them regular mail, money, or gifts. Furthermore, 44% of the children who received an aggressive sexual solicitation online accepted regular mail, money, and/or gifts. Perhaps the most worrisome discovery found in these studies is that more than one third of the aggressive sexual solicitations were not disclosed to parents, teachers, or friends.

Much of the focus of ICAC has been on identifying and apprehending the offenders. However, research about ICAC is almost nonexistent. In the wake of its absence, a new category of victims has emerged: those victimized online. The problem is that online victimization can result in offline consequences, specifically, sexual victimization in real life. Nurses play a pivotal role in providing diagnostic and clinical intervention services to sexually victimized children (Burgess & Holmstrom, 1975). Their biopsychosocial training, as well as their presence in facilities where victims seek services, present a unique opportunity to provide intervention, education, and counseling regarding matters of human sexuality and safety. An understanding of the methods used by sex offenders to exploit and lure children in the context of the Internet is essential for families, law enforcement personnel, nurses, and other healthcare professionals. Knowledge regarding these matters is necessary to develop and provide effective prevention and treatment strategies for child victims and their families in schools, communities, emergency rooms, and pediatric and psychiatric settings.

TECHNOLOGY AND ITS USE IN CHILD SEXUAL VICTIMIZATION

Historically, persons with criminally salacious intentions have been among the first to adopt new technologies (Armagh, Battaglia, & Lanning, 2000; Burgess, 1984; Lanning,

1992; Schultz, 1980; Tyler & Stone, 1985). The introduction of the printing press provided widespread circulation of material offering descriptive tales of the sexual victimization of children. The development of photography introduced pictures of children engaging in sexual activity with adults, other children, and animals as early as 1862 (Schultz, 1980). In the 1980s, the low price and availability of VCRs and home video cameras facilitated and increased the production, distribution, and dissemination of depictions of acts of child sexual victimization (Burgess, 1984; Lanning, 1992; Tyler & Stone, 1985).

The development of new technologies, digital cameras, CD-RW drives, faster connection technologies (cable modems, digital subscriber lines [DSLs]), and better computers exposes the public to a plethora of potential misuses. Beginning in the 1990s, child sex offenders began to use the Internet, which has further facilitated their ability to produce, distribute, and disseminate materials related to the sexual victimization of children. Moreover, the use of the Internet has increased communication among like-minded offenders and given them access to an ever-increasing pool of potential victims.

WHAT EXACTLY ARE THE RISKS?

The Office for Victims of Crime recently released a bulletin identifying the following 4 types of Internet victimization (Office for Victims of Crime, 2001, p. 2):

1. Enticing children through online contact for the purpose of engaging them in sexual acts

2. Using the Internet for the production, manufacture, and distribution of child pornography

3. Using the Internet to expose children to child pornography and encourage them to exchange or "trade" pornography

4. Seducing and enticing children for the purpose of sexual tourism (travel to engage in sexual behavior) for commercial gain and/or personal gratification

Children can now connect with others more quickly and frequently, and from the comfort of their homes, schools, and potentially anywhere. The ease of connectivity that the Internet affords may someday bring all children into the pool of potential victims. The historical pattern of the proliferation of victimization via the misuse of new technologies suggests that as the Internet continues to proliferate its misuse will also flourish (Armagh et al., 2000; Burgess, 1984; Lanning, 1992; Schultz, 1980; Tyler & Stone, 1985). Currently, the population of children accessing the Internet is growing at an exponential rate. The number of children age 2 to 17 years connecting online in the United States has tripled from 8 million in 1997 to 25 million in 2000 (Grunwald Associates, 2000). That statistic reflects an estimated 40% increase in the last year (Grunwald Associates, 2000). In addition, reports from the US Census Bureau found that 25% of children age 6 to 11 years and 48% of children age 12 to 17 years accessed the Internet from home, representing an increase of 9% and 13%, respectively, from 1997 (Newburger, 1999, 2001). Statistics from the National Center for Education reported that in 1999, 95% of public schools were connected to the Internet, reflecting an increase of 60% from 1994 (Williams, 2000). Reports from the CyberTipline of the National Center for Missing and Exploited Children (NCMEC) indicate that the number of children being lured and exploited online is increasing. Since July 1, 1998, there have been 10 751 confirmed cases and 9145 unconfirmed cases of Internet child pornography, 3306 cases of online enticement of children for sexual acts, and 1470 cases of extrafamilial child sexual molestation related to computers reported to the NCMEC (Rabun, 2000). The misuse of the Internet presents unique challenges for parents, professionals, and society.

WHY ARE CHILDREN ATTRACTED TO THE INTERNET?

The Internet possesses several alluring qualities for youth, especially for those disheartened by events in the "real world." The very nature of communities online has afforded each individual the ability to alter his or her social construction of reality (Rheingold, 1993; Turkle, 1995). As Baudrillard (1994) predicted, the simulation of community in an online environment is gaining acceptance as the simulacrum (i.e., reality or hyperreality). Thus, the failure to recognize online communities as "real spaces" for children will place nurses and mental health professionals at a disadvantage when dealing with victims of ICAC. Online communities that facilitate offline criminal behavior produce "real-life" child victims. Therefore, a cursory understanding of these communities and how they operate is essential to comprehend the context of ICAC.

In the science fiction novel *Neuromancer,* the author coined the term **cyberspace** and defined it as follows (Gibson, 1984):

A consensual hallucination experienced daily by billions of legitimate operators, in every nation, by children being taught mathematical concepts . . . . A graphic representation of data abstracted from the banks of every computer in the human system. Unthinkable complexity. Lines of light ranged in the nonspace of the mind, clusters and constellations of data. Like city lights receding . . . (p. 51.)

These cyberspaces and online communities are based on computer-mediated communication and frequently take the form of online bulletin board systems (BBSs); mailing lists (listservs); multiuser dungeons/domains (MUDs); Internet relay chat (IRC), also known as "chat rooms"; and instant messaging (IM). BBSs and mailing lists are some of the earliest forms of online communities that use asynchronous technology (Jones, 1997; Rheingold, 1993; Turkle, 1995). **Asynchronous** means it is up to users to decide if and when they want to respond, similar to e-mail. MUDs are synchronous platforms used for popular types of computer role-playing games, such as SimCity, and can be defined as follows (Rheingold, 1993):

. . . imaginary worlds in computer databases where people use words and programming languages to improvise melodramas, build worlds and all the objects in them, solve puzzles, invent amusements and tools, compete for prestige and power, gain wisdom, seek revenge, indulge greed and lust and violent impulses. (p. 145.)

A significant part of the interest, fun, and fantasy of MUDs is that people connected to the Internet can assume any persona or identity. These personae or identities are known as **avatars**. An avatar, a Hindu religious term, is an incarnation of a deity; an online avatar is the embodiment of an idea or greater reality and is used as a visual pseudonym or display appearance to represent oneself in MUDs (Turkle, 1995). By understanding the concept of MUDs, it is easy to see why cyberspace is alluring to children. The anonymous nature of the Internet allows youth the freedom to experiment with identities and "become" male or female, young or old. Moreover, children are able to indulge in fantasy and see their avatars interact with others.

Another popular form of computer-mediated communication is IRC. These chat rooms are synchronous, with communication occurring in "real time." The absence of a physical social context (i.e., visual cues, voice intonation) in chat rooms requires participants to construct a social context (Rheingold, 1993). Participants in chat rooms communicate and construct contextual cues through the use of acronyms and emoticons, or "smileys" **(Tables 16-1 and 16-2)**.

Older children, in particular, have been found to perceive and embody their own social universe in a distinctive language (Schwartz & Merten, 1967). Through a jargon developed online, these children are able to converse with others while excluding those

Table 16-1. Examples of Chat Room, E-mail, and Instant Messaging Acronyms

Acronym	Meaning
AFAIK	As far as I know
A/S/L?	Age/sex/location?
B4N	Bye for now
BBIAB	Be back in a bit
BBL	Be back later
BRB	Be right back
BTW	By the way
BWTHDIK	But what the heck do I know...?
CU	See you
CUL	See you later
DIKU	Do I know you?
EMFBI	Excuse me for butting in
F2F	Face-to-face
FMTYEWTK	Far more than you ever wanted to know
GIWIST	Gee, I wish I'd said that
GMTA	Great minds think alike
HAK	Hugs and kisses
HTH	Hope this helps
IAC	In any case
IANAL	I am not a lawyer (but)
IIRC	If I recall/remember/recollect correctly
ILU or ILY	I love you
IMing	Chatting with someone online usually while doing other things such as playing trivia or other interactive games
IMO	In my opinion
IOW	In other words
IRL	In real life (i.e., when not chatting)
IYSWIM	If you see what I mean
KFY	Kiss for you
KOTC	Kiss on the cheek
KWIM?	Know what I mean?
LD	Later, dude
LOL	Laughing out loud
MorF	Male or female
MOSS	Member of the same sex
MOTOS	Member of the opposite sex
MUSM	Miss you so much

(continued)

Table 16-1. *(continued)*

ACRONYM	MEANING
MWBRL	More will be revealed later
NAZ	Name, address, zip (also means Nasdaq)
NIFOC	Nude in front of the computer
OLL	Online love
OTOH	On the other hand
P911	My parents are coming in the room!
PAL	Parents are listening
PAN or PANB	Parents are nearby
PAW	Parents are watching
PDA	Public display of affection
PMFJIB	Pardon me for jumping in but...
::POOF::	Goodbye (leaving the room)
POS	Parents over shoulder
ROTFL	Rolling on the floor laughing
RPG	Role-playing games
RSN	Real soon now
SOMY	Sick of me yet?
TA	Teacher alert
TAFN	That's all for now
TMTOWTDI	There's more than one way to do it
TPTB	The powers that be
TTFN	Ta-Ta for now
TTYL	Talk to you later
WDALYIC	Who died and left you in charge?
WFM	Works for me
WIBNI	Wouldn't it be nice if
WT?	What/who the?
WTGP?	Want to go private?
WU?	What's up?
WUF?	Where are you from?
WYRN	What's your real name?
WYSIWYG	What you see is what you get

Adapted from NetLingo. Acronyms & Shorthand. NetLingo, Inc. 2001. Available at: http://www.netlingo.com. Accessed December 10, 2001; TechTarget.com, Inc. 2001. Available at: http://www.whatis.com. Accessed July 12, 2001.

Table 16-2. Examples of Chat Room, E-mail, and Instant Messaging Emoticons

Symbol	Feelings/ Actions/People	Symbol	Feelings/ Actions/People
:-l	Ambivalent/Indifferent	};-*	Kissing
0:-)	Angelic	(-:	Left-handed
}-|	Angry	:-------)	Liar
(::()::)	Band-aid	X:)	Little girl
-)	Bashful	8:-)	Little girl
~===	Birthday/Candle	}:-(	Lonely
:-{}	Blowing a kiss	}:-)}-----<	Male
|-o	Bored	#-)	Parties all night
:-'|	Cold/Flu/Sick	$-)	Rich
{:-)	Confident	@}->--	Rose
:~/	Confused	@}>`--`--	Rose
8-)	Cool	:(	Sad
:'-(	Crying	:-(	Sad
`?-)	Curious	:`-(	Very sad (crying)
{:-)}--8--<	Female	`:-@	Screaming
;-)	Flirting/Winking smile	:-X	Secretive/Lips are sealed
((xoxo))	Giving hugs and kisses	:-O	Shocked
8-)	Glasses	:-@	Sick or "cussing"
(:->--<	Hands up	;-(*)	Sick
:o)	Happy or Goofy	:-p	Silly
:-)	Happy/Smiling	;^)	Smirking
:-D	Very happy	:-`\)	Smoking
(((name)))	Hug	;-w	Speaks with forked tongue
XOXOXO	Hugs and kisses	:-T	Straight face/Tight lipped
((())):**	Hugs and kisses	:-O	Talks too much
%-\	Hung over	X~~~~	Telephone
#-)	Hung over	:-?	Unsure
:-#	Kiss	~=|x|=~	Wants a hug
};-x	Kissing	*<=|:-)	Wizard

Adapted from Dwarfnet Internet Guide. Acronyms and Chat Lingo: Smileys, Faces, Emoticons. Dwarfnet Internet Guide. 2001. Available at: http://www.dwarfnet.com/chat/smileyfaces.shtml. Accessed July 29, 2001; TechTarget.com, Inc. 2001. Available at: http://www.whatis.com. Accessed July 12, 2001.

who are unfamiliar with the language. Thus, it can be difficult for individuals who do not participate in chat rooms to translate and interpret the text of chat room discussions.

Another communication technology fast eclipsing chat and e-mail (especially among adolescents) is IM. IM can be described as a combination of e-mail and chat that allows an individual to "speak" with another person in real time. A report from the Pew Internet and American Life Project found that 73% of children in the 12 to 17 year age bracket use the Internet. Additionally, 74% of these wired teens use IM, compared to only 44% of adults (Lenhart, Rainie, & Lewis, 2001). Clearly, children are adapting to new technologies more quickly than adults.

THE TECHNOLOGICAL GENERATION GAP

Although nurses are proficient and competent with medical technology, few nurses would describe themselves as Internet experts. Other than using the Internet as a tool for research or as a communication device, nurses have not felt the need to develop more adept Internet skills for their clinical practice. This is not surprising because several published reports illustrate a technological generation gap between parents and children (Lenhart et al., 2001; Roper Starch Worldwide, 1999; Turow & Nir, 2000).

In a report published about the Internet and the family, differing results from the perspectives of parents and children have been found (Turow & Nir, 2000). Turow and Nir (2000) presented a scenario in which children and parents were asked if they would answer questions about their likes and dislikes and disclose personal information, such as their name and home address, to receive a free gift. Initially, 22% of children reported that they would disclose this information. If a child responded "it depends," the follow-up question was, "What if the product was worth $25?" A "no" to that question led to a raising of the gift's value to $50, then to $100 (Turow & Nir, 2000, p. 27). By $50 the number of children willing to disclose personal information was 38%, and by $100 it was 45%. That statistic is alarming in light of recent media stories portraying predatory child sex offenders on the Internet (Andrews, 2000; Jabs, 2000; Nordland & Bartholet, 2001). Prior research demonstrates that child sex offenders often use the strategy of offering material goods or gifts to entice children into sexual activity (Budin & Johnson, 1989; Burgess & Holmstrom, 1975, 1978; Christiansen & Blake, 1990; Elliott, Browne, & Kilcoyne, 1995; Groth & Birnbaum, 1978).

The technological generation gap can make it difficult for parents and professionals to protect children. From a lack of understanding, an overreaction can occur. The answer is not to disconnect the computer or forbid access to the Internet. To be truthful, this will not prevent possible victimization. The Internet has become pervasive in the lives of children; if they are disconnected at home, they will still be able to get online at a friend's house, at school, at the mall, or at the public library. Therefore, it is essential to communicate online risks to children. However, having a one-time discussion with children will not suffice. It is incumbent upon parents and professionals to take an active role and become more knowledgeable about the Internet to minimize online risks.

HOW THE INTERNET CAN BE A POTENTIALLY DANGEROUS PLACE: PREDATORS ON THE WEB

TRADERS

Law enforcement investigations have verified that child sex offenders are avid collectors of child pornography (Armagh et al., 2000; Burgess, 1984; Lanning, 2001). With the advent of the Internet, these collectors have also become avid "traders." High priority is given to the maintenance and expansion of these collections. Investigators have offered several motives to explain the offenders' compulsive collecting and trading behavior.

Collecting child pornography may help sex offenders to "satisfy, deal with, or reinforce compulsive, persistent sexual fantasies about children" (Burgess, 1984, p. 84). Additionally, trading appears to fulfill needs for camaraderie and behavior validation among these offenders. Trading pictures among like-minded individuals provides strong positive reinforcement for the offender's behavior.

Although no evidence exists that supports a causal link between pornography and sex offenses, experiential information from law enforcement investigations has identified 5 specific uses for child pornography (Lanning, 2001) as follows:

1. Sexual arousal and gratification

2. To lower children's inhibitions

3. Blackmail

4. As a medium of exchange or communication among like-minded individuals

5. Profit

Lanning (2001) posited that child sex offenders frequently use child pornography as a "teaching tool" to engage children in sexual acts. Child pornography used for the purpose of lowering children's inhibitions typically illustrates a child who appears to be having "fun" participating in the sexual activity. Moreover, to lower inhibitions, sex offenders have often used mainstream books that teach sex education to children. These books and pornography have been used as a method to normalize the behavior (Lanning, 2001; Lanning & Burgess, 1989).

Additionally, child sex offenders frequently maintain lists of names, addresses, phone numbers, and e-mail addresses of persons with similar interests. Before the development of the Internet, if a law enforcement officer arrested an individual in the network, the arrest was rapidly communicated to other members of the network through a "phone tree" or regular mail. The Internet has allowed offenders to alert other members of the network even more promptly than before its invention (Armagh et al., 2000).

A further motivation for collecting and trading child pornography is that a child does not stay a child forever. Eventually, a child will outgrow his or her attractiveness for the offender. Therefore, offenders frequently retain pictures of their victims because a picture preserves the child at a specific point in time. In a photograph or digital image, a 9-year-old girl stays young forever. These images serve as souvenirs or trophies of sexual relationships. When an image is scanned and uploaded to the Internet and then downloaded or saved to another person's computer, it is equivalent to producing a copy of the image. Thus, a child originally victimized in the production of pornography can be further victimized years later because the image has been reproduced and traded on the Internet. Consequently, the victim may be subject to reliving the events of the initial trauma because someone has posted an image of his or her experience online.

TRAVELERS

Applying skills of coercion and manipulation, child sex offenders who captivate children in online conversation and journey distances (even crossing state lines) to meet a child face-to-face and engage him or her in sexual activity have been labeled "travelers" (Finkelhor et al., 2000; McLaughlin, 2000; Office for Victims of Crime, 2001). Currently, the prevalence and incidence of traveler cases is unknown. In 2 studies of online victimization, the investigators were unable to detect any serious Internet traveler cases from a sample of 1501 children (Finkelhor et al., 2000; Mitchell et al., 2001). This finding is not unexpected, given that the studies used a telephone interview to collect data and the well-documented premise that sex crimes against children tend to be underreported (Bolen & Scannapieco, 1999; Finkelhor, 1994; Smith, Letourneau, Saunders, Kilpatrick, Resnick, & Best, 2000).

A Traveler Case Example

Donny14 has been in the chat room "#littleboysex" for over 2 hours. In real life, "Donny14" is actually a 35-year-old man. The regulars are on today. He recognizes Rory16 from California, Hot4U from England, and Jafo, a boy-lover from Toronto. Suddenly, a "newbie" enters the room, Billy14, with whom he immediately initiates chat. This conversation goes as follows (McLaughlin, 1998):

Donny14> Hi what's up

Billy14> Notin yet!

Donny14> :) Maybe i can help with that, where ya from

Billy14> NH, u?

Donny14> NY, near Albany. What ya look like

Billy14> 5'6", 128, brn, blue, 5.5 cut, u?

Donny14> wow u sound hot, i am 5'7", 132, blond, blue, 6 cut got a self-pic

Billy14> yea u?

Donny14> yea lets trade

Billy14> ok, sent

Donny14> Man your pic is hot, What u in2

Billy14> kinda new, done cyber, pics and fone a few times, what age guys u like

Donny14> Love 12-15, especially when they first get hair and have clear cum

Billy14> me2 u got pics like that

Donny14> yea u?

Billy14> no i crashed and lost everything, can u help me out

Donny14> yea sure here, start with these

Clearly, Billy14 has entered a dangerous cyberspace, and by the graphic nature of the conversation it appears that this is not his first experience. Billy14 reports that he has done "cyber," which is a chat abbreviation for cybersex. Cybersex in online chat rooms is defined as computer-mediated interactive masturbation in real time and/or computer-mediated telling of interactive sexual stories in real time with the intent of arousal (Hamman, 1996; Lamb, 1998). As the discussion continues, Billy14 confides in Donny14 that he "loves the Internet" and spends 3 or more hours a day online.

One might ask why a 14-year-old boy would visit such a site. Perhaps Billy14 is lonely and depressed, maybe he is curious and experimenting, maybe he is only playing a joke, or perhaps he has been physically sexually victimized in the past. Indeed, the fact that Billy14 admits to engaging in "cyber, pics and fone a few times" demonstrates that he has experienced noncontact abuse, placing him at a higher risk for revictimization (Finkelhor, 1994; Giardino, 2001).

The computer interaction continues, and in less than 10 minutes child pornographic pictures are sent over the Internet (McLaughlin, 1998). As this is occurring, Donny14 starts to experience some sexual arousal and fantasies. In his mind's eye, he begins to imagine what an unclothed Billy14 looks like. He perseverates on these thoughts and fantasies as the conversation continues. In the next 30 minutes, Donny14 spends time recounting his first acts of masturbation through his complete sexual history to Billy14. As this dialogue continues Donny14 is steadily collecting information from Billy14 by asking both explicit and seemingly innocuous questions. He asks Billy14 if he likes soccer and the name of his soccer team. He asks if Billy14 has any other hobbies and how he is doing in school. The purpose of these questions is to establish rapport and elicit more data so that Donny14 can continue to feed his fantasies and "groom" and test Billy14. At times, Donny14 comments about how sexually aroused he is and asks if Billy14 is also experiencing this sensation. At this point in time, he is masturbating as he carries on this discussion. Additional pornographic pictures are sent and e-mail addresses are exchanged. Donny14 now feels confident and decides to "test" Billy14. He asks Billy14 his opinion of guys in their thirties who like guys "their age." Billy14 is not dismissive and suggests that this is "perfectly normal." Donny14 then reveals that he is really 35 years old and now feels comfortable enough to send an actual picture of himself to Billy14. He is tense as he waits for Billy14's response. Upon receiving a favorable response, Donny14 begins to indulge more in his thoughts and fantasies. He begins to think of meeting Billy14 face-to-face and communicates this idea to Billy14. Billy14 is receptive to this idea as long as no one finds out, a condition that Donny14 quickly agrees to. The discussion continues as follows (McLaughlin, 1998):

Donny14> How will u be able to get out for the night without your mom getting suspicious

Billy14> I could tell her i am staying with friends, she never checks

Donny14> ok, sounds kewl

Donny14> where ya want to meet, should be public so u can decide if I am ok

Billy14> how bout McDonalds

Donny14> sounds good, I will be there at 3:00 right after u get out of school

Billy14> how will i know its u

Donny14> I will be driving a red volvo and I will have on a black baseball cap

Billy14> K cya there

In this thread of conversation, Donny14 appears to be "caring" and asks to meet in a public place so that Billy14 can determine if he is "okay." At this point Donny14 prepares to cross state lines to meet Billy14. Donny14 downloads a map and directions to the specified McDonald's from the Internet. As Donny14 awaits the arrival of Billy14 at the agreed upon location, he fantasizes about their sexual interaction (McLaughlin, 1998). Donny14 has come equipped for this encounter with his "sex kit," complete with condoms, lubricants, and a new digital camera purchased especially for the occasion. He eagerly waits with anticipation and anxiety in the parking lot for the scheduled meeting with Billy14. His fantasy is about to become reality.

Case Study Analysis

Clearly, Billy14 displays several risk factors that place him in great physical danger of sexual victimization **(Table 16-3)**. These risk factors include the following:

— He is age 14 years. Older youth (age 14 to 17 years) are more likely to be solicited online because they are often unsupervised when using the computer and are more likely to discuss personal issues online (Finkelhor et al., 2000; Mitchell et al., 2001; Office for Victims of Crime, 2001).

— He spends at least 3 hours a day online, expresses that the Internet is highly important to him, and is highly experienced with using the Internet. Children

Table 16-3. Risk Factors for Children
— Isolated children; the Internet is main source of information and all of child's activities revolve around the Internet
— Curious, rebellious, or "troubled" youth
— Older children (age 13 to 17 years)
— Children from dysfunctional families
— Children confused about their sexual orientation or identity
— Children with poor verbal communication skills

with high Internet use have been found to be at a higher risk for online solicitation (Finkelhor et al., 2000; Mitchell et al., 2001).

— He displays high online risk behavior, meaning he engages in chat room discussions with strangers and he discloses personal information (e.g., where he lives) (Finkelhor et al., 2000; Mitchell et al., 2001).

— He talks about sex with someone he has never met in person, and he purposefully visits "X-rated" websites and chat rooms. Billy14 may be emotionally vulnerable, and he may be dealing with issues of sexual identity (Finkelhor et al., 2000; Mitchell et al., 2001; Office for Victims of Crime, 2001). This may explain his choice of the chat room "#littleboysex."

What are some other risk factors? Although the victim in our scenario is male, research and anecdotal reports indicate that girls are often at a higher risk for online solicitation than boys (Finkelhor et al., 2000; Mitchell et al., 2001). Finkelhor et al. (2000) found that girls were targeted at almost twice the rate of boys. However, this finding must be interpreted cautiously because of the underreporting of male sexual victimization. Moreover, Finkelhor et al. found that 34% of boys were solicited online, which is a sizable number.

Chat rooms and using IM appear to be the primary conduits for soliciting children online. Finkelhor et al. (2000) found that 68% of solicitations occurred in chat rooms and 24% occurred through IM. Additionally, investigators report that children who are classified as "troubled," meaning those who have experienced a death in the family, have moved to a new home, have divorced or separated parents, have a parent who lost a job, have experienced prior physical and/or sexual victimizations, and have symptoms of clinical depression are at a significantly greater risk for online victimization than their peers (Mitchell et al., 2001).

WHAT CAN NURSES AND HEALTH PROFESSIONALS DO TO MINIMIZE RISKS?

To facilitate the prevention of ICAC, nurses must become more proactive. Nurses care for children and families in a variety of settings and are, therefore, afforded the opportunity to provide education and counseling.

FILTERS

Currently, to protect children online, parents and professionals should make use of filtering devices to protect children from inappropriate online content. In a study testing 4 popular filtering devices among 200 websites, Hunter (2000) found that

25% of objectionable material was not blocked, whereas 21% of benign material related to sex education, safe sex, and liberal views was blocked. Moreover, a recent report from the Kaiser Family Foundation found that among 76% of 15- to 17-year-olds who sought health information online, 46% reported being blocked from nonpornographic websites by filtering technology (Rideout, 2001). Topics they were attempting to research when blocked included human immunodeficiency virus (HIV), sexually transmitted diseases (STDs), and birth control. Although filtering devices are a useful tool, just as you would not trust a movie rating to keep a child safe from viewing inappropriate content, the best filtering device available remains a parent or responsible adult.

AWARENESS AND RISK ASSESSMENT

Online risks to children must be discussed in an open forum. Parents are more often concerned about these issues than children. Children, especially adolescents, often have a cavalier idea about the Internet (Turow & Nir, 2000). Exploitation and crime do not happen to them—they happen to the "other guy." Online risks to children are a public health concern, and thus, a risk assessment screening should be conducted with parents and children. This risk assessment should include the following:

— Does the child surf the Internet alone?

— Does the child go online daily? If so, does he or she spend more than 2 hours per day online?

— Is the computer in a public space?

— Do the parents have a set of "house rules" regarding Internet use?

— Does the child have an "online profile"?

— What types of Internet services does the child use (e.g., chat rooms, IM, e-mail)?

— If the child participates in chat rooms, what types of chat rooms (e.g., hobbies, sports, music, gaming)?

— What types of websites does the child access (e.g., health information, support groups, hobbies, gaming, music)?

Although this list of questions is by no means comprehensive, answers to these questions can provide valuable insights regarding the level of online risk to children. As previously stated, a child surfing the Internet unsupervised is placed at a higher risk for solicitation. Surfing the Web with a child provides an excellent opportunity for quality time. Additionally, spending time online with children gives them the opportunity to be the "teachers." This can be a fun and educational experience for nurses, parents, teachers, and other professionals. Efforts should be made to balance the amount of time children spend online with offline activities. Even though the Internet can be entertaining and educational, we do not want children to become isolated from their real-life peers. Computers should be located in a public space, such as a living room, recreation room, classroom, or library. In addition, it is beneficial to establish house rules or a contract with children for online safety. Many Internet safety experts recommend posting the rules next to the computer to avoid the "out of sight out of mind" phenomenon (Aftab, 2000; Armagh, 1998). Children should not have online profiles. An online profile is a list of personal information that Internet Service Providers (ISPs) let you post online. This information allows other users to know more about you, such as your name, age, sex, address, hobbies, and interests.

Although children may think having a profile is fun, this is a serious mistake. Online profiles can provide a "shopping list" of information for sexual predators and can be more harmful than helpful. Knowledge of the types of Internet services children use allows providers to assess risk and to devise individual care plans of education for children, parents, and professionals who work with children. In particular, school nurses and public health nurses are in an excellent position to provide education to children, parents, and teachers regarding the nature of online risks.

How to Handle Disclosure of Online and Offline Victimization

The most important thing to remember is to remain calm and nonjudgmental. Often children who are lured online from their homes or schools are not completely naive. Frequently, they are curious, troubled, or rebellious adolescents searching for sexual information or companionship (Lanning, 1998). Regardless of the events, these children have been enticed and manipulated by a shrewd offender, and often they are not fully aware of the consequences of their actions. Patience is essential with these victims. Children who are enticed or duped usually are looking to have their needs for attention and affection met (Lanning, 1998).

As Summit (1983) found, children who are sexually victimized may recant their stories after disclosure. This frequently occurs because the child or others blame him or her for the interaction. Additionally, the child may become embarrassed and ashamed. Therefore, do not blame the child.

The legalities of ICAC and criminal proceedings brought against offenders differ from state to state because of age of consent laws and definitions of sexual assault and statutory rape. For example, if a child victim were 16 years old and engaged in consensual sexual relations with an offender, then in 32 states, the 16-year-old would be at, or older than, the legal age of consent (Phipps, 1997). In these 32 states, offenders can be guilty of crimes such as corrupting the morals of a minor, contributing to the delinquency of a minor, or an equivalent offense because a child or minor is generally considered to be an individual under age 18 years (Toth & McClure, 1998). Typically, the latter crimes are considered misdemeanors and are not treated as seriously as conventional child sex offenses. However, for those child victims in one of the 18 states where the age of consent is 17 or 18, the offender could be charged with more serious criminal sexual offenses (Phipps, 1997; Toth & McClure, 1998). This makes it essential for health providers and nurses to be informed about the applicable statutes in their state of practice. Children mature differently, and despite the legal age of consent, no child deserves to be exploited.

What to Do If You Suspect Online Victimization

If you suspect that a child has been victimized through using the Internet, it is essential to report it. The NCMEC has instituted a special CyberTipline to report the online victimization of children. The CyberTipline can be accessed via the Internet at http://www.cybertipline.com or toll-free at 1-800-843-5678. In addition to the CyberTipline, the NCMEC also provides a variety of free educational materials related to Internet safety for children and adolescents at http://www.missingkids.com. Further Internet safety information can be downloaded from the Federal Bureau of Investigation at http://www.fbi.gov/publications/pguide/pguide.htm. Both of these organizations have materials available in English and Spanish.

REFERENCES

Aftab P. *The Parent's Guide to Protecting Your Children in Cyberspace.* New York, NY: McGraw-Hill; 2000.

Andrews W. *Internet Predators* [television news series]. New York, NY: Columbia Broadcasting System Worldwide. May 22-24, 2000.

Armagh DS. A safety net for the Internet: protecting our children. *Juv Just.* 1998;5:9-15.

Armagh DS, Battaglia NL, Lanning KV. *Use of Computers in the Sexual Exploitation of Children: Portable Guide to Investigating Child Abuse.* Washington, DC: US Dept of Justice; 2000. NCJ 170021.

Baudrillard J. *Simulacra and Simulation.* Glaser SF, trans. Ann Arbor: The University of Michigan Press; 1994.

Bolen RM, Scannapieco M. Prevalence of child sexual abuse: a corrective metanalysis. *Soc Serv Rev.* 1999;73:281-313.

Budin LE, Johnson CF. Sex abuse prevention programs: offenders' attitudes about their efficacy. *Child Abuse Negl.* 1989;13:77-87.

Burgess AW. *Child Pornography and Sex Rings.* Lexington, Mass: Lexington Books; 1984.

Burgess AW, Holmstrom LL. Sexual trauma of children and adolescents: pressure, sex, and secrecy. *Nurs Clin North Am.* 1975;10:551-563.

Burgess AW, Holmstrom LL. Accessory to sex: pressure, sex, and secrecy. In: Burgess AW, Groth AN, Holmstrom LL, Sgroi SM, eds. *Sexual Assault of Children and Adolescents.* Lexington, Mass: DC Heath and Company; 1978:105-124.

Christiansen JR, Blake RH. The grooming process in father-daughter incest. In: Horton AL, Johnson BL, Roundy LM, Williams D, eds. *The Incest Perpetrator: A Family Member No One Wants to Treat.* Newbury Park, Calif: Sage Publications; 1990:88-107.

Dwarfnet Internet Guide. Acronyms and Chat Lingo: Smileys, Faces, Emoticons. Dwarfnet Internet Guide. 2001. Available at: http://www.dwarfnet.com/chat/smileyfaces.shtml. Accessed July 29, 2001.

Elliott M, Browne K, Kilcoyne J. Child sexual abuse prevention: what offenders tell us. *Child Abuse Negl.* 1995;19:579-594.

Finkelhor D. Current information on the scope and nature of child sexual abuse. *Center Future Child.* 1994;4:31-54.

Finkelhor D, Mitchell KJ, Wolak J. *Online Victimization: A Report on the Nation's Youth.* Crimes Against Children Research Center; June 2000. Available at: http://www.missingkids.com/download/nc62.pdf. Accessed June 8, 2000.

Giardino AP. Child Abuse & Neglect: Sexual Abuse. Vol. 2, No. 9. 2001. Available at: http://www.emedicine.com/PED/topic2649.htm. Accessed October 29, 2001.

Gibson W. *Neuromancer.* New York, NY: Ace Books; 1984:51.

Groth AN, Birnbaum HJ. Adult sexual orientation and attraction to underage persons. *Arch Sex Behav.* 1978;7:175-181.

Grunwald Associates. Children, Families and the Internet 2000. Available at: http://www.grunwald.com/survey/survey_content.html. Accessed September 4, 2000.

Hamman RB. *Cyborgasms: Cybersex Amongst Multiple-Selves and Cyborgs in the Narrow-Bandwidth Space of America Online Chat Rooms* [dissertation]. September 30, 1996. Available at: http://www.socio.demon.co.uk/Cyborgasms.html. Accessed August 20, 2001.

Hunter CD. Social impacts: Internet filter effectiveness—testing over- and underinclusive blocking decisions of four popular web filters. *Soc Sci Comput Rev.* 2000;18:214-222.

Jabs C. Sex, lies, and children: what parents don't know about the Internet. *Fam PC.* March 2000;79-88.

Jones SG. *Virtual Culture: Identity & Communication in Cybersociety.* London: Sage Publications; 1997.

Lamb M. Cybersex: research notes on the characteristics of the visitors to online chat rooms. *Deviant Behav Interdiscipl J.* 1998;19:121-135.

Lanning KV. *Child Sex Rings: A Behavioral Analysis.* 2nd ed. National Center for Missing and Exploited Children. April, 1992. Available at: http://www.missingkids.com/download/nc72.pdf. Accessed March 17, 2000.

Lanning KV. Cyber "pedophiles": a behavioral perspective. *APSAC Advis.* 1998;11:12-18.

Lanning KV. *Child Molesters: A Behavioral Analysis.* 4th ed. National Center for Missing and Exploited Children. September, 2001. Available at: http://www.missingkids.com/download/nc70.pdf. Accessed December 21, 2001.

Lanning KV, Burgess AW. Child pornography and sex rings. In: Zillmann D, Bryant J, eds. *Pornography: Research Advances and Policy Considerations.* Hillsdale, NJ: Lawrence Erlbaum Associates; 1989:235-255.

Lenhart A, Rainie L, Lewis O. Teenage Life Online: The Rise of the Instant-Message Generation and the Internet's Impact on Friendships and Family Relationships. Pew Internet & American Life Project. June 20, 2001. Available at: http://www.pewinternet.org/reports.pdfs/PIPS_Teens_Report.pdf. Accessed November 16, 2001.

McLaughlin JF. Technophilia: A Modern Day Paraphilia. Keene Police Department. 1998. Available at: http://www.ci.keene.nh.us/police/technophilia.html. Accessed August 8, 2000.

McLaughlin JF. Cyber Child Sex Offender Typology. Regional Task Force on Internet Crimes Against Children for Northern New England. 2000. Available at: http://www.ci.keene.nh.us/police/Typology.html. Accessed August 8, 2000.

Mitchell KJ, Finkelhor D, Wolak J. Risk factors for and impact of online sexual solicitation of youth. *JAMA.* 2001;285:3011-3014.

NetLingo. Acronyms & Shorthand. NetLingo, Inc. 2001. Available at: http://www.netlingo.com. Accessed December 10, 2001.

Newburger EC. *Computer Use in the United States: October 1997.* Washington, DC: US Census Bureau, Department of Commerce, Economics and Statistics Administration; 1999. Current population reports P20-522.

Newburger EC. *Home Computers and Internet Use in the United States: August 2000.* Washington, DC: US Census Bureau, Department of Commerce, Economics and Statistics Administration; 2001. Current population reports P23-207.

Nordland R, Bartholet J. The Web's dark secret. *Newsweek.* March 19, 2001;44-51.

Office for Victims of Crime. *OVC Bulletin: Internet Crimes Against Children.* Washington, DC: US Dept of Justice, Office of Justice Programs; 2001. NCJ 184931.

Office of Juvenile Justice and Delinquency Prevention. *Internet Crimes Against Children Program.* National Center for Missing and Exploited Children. 1998. Available at: http://www.ojjdp.ncjrs.org/grants/grantprograms/mec2.html. Accessed October 15, 2000.

Phipps C. Children, adults, sex and the criminal law: in search of reason. *Seton Hall Law J.* 1997;22:1-60.

Rabun JB. *Quarterly Progress Report.* Alexandria, Va: National Center for Missing and Exploited Children; 2000. 98-MC-CX-K002.

Rheingold H. *The Virtual Community: Homesteading on the Electronic Frontier.* Reading, Mass: Addison-Wesley; 1993.

Rideout V. Generation Rx.com: How Young People Use the Internet for Health Information. Henry J. Kaiser Family Foundation. 2001. Available at: http://www.kff.org/content/2001/20011211a/GenerationRx.pdf. Accessed December 18, 2001.

Roper Starch Worldwide. The America Online/Roper Starch Youth Cyberstudy. Roper Starch Worldwide Inc. November, 1999. Available at: http://www.corp.aol.com/press/study/youthstudy.pdf. Accessed August 7, 2001.

Schultz LG. *The Sexual Victimology of Youth.* Springfield, Ill: Charles C. Thomas; 1980.

Schwartz G, Merten D. The language of adolescence: an anthropological approach to the youth culture. *Am J Sociol.* 1967;72:453-468.

Smith DW, Letourneau EJ, Saunders BE, Kilpatrick DG, Resnick HS, Best CL. Delay in disclosure of childhood rape: results from a national survey. *Child Abuse Negl.* 2000;24:273-287.

Summit RC. The child sexual abuse accommodation syndrome. *Child Abuse Negl.* 1983;7:177-193.

TechTarget.com, Inc. 2001. Available at: http://www.whatis.com. Accessed July 12, 2001.

Toth P, McClure K. An overview of selected legal issues involved in computer related child exploitation: many questions, few answers. *APSAC Advis.* 1998;11:19-22.

Turkle S. *Life on the Screen: Identity in the Age of the Internet.* New York, NY: Touchstone; 1995.

Turow J, Nir L. The Internet and the Family 2000: The View From Parents, the View From Kids. The Annenberg Public Policy Center of the University of Pennsylvania. May, 2000. Available at: http://www.appcpenn.org/internet/family/finalrepor_fam.pdf. Accessed August 7, 2001.

Tyler RP, Stone LE. Child pornography: perpetuating the sexual victimization of children. *Child Abuse Negl.* 1985;9:313-318.

Williams C. *Internet Access in U. S. Public Schools and Classrooms: 1994-99.* Washington, DC: National Center for Education Statistics; 2000. Stats in Brief NCES-2000-086.

Chapter 17

PREVENTION OF CHILD ABUSE AND NEGLECT: APPROACHES AND ISSUES

Eileen R. Giardino, PhD, RN, CRNP

Child abuse and neglect are multifaceted problems and require individual, professional, and community resources to intervene and prevent the circumstances that lead to the occurrence of the phenomena. Some initiatives developed by nurses and other social work and healthcare professionals have focused on preventing abuse by educating families to be aware of potential problems that may lead to maltreatment and how to deal more effectively with the causative issues. Other programs are designed to provide specific services to at-risk families in an effort to keep further abuse from occurring once the problem has been identified. The dynamics of physical abuse, sexual abuse, and neglect differ. Thus, it is reasonable to expect that prevention efforts to address the separate types of maltreatment will also vary.

Long-term effects of child abuse and neglect that are detrimental to the well-being of the child manifest during adolescence and adulthood. Psychological, physical, developmental, and behavioral problems emerge that are consequences of poor parenting and abuse (Glod, 1993; National Research Council, 1993). Physical injuries, permanent brain damage, low self-esteem, difficulty forming relationships, learning disorders, and aggressive behavior are often seen in survivors of child abuse and neglect. Some experience depression, conduct problems, and posttraumatic stress disorder (PTSD), while others manifest problems through drug dependence, delinquency, teen pregnancy, and poor academic achievement (Kelley, Thornberry, & Smith, 1997; National Clearinghouse on Child Abuse and Neglect Information, 1998; Widom, 1992). The personal costs to the individual coupled with the financial costs to society indicate that it is in the best interest of all involved to prevent child abuse and neglect. Prevention is achieved through individual interactions and formalized programs focused on educational programs and family support in a variety of ways.

The focus of this chapter is on the role of nurses in collaboration with community resources and in the prevention of child maltreatment through prevention efforts and effective initiatives developed by nurses and other professionals.

OVERVIEW OF PREVENTION

Prevention of child abuse is often difficult to achieve, because there are a multitude of reasons explaining the phenomenon. Some would say that prevention of abuse in all cases is almost improbable (Melton, 1992). No matter what the obstacles may be, good clinical practice suggests that children, adults, and healthcare professionals should be educated in issues surrounding child physical abuse, sexual abuse, and neglect prevention.

Prevention efforts are focused at 3 different levels, with each level geared toward different goals and activities:

1. Primary prevention activities raise the awareness of the general public, service providers, and decision makers about the scope and magnitude of the problems associated with child maltreatment.

2. Secondary prevention relates to programs and initiatives geared toward children and families known to be at higher risk for maltreatment. The focus is on resources to address those who have known risk factors for abuse and neglect, such as substance abuse, young maternal age, developmental disabilities, and poverty.

3. Tertiary prevention activities focus on families in which abuse or neglect has already occurred. Tertiary programs attempt to prevent the recurrence of maltreatment and the reduction of the longer-term consequences associated with maltreatment, such as poor family functioning, emotional and social problems in children, and lower academic achievement. Communities must provide a continuum of primary, secondary, and tertiary prevention services to decrease the devastating effects of child maltreatment. Toward this goal, nurses have opportunities to talk with their clients about abuse issues, ask questions about abuse, and develop and implement programs that decrease the effects of maltreatment (Finkelhor, 1986a).

Primary Prevention: Increasing Awareness

Primary prevention of child maltreatment involves strategies that educate the public to understand what abuse is and how it can be prevented. Child abuse programs focus on educating parents, children, and the public about situations and behaviors indicative of abuse (Daro, 1994; Kitzman et al., 1999). Types of primary prevention activities include parent education programs to teach parents developmentally appropriate expectations of the child, public awareness campaigns to raise awareness and increase the reporting of abuse and neglect, and radio or television announcements to encourage nonviolent forms of discipline. It is important to strengthen a parent or adult's understanding of factors that contribute to unsafe and abusive situations and relationships so they can protect the child more fully. Effective prevention programs have been instituted in elementary and secondary schools, community agencies and organizations, and public and mental health departments. Overall discussion on the effectiveness of child abuse prevention programs indicates that prevention programs may have the desired effect of decreasing the incidence of abuse because the trends in absolute number of reports made and those reports that are substantiated have decreased (Gibson & Leitenberg, 2000). The more the public knows about the incidence, causes, and interrelationship with other forms of violence, the better the prevention of child abuse and neglect will be.

Secondary Prevention: Nursing's Role in the Detection of Abuse

The focus of secondary prevention is on the early recognition of those situations that place the child at high risk for maltreatment. Nurses interact with families and children in many settings and often observe children who have been maltreated or those families who may be at greater risk for abuse. Nurses are also involved in the early recognition of abuse and neglect when they know signs of abuse, ask the right questions, and intervene appropriately in situations of suspected child abuse and neglect. Therefore, providing services to at-risk individuals and families is an important aspect of nursing care and appropriate nursing intervention. Secondary prevention programs include parent education for teen mothers in high schools, substance abuse treatment for mothers and families with young children, respite care for families with special needs children, and family resource centers, to name a few.

There are factors indicative of at-risk children that manifest in parental characteristics, environmental situations, and child-specific signs (Chiocca, 1998). Knowledge of early recognition signs in different age categories may help nurses identify potential victims of child abuse or neglect. For example, a behavioral manifestation in a preschool-age child for possible sexual abuse includes overt, age-inappropriate sexual behavior (Slusser, 1995). Other child behavioral indicators include sudden school difficulties and vague somatic complaints (Bourne, Chadwick, Kanda, & Ricci, 1993). Whatever the age-related manifestations, it is important for nurses to be able to identify behaviors that may be indicative of an at-risk situation for possible maltreatment and then arrange for services directed at preventing the maltreatment before it occurs.

TERTIARY PREVENTION: HELPING THOSE ALREADY HARMED

Tertiary prevention interventions in child abuse involve the restoration of optimal levels of health and wellness to the child and family who have experienced maltreatment. This is done in the format of counseling children and their parents and caregivers in an effort to work through the aftermath of difficult feelings and related issues. Restoration also involves working with families to prevent further abuse. Tertiary prevention programs include services such as parent mentor programs, family preservation interventions, and programs to improve family communication and functioning. Because this type of prevention occurs after a case of abuse or neglect is identified, many of the services are delivered under the auspices of child protective services (CPS) or by court order. In these situations, the nurse balances the health promotion role with the child advocacy role of ensuring the involved child or children remain safe while services are delivered.

CHILD ABUSE PREVENTION STRATEGIES FOR CHILDREN, ADULTS, AND NURSING PROFESSIONALS

The focus of prevention programs is usually targeted to specific populations. These include children, families or parents, and professionals. Each target group requires a different approach to the prevention strategy because of differences in background and training, as well as differences in focus regarding the children involved. The following discussion gives examples of prevention programs developed for specific target groups.

CHILD-FOCUSED ABUSE PREVENTION PROGRAMS

Child programs focus on education concerning the problem, how to determine whether behaviors of others, both children and adults, are appropriate (as in Good Touch/Bad Touch programs), and what a child can do if abuse occurs. The abuse prevention approach to children is varied, depending on the age and developmental level of the child. Workshops and media programs for children focus on the awareness of people and behaviors children can avoid. For example, the Good Touch/Bad Touch program is a prevention education curriculum developed for kindergarten through sixth grade (DeYoung, 1988). The Good Touch/Bad Touch curriculum focuses on personal safety issues, including sexual victimization, aggression, coercion, manipulation, and disclosure issues, along with "nontouching" sexual abuse, self-esteem, and self-image issues. This program exemplifies an effective approach to reaching children of all ages. Other prevention programs for children address topics such as defining sexual abuse, identifying offenders, and highlighting actions that the child can take to avoid, resist, or escape situations (Finkelhor, 1986b; Hebert, Lavoie, Piche, & Poitras, 2001).

SCHOOL-BASED PREVENTION PROGRAMS

Nurses are involved in the development and implementation of child abuse prevention programs based in elementary and high schools. School-based prevention programs start the learning process about abuse issues at an early age in preschool and continue into high school. Programs empower children to learn victimization prevention concepts, be aware of age-appropriate interactions, and help children resist physical or sexual abuse (Oldfield, Hays, & Megel, 1996). The goal of such programs is to teach children strategies to protect themselves and understand some issues that lead to dangerous or abusive situations. The hope is for long-term effects in the lives of those who participate in the programs. Studies indicate that children who participated in abuse prevention programs have shown a trend toward better preventive skills and knowledge about abuse after exposure to the program (Hebert et al., 2001).

A nurse-initiated child maltreatment prevention program taught in health classes in a high school setting found positive results on parenting attitudes in many of the participants as a result of the program curriculum (Marshall et al., 1996). The student participants learned about child abuse, normal development, and positive parenting techniques. Although long-term attitude changes were not measured, such a program provided a basis for positive ideas and values in the treatment of children. Other study findings suggest that as a result of a school-based program, children were more likely to use self-protection strategies when victimized or threatened, such as yelling, insisting on being left alone, or threatening to or actually telling about abuse (Finkelhor, Asdigian, & Dziuba-Leatherman, 1995a, 1995b).

Programs geared toward a child's knowledge of sexual assault prevention concepts are helpful to increase awareness of appropriate touch from adults in their lives (Hayward & Pehrsson, 2000). The long-term goal for school-based programs is that children carry what they have learned into adolescence and adulthood. To that end, a study of college-age women found that school-based child sexual abuse prevention programs were associated with a reduced incidence of child sexual abuse (Gibson & Leitenberg, 2000).

ADULT-FOCUSED PREVENTION PROGRAMS

Adult-focused prevention programs have been developed to increase public awareness of the problem of child abuse and neglect and the resources available to caregivers to support them in parenting issues. A vast number of educational materials exist for the general public focused on child abuse prevention and healthy parenting. Some of the educational programs include local and national public awareness campaigns, complete with posters and public service announcements to increase community awareness. One example of a campaign is a program called *Project Prevent* that was developed to help prevent abuse and neglect of young children with disabilities. The Council on Child Abuse and Neglect in South Carolina identified that children with disabilities and special needs were at a higher risk for maltreatment than other children and developed a program to help communities build stronger partnerships between child welfare and disability professionals and families of special needs children (Caceres & Mayfield-Smith, 1999). The outcome of the program was an increase in community awareness of the problem and the development of church- and community-based resource programs to help build bridges and offer support to families of children with disabilities, thereby contributing to abuse prevention.

Home Visiting Programs

Home visiting programs have existed since the late 19th century as implemented by public health nurses in Europe and the United States. The goal of nurses visiting families in the home has always been to meet people where they live and teach about the health and well-being of children and families, and then identify and treat health concerns of families. Home visiting programs that have an emphasis on abuse prevention stress the education of individuals about issues related to child abuse and neglect. Nurses address issues such as problems related to social isolation that might lead to abuse and neglect and the need for family support services (Larner, Stevenson, & Behrman, 1998). Home visiting programs provide services to families identified as at high risk for abuse or neglect (Christensen, Schommer, & Velasquez, 1984; Roberts, 1997; Wallach & Lister, 1995) by improving parenting skills and compliance with prevention services (Hardy & Streett, 1989). Risk factors found to be indicators of potential for child abuse or neglect are those that can be identified at an early stage and have a possibility for intervention in a home-based population of mothers with infants and small children. Such risk factors include the characteristics of adolescent motherhood, previous reports of abuse, mothers who have themselves been placed in foster homes or institutions, and high scores on stress indices (Christensen et al., 1984; Roberts, 1997).

The goal of most home visiting programs is to enhance a caregiver's understanding of child development, improve parenting skills, and help people cope with stressors of everyday life. Shorter postpartum hospital stays make it difficult to educate mothers to the many details of infant care, and it is not feasible to teach all that should be known in any hospital stay (Chiocca, 1998). Nurses have proven to be competent home visitors accustomed to working with families and individuals on issues of health, child development, and family concerns (Kitzman et al., 1999; Leventhal, 2001). Nurse-developed programs are often multidisciplinary in focus to include child welfare, social services, mental health, and law enforcement specialists (Onyskiw, Harrison, Spady, & McConnan, 1999). Home visitors are able to observe the family in their own environment. Thus, it is possible for the nurse to gear teaching and interventions to specific issues uncovered by observing nurse, child, and family interactions (O'Toole, O'Toole, Webster, & Lucal, 1996). Furthermore, home visitors usually provide more than just education about childcare or parenting skills because they are called upon to address day-to-day crisis situations that a mother with minimal economic resources may face. These situations include eviction and lack of heat, food, clothing, and money for transportation. The home visitor often must help solve such problems in the midst of providing education on which the home visit was based (Hardy & Streett, 1989).

Home visiting programs often offer family-focused services to pregnant mothers and families with new babies. Activities include structured visits, informal visits, and telephone calls to provide added support to the mother. Topics discussed at home visits may include child development, positive parenting skills, appropriate discipline techniques, and how to access community support and resources. Also addressed are healthcare concerns of the baby and mother and accident prevention strategies for the home. Participants in a Nashville program for pregnant women at high risk for possible difficulties with parenting issues were offered psychological support, self-care education, and education about healthy behaviors by nurses, midwives, home visitors, and other healthcare professionals. Although the results of the control group versus the intervention group were varied for several reasons, the researchers felt that having the mothers in the healthcare system for longer periods of time before and after the birth helped healthcare professionals to see the positive and negative parenting skills and have participants seek help earlier when necessary (Brayden et al., 1993).

Studies of nurse home visiting programs indicate that clients value the interactions and the emotional and physical support of the visitors (Byrd, 1997). The underlying assumption of home visits is that parents who know more about parenting concerns are less likely to abuse or allow abuse to occur within the family system. Home visits provide emotional support and physical care to pregnant women and young mothers as well as instruction for women toward development, supportive relationships, and links to community resources (Olds, Henderson, Kitzman, & Cole, 1995; Williams-Burgess, Vines, & Ditulio, 1995). Nurse home visitors can help families network with other healthcare services (Olds, Hill, Mihalic, & O'Brien, 1998). Furthermore, connections with support systems and social services in communities may help parents feel less isolated and, in turn, improve their ability to parent effectively. Efforts in abuse prevention programs are often collaborative to include mental health, social services, and law enforcement. According to research studies, home visits can reduce the incidence of abuse and neglect, and the effects have been observed up to 15 years after the intervention (Eckenrode et al., 2000; Olds, Eckenrode, & Henderson, 1997; Olds, Henderson, Tatlebaum, & Chamberlain, 1986b; Wallach & Lister, 1995).

Nurses provide home-based family support through educational programs that focus on improving prenatal health behaviors, reduction of pregnancy complications, child development, and aspects of parenting and maternal care (Onyskiw et al., 1999; Olds, Henderson, Chamberlain, & Tatlebaum, 1986a; Olds et al., 1998). There has been a significant decrease in reports of child maltreatment in which nurses followed families at home and provided teaching about child development and care over an extended time period (Eckenrode et al., 2000). Nurses are often the mainstay of home visiting services after delivery and have experience in working with mothers. Therefore, it is an understandable connection with usual postpartum visits to include an approach directed at education on child abuse issues and helping mothers find needed support systems in the family and community. One nurse home visiting program that visited women during the pregnancy and continued through the child's second birthday reported long-term success in specific areas related to maltreatment. The program was successful in reducing the following: child abuse, neglect, and injuries to children as evidenced by review of medical records; mother's behavioral problems resulting from substance abuse and criminal behavior; and criminal and antisocial behaviors of the children born into the study, as indicated by fewer arrests, convictions/violations of parole, and alcohol consumption (Olds et al., 1998). Home visiting programs that provide support and education to mothers in the postnatal period are cost effective and show significant decreases in indices of neglect and abuse (Brooten et al., 1986; Huxley & Warner, 1993; Olds et al., 1998; Velasquez, Christensen, & Schommer, 1984).

A major challenge associated with home visiting programs, including those run by nurses, is finding the funds necessary to provide large-scale services over an extended time period. The costs to provide such programs may exceed the amount of money available in most state or federal budgets (Leventhal, 2001). However, the long-term costs of child maltreatment to society are great because there is a need for child welfare services, foster care, physical and mental health services, and legal services in regard to the occurrence of maltreatment (Collaborative Studies Coordinating Center, 2001). A 1988 study estimated the loss of future productivity of severely abused children was in the range of $658 million to $1.3 billion annually (Daro, 1988).

Creative resolutions to the funding challenge are still underway. Studies consistently demonstrate that in terms of government spending, prevention programs are most effective at the societal level. Typically, for every dollar spent on a prevention program, subsequent program spending for handling the effects of maltreatment are decreased by at least $4 over the child's lifetime (Olds et al., 1998) A well-studied nurse home visiting program in a semirural county in New York performed a cost analysis of the program outcomes to determine whether prevention services provided to women and children caused any overall savings to government expenditures over a period of time. The study showed that the cost of the program is recovered in terms of government spending by the time the child reaches age 4 years, and savings to government and society then exceed the cost of the program over the lifetime of the child generated by improvements in maternal and child health (Olds, Henderson, Phelps, Kitzman, & Hanks, 1993; Olds et al., 1998).

Pregnancy and Abuse

The incidence of abuse toward pregnant women is high, with 20% to 45% of battered women abused during pregnancy (Gaines, 2000; McFarlane & Wiist, 1997). Maternal rates of depression, substance abuse, and suicide attempts are higher in women who have been abused during pregnancy (McFarlane, Parker, & Soeken, 1996). Therefore, screening for abuse during pregnancy and appropriate intervention may help in the prevention of child abuse and neglect in the postpartum period. Nurses and healthcare professionals are in contact with pregnant women through the duration of the pregnancy and have multiple opportunities to observe, ask questions concerning abusive behaviors, and discuss risks to the woman and her family. Disclosure of abuse often occurs after trust is achieved in the patient-nurse relationship, so consistent discussion on the part of the nurse is often helpful.

PROFESSIONAL-FOCUSED PREVENTION PROGRAMS

There are child abuse prevention efforts geared toward professionals who interact with children to increase awareness and knowledge about abuse issues. Professionals, including teachers, nurses, physicians, police, and mental health personnel, are in situations in which they observe the behaviors of children and adults and can see signs that might signify abuse (Finkelhor, 1986a). In many professional programs, little formal education exists about abuse issues in general. Therefore, it is easy for professionals to overlook signs of abuse when they have no knowledge or experience in what to observe or how to approach the situation when identified.

Formal professionally oriented educational programs about child maltreatment help ensure baseline knowledge of abuse issues. Nurses have a responsibility to advocate healthy relationships for their clients and are in a good position to help those who are both past and present victims of abuse (Long & Smyth, 1998). They should be able to understand the many issues surrounding the different types of abuse and help the children and their families deal with those issues. Specifically, mental health nurses are able to develop therapeutic relationships for children and caregivers because they deal with the longer-term issues of experiencing abuse (Long & Smyth, 1998).

Mandated Reporting of Abuse

Nurses are mandated reporters of child abuse and, therefore, responsible to notify appropriate state authorities when there is reason to suspect that neglect or abuse has occurred. Reporting abuse is an intervention and a prevention strategy because the identification of abuse by a healthcare professional may be the first step in helping the child victim. To be effective in the reporting process, the nurse must know ethical issues related to reporting or nonreporting, as well as intervention protocols, legal parameters, and to whom to report (Greipp, 1997). It is important to understand the responsibility associated with being a mandated reporter (O'Toole et al., 1996) because the nurse could be held civilly responsible if failure to report was willful or knowing (Freed & Drake, 1999). However, states have laws that protect nurses against liability for making a false report if reported in good faith (Rhodes, 1996).

There is an incidence of nonreporting of suspected cases for various reasons (Zellman, 1991). Nurses and other healthcare professionals sometimes doubt their instincts or findings and are concerned about the consequences on the caregiver when they report to CPS. In the event that a mandated reporter is unsure of whether to report an incident, he or she should collaborate with others on the multidisciplinary team to determine his or her responsibility (Greipp, 1997).

Abuse Prevention

The long-term negative effects of physical and sexual abuse on the child are well documented and manifest in such symptoms as hostility, depression, poor self-esteem, and revictimization (Finkelhor, 1986a). Nurses are in contact with survivors of abuse in all areas of clinical practice and intervene to provide physical and psychological care to child and adult survivors. The spectrum of sequelae range from the more severe, such as multiple personality disorder and refractory psychosis, to chronic physical reactions, such as headaches and pelvic pain (Glod, 1993). Prevention efforts for abuse begin with a thorough understanding on the part of nurses and other healthcare professionals of how and why abuse occurs and then knowing how to effectively communicate such information to individuals and families (Flournoy, 1996).

School Nurses

School nurses affect the lives of many children in direct and indirect ways. They work directly with children through daily interaction with those who become sick or those with special needs who require daily input. School nurses provide indirect care to children by working with faculty and administrators to teach them about special topics of interest to the school community such as child abuse. They can also provide programs to students about abuse topics (Marshall et al., 1996).

Many reports of child abuse and neglect emanate from the public school system (O'Toole et al., 1996). But despite the many interactions that nurses in schools have with children, estimates of unreported cases remain high (O'Toole et al., 1996). School nurses are in an ideal situation to see potential signs of abuse and maltreatment (Pakieser, Starr, & Lebaugh, 2000). They become better at preventing child abuse when they provide prevention programs, know how to intervene appropriately, and understand the signs as manifested in children of all ages. School nurses may be in an ambiguous position when they voice concerns about making a report. However, the school principal or administrator may be unclear about the nurses' mandated reporter role (DePanfilis & Salus, 1992). Policies and procedures in the school must be clear about the mandated role nurses have to report suspicions of abuse.

NURSES AS COLLABORATORS ON THE HEALTHCARE TEAM

Nurses collaborate with other professionals in the areas of mental health, medicine, and law enforcement in the prevention of child abuse and neglect. They partner to provide appropriate referrals and accomplish the multiple professional system tasks involved when a child is suspected of abuse. A Community Infant Project in Boulder, Colorado, consisted of an intervention team of public health nurses, paraprofessional volunteers, mental health professionals, and a psychiatrist who worked together to provide highly effective support and services to high-risk families (Huxley & Warner, 1993).

Nurses refer adults and children identified as at-risk clients to services within communities geared at decreasing child abuse and maltreatment. Such services include family support groups and child crisis care programs. An Iowa crisis care program that provided a safe environment for children when parents faced a crisis found a decrease in the incidence of child abuse in the counties offering the service (Cowen, 1998). Nurses are instrumental in identifying the at-risk families and providing appropriate referrals to such programs.

Summary

Nurses intervene in all areas of practice to prevent child maltreatment. Nurses develop and implement educational programs focused on children, adults, and other healthcare professionals. Such programs are a mainstay of prevention efforts, as well as interventions to detect abuse and efforts to help children and families when abuse has occurred. It is important for nurses to have a strong knowledge base of the issues involved in child abuse to care for children and their families who are at risk for abuse. The nurse can provide a holistic approach to the many issues involved in the evaluation and treatment of child sexual abuse at all levels of prevention.

References

Bourne R, Chadwick D, Kanda M, Ricci L. When you suspect child abuse. *Patient Care*. 1993;27:22-35.

Brayden R, Altemeier W, Dietrich M, et al. A prospective study of secondary prevention of child maltreatment. *J Pediatr*. 1993;122:511-516.

Brooten D, Kumar S, Brown L, et al. A randomized clinical trial of early hospital discharge and home follow-up of very-low-birthweight infants. *N Engl J Med*. 1986;315:934-939.

Byrd M. A typology of the potential outcomes of maternal-child home visits: a literature analysis. *Public Health Nurs*. 1997;14:3-11.

Caceres S, Mayfield-Smith K. *Project Prevent: Building Bridges for Young Children With Disabilities*. Columbia: Prevent Child Abuse South Carolina; 1999.

Chiocca E. The nurse's role in the prevention of child abuse and neglect: Part II. *J Pediatr Nurs*. 1998;13:194-195.

Christensen M, Schommer B, Velasquez J. An interdisciplinary approach to preventing child abuse. *Matern Child Nurs*. 1984;9:108-112.

Collaborative Studies Coordinating Center. LONGSCAN: Longitudinal Studies of Child Abuse and Neglect. Consortium for Longitudinal Studies in Child Abuse and Neglect. 2001. Available at: http://www.cscc.unc.edu. Accessed July 28, 2001.

Cowen P. Crisis child care: an intervention for at-risk families. *Issues Compr Pediatr Nurs*. 1998;21:147-158.

Daro D. *Confronting Child Abuse: Research for Effective Program Design*. New York, NY: The Free Press; 1988.

Daro D. Prevention of child sexual abuse. *Future Child*. 1994;4:198-223.

DePanfilis D, Salus MK. *Child Protective Services: A Guide for Caseworkers*. Washington, DC: US Dept of Health & Human Services; 1992.

DeYoung M. The good touch/bad touch dilemma. *Child Welfare*. 1988;67:60-68.

Eckenrode J, Ganzel B, Henderson C, et al. Preventing child abuse and neglect with a program of nurse home visitation. *JAMA*. 2000;284:1385-1391.

Finkelhor D. *A Sourcebook on Child Sexual Abuse*. Beverly Hills, Calif: Sage Publications; 1986a.

Finkelhor D. Prevention: a review of programs and research. In: Finkelhor D, ed. *A Sourcebook on Child Sexual Abuse*. Beverly Hills, Calif: Sage Publications; 1986b:224-254.

Finkelhor D, Asdigian N, Dziuba-Leatherman J. The effectiveness of victimization prevention instruction: an evaluation of children's responses to actual threats and assaults. *Child Abuse Negl*. 1995a;19:141-153.

Finkelhor D, Asdigian N, Dziuba-Leatherman J. Victimization prevention programs for children: a follow up. *Am J Public Health*. 1995b;85:1684-1689.

Flournoy J. Incest prevention: the role of the pediatric nurse practitioner. *J Pediatr Health Care*. 1996;10:246-254.

Freed P, Drake V. Mandatory reporting of abuse: practical, moral, and legal issues for psychiatric home health nurses. *Issues Ment Health Nurs*. 1999;20:423-436.

Gaines K. Part II: Abuse and pregnancy: what every childbirth educator/nurse should know. *J Perinat Educ*. 2000;6:28-35.

Gibson LE, Leitenberg H. Child sexual abuse prevention programs: do they decrease the occurrence of child sexual abuse? *Child Abuse Negl*. 2000;24:1115-1125.

Glod C. Long-term consequences of childhood physical and sexual abuse. *Arch Psychiatric Nurs*. 1993;7:163-173.

Greipp M. Ethical decision making and mandatory reporting in cases of suspected child abuse. *J Pediatr Health Care*. 1997;11:258-265.

Hardy J, Streett R. Family support and parenting education in the home: an effective extension of clinic-based preventive health care services for poor children. *J Pediatr*. 1989;115:927-931.

Hayward K, Pehrsson D. Interdisciplinary action supporting sexual assault prevention efforts in rural elementary schools. *J Community Health Nurs*. 2000;17:141-150.

Hebert M, Lavoie F, Piche C, Poitras M. Proximate effects of a child sexual abuse prevention program in elementary school children. *Child Abuse Negl*. 2001;25:505-522.

Huxley P, Warner R. Primary prevention of parenting dysfunction in high-risk cases. *Am J Orthopsychiatry*. 1993;63:582-588.

Kelley B, Thornberry T, Smith C. *In the Wake of Childhood Violence*. Washington, DC: National Institute of Justice; 1997.

Kitzman H, Olds D, Sidora K, et al. Enduring effects of nurse home visitation on maternal life course. *JAMA*. 1999;283:1983-1989.

Larner M, Stevenson C, Behrman R. Protecting children from abuse and neglect. *Future Child*. 1998;8:4-22.

Leventhal J. The prevention of child abuse and neglect: successfully out of the blocks. *Child Abuse Negl*. 2001;25:431-439.

Long A, Smyth A. The role of mental health nursing in the prevention of child sexual abuse and the therapeutic care of survivors. *J Psychiatr Ment Health Nurs*. 1998;5:129-136.

Marshall E, Buckner EJ, Perkins J, et al. Effects of a child abuse prevention unit in health classes in four schools. *J Community Health Nurs*. 1996;13:107-122.

McFarlane J, Parker B, Soeken K. Physical abuse, smoking, and substance use during pregnancy: prevalence, interrelationships and effects on birthweight. *J Obstet Gynecol Neonat Nurs.* 1996;25:313-320.

McFarlane J, Wiist W. Preventing abuse to pregnant women: implementation of a "mentor mother" advocacy model. *J Community Health Nurs.* 1997;14:237-249.

Melton G. The improbability of the prevention of sexual abuse. In: Willis D, Holden E, Rosenberg M, eds. *Prevention of Child Maltreatment: Developmental and Ecological Perspectives.* New York, NY: John Wiley & Sons; 1992:168-192.

National Clearinghouse on Child Abuse and Neglect Information. *Prevention Pays: The Costs of Not Preventing Child Abuse and Neglect.* Washington, DC: US Dept of Health & Human Services; 1998.

National Research Council. *Understanding Child Abuse and Neglect.* Washington, DC: National Academy Press; 1993.

Oldfield D, Hays BB, Megel ME. Evaluation of the effectiveness of project trust: an elementary school-based victimization prevention strategy. *Child Abuse Negl.* 1996;20:821-832.

Olds D, Eckenrode C, Henderson HK. Long-term effects of home visitation on maternal life course and child abuse and neglect. *JAMA.* 1997;278:637-643.

Olds D, Henderson C, Chamberlain R, Tatlebaum R. Preventing child abuse and neglect: a randomized trial of nurse home visitation. *Pediatrics.* 1986a;78:65-78.

Olds D, Henderson C, Kitzman H, Cole R. Effects of prenatal and infancy nurse home visitation on surveillance of child maltreatment. *Pediatrics.* 1995;95:365-372.

Olds D, Henderson C, Phelps C, Kitzman H, Hanks C. Effect of prenatal and infancy nurse home visitation on government spending. *Med Care.* 1993;31:155-174.

Olds D, Henderson C, Tatlebaum R, Chamberlain R. Improving the life course development of socially disadvantaged mothers: a randomized trial of nurse home visitation. *Am J Public Health.* 1986b;78:1436-1445.

Olds D, Hill PL, Mihalic SF, O'Brien RA. Prenatal and infancy home visitation by nurses. In: Elliott DS, ed. *Blueprints for Violence Prevention: Prenatal and Infancy Home Visitation by Nurses.* Boulder: Institute of Behavioral Science, Regents of the University of Colorado; 1998.

Onyskiw J, Harrison M, Spady D, McConnan L. Formative evaluation of a collaborative community-based child abuse prevention project. *Child Abuse Negl.* 1999;23:1069-1081.

O'Toole A, O'Toole R, Webster S, Lucal B. Nurses' diagnostic work on possible physical child abuse. *Public Health Nurs.* 1996;13:337-344.

Pakieser R, Starr D, Lebaugh D. Nebraska school nurses identify emotional maltreatment of school-age children: a replication of an Ohio study. *J Soc Pediatr Nurs.* 2000;3:137-145.

Rhodes A. Immunity for reporting child abuse. *Am J Matern Child Nurs.* 1996;21:169.

Roberts R. Preventing child abuse and neglect through home visiting: informing practice with research. *APSAC Advisor.* 1997;10:7-10.

Slusser M. Indicators of child sexual abuse: children at risk. *Issues Ment Health Nurs.* 1995;16:481-491.

Velasquez J, Christensen M, Schommer B. Intensive services help prevent child abuse. *Matern Child Nurs.* 1984;9:113-117.

Wallach V, Lister L. Stages in the delivery of home-based services to parents at risk of child abuse: a Healthy Start experience. *Sch Inq Nurs Pract.* 1995;9:159-173.

Widom C. *The Cycle of Violence.* Washington, DC: National Institute of Justice; 1992.

Williams-Burgess C, Vines S, Ditulio M. The parent-baby venture program: prevention of child abuse. *J Child Adolesc Psychiatric Nurs.* 1995;8:15-23.

Zellman GL. Report decision-making patterns among mandated child abuse reporters. *J Pediatr Health Care.* 1991;14:258-265.

Index

A

AAP; *see* American Academy of Pediatrics
Abandonment, 252
Abdominal injury
    nonaccidental, 25
    physical examination of, 90-91, 92
Abrasion, genital, 109
Abscess
    Bartholin's, 179
    tubo-ovarian in pelvic inflammatory disease, 185
Abuse
    child; *see* Child abuse
    drug/alcohol
        date and acquaintance rape and, 335
        domestic violence and, 414
        permitted, as form of neglect, 253
    physical; *see* Physical abuse
    psychological; *see* Psychological abuse
    sexual; *see* Sexual abuse
    spousal, as form of neglect, 253
Abuse and neglect forms, 124-129, 303-305
Accidental disclosure of sexual abuse, 12-13
Accidental injury
    bruising as, 216, 217
        anogenital, 238
    burn as, 221
    to child witnessing domestic violence, 416
    fracture as, 223
    inflicted injury *versus,* 75-76
        in burn injury, 82-83, 84-85
    sites of, 24, 25
ACEP; *see* American College of Emergency Physicians (ACEP)
Acid phosphatase analysis, 144, 149
Acidosis, renal tubular, growth problems associated with, 235
Aciduria, glutaric, retinal hemorrhage associated with, 230
Acquired immunodeficiency syndrome (AIDS), 166-167, 205, 207-209, 341, 342
    growth problems associated with, 234
    retinal hemorrhage associated with, 230
    serology testing for, 152
Acronym
    chat room, e-mail, and instant messaging, 432-433
    HELP, expert testimony and, 396-397
Activities to lessen stress in child related to court involvement, 396, 397
Acyclovir, 197
Adhesions, labial, 242
Adolescent
    blood samples from, 142
    sexual abuse of, 331-348
        dating violence in, 334-335
        epidemiology of, 331
        laboratory evaluation of, 340-343
        of males, 335
        medical evaluation of, 335-340, 343, 344, 345
        prevention of and anticipatory guidance in, 346
        questioning of in suspected cases of, 64-65
        risk-taking behaviors and, 332-334
        sequelae of, 343-345
        sexual maturity and, 331-332, 333, 334
    sexually transmitted disease in
        asymptomatic *versus* symptomatic infection in, 167-168, 176
        chlamydial infection, 178-179, 180
        gonorrhea, 183-184
        herpes simplex virus, 194-195, 196
        human papillomavirus, 190-191
        trichomoniasis, 198
    vaginal specimen collection from, 141
Adoption 2002, 363
Adoption and Safe Families Act of 1997 (ASFA), 363
Adult-focused prevention program, 448-451
Advanced practice nurse, 22
Age factors
    in abuse fractures, 88
    in head injury deaths, 91
Aggressive pattern in posttraumatic stress disorder, 321

G

Galactosemia
>growth problems associated with, 234-235
>retinal hemorrhage associated with, 230

Gardnerella vaginalis, 164-165, 168, 338; *see also*
>>Bacterial vaginosis

Gastroesophageal reflux, growth problems associated with, 234

Gastrointestinal system
>disorders of associated with growth problems, 234
>examination of in suspected poisoning victim, 99

GEDS; *see* Genital examination distress scale (GEDS)

General appearance assessment, 75
>in child neglect, 268
>>documentation of, 293

Generic neglect screening, 53-54, 268, 269, 270, 272-273

Genetic disorders, skin lesion of, 28

Genital examination, 109-113, 114, 116-118
>of adolescent, 336-337, 339
>>documentation of, 340
>colposcopic, 107-108, 109, 110
>differential diagnosis for, 235-243
>>in bleeding and/or vaginal discharge, 240-242
>>in bruising, 238-240
>>in erythema, excoriation, and pruritus, 236-238, 239
>goals and focus of, 70-71
>positioning of child for, 107-108, 109, 110, 114
>preparation of child for during interview process, 62
>presence of caregiver during, 57
>protocol script for, 120-122
>specimen collection during, 141
>during well-child check-up, 39

Genital examination distress scale (GEDS), 105, 123

Genital herpes, 164-165, 192-196, 197
>specimen collection for testing for, 152

Genital warts, 166-167, 188-191, 192, 193-194

Genitalia
>anatomy and terminology of, 108-109
>bruising of from straddle injury, 41-42
>colposcopic visualization of, 108, 110
>erythema of, 39
>exposing of in sexual interaction phase of sexual abuse, 12
>nonspecific complaints of in sexual abuse, 39-42
>physical examination of, 109-110
>as possible nonaccidental injury site, 24

Genitourinary system
>anomalies of, vaginal discharge associated with, 99, 242
>examination of in suspected poisoning victim, 99

Gentamicin, 189

Geometric markings, 25, 26, 78

Georgia
>definition of neglect in, 260
>mandatory reporting in, 401

Giemsa stain in adolescent vaginal discharge evaluation, 338

Glans penis, genital warts on, 190-191

Glasgow Coma Scale, 95

Glutaric aciduria, retinal hemorrhage associated with, 230

Gluteal coitus, 114

Gluten intolerance, growth problems associated with, 234

Gonorrhea, 161, 180-185, 186-187, 340-341, 342

pelvic inflammatory disease in, 185
>prophylaxis for, 341
>specimen collection for testing for, 151
>vaginal discharge in, 40-41, 338

Good Touch/Bad Touch program, 447

Grab marks, 78

Gram's stain smear, 151, 338

Graves' disease, growth problems associated with, 234

Greenstick fracture, 86

Grooming assessment in child neglect, 268

Group A beta-hemolytic streptococci, 240

Growth failure, 267; *see also* Failure to thrive
>differential diagnosis for, 231-235

Growth hormone deficiency, 233

Gums, examination of, 96

H

Haemophilus vaginalis in nonspecific vaginitis, 237

Hair brush injury, 26

Hair samples, collection of, 142

Hairline fracture, 86

Hair-thread tourniquet syndrome, 243

Hand
>imaging of in skeletal survey, 91
>patterned bruising seen in injury using, 26

Handprint
>on face, 80
>on leg, 80

Handwriting, legibility of on medical record, 290

Hanger injury, 25

Harm Standard for physical neglect, 264

Hawaii, mandatory reporting in, 401

HBIG; *see* Hepatitis B immune globulin (HBIG)

HBsAg; *see* Hepatitis B surface antigen (HBsAg)

HBV; *see* Hepatitis B virus (HBV)

Head, imaging of in skeletal survey, 91

Head circumference
>assessment of in child neglect, 268
>failure to thrive and, 231

Head injury
>physical examination in, 91-96
>presentations and overview of, 30-33

Headache as manifestation of abuse and neglect, 10

Healing, religious, 257-258

Health status, obtained from caregiver in suspected cases of
>>sexual abuse, 56, 57

Healthcare, refusal of or delay in seeking, 252, 267

Healthcare interview; *see* Interview

Healthcare provider
>difficulty identifying normal prepubescent anatomy by,
>>104-105
>expertise of in sexual abuse examinations, 104-105
>healthcare evaluation *versus* investigation by, 71
>maintaining objectivity during sexual abuse interviews, 57
>mandatory reporting by; *see* Mandatory reporting
>as member of investigative team, 72, 365-366
>in minimizing internet crimes against children, 439-441
>prevention and, 451-452
>testifying in court by, 65, 396-397, 398-399
>views of on neglect, 263

I

M

N

O

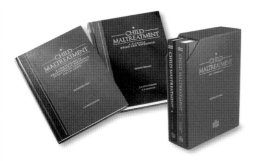
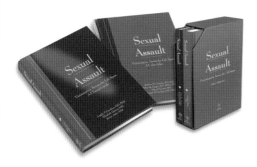
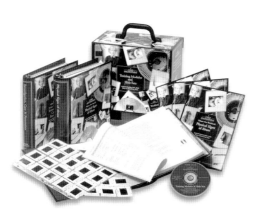

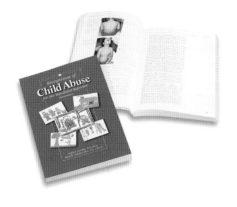

Recognition of Child Abuse for the Mandated Reporter

This text incorporates proven approaches for distinguishing possible abuse from conditions that mimic abuse, conducting necessary interviews and examinations, documenting findings and preparing reports, making appropriate referrals, and joining with other caring professionals to prevent child maltreatment.

Third Edition
Angelo P. Giardino, MD, PhD
Eileen R. Giardino, PhD, RN, CRNP
466 pages, 80 images, 21 contributors
ISBN 1-878060-52-X

$46.95

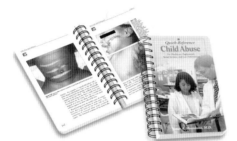

Child Abuse Quick Reference

The perfect comprehensive field guide for identifying child abuse and documenting an investigation.

For Healthcare, Social Service, and Law Enforcement Professionals
James A. Monteleone, MD
340 pages, 186 images, 19 contributors
ISBN 1-878060-28-7

$44.95

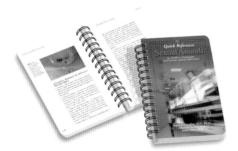

Sexual Assault Quick Reference

An invaluable resource for physicians, emergency room staff, EMTs, social service personnel, attorneys, law enforcement personnel, and anyone else who may be confronted with a sexual assault victim of any age.

For Healthcare, Social Service, and Law Enforcement Professionals
Angelo P. Giardino, MD, PhD; Elizabeth M. Datner, MD; Janice B. Asher, MD; Barbara W. Girardin, RN, PhD; Diana K. Faugno, RN, BSN, CPN, FAAFS, SANE-A; Mary J. Spencer, MD
550 pages, 150 images, 80 contributors
ISBN 1-878060-38-4

$49.95

FORTHCOMING

Abusive Head Trauma in Infants and Children
ISBN 1-878060-40-6; **$229.95**

Medical & Legal Aspects of Child Sexual Exploitation
ISBN 1-878060-37-6; **$229.95**

Child Fatality Review
ISBN 1-878060-58-9; **$229.95**

Abusive Head Trauma Quick Reference
ISBN 1-878060-57-0; **$44.95**

Child Sexual Exploitation Quick Reference
ISBN 1-878060-21-X; **$44.95**

Child Fatality Review Quick Reference
ISBN 1-878060-59-7; **$44.95**

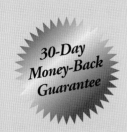

30-Day Money-Back Guarantee

FIVE WAYS TO ORDER

Mail

G.W. Medical Publishing, Inc.
77 Westport Plaza, Suite 366
St. Louis, MO 63146

Toll-Free

1-800-600-0330
8:30 am – 4:30 pm CST

Please have your credit card
ready when you call.

Fax

314-542-4239

Fax this completed form with
your company purchase order
or credit card information.

E-mail

orders@gwmedical.com

Web site

www.gwmedical.com

Yes, I'd like to order

Quantity	Title/Description	ISBN	Unit	Shipping
	Child Maltreatment Training Modules and Slide Sets Select (1) one: ☐ CD-ROM ☐ 35 mm Slide format ☐ Both (additional $125.00)	1-878060-29-5	$469.95	$14.00
	Child Maltreatment Two-Volume Set Second Edition	1-878060-26-0	$229.95	$11.15
	Child Abuse Quick-Reference	1-878060-28-7	$44.95	$6.75
	Recognition of Child Abuse for the Mandated Reporter Third Edition	1-878060-52-X	$46.95	$6.75
	A Parent's & Teacher's Handbook on Identifying and Preventing Child Abuse	1-878060-27-9	$19.95	$6.75
	Sexual Assault Victimization Across the Life Span Two-Volume Set	1-878060-62-7	$229.95	$11.50
	Sexual Assault Quick-Reference	1-878060-38-4	$49.95	$6.75
	Nursing Approach to the Evaluation of Child Maltreatment	1-878060-51-1	$49.95	$6.75
	Abusive Head Trauma in Infants and Children: Medical, Legal, and Forensic Issues Two-Volume Set	1-878060-40-6	$229.95*	$11.15
	Abusive Head Trauma Quick-Reference	1-878060-57-0	$44.95*	$6.75
	Medical & Legal Aspects of Child Sexual Exploitation: A Comprehensive Review of Child Pornography, Child Prostitution, and Internet Crimes Against Children Two-Volume Set	1-878060-37-6	$229.95*	$11.15
	Child Sexual Exploitation Quick-Reference	1-878060-21-X	$44.95*	$6.75
	Child Fatality Review: Evaluation of Accidental and Inflicted Child Death Two-Volume Set	1-878060-58-9	$229.95*	$11.15
	Child Fatality Review Quick-Reference	1-878060-59-7	$44.95*	$6.75

*Tentative Price

Please send my books to

Name _____ Title _____

Company / Organization _____

Address _____

City / State / Zip _____

Phone (____) _____ Fax (____) _____

E-Mail Address _____

I'd like to pay by

Credit Card ☐ Visa ☐ MasterCard

Cardholder's Name _____

Card Number _____ Exp. Date _____

Signature of Cardholder _____

☐ Check Enclosed in U.S. funds (Make payable to G.W. Medical Publishing, Inc.)

☐ Purchase Order No. (This order form must be attached to your company P.O.) Net 10 days after receipt of book(s)

Terms

Please pay personal orders by check or credit card. Make checks payable to G. W. Medical Publishing Inc. All international orders must be prepaid in U.S. funds. Inquire on shipping costs. Please allow 2-4 weeks for shipping.

All orders are billed for postage, handling, and state sales tax where appropriate. All prices subject to change without notice.
If using a purchase order, please attach it to this form. **30-Day Money-Back Guarantee:** If you are not 100% satisfied, simply return the book(s) within 30 days in the original shipping carton, by a traceable source. Your money will be promptly refunded without question or comment less a 15% restocking fee.